# Occupational Health
## Recognizing and Preventing
## Work-Related Disease

# Occupational Health
## Recognizing and Preventing
## Work-Related Disease

**Third Edition**

Edited by
**Barry S. Levy, M.D., M.P.H.**
Adjunct Professor of Community Health, Tufts
University School of Medicine, Boston; Barry S. Levy
Associates, Sherborn, Massachusetts

**David H. Wegman, M.D., M.S.**
Professor and Chair, Department of Work
Environment, College of Engineering, University of
Massachusetts Lowell, Lowell, Massachusetts

Foreword by
Christer Hogstedt, M.D.
Swedish National Institute of Occupational Health and
Karolinska Hospital

Little, Brown and Company
Boston/New York/Toronto/London

**Library of Congress Cataloging-in-Publication Data**

Occupational health : recognizing and preventing work-related disease
    / [edited by] Barry Levy, David H. Wegman.—3rd ed.
        p.   cm.
    Includes bibliographical references and index.
    ISBN 0-316-52271-6
    1. Medicine, Industrial.   I. Levy, Barry S.   II. Wegman, David H.
    [DNLM: 1.  Occupational Diseases—prevention & control.   WA 440
0149 1994]
    RC963.022   1994
    616.9′803—dc20
    DNLM/DLC
    for Library of Congress                                    94-13146
                                                                    CIP

Editorial: Laurie Anello
Production Editor: Karen Feeney
Copyeditor: Libby Dabrowski
Indexer: Deana Fowler
Production Supervisor: Louis C. Bruno, Jr.
Cover Designer: Louis C. Bruno, Jr.

# Contents

v

## Appendixes

# Foreword

Most workers in preventive medical disciplines have to interact with nonmedical authorities in order to undertake major preventive actions (e.g., in the areas of sanitation, nutrition, pollution, and work environment). During the 1990s a healthy work environment has become an integrated part of the quality assurance process of products as well as services. This increasing awareness gives work environment specialists new opportunities to put forward preventive strategies and aspects but also dramatically increases the need for technical, economic, ergonomic, and production system knowledge and cooperation. Therefore, modern occupational health specialists must learn about many things besides occupational hygiene and occupational disorders. As a consequence, *Occupational Health: Recognizing and Preventing Work-Related Disease* has a preventive and social approach. It puts occupational health into the perspective of economic and social systems, public health issues, regulations, and training. The many photographs forcefully remind the reader of realistic work situations.

The regular revision of this textbook makes it particularly useful as so much has changed within the last 6 years. These changes include the increased understanding of toxicologic modeling in industrial hygiene, the greatly enhanced importance of epidemiology in the study of occupationally related musculoskeletal disorders, new principles for regulation, increasing awareness of the importance of psychosocial conditions for many types of disorders, and more knowledge about women and work. This third edition also has added new sections that address the important role of shiftwork and psychological factors on worker health, the importance of conditions in modern buildings as a source of illness in office workers, and the variety of special work hazards and disease among construction workers.

Drs. Levy and Wegman have been active in the international field of occupational health and in this new edition have made a deliberate attempt to provide examples and references from other parts of the world. Indeed, many of the traditional occupational health risks are becoming increasingly frequent in the developing countries.

It is with great pleasure that I recommend this improved edition of a textbook that already, in its earlier editions, has proved to be the most universally appreciated among introductory texts, a tool to recognize and prevent work-related diseases in their social context.

Christer Hogstedt, M.D.

To our wives  and our children
*Nancy, Laura, and Benjamin Levy*
*Peggy, Marya, and Jesse Wegman*
for their never-ending
encouragement and support

# Preface

When we chose to undertake a third edition of *Occupational Health: Recognizing and Preventing Work-Related Disease,* it was in response to suggestions that both we and our publishers had received that there continued to be a high level of interest among health professionals about the variety of ways that work impacts on health. By developing this textbook, we wanted to reaffirm our view that the most important distinguishing feature of occupational diseases and injuries is that they are preventable. In order to take full advantage of this opportunity for disease prevention, we continue to direct attention not only to medical students and physicians, but also to nursing students and practicing nurses and to medical students and practitioners who strive to prevent work-related illness and injury.

In planning this edition we took note of a number of important developments that affect work environments today. We are aware that work in the United States and around the world has undergone substantial change in the interval between the first edition (1983) and the third edition (1995) of this textbook. Dramatic transformations of governments and national boundaries, immense alterations in the international economy, and critical developments in the understanding of the relationships between our general environment and economic growth have irrevocably changed the way we live and work and the opportunities that we have to achieve better health. Associated with the unfolding of these events have been alterations in and a restructuring of work environments. A number of these changes affect the way health care professionals and occupational health experts need to look at the relationships between work and health.

As an example, in the United States during the past 10 years, we have observed a striking shift in employment from manufacturing to the service sector. In addition, reduction in certain legal constraints, along with a revolution in information technology, has led to a return to cottage industry; many more individuals are performing all or part of their jobs at home. While these developments have the advantage of flexible working hours and self-paced work, they also isolate individual workers from the social and organizational advantages of sharing work among a group of workers. They have also brought the hazards of work—both toxic and psychosocial—into the home. Another development is the striking increase in work performed by children under the age of 18. Yet another development is an increasing emphasis on productivity, which places high demands on the individual, often without sufficient attention to the natural limitations on human capacity or to the opportunities to utilize fully the skills and intelligence of workers.

Many of these developments are not unique to the United States. For example, the increase in home-based work has occurred internationally and the increasing use of workers under 18 years old has led the International Labor Organization to target the reduction or elimination of child labor as one of its highest priorities. In addition, developing nations seeking to compete on a global scale are experiencing unprecedented industrial growth; this growth has been accompanied by the introduction of a variety of work risks to these countries, where workplace controls and national laws and regulations are less developed and often inadequately implemented.

With these developments in mind, we set out to revise our textbook to address a more global audience of health care workers. We believe that it is important to recognize that workers' health in one country should not be achieved at the cost of workers' health in another. We, therefore, have integrated international aspects of occupational health throughout the book. Some chapter authors have identified new co-authors who bring a non-U.S. perspective to the revised chapter. In general, authors have included examples or case studies that represent a range of different experiences and settings. As a result, we hope that this book effectively communicates the basic message that occupational health problems do not respect national borders.

The chapter on the social context of work has been completely revised and expanded in an attempt to characterize more clearly the interplay between society, work, and disease as well as the importance of presenting prevention activity in a broad context. Our own chapters on recognition and on prevention of occupational disease and injury have been revised in an effort to provide more prevention-oriented guidance to the reader. These revisions call attention explicitly to approaches for primary, secondary, and tertiary prevention and include a more comprehensive set of examples. The chapter on regulation still focuses on the United States, but the author has provided some examples of regulatory activity from outside the United States to illustrate some important alternative approaches. The revision of the chapter on infectious disease calls better attention to work-related infectious disease in developing countries as well as to the increasing importance of such infectious diseases as AIDS and tuberculosis. The chapter on occupational stress has been expanded to include recent developments in understanding of the rela-

tionships between stress and work organization as they affect opportunities for prevention activity. Finally, the chapters on work-related risks to the reproductive and renal or urinary tract systems have each been substantially revised as has the chapter on agricultural work, an important subject in most countries.

For this edition we have decided to add chapters on several new topics, including shift work, building-related problems, and health and safety of construction workers. We believe that each of these topics is of sufficient importance that even the reader new to this field should be well aware of their impact. At the same time, we recognize that there are a number of topics that we have not been able to include. We urge interested readers to go beyond this book to one of the more comprehensive reference works identified in the bibliography of Chapter 1.

We have retained the basic organization of the book. Parts I and II focus on the context of work and health and on approaches to recognizing, responding to, and preventing the consequences of work-related health problems. Part III is organized around hazardous exposures and their effects and Part IV around occupational disorders by organ system. Part V focuses on workers. Related chapters address occupational health issues related to women and minority workers. There is a separate examination of the role labor unions can play in bringing attention to work risks. Finally, there are chapters that provide an integrated approach to two areas of work that are important throughout the world: agriculture and construction.

We hope readers find that this third edition continues to achieve our original objective of providing students and health professionals with the basic information necessary to improve the health and quality of life for working people throughout the world.

B.S.L.
D.H.W.

# Acknowledgments

We greatly appreciate the assistance and support of many people in the development of the third edition of *Occupational Health*. We thank the many chapter authors, whose work is appropriately credited within the text. In addition, there have been many other people working behind the scenes, to whom we are deeply grateful and appreciative.

Several people in the Professional Division of Little, Brown and Company deserve credit for their outstanding work. We are especially grateful for the assistance of our editor, Laurie Anello, our production editor, Karen Feeney, and also to Priscilla Hurdle.

The illustrative materials throughout the book are included to offer understanding and insights not easily gained from the text. We call special attention to the work of Earl Dotter, who provided many outstanding photographs of workers and workplaces. We were also provided excellent new photographs by Marvin Lewiton and again used photographs by Marilee Caliendo, Christer Hogstedt, Nick Kaufman, and Ken Light. We also thank artist Nick Thorkelson for sharing his talent and perspective in a series of creative drawings that convey concepts and perspectives that are difficult to capture in words or photographs. We are grateful to the following individuals, who critically reviewed draft chapters and made helpful comments and contributions that were incorporated into the final text: Beverly Johnson, Steve Sauter, Robert Mullin, Greg Wagner, Bob Herrick, Linda Rosenstock, Jerry Sherwood, Harvey Checkoway, Frank Mirer, Tage Kristensen, Bill Burgess, Robert McCunney, Joan Roberts, and Marshall Kaplan. Figures 2-1, 2-2, and 2-4 are photographs by Marvin Lewiton. Figure 2-3 is a photograph by Earl Dotter. The section on psychiatric disorders by Richard Schottenfeld was adapted from his chapter in the book *Occupational Medicine* edited by Linda Rosenstock and Mark Cullen.

We wish to thank Deana Fowler for her excellent work in developing a practical and functional index and both Susan Zalot and Nell Switzer for their substantial technical assistance.

While the third edition of this textbook is improved over the first two editions by updating and some expansion, it draws heavily on the first two editions in terms of content and style. We express our appreciation to the many people who made important contributions to the first two editions. We also again acknowledge Curtis Vouwie and Robert M. Davis, who assisted, as editor and production editor, with the first edition over 10 years ago.

Finally, D.H.W. acknowledges his parents Isabel and Myron Wegman and B.S.L. his parents Bernice and Jerome Levy for their long-term and dedicated support.

B.S.L.
D.H.W.

# Contributors

**Torbjorn Akerstedt, Ph.D.**
Adjunct Professor of Clinical Neuroscience, Karolinska Institute; Professor, Work Environment Unit, National Institute of Psychosocial Factors and Health, Stockholm, Sweden
*20. Shiftwork*

**Gunnar B.J. Andersson, M.D., Ph.D.**
Professor and Acting Chairman of Orthopedics, Rush Medical College of Rush University; Senior Attending Physician, Department of Orthopedics, Rush-Presbyterian-St. Luke's Medical Center, Chicago
*23. Musculoskeletal Disorders*

**Kenneth A. Arndt, M.D.**
Professor of Dermatology, Harvard Medical School; Chief, Department of Dermatology, Beth Israel Hospital, Boston
*24. Skin Disorders*

**Nicholas A. Ashford, Ph.D., J.D.**
Professor of Technology and Policy, Center for Technology, Policy, and Industrial Development, Massachusetts Institute of Technology, Cambridge, Massachusetts; and Lecturer, Harvard School of Public Health, Boston
*9. Government Regulation of Occupational Health and Safety*

**Dean B. Baker, M.D., M.P.H.**
Professor and Director, Occupational Health Center, University of California, Irvine, College of Medicine, Irvine, California
*19. Occupational Stress*

**Edward L. Baker, Jr., M.D., M.P.H.**
Director of Public Health Practice Program Office, Centers for Disease Control and Prevention, Atlanta
*26. Disorders of the Nervous System*

**Michael Bigby, M.D.**
Assistant Professor of Dermatology, Harvard Medical School, Boston
*24. Skin Disorders*

**Leslie I. Boden, Ph.D.**
Professor of Environmental Health, Boston University School of Public Health, Boston
*10. Workers' Compensation*

**Marianne Parker Brown, M.P.H.**
Director, UCLA Labor Occupational Safety and Health (LOSH) Program, Los Angeles
*Appendix B. Other Sources of Information*

**Marilee A. Caliendo, M.P.H.**
Occupational Health Program Coordinator, University of California at Los Angeles Labor Center, Los Angeles
*Photographs*

**David C. Christiani, M.D., M.P.H., M.S.**
Associate Professor of Environmental Health, Harvard School of Public Health, and Department of Medicine, Harvard Medical School; Director, Center for Occupational and Environmental Medicine, and Associate Physician, Pulmonary and Critical Care Unit, Massachusetts General Hospital, Boston
*22. Respiratory Disorders*

**Serge A. Coopman**
*24. Skin Disorders*

**Letitia Davis**
*9. Government Regulation of Occupational Health and Safety*

**Morris E. Davis**
Attorney-Arbitrator, Oakland, California
*33. Minority Workers*

**Robert I. Davis**
Auditory Research Laboratories, State University of New York at Plattsburgh, Plattsburgh, New York
*16. Noise and Hearing Impairment*

**Charles D. DelTatto, B.S., P.T.**
Program Specialist, The Return to Work Center, Industrial Rehabilitation, Associates, Easthampton, Massachusetts
*11. Ability to Work and Disability Evaluation*

**Earl Dotter, B.A.**
Adjunct Assistant Professor of Community Medicine, West Virginia University School of Medicine, Morgantown, West Virginia
*Photographs*

**Ellen A. Eisen, Sc.D.**
Associate Professor of Work Environment, University of Massachusetts Lowell, Lowell, Massachusetts
*5. Epidemiology*

**Anders Englund**
*36. Construction Workers*

**Richard Fenske, Ph.D.**
Associate Professor of Environmental Health, University of Washington School of Medicine, Seattle
*35. Agricultural Workers*

**Lawrence J. Fine, M.D., Dr.P.H.**
Director, Division of Surveillance, Hazard Evaluations, and Field Studies, National Institute for Occupational Safety and Health, Cincinnati
*23. Musculoskeletal Disorders*

**David Fram**
*11. Ability to Work and Disability Evaluation*

**Howard Frumkin, M.D., Dr.P.H.**
Director of Environmental and Occupational Health, Emory University School of Medicine; Director, Environmental and Occupational Medicine Program, The Emory Clinic, Atlanta
*1. Occupational Health in the Global Context: An American Perspective; 13. Toxins and Their Effects; 14. Carcinogens*

**Nelson M. Gantz, M.D.**
Clinical Professor of Medicine, Pennsylvania State University College of Medicine, Hershey; Chairman, Department of Medicine, and Chief, Division of Infectious Diseases, Polyclinic Medical Center, Harrisburg, Pennsylvania
*18. Infectious Agents*

**Kenneth Geiser, Ph.D.**
Director, Toxics Use Reduction Institute, University of Massachusetts Lowell, Lowell, Massachusetts
*4. Preventing Occupational Disease*

**Bernard D. Goldstein, M.D.**
Director, Environmental and Occupational Health Sciences Institute (EOHSI), University of Medicine and Dentistry of New Jersey-New Jersey Medical School, Newark, New Jersey
*29. Hematologic Disorders*

**William Halperin, M.D., M.P.H.**
Associate Director for Surveillance, Division of Surveillance, Hazard Evaluations, and Health Studies, National Institute for Occupational Safety and Health, Cincinnati
*3. Recognizing Occupational Disease*

**Roger P. Hamernik, Ph.D.**
Professor of Physics, State University of New York at Plattsburgh, Plattsburgh, New York
*16. Noise and Hearing Impairment*

**Jay S. Himmelstein, M.D., M.P.H.**
Associate Professor of Family and Community Medicine, University of Massachusetts Medical School; Director, Occupational Health Program, University of Massachusetts Medical Center, Worcester, Massachusetts
*11. Ability to Work and Disability Evaluation*

**Howard Hu, M.D., M.P.H., Sc.D.**
Associate Professor of Environmental Health, Harvard School of Public Health; Associate Physician, Department of Medicine, Brigham and Women's Hospital, Boston
*1. Occupational Health in the Global Context: An American Perspective; 17. Other Physical Hazards and Their Effects*

**Stephen Kales, M.D., M.P.H.**
Instructor of Medicine, Harvard Medical School, Boston; Attending Physician, Division of Occupational and Internal Medicine, The Cambridge Hospital, Cambridge, Massachusetts
*17. Other Physical Hazards and Their Effects*

**Robert A. Karasek, Ph.D.**
Professor, Department of Work Environment,
University of Massachusetts Lowell, Lowell,
Massachusetts
*19. Occupational Stress*

**Nick Kaufman**
Producer/Director, Nick Kaufman Productions,
Newtonville, Massachusetts
*Photographs*

**W. Monroe Keyserling, Ph.D.**
Associate Professor of Industrial and Operations
Engineering and Environmental and Industrial Health,
University of Michigan Medical School, Ann Arbor,
Michigan
*7. Occupational Safety: Prevention of Accidents and
Overt Trauma; 8. Occupational Ergonomics:
Promoting Safety and Health Through Work Design*

**Howard M. Kipen, M.D., M.P.H.**
Associate Professor of Environmental and Community
Medicine, University of Medicine and Dentistry of
New Jersey—Robert Wood Medical School; Medical
Director, Environmental and Occupational Health
Sciences Institute, Piscataway, New Jersey
*29. Hematologic Disorders*

**Anders Knutsson**
*20. Shiftwork*

**Kathleen Kreiss, M.D.**
Associate Professor of Preventive Medicine and
Biometrics, University of Colorado School of
Medicine; Director, Division of Occupational and
Environmental Medicine, National Jewish Center for
Immunology and Respiratory Medicine, Denver
*21. Building-Related Factors: An Evolving Concern*

**Philip J. Landrigan, M.D., M.Sc.**
Ethel H. Wise Professor and Chair of Community
Medicine, Mount Sinai School of Medicine of the City
University of New York, New York
*31. Renal and Urinary Tract Disorders*

**Nancy Lessin**
Senior Staff for Strategy and Policy, Massachusetts
Coalition for Occupational Safety and Health;
President, United Steelworkers of America, Local
9267, Boston
*4. Preventing Occupational Disease*

**Charles Levenstein, Ph.D., M.S.**
Professor of Work Environment, University of
Massachusetts Lowell, Lowell, Massachusetts
*2. The Social Context of Occupational Health*

**Barry S. Levy, M.D., M.P.H.**
Adjunct Professor of Community Health, Tufts
University School of Medicine, Boston; Barry S. Levy
Associates, Sherborn, Massachusetts
*1. Occupational Health in the Global Context: An
American Perspective; 3. Recognizing Occupational
Disease; 4. Preventing Occupational Disease*

**Marvin Lewiton**
*Photographs*

**Ken Light, B.G.S.**
Former Photographer and Filmmaker, Labor
Occupational Health Program, University of California
at Berkeley, Berkeley, California
*Photographs*

**Ruth Lilis, M.D.**
Professor Emeritus of Community Medicine, Mount
Sinai School of Medicine of the City University of New
York; Attending Physician, Community Hospital and
Mount Sinai Medical Center, New York
*31. Renal and Urinary Tract Disorders*

**James Melius, M.D., Dr.P.H.**
Professor of Environmental Health and Toxicology,
School of Public Health; Director, Division of
Occupational Health and Environmental
Epidemiology, New York State Department of Health,
Albany, New York
*13. Toxins and Their Effects*

**David Michaels, Ph.D., M.P.H.**
Associate Professor of Epidemiology, The City
University of New York Medical School, New York
*Appendix A. How to Research the Toxic Effects of
Chemical Substances*

**Maureen Paul, M.D., M.P.H.**
Associate Professor of Obstetrics and Gynecology, and
Family and Community Medicine, University of
Massachusetts Medical School; Director, Occupational
and Environmental Reproductive Hazards Center,
University of Massachusetts Medical Center,
Worcester, Massachusetts
*27. Reproductive Disorders*

**John M. Peters, M.D.**
Professor of Preventive Medicine, University of
Southern California School of Medicine, Los Angeles
*1. Occupational Health in the Global Context: An
American Perspective*

**Glenn S. Pransky, M.D., M.Occ.H.**
Associate Professor of Family and Community
Medicine, University of Massachusetts Medical School;
Chief of Clinical Services, Occupational Health
Program, University of Massachusetts Medical Center,
Worcester, Massachusetts
*11. Ability to Work and Disability Evaluation;
30. Hepatic Disorders*

**Laura Punnett, Sc.D.**
Associate Professor of Work Environment, University
of Massachusetts Lowell, Lowell, Massachusetts
*27. Reproductive Disorders; 32. Women and Work*

**Margaret Quinn, Sc.D.**
Associate Professor of Work Environment, University
of Massachusetts Lowell, Lowell, Massachusetts
*4. Preventing Occupational Disease; 32. Women
and Work*

**Robert G. Radwin, Ph.D.**
Associate Professor of Industrial Engineering,
University of Wisconsin Medical School,
Madison, Wisconsin
*8. Occupational Ergonomics: Promoting Safety and
Health Through Work Design*

**Kathleen M. Rest, Ph.D., M.P.A.**
Assistant Professor of Occupational Health,
University of Massachusetts Medical School,
Worcester, Massachusetts
*12. Ethics in Occupational and Environmental Health*

**Knut Ringen, Dr.P.H.**
Director, Center to Protect Workers' Rights,
Washington, D.C.
*36. Construction Workers*

**Beth Rosenberg, M.P.H.**
Doctorial Candidate, Department of Work
Environment, University of Massachusetts at Lowell,
Lowell, Massachusetts
*2. The Social Context of Occupational Health;
32. Women and Work*

**Andrew S. Rowland**
*33. Minority Workers*

**Thomas Schneider**
Director of Industrial Hygiene, National Institute of
Occupational Health, Copenhagen, Denmark
*6. Occupational Hygiene*

**Richard S. Schottenfeld, M.D.**
Associate Professor of Psychiatry, Yale University
School of Medicine; Director, Substance Abuse
Treatment Unit, Connecticut Mental Health Center,
New Haven, Connecticut
*26. Disorders of the Nervous System*

**Cathy Schwartz**
*32. Women and Work*

**Jane Seegal, M.A., M.S.**
Center to Protect Workers' Rights, Washington, D.C.
*36. Construction Workers*

**Barbara Silverstein, Ph.D., M.P.H.**
Special Assistant for Ergonomic Programs, U.S.
Department of Labor, Occupational Safety and Health
Administration, Washington
*23. Musculoskeletal Disorders*

**Michael Silverstein, M.D.**
Director of Policy, U.S. Department of Labor,
Occupational Safety and Health Administration,
Washington, D.C.
*34. Labor Unions and Occupational Health*

**Nancy J. Simcox, M.S.**
Research Industrial Hygienst, Environmental Health,
University of Washington School of Medicine, Seattle
*35. Agricultural Workers*

**David H. Sliney, Ph.D.**
Associate Professor of Environmental Health
Engineering, Johns Hopkins University School of
Hygiene and Public Health, Baltimore; Chief, Laser
Branch, U.S. Army Environmental Hygiene Agency,
Aberdeen Proving Ground, Maryland
*25. Eye Disorders*

**Thomas J. Smith, Ph.D.**
Professor of Industrial Hygiene, Harvard School of
Public Health, Boston
*6. Occupational Hygiene*

**Edward C. Swanson, M.B.A., P.T.**
Program Specialist, The Return to Work Center, Industrial Rehabilitation Associates, Easthampton, Massachusetts
*11. Ability to Work and Disability Evaluation*

**Andrea Kidd Taylor, Dr.P.H.**
Industrial Hygienst, United Automobile Workers Health and Safety Department, Detroit
*33. Minority Workers*

**Gilles P. Thériault, M.D.**
Chairman of Occupational Health, McGill University Faculty of Medicine, Montreal
*28. Cardiovascular Disorders*

**Nick Thorkelson, B.A.**
*Illustrations*

**Patricia Hyland Travers**
*1. Occupational Health in the Global Context: An American Perspective*

**Arthur C. Upton, M.D.**
Clinical Professor of Pathology and Radiology, University of New Mexico School of Medicine, Albuquerque, New Mexico
*15. Ionizing Radiation*

**Paul F. Vinger, M.D.**
Associate Clinical Professor of Ophthalmology, Tufts University School of Medicine; Director of Vision Performance and Safety Service, New England Medical Center, Boston
*25. Eye Disorders*

**Bailus Walker, Jr., Ph.D., M.P.H.**
Dean and Professor of Public Health, University of Oklahoma, Oklahoma City, Oklahoma
*33. Minority Workers*

**James L. Weeks, Sc.D.**
Research Scientist of Occupational and Environmental Medicine, George Washington University School of Medicine and Health Sciences, Washington, D.C.
*9. Government Regulation of Occupational Health and Safety*

**David H. Wegman, M.D., M.S.**
Professor and Chair, Department of Work Environment, University of Massachusetts Lowell, Lowell, Massachusetts
*1. Occupational Health in the Global Context: An American Perspective; 3. Recognizing Occupational Disease; 4. Preventing Occupational Disease; 5. Epidemiology; 22. Respiratory Disorders*

**John Wooding, Ph.D.**
Assistant Professor of Political Science, University of Massachusetts Lowell, Lowell, Massachusetts
*2. The Social Context of Occupational Health*

**Susan R. Woskie, Ph.D.**
Assistant Professor, Department of Work Environment, University of Massachusetts Lowell, Lowell, Massachusetts
*32. Women and Work*

**Stephen Zoloth**
*Appendix A. How to Research the Toxic Effects of Chemical Substances*

# I
# Work and Health

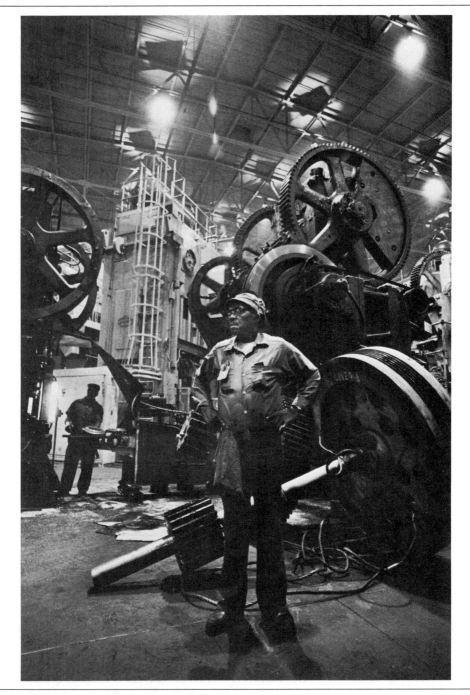

**Fig. 1-1.** While a declining percentage of workers in the United States work in heavy manufacturing, it still represents a major part of the economy and a source of many occupational health and safety hazards. (Photograph by Earl Dotter.)

# 1
# Occupational Health in the Global Context: An American Perspective

Barry S. Levy and David H. Wegman

A pregnant woman who works as a laboratory technician asks her obstetrician if she should change her job or stop working because of the chemicals to which she and her fetus are exposed.

A middle-aged man sees an orthopedic surgeon and states that he is totally disabled from chronic back pain, which he attributes to lifting heavy objects for many years as a construction worker.

A long-distance truck driver asks a cardiologist how soon after his recent myocardial infarction he will be able to return to work and what kinds of tasks he will be able to perform.

A chemical manufacturer, aware that a pesticide that he produces is carcinogenic and has recently been banned from sale in the United States, makes arrangements for the export of the pesticide for sale and use in developing countries.

A former asbestos worker with lung cancer asks his surgeon if he can submit a claim for workers' compensation for his disease.

An oncologist observes an unusual cluster of bladder cancer cases among middle-aged women in a small town.

The vice president of a small tool and die company asks his local family physician to advise his company regarding prevention of occupational disease among his employees.

A pediatric nurse practitioner diagnoses lead poisoning in a young child and wonders if the source of the lead may be dust brought home on the workclothes of the father, who works in a battery plant.

A U.S.-based physician epidemiologist visits a developing country to advise its occupational health program on identifying and controlling workplace hazards.

And three women who work for a plastics company, all complaining of severe rashes on their hands and forearms, consult an internist, who believes their problems may be work-related.

These are but a few examples of the numerous occupational health challenges facing health professionals. Virtually all health professionals need to be able to deal with these challenges effectively. They therefore need to be able to recognize, manage, and prevent work-related injuries and diseases.

## The United States Workforce

Work and the work ethic are basic to life throughout the world. Most adults in the U.S. spend almost one-fourth of their time at work, and despite the high degree of automation and computerization of American industry, many workers are exposed to dust, chemicals, noise, and other workplace hazards. Table 1-1 categorizes workers in the United States by industry, and Table 1-2 by occupation (Fig. 1-1). Over 40 percent of American workers are women (Fig. 1-2). These statistics

3

**Table 1-1.** Employed civilians in the United States, by industry (1993)

| Industry | Size of workforce (in millions) |
|---|---|
| Agriculture | 3.1 |
| Mining | 0.7 |
| Construction | 7.2 |
| Manufacturing | 19.6 |
| Transportation and public utilities | 8.5 |
| Wholesale and retail trade | 24.8 |
| Finance, insurance, real estate | 8.0 |
| Services | 41.8 |
| Public administration | 5.8 |
| Total | 119.3* |

*Because of rounding, the sum of the components does not add up to the total.
Source: Bureau of Labor Statistics, U.S. Department of Labor, 1994.

**Table 1-2.** Employed civilians in the United States, by occupational category (1993)

| Occupational category | Number of workers (in millions) |
|---|---|
| Executive, administrative, and managerial workers | 15.4 |
| Professional workers | 16.9 |
| Technicians and related support workers | 4.0 |
| Sales workers | 14.2 |
| Administrative support workers, including clerical workers | 18.6 |
| Precision production, craft, and repair workers | 13.3 |
| Operators, fabricators, and laborers | 17.0 |
| Service workers | 16.5 |
| Farming, forestry, and fishing industry workers | 3.3 |
| Total | 119.3* |

*Because of rounding, the sum of the components does not add up to the total.
Source: Bureau of Labor Statistics, U.S. Department of Labor, 1994.

overlook full-time homemakers, who are usually not included in data on the U.S. workforce. Approximately 14 percent of American workers belong to unions, a lower percentage than in most industrialized nations. Most U.S. workers are employed by small or moderate-sized firms that do not employ physicians or other health professionals to provide health and safety programs.

Only about 2,000 occupational health physicians who have been certified by the American Board of Preventive Medicine practice in the United States. Therefore, most workers with work-related medical problems are treated by physicians who have little or no training in occupational health. Similar shortages exist for qualified occupational health nurses and other personnel in the field.

While the workforce in other developed countries in Western Europe, Canada, and Japan has many similarities to the workforce in the United States, the same is not true for the workforce of developing countries—in the aggregate potentially much larger than the workforce of the developed world.

In developing countries, the workforce has several distinct characteristics:

1. Most people who are employed work in the informal sector of the economy, mainly in agriculture, or in small-scale industries, in which they are often self-employed or working in a small workplace.
2. There are high rates of unemployment, sometimes reaching 25 percent or higher, and in many developing countries the rates of unemployment—and underemployment—are increasing each year.
3. In general, workers are at greater risk of occupational hazards for a variety of reasons, including lower rates of education and literacy; unfamiliarity with work processes and exposures, in part due to inadequate training; pre-

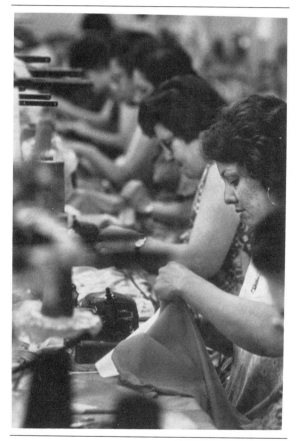

**Fig. 1-2.** The garment industry, largely unchanged in this century, is a major employer of women, who constitute over 40 percent of the U.S. workforce. (Photograph by Earl Dotter.)

disposition not to complain about working conditions or exposures because jobs, whether or not they are hazardous, are relatively scarce; high prevalence of endemic (mainly infectious) diseases and malnutrition; and inadequate infrastructure and human resources to diagnose, treat, and prevent work-related illnesses and injuries.

4 Wages are low; annual per capita income in many developing countries is $500 (U.S.) or less per year.

5. Groups that comprise vulnerable populations in any country are at even greater risk, including:
   • Women, who make up a large proportion of the workforce in many developing countries and often face significant physical and psychological hazards in their work, in addition to the physical and psychological stresses of being homemakers and mothers. In the rural areas of many developing countries, from which men have left to seek jobs in the cities, women often do most of the physical labor in raising crops on small plots of land, in addition to raising children and maintaining their households.
   • Children, sometimes even very young children, who account for a significant part of the workforce in many developing countries and often undertake some of the most hazardous tasks at work. In many of these countries, primary education is not required and there are no legal protections against child labor.
   • Migrants, both within countries and between countries, who, for a variety of reasons (such as uncertain legal status and unfamiliarity with the culture in and around the workplace), face significant health and safety hazards at work.

## Magnitude of the Problem

Workers are exposed to a wide range of occupational health and safety hazards (Figs. 1-3, 1-4, 1-5, and 1-6; see box on p. 10). An estimated 20 million work-related injuries and 390,000 new work-related illnesses occur each year in the United States. However, the number of occupational diseases and injuries reported each year is much lower. Analyses of reported injuries by industry and reported illnesses by category are shown in Tables 1-3 and 1-4. In addition, it is estimated that there may be 100,000 or more work-related deaths in the United States each year. According to the National Institute for Occupational

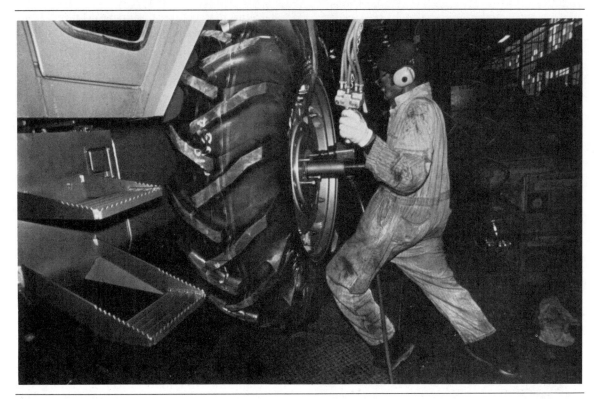

**Fig. 1-3.** Mixed occupational hazards occur in many jobs. This worker is exposed to loud noise and risk of low back injury. (Photograph by Earl Dotter.)

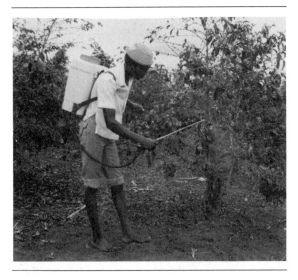

**Fig. 1-4.** Agricultural workers in developing countries are at high risk of poisoning from pesticides, including those banned or restricted in the developed world. (Photograph by Barry Levy.)

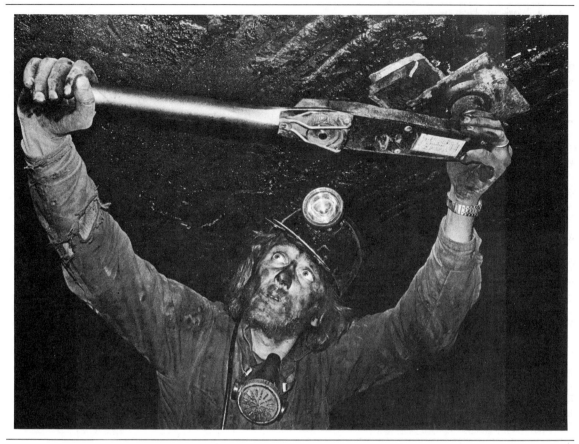

**Fig. 1-5.** Roof bolting in coal mines is essential to prevent roofs from collapsing. Miners face many other injury risks as well. (Photograph by Earl Dotter.)

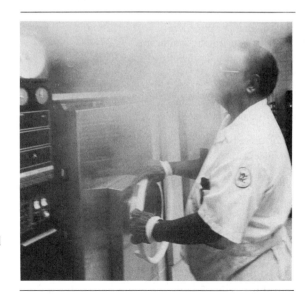

**Fig. 1-6.** Hospital worker, while opening an autoclave, is exposed to carcinogenic ethylene oxide gas. Hospital workers are exposed to chemical, biologic, and physical hazards as well as psychological stress at work. (Photograph by Earl Dotter.)

Table 1-3. Nonfatal occupational injury incidence rates in the United States, by industry, private sector (1992)

| Industry | Number of nonfatal injuries per 100 full-time workers |
|---|---|
| Construction | 12.9 |
| Agriculture, forestry, and fishing | 11.0 |
| Manufacturing | 10.8 |
| Transportation and public utilities | 8.8 |
| Wholesale and retail trade | 8.2 |
| Mining | 7.0 |
| Services | 6.8 |
| Finance, insurance, and real estate | 2.7 |
| Average | 8.3 |

Source: Bureau of Labor Statistics, U.S. Department of Labor, 1993.

Table 1-4. Distribution of new cases of reported occupational illnesses in the United States, by category of illness, private sector (1991)

| Category of illness | Number[a] | Percent |
|---|---|---|
| Disorders associated with repeated trauma | 459,300 | 61 |
| Skin diseases or disorders | 120,800 | 16 |
| Disorders due to physical agents | 37,400 | 5 |
| Respiratory conditions due to toxic agents | 36,900 | 5 |
| Poisoning | 13,400 | 2 |
| Dust diseases of the lungs | 4,800 | 1 |
| All other occupational illnesses | 86,800 | 11 |
| Total | 759,400 | 100 |

[a]Excludes farms with fewer than 11 employees.
Source: Bureau of Labor Statistics, U.S. Department of Labor, 1993.

Safety and Health (NIOSH) National Traumatic Occupational Fatality database, approximately 7,000 *traumatic* occupational fatalities occur in the United States each year; the highest rates are in mining (30 per 100,000 workers per year), con-struction (23 per 100,000) (see Chap. 36), and agriculture (20 per 100,000) (see Chap. 35). While these statistics provide some idea of the scope and types of occupational medical problems, they grossly underestimate the role of the workplace in causing new diseases and injuries and exacerbating existing ones. In addition, statistics do not represent the relative distribution of various work-related diseases. For example, because skin disorders are easy to recognize and to relate to working conditions, their representation in Table 1-4 exaggerates their relative importance.

As indicated in the box on page 9, myths about work-related disease impede the identification of occupational health problems.

The difficulty in obtaining accurate estimates of the frequency of work-related diseases is due to several factors, as indicated below and as shown in Fig. 1-7.

1. Many problems do not come to the attention of health professionals and employers and, therefore, are not included in data collection systems. A worker may not recognize a medical problem as being work-related, but even when the connection is obvious, a variety of disincentives may deter the worker from reporting such a problem, the greatest being fear of losing a job. Training workers about both occupational hazards and legal rights has been helpful.

2. Many occupational medical problems that do come to the attention of physicians and employers are not recognized as work-related. Recognition of work-related disease is often difficult because of the long period between initial exposure and onset of symptoms (or time of diagnosis), making cause-effect relationships difficult to assess. It is also difficult because of the many and varied occupational and nonoccupational hazards to which most workers are exposed. Training of health professionals in occupational health has begun to improve health care providers' knowledge of these factors, resulting in increased recognition of the work-relatedness of diseases and chronic injuries.

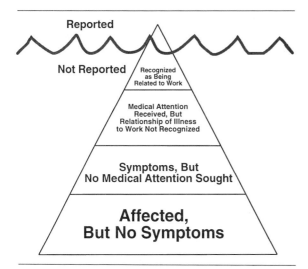

**Fig. 1-7.** The "iceberg" of occupational disease.

3. Some medical problems recognized by health professionals or employers as work-related are not reported because the association with work is equivocal and because reporting requirements are not strict. The initiation of occupational disease surveillance activities by federal and state governments has begun to address this problem.
4. Because many occupational medical problems are preventable, their very persistence implies that some individual or group is legally and economically responsible for creating or perpetuating them.

There are few good statistics on the occurrence of occupationally related illnesses and injuries in developing countries, or on the magnitude or degree of health and safety hazards at work. This inadequacy is a function of the inadequate infrastructure and human resources for occupational health and safety in developing countries as well as the inherent difficulty in diagnosing and obtaining data on work-related health problems.

In those situations for which data are available, there is evidence that the occurrence of occupational illnesses and injuries in developing countries

12 MYTHS ABOUT WORK-RELATED DISEASE
John M. Peters
1. "It can't be a bad place to work. Joe has been working here for 45 years and there is nothing wrong with him."
2. "It is only statistical, so it is of no clinical significance."
3. "Our working population is healthier than the average population."
4. "There is no problem—the exposure level is below the standard."
5. "It will cost too much to control the problem; it will put us out of business."
6. "It is only a mortality study and you know how inaccurate death certificates are."
7. "Okay, there is a problem, but it is not the occupational exposure. It is all the smoking and drinking the workers do."
8. "Exposures are good for people because they keep up their defenses. If we stop exposing them, their defenses will break down."
9. "If there is a problem, it is because of all the old exposures that do not exist any longer."
10. "We have this party for retired people and they all look great."
11. "Don't tell the workers; they will only worry."
12. "If there is a problem, the nurses and doctors in the clinic would know about it because the workers would tell them."

is much higher than in developed countries. The International Labour Organization (ILO), for example, collected data on annual rates of fatal injuries in 24 developing countries from 1971 to 1975 and 1976 to 1980. While rates of fatal injuries at work were decreasing in developed countries during the 1970s, these rates stayed the same, or even increased, in developing countries; in almost half of these 24 countries that ILO studied, the rates increased between the first half and the

# VIOLENCE IN THE WORKPLACE

By 1990, occupational health and safety experts realized that the role of violence as a cause of work-related injury and death had been seriously underestimated. This silent epidemic had been largely overlooked until the National Institute for Occupational Safety and Health (NIOSH) began its National Traumatic Occupational Fatality Surveillance System (NTOF).

Reviewing death certificate data for the 1980s, NIOSH has shown that about one in eight work-related fatalities in the U.S. are homicides. Among women, homicide is the largest single cause of death in the workplace, accounting for almost half of these deaths. Victims of occupational homicide are young (primarily 25 to 44 years old). Although 75 percent are white, the rate of occupational homicide among African-Americans and other minority workers is twice that for whites.

Due to the availability of death certificates, the discovery of the importance of violence was primarily based on the surveillance of occupational fatalities. However, these data probably *underestimate* occupational homicide. The problem is clearly more widespread when one considers nonfatal effects of violence, ranging from injuries due to violent acts to sexual harassment on the job. An estimated one in four workers in the U.S. (over 25 million) is harassed, threatened, attacked, or injured violently each year; of these, about 2 million workers are physically attacked at work. Data from Great Britain indicate that 1 in 8 health care workers suffer a physical attack each year. Studies in the U.S. suggest that those responsible for nonfatal violent events are most commonly coworkers (as many as one-half), while in Sweden some industries have reported that as many as 14 percent of the workforce are subjected to *chronic* harassment by coworkers. Customers are also a common cause of violent events, whereas strangers account for only a small portion.

The typical victim of occupational homicide is a regular worker employed in a work setting that allows continued exposure to hazards of crime and violence. Retail trade and service workers are those most frequently killed by violent acts at work; these workers accounted for 54 percent of occupational homicides in the 1980s. In this context, some of the most hazardous workplaces were taxicabs, liquor stores, gas stations, detective/protective services, and justice/public order establishments; some workers with the most hazardous occupations were taxicab drivers (with 21 times greater than average risk of occupational homicide), law enforcement officers, hotel clerks, gas station workers, stock handlers/baggers, store owners/managers, and bartenders.

Efforts to understand the circumstances of these fatalities include robbery as a primary motive, with some being caused by disgruntled workers and clients. NIOSH has summarized the major risk factors known to increase probability for occupational homicide: (1) exchange of money with the public, (2) working alone or in small numbers, (3) working late-night or early-morning hours, (4) working in high-crime areas, (5) guarding valuable property or possessions, and (6) working in community settings, as taxicab drivers and police do (Fig. 1-8).*

NIOSH has recommended preventive measures that can be quickly introduced to reduce the risk of occupational homicides, especially in high-risk establishments and occupations:

- Make high-risk areas visible to more people and install good external lighting
- To minimize cash on hand, use drop safes, carry small amounts of cash, and post signs stating that limited cash is on hand
- Install silent alarms and surveillance cameras
- Increase the number of staff on duty and have police check on workers routinely
- Provide training in conflict resolution and nonviolent response as well as the importance of avoiding resistance during a robbery
- Provide bullet-proof barriers or enclosures
- Close establishments during high-risk hours (late at night and early in the morning)

*NIOSH. Alert: Request for Assistance in Preventing Homicide in the Workplace. DHHS (NIOSH) publication no. 93-109, September 1993.

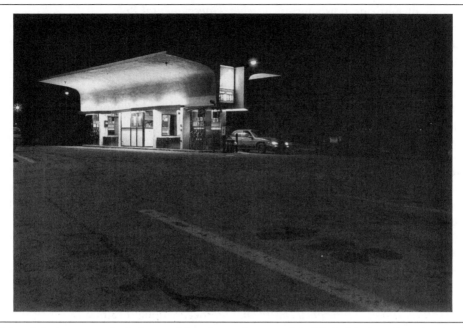

**Fig. 1-8.** Violent injuries are particularly a problem for workers employed in isolated work settings such as this gas station. (Photograph by Marvin Lewiton.)

second half of the decade. In addition, ILO found that in 21 developing countries, nonfatal occupational injury rates rose 5.3 percent during the 1976 to 1980 period, while they were declining elsewhere.

There are a variety of reasons for the poor occupational *safety* situation in developing countries, including use of outdated machinery, often imported used from more developed countries; poor maintenance and little safety guarding of machinery; inadequate training of workers; poor design of equipment and workstations; and lack of personal protective equipment, which, even when available, may be difficult to wear because of working conditions or workers' health status. In addition, workers' underlying health may be compromised by endemic diseases, poor housing and sanitation, and inadequate nutrition.

The same picture is true for occupational *health* hazards in developing countries, and resultant oc-

cupational diseases. Pesticide exposures, often to highly toxic or carcinogenic pesticides that have been banned or restricted in developed countries that produce them and then export them to developing countries, and resultant cases of acute and chronic poisoning are a major problem. This problem is exacerbated by intensive use of pesticides, especially on coffee, cotton, and other "cash crops"; inadequate labeling on pesticide containers; inadequate training of workers on pesticide safety; inadequate personal protective equipment; and inadequate knowledge of health care providers on the diagnosis, treatment, and prevention of pesticide poisoning. In addition, pesticide formulation, mixing, and application are often done by small groups or individual workers, making control of this hazard even more difficult. A number of studies have confirmed the seriousness and the magnitude of pesticide poisoning in developing countries.

The problems of pesticide poisoning in developing countries are multiplied by the numerous other chemicals and other occupational health hazards to which workers are exposed in these countries. Exposure to organic and inorganic dusts, organic solvents, heavy metals, and other chemicals represents a serious problem; in some countries, for example, miners experience 10 to 12 percent rates of pneumoconiosis, or higher. Physical hazards, such as noise, biologic hazards related to exposure to infectious agents (see box on Infectious Diseases in Developing Countries, Chap. 18), and psychosocial problems directly related to work (such as work stress) and indirectly related to work (such as alcoholism) are also usually much more prevalent in developing countries than in developed ones.

Two important aspects of occupational disease distinguish it from other medical problems: (1) *Recognition of work-related medical problems is almost totally dependent on obtaining occupational information in the medical history.* The health professional must know when to suspect work-related medical problems and what questions to ask in an occupational history to evaluate the work-relatedness of that problem (see Chap. 3). (2) *In contrast to many nonoccupational diseases, occupational diseases can almost always be prevented.* Most occupational medical problems can be alleviated by a variety of preventive approaches in which professionals in health, safety, and other fields play vital roles (see Chap. 4).

## Illustrative Occupational Health Issues

Legislation, social activism, educational activities, and other developments have contributed to increased interest in work-related medical problems in recent years. Some of these developments are summarized below.

### Governmental Role

With the passage of the Federal Coal Mine Safety and Health Act of 1969 and the Occupational Safety and Health Act (OSHAct) of 1970, the federal government began taking a more active role in the creation and enforcement of standards for a safe and healthful workplace (see Chap. 9). In addition, the OSHAct established NIOSH, which (1) has greatly expanded epidemiologic and laboratory research into the causes of occupational diseases and injuries and the methods of preventing them; and (2) is strengthening the training of occupational health and safety professionals.

### Occupational Safety and Health Education

A variety of factors have contributed to a recent growth in education and training opportunities for workers, employers, health professionals, and others. Unions have recently directed more attention to occupational health and safety through collective bargaining agreements, hiring of health professionals, workplace health and safety committees, educational programs, and support of epidemiologic studies. Worker education has been facilitated by Right-to-Know laws and regulations, independent coalitions for occupational safety and health (COSH groups; see Appendix B), employer-sponsored programs, and academic institutions concerned with occupational health and safety. When available, government funds for medical student, resident, and other professional training programs in occupational health have improved existing professional training opportunities and created new ones. Furthermore, alerted to the critical problems associated with asbestos, lead, pesticides, and ionizing radiation, the mass media have made the public aware of many workplace hazards.

### Social and Ethical Questions

Serious social and ethical problems have arisen in recent years concerning such subjects as allegiance of occupational physicians who are employed by management, workers' "Right to Know" about job hazards, confidentiality of workers' medical records kept by employers, and restricting female workers of childbearing age from certain jobs (see Chaps. 2 and 13). Controversies relating to such subjects will eventually be settled by labor-management negotiations and by the deliberations of the courts and legislative and executive bodies of government. As an example, in 1980 the United States Supreme Court upheld a worker's right to refuse hazardous work; it ruled that a worker could not be discharged or discriminated against for exercising his or her right not to work under conditions he or she reasonably believed to be very dangerous.

### Workplace-Related Health and Medical Programs

Health care is increasingly available in or near the workplace. Increasingly the emphasis is on prevention programs focused on education and screening. Some programs deal not only with specific occupational medical problems, but also with problems such as hypertension and smoking that may be a function of the personal lifestyles of workers. In recent years, there has been substantial growth in both academic-oriented occupational health clinics and free-standing, or hospital-based, community clinics providing occupational medicine services. A number of hospital-based programs have been designed primarily for financial reasons; the impact of these on occupational disease and injury prevention is not yet clear.

### Liability

An extremely controversial force in occupational health is the product liability suit. Workers, barred from suing their employers under workers' compensation laws and unhappy about deregulation of the workplace, have increasingly turned to "third-party," or product liability, suits as a means of getting redress for occupational disease. Liability suits are not a particularly effective way to ensure compensation on a general scale because of the uncertainty of the jury system. However, the fear of liability suits has driven many employers to focus on preventive activities. Although such suits currently play an important role in directing attention to prevention of some diseases, the method is cumbersome and inequitable. (It is hoped that in the future these problems can be dealt with in a more rational way.) Recently, some jurisdictions have turned to criminal prosecution of the most egregious health and safety offenders.

### Advances in Technology

Recent advances in technology have facilitated the identification of workplace hazards and potential hazards. Most notable are in vitro assays to determine mutagenicity (and to suspect carcinogenicity) of substances, improvements in ways of determining the presence and measuring the levels of workplace hazards, and new methods of monitoring concentrations of hazardous substances in body fluids and the physiologic impairments they cause (see Chaps. 6, 13, and 14).

### The Environmental Movement

Public concern for a safe and healthful environment—from protecting air, soil, and water from contamination to ensuring safety in consumer products—extends to the workplace. When considering asbestos or pesticides, noise or radiation, there is a continuum of exposures that extends from the workplace to the general environment.

### Additional Challenges in Developing Countries

While all of these issues are important in developing countries as well, these countries face the following additional challenges:

*Export of hazards.* Developed countries often export their most hazardous industries, as well as hazardous materials and hazardous wastes, to developing countries, where laws and regulations concerning these substances are more lax or nonexistent and workers may be less aware of these hazards.

*Inadequate infrastructure and human resources.*
In developing countries, there are far fewer
numbers of adequately trained personnel to
deal with the diagnosis, treatment, and prevention of occupational health problems.
Governments and often employers have far
fewer resources to devote to occupational
health, and labor unions, facing other challenges such as low wages and high unemployment rates, may give little attention to occupational health.

*Transnational problems.* Occupational—and environmental—health problems in the developing world often involve a number of countries in the same region, requiring transnational, regional, or global approaches to the
problem, such as development and implementation of transnational standards.

*Relationships between work and the environ-
ment.* In developing countries, where so many
people work in or near their homes, the distinction between workplace and the general
environment is blurred. As a result, family
members may often be exposed to workplace
hazards.

*Economic development.* Governments of developing countries often give high priority to
economic development, sometimes even over
the health of their people. In the context of economic development, and accompanying rapid
industrialization and urbanization, there is
often pressure to overlook occupational and environmental health issues, given limited resources and the fear that attention to these issues may drive away potential investors or
employers.

*Occupational health services and primary
health care.* Given limited resources and infrastructure, opportunities are recognized to integrate an occupational health survey with primary medical care and public health. While
some successes have been achieved with this
approach, there remains much untapped potential in fully achieving this integration.

## Conclusion

Many readers of this text will at some time work
with management, labor, or government, and a
few will become full-time occupational health
professionals. Almost all health professionals who
read this book, however, will at times have to deal
with work-related medical problems. Pulmonary
disease specialists see asbestosis and occupational
asthma; ophthalmologists diagnose and treat work-
related conjunctivitis and foreign bodies in the eye;
orthopedic surgeons frequently evaluate work-related musculoskeletal disorders; and providers of
primary care are confronted with a wide range of
medical problems that either are work-related—
such as trauma, back and skin problems, and toxic
reactions—or have a critical impact on the patient's capacity to work. Clearly, all types of health
professionals have a vital role in recognizing and
preventing work-related disease.

## Bibliography (Suggested Books for Beginning an Occupational Health Library)

Ashford NA, Caldart CC. Technology, law, and the
working environment. New York: Van Nostrand
Reinhold, 1991.
*An in-depth analysis of the technical, legal, political,
and economic problems in occupational health and
safety.*

Brodeur P. Expendable Americans. New York: Viking,
1974.
*A detailed account of the sociopolitical forces that
have worked against dissemination of research information on occupational hazards and effective enforcement of occupational health and safety laws. Focus on asbestos.*

Burgess W. Recognition of health hazards in industry: A
review of materials and processes. 2nd ed. New York:
Wiley, 1995.
*An excellent summary of industrial hazards, updated,
made more comprehensive, and well illustrated with
photographs, drawings, and graphs in this second edition.*

Environmental Health Criteria Series, Environmental
Program, World Health Organization, Geneva.

*This is a collection of monographs, each of which provides a succinct and comprehensive review of the relevant literature on the human health effects due to exposure to over 100 individual chemical substances. This is an excellent starting point for anyone investigating the health impact of chemical exposures.*

Hamilton A. Exploring the dangerous trades; an autobiography. Boston: Little, Brown, 1943.
*A classic historical reference.*

Hathaway GJ, Proctor NH, Hughes JP. Chemical hazards of the workplace. 3rd ed. Philadelphia: Lippincott, 1991.
*Brief summaries on 542 chemical hazards, including basics about their chemical, physical, and toxicologic characteristics; diagnostic criteria, including special tests; and treatment and medical control measures.*

Raffle A, et al. The diseases of occupations. 8th ed. London: Hodder & Stoughton, 1994.
*A comprehensive but somewhat dated review of the history and related literature of occupational health. Excellent description of many classic occupational diseases.*

Rom W, ed. Environmental and occupational medicine. 2nd ed. Boston: Little, Brown, 1992.
*An excellent in-depth textbook.*

Rosenstock L, Cullen M. Textbook of clinical occupational and environmental medicine. Philadelphia: Saunders, 1994.
*An excellent comprehensive clinical reference that covers all aspects of occupational and environmental medicine with special attention to the opportunities for prevention that rest in the hands of the health care provider caring for individual workers.*

Schilling RSF, ed. Occupational health practice. 2nd ed. London: Butterworth, 1981.
*A general overview of occupational disease and health services with a British orientation.*

Weeks JL, Levy BS, Wagner GR, eds. Preventing occupational disease and injury. Washington, D.C., American Public Health Association, 1991.
*A systematically organized handbook that presents a summary of the key diagnostic characteristics and the approaches to prevention of a wide range of occupational disease and injuries (both acute and chronic). The book is written for the general health care provider and public health worker as a resource for guiding occupational health and safety activity that emphasizes prevention.*

Zenz C, ed. Occupational medicine. 3rd ed. Chicago: Year Book, 1994.
*Broad and detailed review designed for occupational health physicians.*

## Selected Periodical Publications in Occupational Health Disciplines

### Occupational Health and Occupational Medicine

*American Journal of Industrial Medicine,* published monthly by John Wiley and Sons, Inc., 205 Third Avenue, New York, NY 10003.

*Journal of Occupational Medicine,* published monthly by the American College of Occupational and Environmental Medicine, 55 W. Seegers Road, Arlington Heights, IL 60005.

*New Solutions: A Journal of Occupational and Environmental Health Policy,* published by the Alice Hamilton Institute, P.O. Box 281200, Lakewood, CO 80228-8200.

*Occupational and Environmental Medicine,* published monthly by the British Medical Association, Tavistock Square, London WC1H 9JR, United Kingdom.

*Scandinavian Journal of Work, Environment & Health,* published bimonthly by occupational health agencies and boards in Finland, Sweden, Norway, and Denmark; address: Topeliuksenkatu 41A, FIN-00250, Helsinki 29, Finland.

*State of the Art Reviews: Occupational Medicine,* published quarterly by Hanley & Belfus, Inc., 210 S. 13th Street, Philadelphia, PA 19107.

### Occupational Health Nursing

*American Association of Occupational Health Nurses Journal,* published monthly, 50 Lenox Pointe, Atlanta, GA 30324.

### Industrial Hygiene

*American Industrial Hygiene Association Journal,* published monthly by the American Industrial Hygiene Association, 2700 Prosperity Ave., Suite 250, Fairfax, VA 22031.

*The Annals of Occupational Hygiene,* published 6 times a year by Elsevier Science, 660 White Plains Road, Tarrytown, NY 10591-5153 (alternate address: The Boulevard, Langford Lane, Kidlington, Oxford, United Kingdom OX5 1GB).

*Applied Industrial and Environmental Hygiene,* published monthly by Applied Industrial Hygiene, Inc., a subsidiary of the American Conference of Governmental Industrial Hygienists, 1330 Kemper Meadow Drive, Cincinnati, OH 45240.

### Occupational Safety

*Professional Safety,* published monthly by the American Society of Safety Engineers, 1800 E. Oakton Street, Des Plaines, IL 60018-2187.

*Safety and Health,* published monthly by the National Safety Council, 1121 Spring Lake Drive, Itasca, IL 60143-3201.

### General News and Scientific Update Publications

*BNA Occu Safety and Health Reporter,* published weekly by the Bureau of National Affairs, 1231 25th Street N.W., Washington, DC 20037.

*Occupational and Environmental Health Report,* published monthly by Curtis Vouwie, 55 Tozer Road, Beverly, MA 01915.

---

APPENDIX

# Training and Career Opportunities

Howard Frumkin, Howard Hu,
and Patricia Hyland Travers

---

## Education and Training

Few medical schools and training programs teach occupational health in anything more than a cursory fashion. The same is true for most nursing schools and other clinically oriented health professional schools.

Some medical and nursing schools have developed formal courses, and others include occupational health in their basic science and clinical curricula, often as the result of student efforts. Many students find it easier to incorporate occupational health into existing courses, rather than to add extra courses to already crowded schedules.

Students can also participate in full-time structured programs that include occupational health field work. In such programs students learn the fundamentals of recognizing occupational disease, occupational history taking, and work process analysis. They visit various worksites and conduct health evaluations, sometimes designing and implementing specific projects. Students can also participate in a wide variety of extracurricular activities, some of which are acceptable for elective credit by medical schools. Examples include work with public interest organizations, labor unions, companies, and academic research groups.

Those who seek training at the postgraduate level will find a variety of opportunities available. A good source for information on current training programs is the Division of Training at NIOSH (800-356-4674). The most complete programs are located at the NIOSH Educational Resource Centers (ERCs). As of 1993, there were 14 ERCs in the United States aiming to provide full- and part-time academic career training, cross-training of occupational health and safety practitioners, mid-career training in the field of occupational safety and health, and access to relevant courses for students pursuing various degrees. The ERCs are listed in Appendix B.

ERCs have developed core areas of instruction for graduate and postgraduate students and continuing education programs for professionals. Areas of study include epidemiology and biostatistics, toxicology, industrial hygiene, safety and ergonomics, policy issues, administration, and clinical occupational medicine. Many ERCs are located at schools of public health, where they draw on the strength of departments in related disciplines. Emphasis is placed on training occupational physicians, industrial hygienists, occupational health nurses, and other professionals to work as a team in preventing occupational disease and injury.

The schools of public health that house ERCs, and many others as well, offer masters and doctoral programs that focus on occupational health. Some medical students earn master of public health (M.P.H.) or equivalent degrees during medical school elective time or during time off from medical school. Interested professionals may enroll in public health programs after completing other professional study; some have done so after many years of practice.

Both occupational health specialists and other physicians can seek continuing education credits in occupational health by attending appropriate seminars and short courses. These are frequently offered by ERCs. Another source is the American College of Occupational and Environmental Medicine, through both its national office and its regional affiliates. Announcements appear in its *Journal of Occupational Medicine* and other journals in the field.

Finally, physicians—and a few nonphysicians—who seek full-time on-the-job training may join a 2-year program administered by NIOSH in conjunction with the Epidemic Intelligence Service (EIS) of the Centers for Disease Control and Prevention (CDC). Members of this program learn occupational disease epidemiology through rigorous field studies, data analyses, and seminars. Information may be obtained from NIOSH, Centers for Disease Control and Prevention, Atlanta, GA 30333.

## Career Opportunities

The following is an overview of career opportunities available to professionals in occupational health with personal examples of career pathways.

### Physicians Employed by Companies

Industry has traditionally provided most employment in occupational medicine. Those employed by companies have responsibilities in three general areas: prevention and early detection of occupational disease and injury; diagnosis and treatment

---

BOARD CERTIFICATION IN
OCCUPATIONAL HEALTH
FOR PROFESSIONALS

Physicians may pursue board certification in occupational medicine. Eligibility is based on academic training, clinical training, and practical experience. A current list of approved academic and field-training programs and criteria for board certification may be obtained from the American Board of Preventive Medicine, 9950 West Lawrence Avenue, Suite 106, Schiller Park, IL 60176 (telephone: 708-671-1750).

Certification for industrial hygienists is based on academic preparation, experience, and written examination. Further information, including a list of training programs that has been compiled by the American Industrial Hygiene Association, can be obtained from the American Board of Industrial Hygiene, 4600 West Saginaw, Suite 101, Lansing, MI 48917 (telephone: 517-321-2638).

Certification for industrial safety professionals is also based on academic preparation, experience, and written examinations. Further information, including a list of training programs, can be obtained from the Board of Certified Safety Professionals, 208 Burwash Avenue, Savoy, IL 61874 (telephone: 217-359-9263).

The designation of Occupational Health and Safety Technologist is a joint certification offered by the American Board of Industrial Hygiene and the Board of Certified Safety Professionals (BCSP). Further information can be obtained from the BCSP.

Board certification is available for occupational health nurses and requires passing a written examination, 5,000 hours of occupational health nursing practice over a five-year period, current in employment in occupational health nursing, and 75 contact hours of continuing education. (As of 1996, it will also require a baccalaureate degree in nursing.) Information on board certification can be obtained by contacting the American Board for Occupational Health Nurses, 10503 North Cedarburg Road, Mequon, WI 53092 (telephone: 414-242-0704).

of occupational disease and injury (emphasizing return of workers to their jobs); and diagnosis and treatment of nonoccupational disease or injury in emergency situations or when community resources are unavailable.

Physicians who work at the upper management level are more involved in questions of policy, whereas those at the plant level are more involved in clinical duties. David C. Logan, M.D., M.P.H., Clinical Toxicologist for the Mobil Oil Corporation, writes:

I provide guidance and technical assistance to the company on issues pertaining to the health and safety of our processes and products. One of my responsibilities is to review the company's existing medical surveillance programs. I am called upon to develop medical department procedures to ensure compliance with company standards for workplace and product safety and the medical requirements of OSHA and other federal and state regulations. I respond to customer and employee concerns regarding the health and safety of our operations, such as the safety of video display terminals and the use of contact lenses in our various work environments.

My office works very closely with environmental affairs, toxicology, industrial hygiene, and product safety professionals in performing risk assessments, setting internal exposure standards, planning our toxicology testing programs, providing recommendations concerning the medical information to be included on labels and material safety data sheets, and evaluating adverse effect allegations received by the company. Recent areas of review have included the potential toxicity of ceramic fiber insulation and the thermal degradation products of plastics commonly referred to as "blue haze." I participate as a member of the company's Product Safety Emergency Response Team and in disaster preparedness activities of the company.

My group has also had a role in developing a process for evaluating the reproductive risks of our operations.

Providing assistance to our attorneys has become another important responsibility. I am frequently called upon to review medical records related to lawsuits against the company and to provide recommendations and opinions.

I also contribute to policy development, program planning and the administration of the Medical Depart-

ment. For example, my office has helped in developing the Medical Department role in the company's Alcohol and Drug Control Program.

Finally, I represent the company in outside professional organizations and teaching activities.

### Physicians Employed by Labor Unions

Physicians employed by labor unions work closely with other members of their unions' health and safety departments. Their job responsibilities are generally less well defined and more flexible than those of company physicians and nurses. Responsibilities may include worker education, health hazard evaluation, participation in contract negotiations, research, and maintenance of disease registries.

Health care providers employed by labor unions may function as worker advocates. This perspective is described by one physician, Dr. Michael Silverstein, who formerly worked for the United Auto Workers union (UAW):

The basic thrust of the union's health and safety program is to identify hazardous plant conditions and eliminate them before damage has been done to workers' health. In situations of uncertainty, the benefit of the doubt goes to the worker. In other words, it is assumed that an exposure or condition is hazardous until and unless we can demonstrate otherwise.

I spent my time responding to requests for service and assistance from local unions; providing education and training as well as developing educational materials on health and safety issues; participating in collective bargaining concerning specific issues in which we have particular expertise, such as guarantees to members of certain rights to health and safety protection of various types; and helping in defining and implementing the union's public posture and activity in the area of health and safety, including work on health and safety legislation, OSHA standard setting, and workers' compensation reform.

Within this framework, I have found myself able to apply a substantial portion of my medical skills and resources to a diversified set of problems in a manner that has been professionally challenging and politically satisfying. I fall among those who approach occupational medicine as a public health discipline rather than an internal medicine specialty.

### Federal Government Physicians

Physicians work with NIOSH and have worked with OSHA, assisting in the functions of these two agencies (see Chaps. 4 and 9). Since NIOSH is primarily a research agency, its medical staff is devoted primarily to research. This research may take the form of health hazard evaluations or field investigations, or it may involve basic scientific or epidemiologic investigation.

Dr. Paul Seligman has worked in the Hazard Evaluation Program and in the Surveillance Branch. He writes:

During my time at Hazard Evaluation I worked on: outbreaks of phytophotodermatitis in grocery workers; cumulative trauma disorders in machine operators in the bookbinding and wire die industries and among police transcribers; breast cancer and spontaneous abortion clusters among women exposed to radiofrequency heat sealers in the manufacture of loose-leaf binders; lead and arsenic exposures in a copper smelter; health effects among firefighters exposed to polychlorinated biphenyls (PCBs) and PCB pyrolysis products during a dumpsite fire; skin sensitization and restrictive lung disease in workers exposed to hard metals in the manufacture of hardened blade tips; control of ethylene oxide (EtO) exposures in hospitals; acute neuropathy and cataracts in EtO-exposed workers in the manufacture of hospital supplies; an assessment of carboxyhemoglobin levels in workers exposed to methylene chloride in the electronics industry; health effects from exposure to chlordane following a misapplication; and eye irritation associated with use of soft contact lenses among university biochemists.

I have also responded to numerous telephone calls and letters from workers and/or their families requesting information and advice concerning workplace exposures and their potential health effects, and to requests for information from the media, other governmental agencies, and Congress.

Later, I worked on surveillance and studied workers' compensation claims in Ohio, as a source for describing the epidemiologic characteristics of occupational lead poisoning, skin disease, cumulative trauma disorders, and work-related violent crime injuries. Work in surveillance has offered me the opportunity to learn how to use data sets to create surveillance systems for the identification and follow-back of companies with lead exposure, skin disease, or cumulative trauma problems, and to generate hypotheses relating disease outcomes with industries at high risk. This work is very satisfying in that it allows me to work in the area where policy planning, epidemiology, and health overlap.

Dr. Seligman counts as the advantages of his job: the NIOSH mission to promote worker safety and health, the access to workplaces for study purposes, the variety of problems he confronts, the freedom and responsibility it entails, the opportunity for interdisciplinary collaboration, and the opportunity to publish. He notes that work at NIOSH offers little opportunity for clinical practice.

Other federal agencies that employ physicians may also become involved in occupational health issues. For example, a medical epidemiologist at the National Cancer Institute might study mortality patterns among certain occupational groups, or a staff physician at the Office of Technology Assessment of the U.S. Congress might review the health effects of certain occupational exposures.

### State and Provincial Government Physicians

Some states and provinces that are active in occupational health and safety regulation employ physicians. In some cases, physicians work in environmental health or cancer prevention programs and naturally become involved with issues of occupational safety and health.

Dr. Rose Goldman, an occupational hygiene physician for Massachusetts, describes her work as follows:

The Division of Occupational Hygiene inspects workplaces and assists employers and employees in correcting health hazards and improving working conditions. It also publishes recommended exposure limits and safe practice bulletins. I participate in worksite health hazard evaluations, conduct small-scale epidemiologic projects, perform educational activities, answer telephone inquiries, and supervise a full-time occupational hygiene nurse who surveys health programs in industrial plants.

For workplace evaluations, I work with an industrial hygienist to assess health hazards and evaluate workers. We usually make recommendations to eliminate or diminish the hazard; sometimes we recommend a program of ongoing medical surveillance. For example, in evaluating workers at a sewage treatment plant with possible lead and chromate exposure, I administered brief questionnaires, performed physical examinations, and obtained blood analyses for chromium and lead. We were able to determine that the current control measures usually limited exposure and protected workers, but that in a few parts of the work process additional control measures were warranted.

The opportunity for plant access provides the potential to perform epidemiologic surveys, such as a recent survey of automobile radiator repair shops and workers for lead poisoning. Previous state occupational hygiene physicians in Massachusetts have performed important studies of the health effects of beryllium, cadmium, toluene diisocyanate (TDI), lead, and talc, which have often led to important preventive measures.

I also educate employers and employees daily on hazardous exposures and control measures, update and write the medical aspects of safe practice guides and material safety data sheets, supervise medical residents and industrial hygiene students learning about worksite evaluations, and participate in preparing state regulations and proposed statutes. I am also a member of a state interagency task force that is developing methods for surveillance and intervention of occupational health problems.

Although a strong national program is integral to controlling workplace hazards, state agencies perform additional important functions: They provide services more readily to local small plants not covered by OSHA, respond quickly to emergencies, provide enforcement on problems not covered by OSHA, help employers comply with OSHA standards, and respond to complaints.

### Occupational Medicine in the Community Setting

A growing number of opportunities to practice occupational medicine can be found in clinical set-

tings in the community. In some cases occupational medical clinics exist as independent contractors that sell to client companies such services as preplacement and return-to-work evaluations, drug screening, and trauma care. Alternatively, some clinical occupational medicine units exist as parts of hospital staffs, usually within departments of medicine or family practice. Dr. John Davis, Chief of Occupational Health at Norwood Hospital in Norwood, Massachusetts, reports that both community hospitals and companies have an interest in such arrangements, the former, in part, to increase revenues and the latter to cope with regulatory demands and workers' compensation costs. Dr. Davis indicates that a wide range of options may be available in the community hospital setting, including extension of emergency services that triage the injured worker, extension of employee health services, development of free-standing occupational health departments, and development of satellite sites.

Dr. Davis reports that his clinical practice is a combination of general internal medicine and office orthopedics. He performs "complex injury management," evaluates patients for insurance companies, manages an active executive health and wellness program, and establishes medical surveillance programs on a consultative basis, subcontracting with industrial hygiene and clinical laboratory facilities when appropriate. He notes that one potential controversy is that some community physicians might feel threatened by an occupational medicine service if they have been previously performing such duties on an informal basis.

### Nurses in Occupational Health

Occupational health nursing has undergone a metamorphosis since its beginnings in the late 1800s, when nurses were employed by industries to care for ailing workers and their families. Attention in the field of occupational health nursing has shifted from a narrow focus on communicable disease, maternal and child health issues, and emergency treatment of injured workers to a much broader focus today. Presently, the occupational health nurse (OHN) applies public health principles to meet the needs of workers in an ever-changing work environment. The focus of the OHN has thus expanded to include integration of many areas, including epidemiology, industrial hygiene, environmental health, toxicology, safety, management, health education, early disease detection, disease prevention, health promotion, and health and environmental surveillance.

The American Association of Occupational Health Nurses (AAOHN) defines occupational health nursing as:

... the application of nursing principles in conserving the health of workers in all occupations. It emphasizes prevention, recognition, and treatment of illnesses and injuries and requires special skills and knowledge in the fields of health education and counseling, environmental health, and human relations.

Most OHNs work for company medical departments. The OHN, whether employed as a single health care provider at a small plant or as a member of a multidisciplinary health unit, must balance ethical and clinical responsibilities to employees with ethical and administrative responsibilities to management. This balance requires the OHN to assist management in providing a safe and healthful work environment through disease prevention and health promotion activities. Some of the responsibilities include the daily operation of a comprehensive health care program; development of treatment and surveillance protocols; keeping informed about health and safety legislation; maintenance of a toxic substance list; identification of high-risk areas; clinical intervention, including delivery of health care and counseling services; recordkeeping; liaison with managers, workers, and health and safety colleagues; and implementation of health-related programs on a primary, secondary, and tertiary level. (See P. Travers. *A Comprehensive Guide for Establishing an Occupational Health Service.* New York: AAOHN, 1987. Available from AAOHN, 50 Lenox Pointe, Atlanta, GA 30324; 1-800-241-8014.)

Judy H. Manchester, R.N., manager of nursing and health services for the GTE Products Corporation, writes:

I am responsible for overseeing nursing functions and health services for approximately 150 locations throughout the United States, Canada, Puerto Rico, Haiti, and Central America. My responsibilities include performing audits of health services throughout the company, developing policy, arranging for continuing education, and apprising the nurses who report to me of current events in medicine, legislation, health care delivery, and other fields as they relate to employee health and safety. I act as a resource, consultant, and liaison among health services and other areas of the company, and as an advocate for the nurses.

I find occupational health very exciting. In no other area of nursing does one need such a broad base of nursing knowledge or have such a varied role. In no other area of nursing does one have such a captive audience in which to promote health and wellness, or such an opportunity to express individuality and creativity within a practice.

Opportunities for OHNs also exist in other sectors, such as organized labor and government.

### Industrial Hygiene

The practice of industrial hygiene includes the recognition, evaluation, and control of occupational hazards. Most industrial hygienists are employed directly by companies; however, many are also employed by government agencies concerned with regulation, independent consulting groups, and academic institutions. A few are also employed by labor unions. The following is an account by an industrial hygienist that reflects the breadth of opportunities in this field. Barbara Plog, an industrial hygienist with the Labor Occupational Health Program, Northern California Occupational Health Center, University of California at Berkeley, writes:

My job as an industrial hygienist involves the development and implementation of education and training programs on all aspects of industrial hygiene for workers, their representatives, managers, and members of labor-management health and safety committees. This work has included training programs that address basic hazard recognition procedures, hearing conservation, dust exposures (silica and asbestos), chemical exposures, hazardous waste, OSHA standards, ventilation, control measures used in the workplace, ergonomics, and manual materials handling. I also teach in university courses for occupational and environmental health sciences students and in continuing education courses for occupational health professionals at a NIOSH educational resource center. I have trained contractors and workers in asbestos abatement techniques at an EPA asbestos training center.

The creation of written materials has been a key part of my career. I have written a number of slide and videotape training programs and a series of guidebooks on various industrial hygiene topics. I am the editor of the third edition of the *Fundamentals of Industrial Hygiene*, a basic textbook in the field.

Providing technical assistance to workers, managers, and the general public has also been a part of my work. Acting as a technical resource is a large part of industrial hygienists' work, whether they work for industry, labor, academic institutions, or the government.

My career as an industrial hygienist reflects a heavy emphasis on writing and teaching. Many industrial hygienists may find themselves also performing a training and education function, but as a smaller part of their jobs. They may be in the field, performing sampling and evaluations much of the time. These evaluations may cover a wide range of chemical and physical workplace health hazards. Some industrial hygienists specialize in one particular hazard. For example, health physicists specialize in ionizing radiation while other industrial hygienists may specialize in hearing conservation and noise control technologies or in asbestos abatement work.

Government jobs for industrial hygienists include program development, training and education, and compliance inspections and evaluations of worksites.

Industrial hygienists who work for private industry may work mainly as field hygienists, performing daily sampling and evaluation; as trainers and program developers; or as program administrators. The typical job incorporates all of these functions, depending upon the size of the company.

Industrial hygienists in academic organizations typically divide their time between teaching and research functions. Some are program administrators.

The field of industrial hygiene is exciting and challenging. It draws upon many other disciplines (chemistry, biology, toxicology, epidemiology, occupational medicine, health physics, engineering, and health education) to meet its goal of protecting the health of workers.

Leopoldo Yanes, the coordinator of the Graduate Occupational Hygiene Program at the University of Carabobo in Venezuela, writes:

Our graduate program, which was established in 1970, is the first one in Venezuela. Now, there are two other programs in other universities more focused on occupational medicine. Our program is a multidisciplinary program that is oriented principally toward prevention. It is integrated, with engineers, physicians, epidemiologists, and other professionals.

In general, industrial hygienists in Venezuela are limited in their activity in the factories. Only in the larger ones are there occupational health policies, on which industrial hygienists can base preventive activities. Another problem is that access to technical resources is too limited, leading to inadequate quantity and quality of equipment in laboratories. In small- and medium-sized facilities, occupational health and safety problems are greater. Government policies are not structured to improve the work environment. Venezuela has a deficit of over 1,000 industrial hygienists.

My job involves the development and implementation of preventive programs in different areas of industrial hygiene. The most important activity developed is recognition and control programs. Evaluation is limited because we do not have sufficient equipment, laboratories, and other resources. Education and training programs are common activities in my professional practice. We have developed introductory courses in occupational health and industrial hygiene for managers, technical employees, and workers in several industries in our state.

Providing technical assistance to workers, managers, and governmental agencies has also been part of my work. Now, the unions and the manager organizations have begun to take interest in this area, and day to day, more requests for services and technical assistance are arising.

My career as an industrial hygienist reflects a heavy emphasis on teaching and researching, but this is not the most common activity of industrial hygienists in Venezuela. In our program, we develop different educational course levels—introductory, intermediate, and intensive courses in the occupational health—with special emphasis in workers' training programs. We have agreements with unions in our state to provide technical assistance, a priority activity for our work.

Researching is another area of my activity. The possibility of creating a multidisciplinary team in this area is very important, and now we have one. The development of new research models that are adequate for our conditions, and that promote the worker participation, is a policy of our team. We are also developing different research programs—for example, on neurotoxicity and occupational exposures to solvents, mercury, and lead, or new technologies and worker health effects.

### Academic Occupational Health

Many occupational health specialists have faculty appointments at schools of medicine, nursing, public health, or other disciplines. Often these are part-time appointments that complement clinical appointments or employment in other settings.

Academic positions in occupational health entail the same types of duties as do other faculty posts, including research and publication, classroom and clinical teaching, outside consulting, and patient care. Faculty members may specialize further, depending on their interests and training. Many collaborate with statisticians, epidemiologists, toxicologists, and others in their research and with clinicians from other fields in their clinical duties. Specific job responsibilities are variable and are often largely defined by the individual.

Dr. Linda Rosenstock, former Director of the University of Washington Occupational Medicine Program and now Director of NIOSH, writes:

Academic medicine is traditionally described as demanding productivity in three areas: clinical service, teaching, and research. Increasingly, administrative activities are added responsibilities even for junior faculty. Although these expectations may be viewed as overly demanding in some disciplines, they add to the variety and challenge of working in the emerging academic field of occupational medicine. My colleagues and I have responsibility for teaching medical students in the basic science years and providing elective opportunities to them in the clinical years. Residents in internal medicine, family medicine, and occupational medicine also rotate through our program, participating in clinical and research activities and interacting with a multidisciplinary staff of physicians, industrial hygienists, and nurses. Other trainees are also involved, including students in industrial hygiene and occupational nursing.

Our main objective, determining whether an individual's health problem is work-related, is largely carried out in a consultative clinic setting. Here, patients are referred for evaluation by themselves or by physicians, unions, companies, and workers' compensation and other agencies. After our review of medical records and available information about exposures, each patient undergoes a comprehensive interview eliciting information about work and exposure history, a physical examination, and appropriate laboratory tests. It is against this background that a determination about the individual's medical condition and its relation to workplace factors is made. Often this task is relatively straightforward, but sometimes in the process we recognize unexpected or new associations between the workplace and health.

Probably in no other field is there this same potential for discovering and detecting new etiologies and syndromes. But, regardless of the complexity of evaluating disease and its cause in an individual, we are always thinking about the implications of our findings in terms of prevention—for the individual in terms of returning to the workplace and for others who may be similarly affected or at risk.

This process—from initial evaluation to diagnosis and follow-through—is, I think, the most rewarding part of clinical occupational medicine. In our setting all aspects of a patient's situation are discussed by the entire staff in case conferences; these discussions are open and sometimes heated, recognizing that occupational diseases have not only medical, but also social, economic, legal, and political components.

Scholarly investigation and research are also fundamental to our activities and often brought about by problems encountered in the clinic. Occasionally, this leads to basic "bench" research, but the objectives of such inquiry—to provide new knowledge—can also be achieved by describing individual cases or clusters of cases, or by undertaking population-based studies to answer predetermined questions systematically.

We bring a collaborative spirit to all these activities, that they are largely enjoyable (and often fun), and rewarding. It is an opportunity and challenge to work in an evolving field, to be humble in recognizing what we do not know, to be vigilant about opportunities to broaden knowledge, and to recognize that in occupational health we are dealing with the social context of disease, a context that is central to the recognition, determination of causation, and prevention of occupational disease.

Dr. Arthur Frank, Professor and Chairman of the Department of Preventive Medicine and Environmental Health at the University of Kentucky College of Medicine, also describes teaching, research, patient care, and administration as his four duties. He writes:

As an academic occupational health physician, I see to it that our medical students get a reasonable amount of occupational health in their curriculum (with all the usual constraints and competing educational needs). I have started a masters program, on which to base a new residency program in occupational medicine. Patient care activities are in many ways similar to traditional occupational medicine, and patients are seen in the university occupational medicine clinic. In addition, the department operates occupational health programs for several companies in such fields as coal mining and electronics repair, and I have served as medical consultant to Toyota Motor Manufacturing, U.S.A., Inc., as it builds a major new facility near Lexington. My busy program of work at the university is supplemented by regional and national activities; I serve as a board member of several national organizations and as a consultant to NIOSH.

# 2

# The Social Context of Occupational Health

Charles Levenstein, John Wooding, and Beth Rosenberg

Why should scientists and health professionals concern themselves with the social and political context of occupational health and safety problems? Is it not sufficient to learn about the characteristics of risk factors, the diagnosis of occupational disease, and technical approaches to prevention?

- There has been evidence for centuries about the health hazards of lead. Why are workers and children poisoned by lead exposures?
- Pesticides are designed to kill pests, but they are also toxic for other living things. Why do we know so little about the human health effects of most pesticides in use today?
- The textile industry has been the leader of the Industrial Revolution throughout the world. Why did byssinosis, a respiratory disease of cotton mill workers, go unrecognized in the United States until the late 1960s?
- Asphalt fume has been identified as a carcinogen in Denmark. Why is it regulated in the U.S. not as a carcinogen, but only as an "air contaminant"?
- A major transnational automobile company has clear internal guidelines for reviewing possible equipment purchases in order to prevent hearing loss among its employees. Why are these guidelines ignored by plant managers?
- There is less full-time work, more temporary work, more work speed-up, and more shift work, all of which increase physical and psychological health problems. Although there are sci-

entific and technical aspects of this situation that are worth studying, are the solutions solely scientific and technical?
- When hazardous technologies and hazardous substances find their way to developing countries, after being prohibited from use in the developed countries where they originated, what kind of solutions are available?
- What can economically challenged workers or countries do when confronted with the choice between jobs or their health?

The effective understanding of workplace injury and disease requires a full comprehension of the nature of work and the social, political, and economic context of the workplace. Work is a necessary human activity.

People work to survive. Yet work is more than a way to gain an income. Work provides a host of rewards and problems: It can be laborious and numbing, stimulating and satisfying, frustrating and demeaning. All too often it is dangerous and unhealthful.

Work occupies a central place in most people's lives, but the overall context of work is often ignored or poorly understood. To recognize and prevent work-related disease and injury requires that health care providers and other health and safety professionals appreciate the full context of work and workplaces in the world today. This chapter focuses primarily on the U.S. experience, although parallels to other countries are drawn when possible. It is believed that many of the underlying is-

sues being addressed here cross national boundaries.

## The Global Context of Occupational Health

The magnitude and pattern of occupational disease and injury in a particular society are strongly
affected by the level of economic and technological
development, by the societal distribution of
power, and by the dominant ideology of a particular social and political system. These factors bear
on the way in which diseases and injuries are "produced," on the recognition and prevention of these
problems, and on the extent to which workers receive compensation for them. Fully understanding
occupational injury and disease requires, therefore, an understanding of the broad context in
which production takes place. This context includes the economic and technological basis of
production, ideological and cultural factors driving the design and organization of work and the
workplace, and the main social "actors" in decisions that affect the work environment.

### The Social Actors in Occupational Health and the Role of Ideology

The medical/scientific model focuses on disease
and injury causation, using scientific methods to
discover, explain, and solve problems in the work
environment; it rarely addresses the critical economic, social, and political context of work organization. Occupational diseases and injuries are
distinct from other health issues because they are
the direct, although unintended, result of economic activity. The analysis presented here provides a different perspective (Fig. 2-1), one that
places management's control of the workplace,
technological decisions, and the labor process at
the center of occupational health.

The structure in Fig. 2-1 suggests that the key
relationship for understanding the work environment is a "triangle" of control: workers, any potential hazards, and management—and its domi-

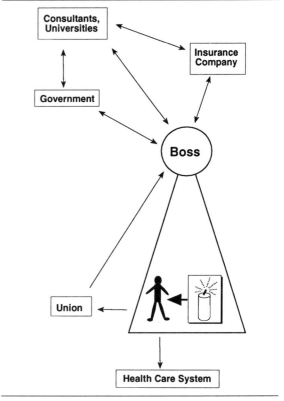

Fig. 2-1. The industrial hygiene system.

nance of the workplace. This relationship exists in
an historical and ideological context, influenced
by a number of other institutions and individuals.
These "actors" include professional consultants,
universities, and research institutes that typically
provide scientific information about workplace
hazards and how to control them. These research
institutes may or may not work in collaboration
with government; government, however, plays a
key role in providing and initiating research about
work environment hazards in most countries.
More specifically, government typically sets and
enforces occupational safety and health standards.

Insurance companies are also key actors. They
provide the economic context in which firms obtain workers' compensation insurance and may, by
"experience rating" premiums, encourage firms to

improve health and safety conditions. Unions provide the collective strength of organized workers. They negotiate working conditions and may provide a counterweight to management's prerogatives. Many unions in the U.S. have their own health and safety staff to provide information and services to workers and workers' representatives. They also push government to act on workplace hazards by lobbying for establishing and enforcing regulations.

The organization of work and the roles played by key actors are deeply influenced by ideology—a set of beliefs, norms, and values. Ideologies of workers, managers, government officials, scientists, and others reflect what they think about society and about themselves. Ideologies also reflect what they expect from work and from employers, government, and each other.

A capitalist, free-market economic system incorporates presumptions about human behavior that most people have come to accept: notions about individual "choice" and "rights," a belief in the primacy of private property, and the efficiency of markets. Americans, in particular, are deeply suspicious of government. It is, therefore, necessary to examine the role of ideology in order to identify the assumptions that determine power relations in the workplace and how they are reflected in the problem of occupational health and safety.

The typical workplace in the U.S. is organized hierarchically. In large workplaces the model is: owner or owners, leading managers, supervisors, and then the workers. Smaller workplaces compress this structure. The hierarchy reflects the distribution of power; owners and managers have complete control over investment decisions, the budget, the structure of production, what is produced, how and when production occurs, hiring and firing of workers, and ultimately controls over the conditions of work.

Labor unions, considered to be a counterweight to this power, have had some success in gaining better wages and working conditions. They have usually been constrained, however, by a number of factors: the strength of the general economy, the level of unemployment, their own economic and political strength, and an ideology that supports the rights of property. Labor's achievements have also depended importantly on the level of government support for protecting and promoting the rights of workers.

In Europe, although the rights of private property remain relatively sacrosanct, the power of unions and workers' parties, as well as the acceptance and expectation of government regulation of working conditions, has led to a greater ability by government to regulate private industry and working conditions than is found in the U.S.

The culture of most liberal democracies, including the U.S., has supported belief in the rationality and apolitical nature of science and technology—a belief that social and public health problems (indeed most societal problems) are amenable to technical solutions. Remarkably enduring has been the ideology of the "technical fix," and the notion that science can be separated from politics and from issues of power and control.

### Economic and Technological Development

Changes in the national and international economic order—growth of new markets and the disappearance of old ones, new technologies, new competitors, demographic shifts, and shifts in investment—all directly affect the structure of production and work.

In contrast to the 20 years following World War II, when American economic power was at its peak, the U.S. now faces fierce competition in heavy manufacturing, in the service sector, and in high-technology production. By 1970 the U.S. found itself confronting a new and highly competitive world economy in which American goods and American companies no longer dominated. In addition, multinational corporations based in Europe and the U.S. began to spread their activities across the globe, setting up production facilities in many developed and developing countries. These multinational corporations invested heavily abroad, seeking new markets and new places of production with lower wages, less regulation, and less taxation. Aided by new communications systems and new opportunities for investment, industry and investment capital has become increasingly mobile. This situation undercuts the ability of advanced industrial countries to regulate domestic industry for fear that this might cause industry to flee regulation. At the same time it spreads hazards, some of which are associated with advanced technologies to countries without the social or scientific infrastructures to protect their citizens.

Some particular economic developments have led to this situation such as the major increase in oil prices by the Oil Producing and Exporting Countries (OPEC) in the 1970s, which led many developing countries to borrow heavily to buy oil. This resulted in a vicious circle for these countries, involving the siphoning-off of domestic savings to service the debt, domestic austerity programs imposed by institutions such as the World Bank and the International Monetary Fund, and a shift to export-oriented production. As a consequence, developing countries had to increasingly accept foreign investment and foreign technologies in order to survive. At the same time, the dire economic situation in these countries forced many of their most productive and mobile citizens to migrate to other countries in search of work, often at substandard conditions in Europe and elsewhere.

By the end of the 1980s, the world economy had undergone a fundamental realignment, with four major effects on the U.S. and developed countries of Europe:

1. Their economies shifted from heavy manufacturing (of chemicals and steel) toward the service sector (banking, insurance, food, and clerical work). American businesses lost approximately 38 million manufacturing jobs during the 1970s and 1980s [1].
2. Their economies became dominated by extremely mobile and mostly large international corporations.
3. In the U.S., ownership of industry has become concentrated in a smaller number of very large

firms. The frequent buying and selling of companies during the 1980s led to the U.S. economy becoming increasingly under the control of the banking and finance sector.
4. With decreasing profitability, management in the U.S. could not afford, and was not willing to accept, the "social contract" with labor—a commitment to maintaining decent wages and working conditions in return for some job security and rising standards of living for most workers—a contract that it had maintained for most of the period since World War II. Companies tried to cut the costs of production by demanding reductions in wages or benefits, and they fought health, safety, and environmental regulation. In Europe, similar economic changes ushered in a period of political conservatism, resulting in the deregulation of the market and a reduction in government control over private industry.

All this had an impact on workers; for example, in the U.S., real wages fell by 17 percent between 1973 and 1988 [1]. Housing, education, and medical costs have all increased at a rate of about 9 percent faster than inflation over this period. By 1994, despite more two-earner families, American workers were much worse off than they had been in 1970.

In addition to these effects, there have been some major technological changes that, throughout the twentieth century, have contributed to the current structure of the work environment. The combination of increasing specialization, the spread of assembly-line production techniques, and the introduction of many chemicals and chemical processes have transformed the workplace.

### Management Theory and the Structure of Work

Although under attack and reconsideration in recent years, the general tendency in management theory from the time of Adam Smith, the father of economic liberalism, to the present has been to divide work into ever more discrete units in order to increase productivity, cheapen the cost of labor, and increase management's control over the labor process (Fig. 2-2). This quest for "efficiency" became more self-conscious and explicit in the early twentieth century with the work of such promoters of "scientific management" as Frederick Winslow Taylor [2, 3]. In Taylor's view, the worker should be treated not as a whole person but rather as a collection of machinelike movements: walk, bend, grasp, sit, depress typewriter key. Such motions can be analyzed, timed, and reassembled into a program for maximum productivity. This "scientific" approach to management was widely accepted, both in capitalist and noncapitalist economies. Taylorism's impact is well illustrated by the following comment by an automobile assembly-line worker [4]:

My father worked in auto for 35 years and he never talked about the job. What's there to say? A car comes, I weld it; a car comes, I weld it; a car comes, I weld it.

One hundred and one times an hour. . . . There is a lot of variety in the paint shop . . . you clip on the color hose, bleed out the old color, and squirt. Clip, bleed, squirt, think; clip, bleed, squirt, yawn; clip, bleed, squirt, scratch your nose. Only now the [company has] taken away the time to scratch your nose.

Taylorism had a wide-ranging impact on the quality of work life. It meant the separation of conception from performance and the division of performance into multiple repetitive tasks. The intrinsic satisfaction of "work," craftsmanship, and the ability to take pride in the whole finished product necessarily diminished. Employers increasingly relied on supervisory hierarchies and monetary rewards and punishment, such as piece rates and bonuses, to motivate workers in a carrot-and-stick fashion[4]:

You're too busy to talk. Can't hear. They got these little guys coming around in white shirts and if they see you running your mouth, "This guy needs more work." A

Fig. 2-2. Automobile assembly-line worker.

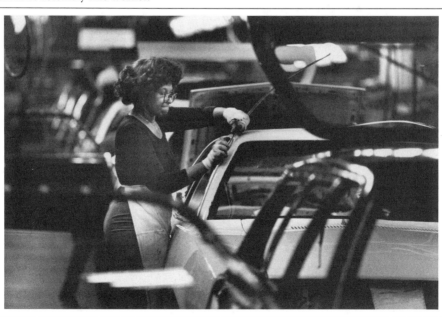

lot of guys who've been in jail they say you don't work as hard in jail. They say, "Man, jail ain't never been this bad."

Another profound influence on modern production and the workplace has been the rapid increase in the use of chemicals, especially since World War II. There are currently 70,000 chemicals in use in the United States, with 1,000 new chemicals introduced each year [5] (Fig. 2-3). A similar number of chemicals and chemical processes exist in most of the industrialized world, and increasingly so in developing countries as production is shifted to them. The vast majority of these chemicals are unregulated and their human health effects unknown. They are used in a variety of production settings to produce a wide range of products, but they are also encountered in a range of occupations not traditionally considered dangerous. From typists and stockroom workers to janitors and artists, workers confront some potentially toxic chemicals on a daily basis.

Technology has increased the speed of production enormously, putting greater pressure on workers to perform rapid and repetitive motions that are damaging to mental and physical health. Stress and related psychological and physiologic illnesses are increasing in industrialized countries, including the U.S., as the pace of work and life increases, as well as pressures to work longer hours in order to compensate for falling wage rates and declining standard of living increases [6]. In some countries, however, such as those in Europe, because of historical and cultural reasons and pressure from powerful trade unions, a shorter work week with reduced working hours has been adopted since World War II. More recently, unemployment pressures have furthered the call for a shorter work week [7].

With speed-up has come automation. Apart from obvious physical hazards associated with use of robots, robotic systems, and highly automated machinery, automation also eliminates jobs and de-skills others, leaving fewer workers responsible

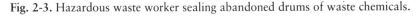

**Fig. 2-3.** Hazardous waste worker sealing abandoned drums of waste chemicals.

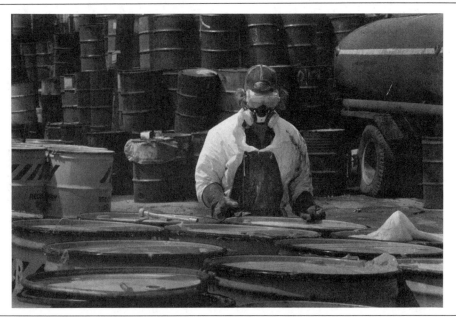

for complex systems. With the help of automation, one worker can do a job that may have required 10 workers before. This advance, however, has been accompanied by greater stress and generally more overtime work. Under these circumstances, rather than achieving the promise that automation would replace grueling mindless labor, it has resulted in more stress, longer hours, and overwhelming responsibility at work [8].

Economic and technological changes go together. The spread of new technologies, the globalization of the world economy, and vast changes in the international division of labor both directly and indirectly affect not only the work environment, but also the general power relations in society. Class, race, and gender are key dimensions in the power relationships in the U.S. that shape substantial aspects of the work environment.

### The Distribution of Power

All societies are composed of classes, of interest groups, of sects and sectarians, of minorities and majorities, with varying degrees of power and influence. The distribution of such political and economic power and influence is another essential factor shaping the work environment. In the most simple formulation, there are "workers" and "owners." In advanced industrial societies, such a formulation cannot capture the complex features of the contemporary class system. In such societies, a middle stratum has developed that is composed of independent professionals, an enduring class of small business owners, and a growing group of government employees with a wide range of social functions and with their own roles, interests, and power. The varying degrees of political power amongst lower, middle, and upper classes set limits on what can happen in a particular workplace or a particular industry. Class and the distribution of power in society, therefore, shape the work environment.

In many liberal democracies, although the stated goal is equality, power in society at large is unevenly distributed along the lines of class, race, and gender. Because the workplace is a microcosm of society, the power relationships in society are reproduced at work. Inequities in the distribution of power have a profound influence on work and health because power determines who does what work and under what conditions, who gets exposed to risks, and what is considered acceptable risk. Furthermore, the people affected are not the people deciding the acceptability of workplace hazards [9]:

All the clichés and pleasant notions of how the old class divisions . . . have disappeared are exposed as hollow phrases by the simple fact that American workers must accept serious injury and even death as a part of their daily reality while the middle class does not. Imagine . . . the universal outcry that would occur if every year several corporate headquarters routinely collapsed like mines, crushing sixty or seventy executives. Or suppose that all the banks were filled with an invisible noxious dust that constantly produced cancer in the managers, clerk and tellers. Finally, try to imagine the horror . . . if thousands of university professors were deafened every year or lost fingers, hands, sometimes eyes, while on their jobs.

Social class and class-based assumptions have been widely discussed from a variety of perspectives: sociologic, economic, and political. Class is clearly related to family background, level of education, occupation, and a variety of cultural factors. The lower the social class of an individual, the less likely that he or she will be to have a range of educational and employment options. Class determines levels of material well-being and health. Because class influences employment options, it affects the probability of becoming ill or injured at work.

### Impact of Racism

In the workplace and in society as a whole, racism plays a role in determining who does what job, how much he or she will be paid for it, and what alternatives are open. For most of its history, the U.S. has depended on minorities to do the least desirable and dangerous work. Immigrant and minority communities have been the major sources of labor to build the railways, pick cotton and weave it in the mills, work in the foundries in the automobile industry, run coke oven operations in the steel industry, sew in the sweatshops, and provide migrant agricultural labor (Fig. 2-4). Minorities are still overrepresented in the most hazardous and least desirable occupations (Fig. 2-5). Minority workers may leave a hazardous work environment only to arrive home to a hazardous community environment. Since the early 1980s, in the U.S., scientific evidence has increasingly pointed to discriminatory environmental practices of certain industries, of state and local governments, and in some instances, of the federal government. One well-documented example is that minority communities have a disproportionate number of toxic threats to health [10].

A social system with strongly racist elements bars members of minority groups from significant positions of power and, consequently, elevates the concerns of dominant racial or national groups. For example, one of the essential reasons for the lack of attention to hazards faced by farmworkers in the U.S. (most of whom are African-American or Latino) is their relative lack of power in the American political system.

### Impact of Sexism

Any discussion of power relations must include the situation of women, whose experience of work is generally different from that of men. Most obviously this is reflected in the wage differentials paid to women for comparable work. Despite a political and legal commitment to equality in the U.S., as of 1991, women were earning 70 cents to every dollar earned by a man and the gap widens as one goes up the career ladder [11]. African-American women and Latinas earn only 50 percent of white men's pay (see Chap. 32) [12].

Even though women frequently work outside the home for as many hours as their spouses, domestic duties are rarely shared equally. Working mothers sleep less, get sick more, and have less leisure time than their husbands. One study finds

**Fig. 2-4.** Migrant workers picking cotton.

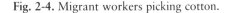

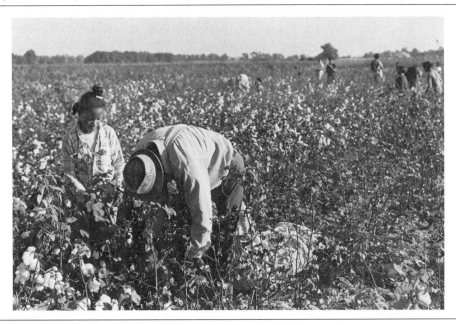

that women who are employed full-time outside the home and whose youngest child is less than five years old spend an average of 47 hours per week on household work, while their male counterparts spend a mere 10 hours [13]. Although the situation may have improved somewhat over the last 10 to 20 years, the stress and fatigue from balancing work life and home life remain a serious problem. The average working woman puts in an estimated 80 hours a week in both job and household work, and up to 105 hours if she has sole responsibility for children.

A proposal from the Italian women's movement (see chapter Appendix) presents recommendations based on an analysis of the profound impact of gender relations on the work environment. The proposed far-reaching reconstruction of work and work relations flows from their conclusion that these gender relations cannot change without fundamental reorganization of all relations in society. The work environment is an integral part of the larger social fabric.

Women are also the main targets of sexual harassment at work. Any unwanted verbal or physical sexual advance constitutes harassment, and this can range from sexual comments and suggestions, to pressure for sexual favors accompanied by threats concerning one's job, to physical assault, including rape. Studies indicate that 40 to 60 percent of women have experienced some form of sexual harassment at work [14]. An estimated one-third of the largest 500 companies in the U.S. spend approximately $6.7 million in dealing with sexual harassment [14].

Gender relations have political, and hence work environment, implications. Cultural assumptions about gender can have strong impact on the distribution of power in society. A strongly patriarchal society that bars women from positions of power is also likely to have a profoundly sex-segregated labor market. As a result, sexual harassment and occupational health in female-dominated retail trade jobs may not be considered important.

**Fig. 2-5.** Worker in a commercial laundry.

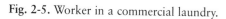

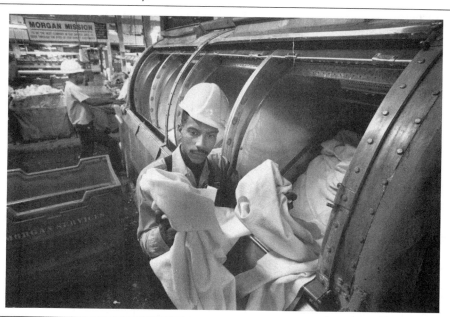

Thus, in addition to the development of the market, the level of technology, ideological considerations, and changes in the global economy, power distribution related to class, race, and gender constitutes the framework in which the actors in an industrial system attempt to create a "web of rules" governing the work environment. Management, labor, and government are constrained in their behavior by these broad social-environmental factors.

## The Micro-context of Occupational Health: Labor-management Relations

### The First Key Actors: Workers

A hundred years ago, when a cobbler woke up in the morning, the decision to make boots or shoes, to buy hides, or to take some of his wares to the neighboring town was under his control. If the cobbler acquired an allergy to a certain polish or was told that it caused cancer, he could choose not to use it. If he found that carving heels bothered his elbow, he could do a few every other day instead of spending a long stretch of time on a bothersome or painful task. Or he could try redesigning the tools or using alternative carving methods that might be better for him. He was his own manager. He set the pace and conditions of his work.

Contrast the cobbler's situation with the working lives of most people today. These options are not open to modern-day shoemakers—or to nurses, auto workers, bank tellers, or employees in countless other occupations. Management controls the work environment; the hours of work, the pace, the tasks, the tools, and the technologies are all determined by someone other than the worker.

In addition to the detrimental effects of lack of control, which by itself causes stress (see Chap. 19), workers' interests conflict with those of management. Management's goal is to maximize profit, labor's goal is a fair wage for a fair day's work. Expenditures on health and safety are often seen by management as limiting profit. As a business school textbook advises [15]:

In making decisions about their workplace, managers have two choices. They can remedy health and safety problems or they can provide risk compensation to workers. If reducing risk is less costly than the additional compensation, then working conditions will be improved. However, if the marginal cost of worker compensation is less than the marginal cost of safety improvements, then the firm will choose the compensation alternative. This outcome represents an efficient allocation of resources in that the firm minimizes its total costs.

Although one would hope that the consciences of managers will go against their training and the incentive system within their businesses, history has shown that it is unwise for workers to depend on the benevolence of management. The sociopolitical structure provides only weak motivation for management to construct a safe workplace. Government regulations exist but they are not always enforced, which is not surprising given that current Occupational Safety and Health Administration (OSHA) resources would allow the federal government to inspect each of 6 million workplaces once every 84 years [16].

Labor-management relations may be particularly problematic when jobs are pitted against improving occupational or environmental conditions. The most frequent example of this contradiction occurs under conditions of "job blackmail," a colloquial term for the problem created when workers are forced to choose between remaining in a hazardous job or finding employment elsewhere [17]. Examples include employers who threaten to fire workers or relocate the plant if workers or regulatory agencies try to impose controls over hazardous production. Job blackmail is found more often in those workplaces where workers have little or no power of control over their jobs as well as in workplaces that are not unionized. Although not unique to minority workers, job blackmail takes a heavy toll on them, because they are more likely than nonminority workers to hold hazardous jobs. Although job blackmail may occur in a variety of direct and indirect ways, the end result is to force workers to choose between being employed or not.

In job blackmail the choices are seldom, if ever, favorable to the worker. The worker who chooses to remain on a hazardous job may, in the short term, avoid unemployment, but may seriously jeopardize his or her future health and safety. The worker who chooses not to question "unfair" compensation will continue to receive a paycheck but will still earn less than she or he is worth. The worker who chooses not to unionize may remain employed, but will likely remain employed in an unjust, unsafe, and unhealthful workplace. Even in those situations in which a worker remains on the job, she or he may be labeled a troublemaker and ostracized to the point of quitting the job anyway.

---

## HISTORY OF A SECONDARY LEAD SMELTER IN AN URBAN ENVIRONMENT

A small smelting company made the news in the early 1980s after OSHA charged the company with administering chelating drugs to employees to lower the level of lead in their blood. The small scrap recycling company, located in Massachusetts, was charged with illegally providing these lead-purging drugs to employees while they continued to work in a lead-contaminated environment. Following the administration of these drugs, two employees became severely ill. One suffered from kidney failure and was ultimately diagnosed with kidney cancer. The other employee died; lead poisoning was listed as a significant contributing factor on his death certificate.

While OSHA cited the company for many serious violations of standards, the fines and some of the charges were significantly reduced after negotiation. The company agreed to clean up the plant and reduce employee lead exposures.

Ten years later, however, not much had changed. One of the first reports of multiple poisonings in a single workplace listed in the state's new adult lead poisoning registry came from employees of the smelting company. Every "shop floor" employee was reported to the registry as having an elevated blood lead level, the average being 40 μg/dl, a level associated with adverse health effects in adults.

Shortly before the registry was established, the employees decided they had been poisoned long enough. A complaint was filed with OSHA and an inspection was conducted. The inspector was told by company officials that they no longer used lead and that there was no need to perform industrial hygiene sampling. The inspector took them at their word.

Frustrated, the employees approached the Massachusetts Coalition for Occupational Safety and Health (MassCOSH), a worker health and safety advocacy group (see COSH groups in Appendix B). There they told their story to staff members of the Latino Workers Project of MassCOSH. They explained that conditions had not changed in years and that employees were routinely sick from processes that were kept secret from regulatory agencies. They described conditions that were not unlike those of smelters from another century.

The workers were mostly non–English-speaking immigrants from Central America, many of whom had entered the U.S. illegally. They worked among family and friends at the plant and were unlikely to find other jobs. But they were not comfortable with their failing health and the daily compromises they were expected to make for a meager living.

The most vocal of the workers was fired after being accused of reporting working conditions to OSHA. The Immigrants' Rights, Advocacy, Training and Education Project (IRATE) became involved in the case and worked with MassCOSH and the employees to establish strategies to improve working conditions. A union organizing drive was initiated with the International Ladies' Garment Workers Union (ILGWU).

By the time the state's Division of Occupational Hygiene investigated the reports of lead poisoning at the plant, the employees' organized struggle was well under way. The inspection revealed years of accumulated lead dust and debris, as well as very high levels of airborne lead from incineration of insulated wire and a process of sifting scrap metal dust and grit. Workers were not given clean washing facilities, and were forced to eat their lunches in a filthy washroom where a microwave oven was set up in a toilet stall. There was no soap, hot water, or towels. Many serious safety hazards were also observed.

OSHA was called back in and this time it found many violations. It cited the company with 48 serious violations and 3 willful violations, accompanied by a fine of more than $200,000.

A review of the Division of Occupational Hygiene files later revealed that the company had a record that extended back to the 1930s with nearly 50 site inspections. Each report was almost identical, with the company saying the process that had once produced lead was no longer practiced and that cleanup was in progress.

Why was the company able to elude the full authority of the regulatory agencies for so many years? What happened that brought about the ultimate rigor of these agencies in this case? The answer appears to be that for the first time in 50 years, the workers were organized. While they finally lost their union election, they did understand their rights and recognized the consequences of their working conditions.

Through the efforts of the advocacy groups, the workers were able to communicate critical information to the health and safety inspectors regarding lead-generating processes, so that inspections could be conducted under typical working conditions. All of the workers were interviewed during inspections in the presence of interpreters. The workers had been empowered to hold the inspectors accountable for workplace health and safety.

In addition to the issues of worker health and safety, for many years community residents had expressed concerns about their exposures to the environmental pollution produced by the plant. Inspections were conducted by the state's Department of Environmental Protection and the company was ordered to halt certain processes and reduce emissions from others. Local oversight by the city's health department was critical in informing the Department of Environmental Protection when conditions worsened, so that unannounced inspections could be conducted.

The conditions at the smelting company were reported to the state attorney general's Environmental Strike Force. Following months of scrutiny by that office, both civil and criminal charges were sought against the company. Under a civil consent order, the company removed all of the lead debris and cleaned the facility. Most of the lead-generating processes were eliminated, although the company still conducts a brisk business in metal scrap recycling.

Under the company's settlement with OSHA, workers' lead exposure is regularly monitored and they are protected against airborne contamination through a combination of engineering controls, personal protective equipment, and safe work practices. Blood lead levels have been significantly reduced.

While the fines from OSHA and the threat of additional fines from the attorney general motivated the cleanup, publicizing the outcome of the criminal investigation is likely to be an effective deterrent to other companies that are exposing their employees to unsafe working conditions.

While unions are a force in spurring companies to attend to health and safety problems—typically through collective bargaining agreements or, where they exist, union-controlled health and safety committees—and government regulation provides a further stimulus, there are two other motivational sources for improving health and safety: (1) corporate reputation ("public relations"), which functions to press management not to appear negligent in its provisions for workplace safety (although this tends to function more effectively for pollution problems and environmental concerns and, more often, in large corporations); and (2) the cost of replacing labor. If a company has invested in developing a skilled and loyal workforce, it is unlikely to want to damage that investment by exposing workers to dangerous conditions. This factor helps to explain why low-skilled, easily replaced workers, such as migrant laborers or poultry workers, are so vulnerable (Fig. 2-6).

***The Changing Structure of Work.*** The economy of the United States and many other developed countries is changing rapidly. The shift from heavy manufacturing toward the service sector affects the structure of work and the work experience for many Americans. In general, in service industries, the most rapidly growing sector of the economy, wages are lower, benefits scanty, job security limited, and unions virtually nonexistent. Much of this work is part-time or temporary.

In response to the shrinking economic pie of the 1980s, employers are increasingly using part-time and temporary workers to cut costs. The average part-time worker earns only 60 percent of a full-time worker on an hourly basis. Fewer than 25 percent of part-timers have employer-paid health insurance compared to nearly 80 percent of full-time workers. Sixty percent of full-time workers have pensions provided by employers, while only 20 percent of part-time workers have this coverage [12]. In 1990, in the U.S., there were 5 million involuntary part-time workers, that is, workers who would prefer to be working full-time but were unable to do so.

In addition to lower pay and fewer benefits, there are other negative aspects to this trend toward temporary and part-time work. Temporary workers live with the stress of not knowing when and for how long they will work. They have little or no job security. Neither part-time nor temporary workers receive equal protection under government laws, including occupational safety and health regulations, unemployment insurance, and pension regulations. Few are represented by unions [12]. A case study commissioned by OSHA of contract labor in the petrochemical industry (usually small contractors of nonunion workers, brought into a plant to do maintenance and other work) shows that contract workers get less health and safety training and have higher injury rates than do noncontract workers [18]. The consequence for occupational health and safety of an increasingly unorganized, temporary, and part-time workforce should not be underestimated.

Another increasingly common characteristic of changes in the structure of work in the U.S. is the rise in home-based industry. In 1949 the U.S. Congress passed a law making industrial home work illegal, largely because it was almost impossible to enforce workplace regulations and labor standards (such as the minimum wage) for home work. The Reagan administration pushed Congress to reverse this policy and to legalize home work. The consequence was a rapid growth of home-based manufacturing and service work throughout the 1980s [12]. A large number of home workers are women, typically garment and clerical workers who are paid on a piece rate system. Piece rate payments encourage speed, increase the risks of accidents, and exacerbate repetitive motion injuries, resulting in numerous ergonomic problems in workplaces not designed for the type of work being undertaken. Chemical exposures also pose a problem. Semiconductor manufacture undertaken at home, for example, not only exposes workers and their families to toxic agents used in the manufacturing process but also may contaminate local sewage systems.

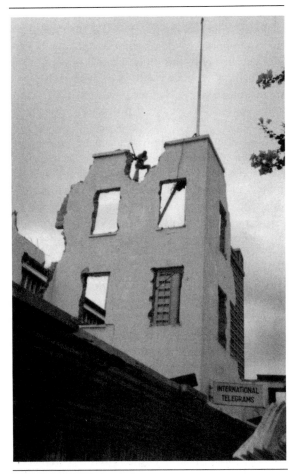

**Fig. 2-6.** Nonunion demolition worker in East Africa. (Photograph by Barry Levy)

***Work and Labor.*** Of the 110 million American workers, approximately 92 percent work for other people. Approximately one-fourth have professional, managerial, or supervisory employment, with varying degrees of partial autonomy and control over their own jobs. These people both work and labor. Most workers, though, only *labor*. They find what jobs they can and, by and large, do what they need to do to keep them. They do not choose what they will make, under what conditions they will make it, or what will happen to it afterward.

These choices are made for them by their employers, the sales and labor markets, and the workings of the economy as a whole. Whatever control most workers have over how much they receive in return for their labor, how long they labor, how hard they labor, and the quality of the workplace environment is acquired in a contractual situation in which the workers' desire for comfort, income, safety, and leisure is continually counterbalanced by the employers' need for profit.

Many workers have profound ambivalence about their jobs. While labor provides an income, workers also seek less tangible satisfactions from their work. For example, an unemployed miner reflected [19]:

Some no doubt will find this a sad thing, the fact of me not having any work, I mean. Others simply won't notice, while still others, with a more fundamental way of looking at things and sadly lacking a working-class consciousness, will utter some such expression as "Lucky bastard!". . . Frankly, I hate work. Of course I could also say with equal truth that I love work; that it is a supremely interesting activity; that it is often fascinating; that I wish I did not have to do it; that I wish I had a job at which I could earn a decent wage . . .

The contradictions in this statement cannot be dismissed as the contrariness of human nature; they correspond to contradictions in the real situation. What workers love about work is the opportunity to guide their own lives, to do meaningful things, or "to get back from the activity not only the physical means to live, but also a confirmation of significance, of the process of being oneself and alive in this unique way" [20]. On the other hand, workers oppose their work being made meaningless by the ways it is organized by others and bleached of integrity, autonomy, and creativity for reasons of efficiency, productivity, and profit.

Modern production and market competition lead employers to seek the highest possible rates of productivity. The normal social interactions among workers, which in a less mechanized and fragmented work process appear as part of the rhythm of work itself, are seen as disruptive of production. Attempts on the part of workers to establish some level of control and sociability in the workplace are often misconstrued. Employers and managers who see such acts as threats to productivity and efficiency consider them to be indications of laziness. Workers, even in nonunion settings, may view them in a similar way or as efforts to protect themselves against the requirements of a fragmented division of labor that treats them as tools rather than as people. These attempts at greater control actually represent, consciously or unconsciously, the individual's desire to replace labor with work. The structure of the contemporary workplace undercuts such acts of rebellion and self-assertion, however.

Innovations such as word-processing technology, computerized recordkeeping, electronic mail, and computer and video monitoring have turned large offices into assembly lines. New forms of work organization have broken the close personal tie that frequently existed between secretaries and their employers, and new technology has downgraded the skills required. With these changes, clerical work becomes subject to the same kind of machine-like analysis and control as factory work.

Similar situations are often found in service, retail, distributive, and other types of work. What is true for the autoworker, the word processor, and the keypunch operator is increasingly the case for the short-order cook, the checkout clerk, and the telephone operator. One young woman describes her sense of powerlessness and alienation as a grocery store cashier [21]:

It was extremely repetitive work. Pushing numbers all day sort of got to me. I used to have dreams, or should I say nightmares, all night long of ringing up customers' orders when it was after closing time. I have even woken up and found myself sitting up in bed talking to customers. That job ended when the whole building exploded one night because of some faulty electrical work. The summer of my senior year in high school I got another job as a cashier in a discount department store, doing the same thing, pushing numbers again. My nightmare of talking to customers in my sleep began again.... This was a job that was an extremely strict one. There was no leeway about anything. They had cameras above the registers watching us to see if we were polite, if we checked inside of containers for any hidden merchandise, checked the tags to see if they were switched, etc. If we failed to do something we were given a written warning. ...

Everyone who worked there, with the exception of the management, was part-time. The schedules were made so that no one had exactly forty hours. I worked for three months, 35 to 38 hours per week. By not giving us those few extra hours, they saved themselves a lot of money by not having to give their employees benefits, insurance, etc. Of course, their hiring, firing, quitting went on week after week. There weren't too many loyal employees.

A fractionated division of labor and "scientific" work discipline are ways of exerting managerial control in the interests of efficiency and profit (Figs. 2-7, 2-8). The experience of alienation and powerlessness on the part of the workers, however, is not limited to workplaces where this type of organization is imposed. Many jobs in small shops—particularly in the service and retail sectors, which employ the largest number of women and youth—are equally unattractive despite their lack of specialization.

The characteristic jobs of a service sector economy tend, therefore, to replicate quite often the alienating, repetitive work once associated with assembly-line production and the monotony of the modern factory. Today, in developed countries, however, improved technology and the ubiquitousness of computers have enormously increased the potential pace of work as well as the ability of the work rate to be monitored. Technology combines with pressures for increased productivity in an increasingly competitive world economy. "Competitiveness" and the drive for productivity have enormous costs to the health and well-being of workers.

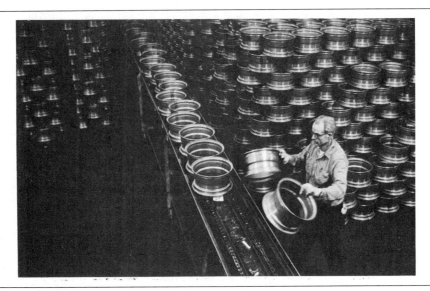

**Fig. 2-7.** There is a surprising amount of isolation in today's work environment. (Photograph by Earl Dotter)

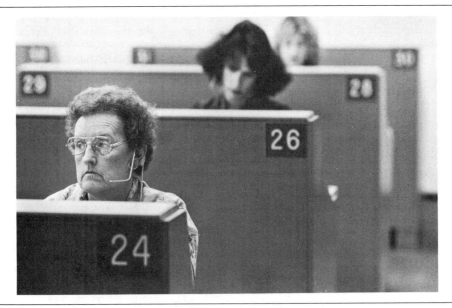

**Fig. 2-8.** Long-distance telephone operators. Monotony characterizes many jobs. (Photograph by Earl Dotter)

The constant demand to do work faster and more efficiently, to "produce" under the whip of being fired or laid off, takes an enormous toll on the mental and physical health of workers. The dignity of work is not evident in the voices quoted above. As American international competitiveness declines further and goods and services enter the U.S. from developing countries where workers get wages little above subsistence and often work in horrendous conditions, there is even greater pressure on domestic manufacturing to "compete." The reality of that competition for most American workers has been demands for wage give-backs, compulsory overtime, work speed-up, and increasingly less attention to workplace health and safety.

*Organized Labor.* Unions are a way to counteract the disempowering, disenfranchising effects of class, race, and gender (see Chap. 32). They provide workers a voice in determining the rules and conditions of work, wage rates, and benefits. They are the collective strength that provides a counterweight to management power and prerogative. Some unions have been deeply involved in health and safety issues but, for most unions, the health and safety issues are only a few among many. In the U.S., given the weakness of unions and the historic antagonism to organized labor, unions have not always been able to give the necessary resources to protect their members from workplace hazards. In Europe, organized labor has been more successful in combating the prerogatives of management and, in a number of European countries, social democratic political parties that have been supported by labor movements have frequently been in power. Even in the U.S., with its relatively weak labor movement and the absence of social democratic or labor parties, unions do offer some protection against arbitrary exercise of power.

Formally, unionized workers try to regain some control over the labor process through collective bargaining—the negotiation of work rules and grievance mechanisms, the institutionalized process for adjudicating individual complaints. How-

ever, only approximately 15 percent of workers in the United States are unionized, and even where grievance mechanisms exist, they are not always respected. Informally, workers seek what escapes they can find or fabricate. They sneak a surreptitious cigarette, they fantasize, they horse around, and they fight. "Anything so that you don't feel like a machine" is a common refrain.

Organized labor in the United States is now weaker numerically and politically than at any time since World War II. This decline began in the 1970s and had worsened by the late 1980s. The decline is evident across the whole range of union activity: loss of negotiating strength, decrease in membership, decline in strike activity, and a vast increase in "concessionary" collective bargaining agreements between unions and industry.

In contrast to the U.S., in Great Britain, 55 percent of workers are in unions and labor governments have ruled the country. In Sweden, more than 95 percent of blue-collar workers are organized, and approximately 75 percent of white-collar employees are in unions. For most of the past 45 years, Sweden has had a labor government and the labor laws reflect that power [22]. In Germany, France, and many other countries, the existence of a labor party (or a social democratic party) has enabled workers to push for and defend significant legislation to control workplace hazards and provide extensive schemes of social insurance and welfare.

The strength of a labor movement determines a host of issues that directly influence worker health, including what information is generated about workplace hazards, who has access to it, what workplace standards are set and by whom they are enforced, the options open to workers encountering a hazard, and the effectiveness of workers' compensation [22].

Unionized workers are more likely to be informed about the presence of health and safety hazards than are nonunion members in the same jobs [23]. In addition to union-sponsored education programs, the union provides a shield against employer discrimination. This shield is extremely important for health and safety because employers may fire a worker for raising concern about health and safety problems.

Unions in the U.S. and elsewhere have fought to create legislation requiring employers to clean up the workplace, to control the employment of women and children, to limit the hours of work, and to set and enforce industrial hygiene standards. In the U.S., where OSHA requires that workers be informed about the hazards associated with the chemicals with which they work, unions have pushed to make sure that employers comply with these "Right-to-Know" regulations. When there was no federal Right-to-Know law, some unions negotiated this right, as well as the right to refuse unusually hazardous work (see Chap. 9).

*Unemployment.* It is striking that, even though unsatisfying jobs produce hostility in many workers, almost all workers would rather have a job than no job at all. One worker says of unemployment: "Lovely life if you happen to be a turnip. . . . One does not willingly opt for near-the-bone life on the dole. My personal problem is easily solved. All I need is work" [24].

Unemployment is more destructive to physical and mental health than all but the most dangerous jobs. Recent studies have even suggested a correlation between unemployment and mortality from heart disease, liver disease, suicide, and other stress-related ailments [25]. Interestingly, changing levels of unemployment have an impact not only on unemployed workers but also on their families. For example, households in which the husband is unemployed or underemployed show rates of domestic violence two to three times greater than households of fully employed men [26]. Many studies have shown that workers internalize the experience of joblessness as personal lack of worth. This sense of worthlessness appears completely unrelated to a worker's actual degree of responsibility in losing his or her job [27].

In the 1980s, the unemployment rate in the U.S. fluctuated between 6 and 11 percent. Some econ-omists have proposed that a 5 percent unemployment rate be considered "full employment." Unemployment has also become a regional and international problem, with the official average unemployment rate among the 12 member states of the European Community almost 13 percent in 1993. Furthermore, these unemployment rates are based only on those actively seeking work; by excluding those jobless who, through discouragement, have stopped looking or never began to look for work, the official data understate the magnitude of the problem. Unemployment figures rarely include the underemployed, those working part-time who seek full-time work, and those women who would be working if good well-paying jobs were available. In the developing world, the percentages of workers who are unemployed or underemployed is often much higher than in the U.S. or Europe.

Unemployment has significant economic effects. The existence of many unemployed people keeps wages down as more people compete for jobs and are willing to take lower wages in the struggle to earn a living. It also makes union organizing extremely difficult. As workers lose jobs in manufacturing—where unions had strength—and as management campaigns against unions, the barriers to encouraging people to join unions or to mount significant organizing drives become larger. All these factors weaken the movements to protect workers from occupational hazards.

### The Second Key Actors: Management

Unquestionably, there are firms that seek to maintain safe and healthy work environments. These are frequently large, profitable companies that have relatively secure markets for their products and that have decided that their continued success depends on a well-motivated, high-quality, and healthy workforce. Frequently these are firms that have a deep commitment to collective bargaining and to negotiating industrial peace. Some firms have decided that the only way that they can attract and keep highly skilled workers is to ensure the quality of working life. Other firms, concerned about product safety because of consumer concerns or the inherent risks of their technology, have attended to worker health and safety virtually as a spillover from their other essential activities.

The remarkable success of Japanese industry in reducing its injury rate, probably as a consequence of its attention to quality in general and its abhorrence of waste, may have beneficial consequences in American and European firms pursuing Japanese-style manufacturing success. Sometimes these company efforts may miss the problems associated with low-level chemical exposures, because they focus primarily on the more obvious safety hazards. Nevertheless, such efforts are to be applauded.

Some small firms pay serious attention to safety and health hazards because the owner or manager came up from the ranks, knows the processes well, and maintains close social contact with the employees. The economic pressures on small companies, however, may undercut even the most decent employer. For small or large firms, the pressures of the market are hard to resist. In these cases, the role of government in enforcing work environment standards is particularly important.

### The Third Key Actor: Government

A third key actor in the complex of workplace health and safety is "government" in the form of regulatory intervention (see Chap. 9). The impact of the state intervening in health and safety is defined by that set of institutions—legislature, executive, judiciary, and civil service—that responds to needs and initiates policy, establishes laws and regulations, and implements them. In this century, social policies created by government have embraced such measures as unemployment benefits, pensions, and medical insurance, and have protected consumers (such as by control of food additives and laws on advertising and product liability), preserved the environment, and promoted public health and safety.

Why should the state in free-market economies interfere in the operation of that market to ensure the achievement of public welfare goals? What prompts the state to ascribe to itself a regulatory role? The effort to protect the health and safety of workers provides an excellent example of the contradictory forces operating on the state.

On the one hand, such regulation helps ensure the continued existence of a healthy workforce capable of continual productivity, resulting in a positive effect for the economy as a whole. By creating national rules and regulations, it equalizes the responsibilities, as well as the penalties, among industries by requiring certain minimum standards in the workplace, thus giving stability and continuity to all forms of production. Further, by establishing the apparently neutral and regulatory role of the state, such intervention increases the legitimacy of the existing political order. The state must respond to public pressures; to demands that it intervene to prevent illness, injury, and death on the job; and to appear to be responsible and responsive to the concerns of trade unions, workers, and public opinion.

On the other hand, such regulation may have enormous costs for capitalism as a whole and for individual firms. By controlling activities at the point of production, such direct state intervention challenges control of the workplace and, by requiring certain levels of safety and minimum health measures, it imposes costs on industry that may affect profitability. In addition, such intervention gives specific rights to workers (for example, the right to refuse unsafe work), which, again, threatens managerial and corporate control of the production process. Of course, the particular ways in which government develops and implements policy are constrained by the constitutional and governing structures of a given country and by the ideological and cultural "mix" arising from history and traditions.

As countries industrialized and factory production became centralized, the issue of working conditions emerged as a serious cause for concern. In England, the state began to develop laws to prevent the worst abuses. In most countries, as modern industrial production became established, the state was forced to take action to improve working

## A SOCIAL AND POLITICAL PERSPECTIVE ON THE HISTORY OF OCCUPATIONAL HEALTH AND SAFETY

Occupational health has rarely received much attention in most societies. Historically, our commitment to economic advance through technology has made us blind to the toll on workers' health. Workers have been engaged in the more pressing task of making a living for their families to pay too much attention to widespread occupational safety and health problems. The labor movement in the United States has not been strong enough to force public attention to these issues on a continual basis. As a result of a number of interrelated historical and ideological factors, relatively little attention has been paid until recently to the problem of occupational illness and injury in the United States.

In most countries, the process of industrialization that resulted in the creation of the factory system radically changed people's experience of work. Forced by economic necessity into the newly created factories of the machine age, workers found themselves controlled by bosses whose sole concern was the maximization of profit. Working in large-scale plants and using the new technology of modern industry, workers confronted a whole new set of conditions; powerless and tied to the speed of the machine they served, facing the ever-present dangers of physical injury from conveyor belts and speeding looms, and exposed to a range of dyes, bleaches, and gases, the workplace became a source of injury, disease, disability, and death.

With the help of social reformers and professionals, workers, newly organized into unions, fought back against these conditions in countries such as Britain and Germany in the middle and end of the nineteenth century, and they were somewhat successful in improving conditions through government regulation. Laws restricting working hours and the employment of women and children, and promoting protection against safety hazards and some hazardous chemical exposures, increased. A system of factory inspection was established in Britain by the mid-nineteenth century, and Germany moved to control working conditions by the beginning of the twentieth century. In Europe, these efforts built on an earlier tradition of occupational medicine, an acceptance of government intervention and paternalism, and a relatively powerful workers' movement. By the twentieth century workers and unions had achieved political representation in the form of labor, socialist, or social democratic parties. This gave workers powers to demand reform and was a major factor in establishing laws to improve working conditions.

In the nineteenth century, the Industrial Revolution brought to the U.S., as it had to Europe, many safety problems and some public concern about these problems. Massachusetts created the first factory inspection department in the United States in 1867 and in subsequent years enacted the first job safety laws in the textile industry. The Knights of Labor, one of the earliest labor unions, agitated for safety laws in the 1870s and 1880s. Social reformers and growing union power did gain, by 1900, minimal legislation to improve workplace health and safety in the most heavily industrialized states. In the U.S., the regulations and the system of inspection were, however, inadequate. Those states that had some legislated protections rarely enforced them and focused largely on safety issues; little was done to protect workers from exposure to the growing number of chemicals in the workplace.

After 1900, the rising tide of industrial accidents resulted in passage of state workers' compensation laws, so that by 1920 virtually all states had adopted these no-fault insurance programs. Britain had passed its Workmen's Compensation Act in 1897 for occupational injuries, and occupational diseases were added in 1906. Germany, too, had a system of compensation in place by the turn of the century.

Throughout the 1920s in the U.S., the rise of company paternalism was accompanied by the development of occupational medicine programs. Much attention was paid to preemployment physical examinations rather than to industrial hygiene and accident prevention. Occasional scandals reached the public eye, like cancer in young radium watch dial painters. However, it was not until the resurgence of the labor movement in the 1930s that there was important national legislation: The Walsh-Healey Public Contracts Acts of 1936 required federal contractors to comply with health and safety standards, and the Social Security Act of 1935 provided funds for state industrial hygiene programs. During this period, the Bureau of Mines was authorized to inspect mines; this helped to a minimal extent to improve working conditions in the mining industries.

The mobilization for World War II required that the U.S. government become involved in the organization of production. Concern for the health of workers increased during this period since a healthy workforce was considered indispensable to the war effort. However, after the war health and safety receded from public attention. An exception to the general neglect of the field was passage of the Atomic Energy Act in 1954, which included provision for radiation safety standards.

Not until the 1960s, when labor regained some political clout under the Democratic administrations of Presidents Johnson and Kennedy, did the issue reemerge as significant. Injury rates rose 29 percent during the 1960s, prompting union concern, but it was a major mine disaster in 1968 in Farmington, West Virginia, when 78 miners were killed, that captured public sympathy. In 1969, the Coal Mine Health and Safety Act was passed and, finally, the first comprehensive federal legislation to protect workers was created when the Occupational Safety and Health Act (OSHAct) became law in 1970.

This brief history illustrates just some of the dimensions of the struggle to provide a safe and healthy workplace. Although many countries provide regulatory protection for workers and unions often demand safe working conditions through collective bargaining agreements, the problems facing workers have increased. New chemicals in the workplace, limits in regulatory enforcement, and the demands of an increasingly competitive global economy exacerbate the need to maintain and improve working conditions.

These problems are global in scope. The globalization of production, trade, and consumption has resulted in occupational and environmental safety and health problems becoming ubiquitous. Workers in developing and newly industrialized countries now face a range of workplace hazards. Stricter environmental regulations in the industrialized countries make it attractive for companies to use countries in Latin America, Asia, and Africa as dumping grounds for toxic waste, and as places to export highly toxic substances and hazardous industries.

Perhaps the most pressing problems in occupational health concern stem from the increasing integration of the world economy. In North America, the development of continental free trade may threaten the more advanced work environment standards of Canada and the United States, while bringing many new hazards to Mexico. In Europe, integration has made the movement of capital and labor across borders much easier; industries can move to countries with less strict occupational and environmental standards. In some cases, this intrusion has led to threats to worker and environmental health; in others, the more advanced standards of some countries are being imposed on the less advanced, improving working and living conditions. In both situations, conflict over standards has arisen. The export of hazardous technologies, hazardous products, and hazardous wastes represents increasing challenges for public health worldwide. On the one hand, our understanding of the nature of health hazards to workers has been improving; on the other hand, however, the restructuring of the world economy may undercut the political will to control these hazards.

conditions. In nearly all cases, legal protections grew in piecemeal fashion, reflecting class pressures as well as moral outrage at working conditions.

Since most countries faced similar problems, the solutions have taken largely the same form. In Britain, the body of laws (until the passage of the Health and Safety at Work Act [HSWAct] in 1974) reflected the incremental progress of legislative action. In Germany, France, Sweden, and some other European countries, specific problems in the field of health and safety were dealt with as information about a given issue became available or as pressures built up to demand legal or administrative action.

In the U.S., the history of health and safety legislation has taken a somewhat different course (see box). Influenced by the federal structure of the country, it was not until the passage of the Occupational Safety and Health Act (OSHAct) in 1970 that the U.S. had a comprehensive federal law to control workplace conditions. The creation of OSHA resulted in extensive debate about the role of the state in the American polity, and the agency has often been stigmatized as a vivid example of too much government (see Chap. 9).

The U.S. case is especially interesting in that, alone among the developed capitalist economies of the West, the commitment to welfarism has remained embryonic. While the characteristic structures and programs of the welfare state are not entirely absent, they remain relatively undeveloped in the U.S., in comparison with Europe.

Since the passage of the OSHAct and the creation of OSHA, the struggle for healthful and safe working conditions has raised issues of control of the workplace and organization of production. Throughout the 1970s intense debates occurred over the role and actions of OSHA, the validity of the scientific evidence on the dangers posed by chemicals, the enforcement of standards, the extent and legitimacy of government regulation, and workers' rights to a hazard-free working environment. From the time the first draft of the OSHAct appeared before Congress, industry associations, chambers of commerce, trade unions, and government agencies all became deeply embroiled in a highly politicized and emotionally charged issue.

In Europe, the existence of government regulatory agencies and the idea of government inspection of workplaces has, on the whole, been less controversial. The U.S., on the other hand, is unique in the openness of its government institutions and the extent of the potential citizen participation in policy-making. Most Western European and former Eastern Bloc countries allow much less public input into policies and provide far fewer channels for public supervision. In principle, unions, representatives of workers, serve as "partners" in policy-making by participating at the highest governmental levels on an equal footing with business and industry. The efficacy of their participation, however, may be diluted in Europe, if unions are numerically and economically weaker than they once were. Community groups and nonunionized workers have also questioned whether union partnerships and involvement with government and business representative bodies may exclude others from having their interests served.

### Science Professionals and the Work Environment

So what about the other actors? What can be said about the importance of understanding the social context of occupational health? First, ideology shapes the way we think about problems and how to solve them. Second, the changing structure of the economy—and, hence, of work—has presented new problems for workers and for people involved with occupational health. Third, the global sociotechnical environment has enormous impact on the work environment. Fourth, the direction of technological development may create new hazards and may set limits on our ability to remedy them. Finally, the distribution of power in the society can have profound impact on the attention given to worker health and safety.

The relationships among major social actors—labor, management, and government—define the rules of the work environment, including health and safety standards and practices as well as boundaries within which health care providers, occupational health specialists, and health and safety advocates operate. While the web of rules sets real limits on reform at the "point of production," changes in the global factors can open up new possibilities to provide a safe and healthful work environment.

*Professionals in the Work Environment*
What is the significance, then, of this analysis for the actual work of health care providers and, in particular, occupational health specialists?

In the United States, the largest group of people working in occupational health are occupational health nurses. Other professionals include occupational health physicians, industrial hygienists and industrial hygiene technicians, safety engineers, ergonomists, health and safety educators, and program administrators. Ideological assumptions determine aspects of scientific investigation and research. Scientific disciplines focus attention on the technical aspects of occupational hazards and underestimate the importance of the macro- and micro-social, economic, and political context. In this regard, some workplaces have worker or union safety stewards and, increasingly, joint labor-management occupational safety and health committees, that is, nonprofessionals who are involved in hazard surveillance as well as injury and illness prevention. These individuals tend not to be imbued with the scientific model of research and hazard control, which, in some circumstances, may be advantageous in dealing with workplace hazards.

Where do these different types of people responsible for occupational health work? Some are blue-collar workers in factories with special assignments on health and safety. Most occupational health professionals work for companies as staff. In most companies, they are part of human resources or labor relations departments or, much less commonly, part of a safety and health department that is directly responsible to top management. With surprising frequency, health is separated from safety, with professionals from the different fields reporting through different hierarchies. Rarely are work environment professionals given direct responsibility and authority over production; they are advisory staff and can be influential, but basic decisions are made typically by "production" managers, even in service industries. One should remember that, in the private market, profit-making production is the prime commitment of the enterprise.

Small companies—where most people in the U.S. and the rest of the world work—rarely have professionals in health and safety on their payrolls. If they do, the professional will most often be an occupational health nurse. Usually, such firms rely on ad hoc consultations with independent professionals or simply on emergency medical services. Occasionally, there may be a relationship with specialist occupational health clinics or services. Such consulting operations must sell their services and are sometimes confronted with ethical difficulties because their clients are companies, not sick or injured workers (or workers at risk because of workplace hazards). Large and small companies buy the services of a wide range of consultants, often without understanding the degree of specialist knowledge and training necessary for effective management of health and safety problems.

In addition, many small firms, and some large ones, rely on professionals employed by workers' compensation insurance carriers. "Loss prevention" departments of the insurance companies, however, may be as concerned with reducing short-term financial losses as reducing injury rates, and they may focus on case management rather than prevention of disease and injury. A new type of consulting firm has recently emerged to reduce workers' compensation costs through "managed care" for injured workers. It is probably too soon to tell whether these firms, working on contract with employers, will attempt to reform the work environment or seek to reduce company expenditures in other ways.

Some professionals in this field work for labor unions (see Chap. 34). Although groups such as the United Mine Workers of America have had health and safety staff members for many years, the real growth of occupational health professionals in labor unions has happened since the 1970 passage of the OSHAct. Nevertheless, the number of physicians, industrial hygienists, and other work environment professionals employed by the labor movement remains quite small and is usually at the national or international level. These individuals generally provide policy assistance rather than direct services to workers. An exception is the government-subsidized growth in the number of health educators working for unions, some providing or facilitating general health and safety education, others working on targeted programs, such as hazardous materials training for emergency responders and other hazardous waste–related workers.

Finally, and perhaps most important, many practitioners, including those in the full range of work environment professions, are employed by government agencies, usually as inspectors, but sometimes as technical advisers to government or industry, or as educators. In the U.S., practitioners are employed by such institutions as the Occupational Safety and Health Administration, the Mine Safety and Health Administration, the Department of Energy, the Environmental Protection Agency, the National Institute for Occupational Safety and Health, and state departments of labor and of health.

## Conclusion

The significance, then, of a social analysis of the fundamental, but often unrecognized, problem facing health care providers and others working in occupational health is that they frequently are in the difficult situation of having responsibilities for worker health while working in organizations with other priorities. Management and government organizations are influenced by economic responsibilities that may compromise worker health and safety. Even labor organizations with their key responsibility to rank-and-file workers may find health and safety low down on a list of concerns and demands. In Fig. 2-1, professionals in occupational health are not separately identified since, because they are not key players, they fall either under or between the listed categories.

Health professionals can be successful in improving the working environment, especially if they understand the social and economic context for their efforts and work toward "win-win" situations. For example, where workers' compensation costs to a company are high it may be possible to improve the economic performance of the company and improve worker health through preventive measures. In cotton textile manufacturing, new equipment increased productivity and reduced cotton dust exposure for mill workers. When OSHA mandated reductions in vinyl chloride exposure, the controls introduced by the companies resulted in increased profits. Some have argued that health and safety regulation may stimulate companies to technological innovation they might not otherwise have considered [28]. Health and safety practitioners need to master economic, as well as humanist, arguments for change.

Sometimes, however, the economic arguments alone are not sufficiently convincing to sway management. Many industrial hygienists are members of regional and local professional groups that exchange technical information. These groups have codes of ethics (see Chap. 12) that can inspire and strengthen efforts to improve the work environment. An important source of support, as well as technical and strategic ideas, for professionals in occupational health and professional education are the professional societies, such as the Association of Occupational Health Nurses, the American College of Occupational and Environmental Medicine, the American Industrial Hygiene Association, the American Conference of Governmental Industrial Hygienists, the Human Factors Society, the American Public Health Association, and the American Society of Safety Engineers.

Professionals in occupational health, however, need to think in broader terms than usual when confronting difficult situations and recalcitrant employers. In many states, occupational health professionals have played important roles in new coalitions of labor activists and environmentalists. Committees or coalitions for occupational safety and health (COSH groups) have engaged in worker education and advocacy since the early 1970s and have been instrumental in establishing Right-to-Know laws in some states, in improving workers' compensation in others, and in focusing the attention of labor unions and the general public on health and safety issues (see Appendix B). These groups represent a grassroots movement that links professionals and concerned citizens in a new way to improve the work environment.

## References

1. Kuhn S, Wooding J. The changing structure of work in the U.S. Part I: The impact on income and benefits. New Solutions 1994; 4:43.
2. Braverman H. Labor and monopoly capital. New York: Monthly Review Press, 1974.
3. Buroway M. Manufacturing consent: Changes in the labor process under monopoly capitalism. Chicago: University of Chicago Press, 1979.
4. Garson B. All the livelong day: The meaning and demeaning of work. New York: Penguin, 1977.
5. Rizer-Roberts E. Bioremediation of petroleum contaminated sites. Boca Raton, FL: CRC Press, 1992, p. 4.
6. Karasek R, Theorell T. Healthy work. New York: Basic Books, 1990.
7. Schor J. The overworked American. New York: Basic Books, 1991.
8. Zuboff S. In the age of the smart machine. New York: Basic Books, 1988.
9. Levison A. The working-class majority. New York: Coward; McGann Geoghegan, 1974.
10. Bullard RD. Reviewing the EPA's Draft Environmental Equity Report. New Solutions 1993; 3:78.
11. Boston Globe, Dec. 17, 1992.
12. Amott T. Caught in the crisis: Woman and the U.S. economy today. New York: Monthly Review Press, 1993, p. 56.
13. Byant WK, Zick CD, Kim H. The dollar value of household work. Ithaca, NY: Cornell, 1992, p. 3.
14. Spangler E. Sexual harassment: Labor relations by other means. New Solutions 1992; 3:24.
15. Peterson HC. Business and government, 3rd ed. New York: Harper & Row, 1989, pp. 429–430.
16. AFL-CIO. Death on the job: The toll of neglect. AFL-CIO Department of Occupational Safety and Health, April 1992.
17. Kazis R, Grossman RL. Fear at work: Job blackmail, labor and the environment. New York: Pilgrim Press, 1982.
18. Managing workplace safety and health. Beaumont, TX: John Gray Institute, Lamar University, July 1991.
19. Keenan J. On the dole. In R Fraser. ed. Work: Twenty personal accounts. Harmondsworth, England: Penguin, 1968.
20. Williams R. The meanings of work. In R Fraser. ed. Work: Twenty personal accounts. Harmondsworth, England: Penguin, 1968.
21. Miller L. Unpublished interview. Southeastern Massachusetts University, 1980.
22. Elling R. The struggle for workers health. Farmingdale, NY: Baywood, 1986.
23. Weil D. Reforming OSHA: Modest proposals for major change. New Solutions 1992; 2:26.
24. Tepperman J. Not servants, not machines: Office workers speak out. Boston: Beacon Press, 1976.
25. Whiteside N. Unemployment and health: An historical perspective. Social Policy 1988; 17:177–194.
26. Leeflag RLI, et al. Health effects of unemployment. Social Science Medicine 1992; 34:351–63.
27. Lerner M. Surplus powerlessness: The psychodynamics of everyday life. Oakland, CA: Institute for Labor and Mental Health, 1989.
28. Ashford NA, Heaton GR Jr. Regulation and technological innovation in the chemical industry. Low Contemp Prob 1983; 46:109–57.

---

APPENDIX

# A Proposal from the Italian Women's Movement*

---

Everyone needs time to study, to work, and to care for others and for themselves. The work of providing care is an activity that enriches rather than penalizes a society. The time spent providing care must be considered "social time," for the benefit of society as a whole, and not just something we do

*A proposal from the Italian women's movement. New Solutions Spring 1993. Translated by Margaret M. Quinn and Eva Buiatti.

in our personal lives. We think that a law will be useful to give a voice and force to the idea of reorganizing time to allow for caring relationships. We do not believe that modes of thought and behavior in private lives will change by decree but we think that a law enacted by popular initiative can be a vehicle for ideas; it provides a mechanism for men and women to confront and to crystallize their thinking about the cultural issues. If it is successful, perhaps the law can encourage individual and social change. There is, however, another important reason why we have chosen to put this question into the legislative arena. This is the time for women to become a full and autonomous political force; not to renounce their needs, but to participate with their valid experience. The choice to involve the government is one to claim a place in the mainstream of democratic action.

To become the boss of our own time, to value all of the phases of our lives and to extend the work of care giving to both men and women is to give substance to the idea of a democracy of daily life. This everyday democracy can only be achieved by rethinking many behaviors and parts of our lives that are now considered natural or inevitable, such as the organization of time into public (masculine) and private (feminine) parts; even the organization of the cycle of our lives. Achieving a democracy of daily life also would mean redefining our relationship to work and transferring resources and power from single or small groups of individuals to all who participate in the work.

We are starved for time. Nurses work around the clock even on holidays; university faculty and researchers teach and work nights and weekends to publish; factory workers and managers and employees of private businesses do shift work; store employees get out of work when everything else is closed. And then women add thousands of other jobs for the home, children, elderly, other family members and friends. We are employed in many hours of domestic work and the care of others including having a major role in the education of our children.

We need more day care centers with the characteristics and schedules that suit our needs; full-time programs; places and organized activities for our children to meet after school; social centers for the elderly; more vacation time and domestic assistance. But even with all of these social services, part of the job of providing care to others still remains and cannot be covered through social institutions and services. And there often are times when taking care of others gives us joy and satisfaction. However, there is no time to do it: not because we don't know how to organize our time well, but because our time depends on others, on work, the hours that stores and services are open, on school hours, on traffic and means of transportation. Only rarely can we really decide how to use our time. We are calling for a way to reconcile all of the different types of work that we do and we are asking that all of the jobs, including "women's work," be shared by men.

## Introduction to the Bill: The Cycle of Our Lives

Our entire life is conditional on a model that does not take into account the fact that we are women. Is it really natural that while we are young we are involved in school, the university or other formative activities and then—if we are fortunate enough to find work—we work all day, all week for 11 months for 25 to 40 years until we retire? We are beginning to think not; to realize that this model, in reality, was thought of and made by men for men, and it doesn't suit us well. In the past, and still today, many women abandon work when they have children and then look for it again (often in vain) when their children are grown. Or else many women today do not leave their work or their cultural commitments but become acrobats trying to do it all. Many others begin to get established in their careers or public life or acquire seniority at work and then must choose whether or not to have children or to postpone maternity to a biologically advanced age with lower fertility and more risks for the pregnancy and the newborn. These examples demonstrate how the model of social and workplace organization truly violates the biological clock of women.

Is it any wonder then that some women refuse to live like men or to take on the great effort of a double job and choose to work in the home even if this choice costs in terms of reduced income and personal autonomy? One can count the rhythm of life in a way that is more consonant with all the needs of humans because all that goes well for women can improve everybody's life, including men's lives: to study, to work, to have time for oneself, to love and care for others, to enrich our life experiences and knowledge, to do sports, to travel, to participate in cultural life, and to be involved socially and politically. One life with many dimensions and not just a life of work. We know that to accomplish this proposal would take a cultural revolution. Businesses would have to think about an organization of work that is not modeled exclusively on the needs of productivity and profit or on the idea that employees should be available totally to the company without obligations other than to work and to earn. This means a new relationship of people to their work.

The state must adjust the allocation of resources to provide care in a way that recognizes not only the time needed for care-giving but also the autonomous rights of children, the elderly, and women by constructing the necessary social services for them. Therefore we propose a policy called the "new cycle of life" that combines periods of work during the school years and provides time for personal and professional development and study, parental and family leaves during our working lifetime. We want to make it possible for men and women to take temporary leaves from their work to study, to play with a child, to give companionship to an elderly or sick person, to gain new professional qualifications or simply to reflect on their own lives. This should be possible while maintaining a position at work, without greatly decreased salary, without losing health and other benefits and without compromising one's career.

## Excerpts from the Proposal

We propose that every working person have the right to parental leave: a period of leave from work up to a maximum of 12 months which can be taken together or in portions until the child is 11 years old. In families with a handicapped child or with only one parent, the duration of the leave is extended to 24 months.

To address family emergencies such as a child in adolescent crisis, an elderly or seriously sick person, a death, all of the situations that require emotional care, we propose a leave for family reasons. This is the right to be absent from work for a period of not more than 30 days for every two years of work.

Whether the leave is for parental or family reasons, there should be some form of recognition that the time taken to provide care is socially useful—as productive as commercial work. For this, we think that one should have a salary during the leaves with one part paid by the state and another by the employers.

During the leaves, workers should receive a minimal, guaranteed salary equal to 50 percent of the national average salary for their occupation. In addition, if a worker wants, he or she should be permitted to have up to 100 percent of the normal salary during the year just prior to the leave, drawing on money which will be received upon leaving work—a type of severance pay. (In Italy, a worker gets a significant sum of money, in addition to his or her monthly pension, upon leaving work. The amount of severance pay is based on the amount earned during the working lifetime.)

If the time for providing care has a value for all of society, then the care given by men and women who do not have wage-earning work, such as the unemployed, students, housewives, or those who are self-employed, such as artists, trades people, shopkeepers, farmers or professionals, should be recognized also. The first group has the time to provide care, but doesn't have a corresponding salary. The second may be able to decide to suspend work temporarily, but also will not have a salary. We propose that all members of our community, including immigrants, who do not have full-time jobs, also have the same rights to a guaranteed minimum income distributed by the state for parental leave.

We know very well that a law will not be enough to redistribute the work of care-giving between the sexes: how many men will ask for parental or family leave? As we have already said, this will take a cultural revolution. A decisive role in the new socialization could be developed by the schools. In addition, other traditionally masculine institutions could be employed. For example, the military service or alternative service could be used to provide care. Young men in the military service could satisfy part of their duty with a certain number of months (three) spent in care-giving activities such as infant and child care, domestic assistance, care of the elderly, assistance in preventive and medical services and in recognized community organizations.

Above all, a different cycle of life means being able to use time for oneself without having to wait until retirement. There are dead-end jobs such as in the fast-food service sector, and then there are jobs—such as a pre-school, kindergarten, or secondary school teacher—which, although they may be gratifying, nevertheless become exhausting after many years. We propose that all employees, after working at least seven years, be eligible for a one-year sabbatical. Workers should be able to request the leave without specifying the reasons and the job positions would be held for them. The sabbatical would not be a concession of the employer, but a right of the employee. However, the employee would have to replace the time taken by delaying retirement age and working an additional year for every year of personal leave. The idea is that we could work longer when we are older in

order to have time for ourselves when we are younger. The restitution of time in later years is important to make it clear that the sabbatical is time for oneself and it is the responsibility of the person who takes it. The time cannot be viewed as a gift from the state or the employer nor can the time be used to assume another salaried job. During the sabbatical, the person would receive part of the pension and severance pay settlement and it would be repaid with interest.

## Work Time

Legislators, employers and union officials think only of three times: the times for work, rest and "free time." For decades, the objective of workers has been to have eight hours of work, eight hours of rest and eight hours of free time per day. However, the time for care-giving has never been explicitly included in the daily schedule and for this, women have never had free time—it is full of other work. For this, we propose a work week limited by law to 35 hours. The daily work schedule should be flexible and the hours should be established in a contract between the employer and the employee which acknowledges not only the demands of production but also the private life of the employee. We want to avoid having a discrepancy between the "real" hours required for the job and those set by law. It is essential that work time over the legal limit be viewed as truly extraordinary— not the norm, but the exception. Therefore overtime work must be voluntary and must not exceed two hours per day and eight hours per week. In each case, the employee should have the right to recover the extra time. In both small and large workplaces, public and private, each employee should have the right to four paid weeks of vacation with at least two of those weeks chosen by the employee.

There are certain jobs, such as public utilities, hospital work, transportation, and so forth that must be conducted 24 hours a day. However, work should be confined to the day shift whenever possible. This especially refers to stores. Those workers who cannot work the night shifts because they have to provide care should have the right to refuse. Those who work the night shift or Sundays and holidays should be given 20 percent extra time off for every eight hours worked. Those who do very demanding work should have some compensation in time, rather than money, as well as the possibility of an early retirement or pension. Compensation in time instead of money is emphasized to make it explicit that extenuating work conditions take time from the provision of care and that the time for care is valuable. The purpose of this aspect of the law is to provide minimum, guaranteed rights. This should not preclude unions from negotiating even better conditions.

All of these proposals liberate time and they also create new positions for those seeking employment. We have chosen solutions that limit the time at work for all workers. There are those who are proponents of other solutions, such as part-time work and job-sharing. To us, these do not seem like good solutions because they are voluntary and because they are not imposed evenly throughout the workplace. It is also difficult to provide adequate benefits and union coverage. When permitted at all, these forms of work are used in an uneven fashion throughout workplaces and, overall, it is women who use them. It has become a way to reconcile "women's work" in the home with wage-earning work. Thus the idea of women as not really serious about their jobs. It also prevents or limits the redistribution of work between the sexes and the social recognition of the value of time spent care-giving. In this way, it may be viewed as a means for not having to create so many social services outside the home. It is for these reasons that, in our opinion, the best way to address time in the workplace is to reduce the work schedules for all, men and women.

### Time in the Community

The schedules of services and store hours seem made as if to play a nasty trick on us! For many of us, when we have to leave work, the banks, post offices, doctors' offices, state administrative services and often even the stores are closed. As women continue to enter the workplace in even greater numbers, there is no one at home during the day to attend to all the services necessary to sustain a family. Upon reflection, we think that the schedule of the city is set on a model developed by men, of a city made for the "producers," a city in which women and their work are invisible, erased. For this, we propose that the city council be entrusted with developing a plan to coordinate the schedules of the city. This should be established in accord with the employers, employees, and with the users of the services. Instead of paying more taxes to plan these improved services, perhaps members of a community could donate time to the town government.

And finally, there is the time that is stolen from us: the time having to deal with various aspects of public administration. We call for the community to make the bureaucracy simpler.

# II
# Recognition and Prevention of Occupational Disease

# 3
# Recognizing Occupational Disease

David H. Wegman, Barry S. Levy, William E. Halperin

For effective prevention of occupational illness and injury, health care providers must know how to recognize relevant conditions, not only in workers who present with symptoms, but also in those workers who are presymptomatic and in those for whom individual and group health information is available. If one's approach is systematic, then all aspects of prevention—primary, secondary, and tertiary—will be considered in reducing or eliminating occupational hazards.

This chapter is organized into three sections in order to highlight the three levels of recognition that serve the three levels of prevention. The correct diagnosis and approach to treatment of a worker suffering from an occupational illness or injury are essential to maximize opportunity for tertiary prevention, and can also promote primary and secondary prevention. The selection and use of medical screening and monitoring tests that are appropriate to identified workplace risks will promote secondary prevention. A carefully designed occupational surveillance program, using both case- and rate-based approaches, will promote primary prevention.[1]

---

[1]*Primary prevention* is based on measures designed to promote general optimum health or specific protection against disease agents or the establishment of barriers against agents in the environment. *Secondary prevention* is prompt and adequate treatment of the pathogenic process as soon as it is detectable. *Tertiary prevention* is corrective therapy, when the disease has advanced beyond its early stages, in order to prevent sequelae and limit disability, or, if too advanced, to address rehabilitation needs. (From HR Leavell and EG Clark. Preventive medicine for the doctor in his community. New York: McGraw-Hill, 1958.)

When properly planned and integrated, these approaches will contribute to: (1) controlling risks at the source, (2) identifying new risks at the earliest possible time, (3) delivering the best level of therapeutic care and rehabilitation for workers who are ill or injured, (4) preventing recurrence of disease and injury of affected workers and occurrence of disease and injury in other workers who are exposed to similar risks, (5) assuring that affected workers receive economic compensation legally due them, and (6) discovering new relationships between work exposures and disease.

The remainder of this textbook provides necessary information needed to recognize and prevent occupational disease and injury. This chapter introduces a systematic approach for the health care provider to recognize occupational disease and injury, with an eye toward prevention.

## Diagnosis of Symptomatic Workers

Proper diagnosis of illness or injury related to work requires information from a variety of sources. In fact, an important impediment to proper diagnosis of these conditions has been the mistaken belief that they are uniquely caused by work and are, therefore, uncommon. The World Health Organization has attempted to correct this misimpression by making the distinction between occupational and work-related disease (see box).

Using this distinction, it can be understood that two complicating features of recognizing the role of work in the etiology of illness and injury, par-

WORLD HEALTH ORGANIZATION
DISTINCTION BETWEEN
OCCUPATIONAL AND
WORK-RELATED DISEASES

The World Health Organization (WHO) has advocated the following use of the terms *occupational* and *work-related* diseases. Although we use these terms interchangeably in this book, we expect that this distinction will become increasingly useful in understanding the full range of the impact of work on health, and that it could have important implications in the future for diagnosis and treatment of workers, as well as for research.

WHO[*] has stated:

Occupational diseases . . . stand at one end of the spectrum of work-relatedness where the relationship to specific causative factors at work has been fully established and the factors concerned can be identified, measured, and eventually controlled. At the other end (are) diseases (that) may have a weak, inconsistent, unclear relationship to working conditions; in the middle of the spectrum there is a possible causal relationship but the strength and magnitude of it may vary.

Work-related diseases may be partially caused by adverse working conditions. They may be aggravated, accelerated, or exacerbated by workplace exposures, and they may impair working capacity.

Personal characteristics and other environmental and socio-cultural factors usually play a role as risk factors in work-related diseases, which are often more common than occupational diseases.

[*]World Health Organization. Identification and control of work-related diseases. Technical Report no. 174. Geneva: WHO, 1985.

depends critically on a comprehensive appropriate patient history that adequately explores the relationship of the illness to the occupation.

The more specialized use of the laboratory for biomonitoring and clinical testing, the need for proper environmental exposure assessment, and the important concerns with ethical, legal, and socioeconomic factors are appropriately addressed in subsequent chapters. In this section, attention is devoted exclusively to the task of obtaining and interpreting the occupational history.

### The Occupational History

Consider the following four cases:

A woman who worked in a high-technology manufacturing plant had numbness in the distal arms and legs that her physician attributed to her diabetes.

A machinist was noted by his supervisor to have loss of balance on the job and was diagnosed at a nearby emergency department as being acutely intoxicated with alcohol.

A garment worker was told by her primary care physician that the numbness and weakness in some of her fingers were due to her rheumatoid arthritis.

A man working at a bottle-making factory was told by his internist that the worsening of his chronic cough was due to cigarette smoking.

In each of these situations, the physician made a reasonable and considered evaluation and diagnosis. The facts fit together and resulted in a coherent story, leading each physician to recommend a specific therapeutic and preventive regimen. In each of the cases, however, the physician made an incorrect diagnosis because of a common oversight—failure to take an occupational history.

The first patient had a peripheral neuropathy and the second, acute central nervous system (CNS) intoxication, both caused by exposure to solvents at work. The garment worker had carpal

ticularly chronic conditions, are that most of the conditions are multifactorial in origin and that most will resemble conditions that are unrelated to work. Consequently, the successful identification of the work association rarely results from a single laboratory test or diagnostic procedure, but rather tunnel syndrome, possibly caused by some combination of her rheumatoid arthritis and the strenuous repetitive movements she performed with her hands and wrists hundreds of times an hour. The man working in the bottle-making factory had worsening of his chronic cough and other respiratory tract symptoms as a result of exposure to hydrochloric acid fumes at work.

This is not to say that the associations noted by the physicians were unrelated to the conditions diagnosed. They were probably contributory in at least the first, third, and fourth cases, but without the occupational history, proper therapy and prevention could not be planned.

The identification of work-related medical problems depends most importantly on the occupational history. Physical examination findings and laboratory test results may sometimes raise suspicion or help confirm that a disease or injury is work-related, but ultimately it is information obtained from an occupational history that determines the likelihood that a medical problem is work-related. A phrase or two in the psychosocial section of the medical history is not enough; the physician should obtain data on the current and the two major past occupations for all patients. The extent of detail will depend largely on the physician's level of suspicion that work may have caused or contributed to the illness. The history should be recorded with great care and precision so that the data can be used for legal or research purposes.

> OUTLINE OF THE OCCUPATIONAL HISTORY
> 1. Descriptions of all jobs held
> 2. Work exposures
> 3. Timing of symptoms
> 4. Epidemiology of symptoms or illness among other workers
> 5. Non-work exposures and other factors

*What Questions to Ask.* The occupational history has five key parts (see box): (1) a description of all of the patient's pertinent jobs—past and present, (2) a review of exposures faced by the patient in these jobs, (3) information on the timing of symptoms in relation to work, (4) data on similar problems among coworkers, and (5) information on non-work factors, such as smoking and hobbies, that may cause or contribute to disease.

Some hospitals or clinics have standardized forms for recording the occupational history, which can expedite taking and recording this information. Ideally, such forms should include a grid, with column headings for job, employer, industry, major job tasks, dates of starting and stopping jobs, and major work exposures. (Asking questions about whether the patient has had any exposures to hazardous substances or physical factors, such as noise or radiation, from a list prepared in advance may be helpful.) On such an occupational history form (Fig. 3-1), the rows of the grid should be completed with information on each job, starting with the current or most recent job.

Further elaboration on each of the key parts of an occupational history may be helpful.

*Descriptions of All Jobs Held.* The history should include descriptions of all jobs held by the patient; in some cases, it may be important also to obtain information on summer and part-time jobs held while the patient attended school. (Generally, details of these jobs are sought only on second interviews.) Job titles alone are not sufficient: An electrician may work in a plant where lead storage batteries are manufactured, a clerk may work in a pesticide-formulating company, or a physician may perform research with hepatitis B virus. It is important to remember that workers in heavy industry are not the only ones prone to occupational diseases—so are clerks, electronic equipment assembly workers, domestic workers, food service employees, and virtually all other types of workers. To learn exactly what the patient does at

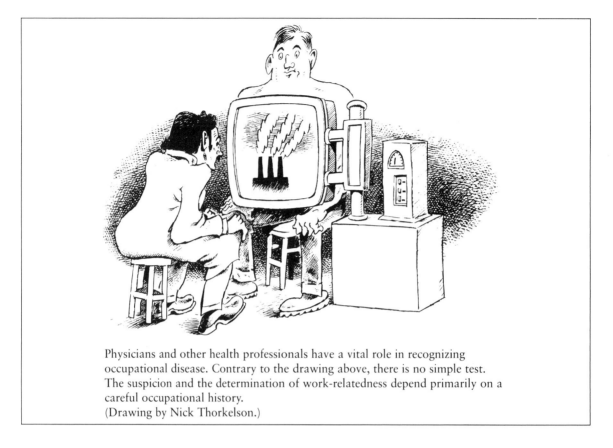

Physicians and other health professionals have a vital role in recognizing occupational disease. Contrary to the drawing above, there is no simple test. The suspicion and the determination of work-relatedness depend primarily on a careful occupational history.
(Drawing by Nick Thorkelson.)

work, it may be useful to have the patient describe a typical work shift from start to finish and simulate the performance of work tasks by demonstrating the body movements associated with them. A visit to the patient's workplace by the physician may be necessary and is always informative.

The history should describe routine tasks (unless the job title is self-explanatory); unusual and over-time tasks, such as cleaning out tanks, should also be noted since they may be the most hazardous in which a patient is involved. It is important to ask about second or part-time jobs, the patient's work in the home as a homemaker or parent, and service in the military.

*Work Exposures.* The patient should be carefully questioned about working conditions and past and present chemical, physical, biologic, and psy-chological exposures. As in other parts of a medical history, in order to avoid limiting the responses, it is wise to initially use open-ended questions such as, "What have you worked with?" Then ask more specific questions such as "Were you ever exposed to lead? Other heavy metals? Solvents? Asbestos? Dyes?" Some knowledge of the most likely exposures in the jobs listed can help focus additional questions, and it is important to remember that tasks performed in adjacent parts of the workplace can also contribute to a worker's exposures. It is often worthwhile to repeat these questions in a somewhat different manner at two points in the interview because patients will sometimes recall, on repeat questioning, exposures that they initially overlooked. It is also wise to inquire about unusual accidents or incidents, such as spills of hazardous material, that may be related to the

1. Please provide the following information on your work history.

| Job | Employer | Industry | Major job tasks | Dates of starting | stopping | Major work exposures* |
|---|---|---|---|---|---|---|
| CUSTODIAN | City of Boston | Day Care | Repair, cleaning | 10/91 | → | Flu, kids' infections, asbestos, cleaners |
| GRINDER | Hudson Engine | Engine Mfg. | metal machining | 10/86 | 10/91 | Oil mist, |
| LATHE OPER. | Nash Engine | Engine Mfg. | metal machining | 10/76 | 10/86 | Noise, |
| BORE MACHINE OPERATOR | Kaiser | Die Making | Cutting metals | 10/70 | 10/76 | Lifting/Twisting |
| VOLUNTARY FIREFIGHTER | Town of Salem | — | Fighting House Fires | 10/68 | 10/79 | Fumes, gases |
| STUDENT | — | — | mechanic Student | 4/68 | 9/70 | Noise, oils |
| Military? YES | US Air Force | Helicopter Mech. | motor Repair | 1/67 | 1/68 | Noise, Stress |
| Part-time work? | Town General Store | Retail Food | Checkout Clerk | 1/64 | 1/67 | Repetitive motion |

2. Have you had any possibly hazardous exposures outside of work? __Yes__ If yes, complete the following.

| Major exposures | Associated activity | Location | Dates of starting | stopping |
|---|---|---|---|---|
| Wood dust | Cabinet making | Home | ~1971 | → |
| | | | | |
| | | | | |

3. Have you ever smoked cigarettes? __Yes__ If yes, please answer the following questions.
How old were you when you started smoking? __18__
On average, how many packs have you smoked a day? __1/2__
Do you currently smoke? __No__ If no, how old were you when you stopped smoking? __31__

*Such as chemicals, fumes, dusts, vapors, gases, noise, and radiation.

**Fig. 3-1.** Sample occupational history form. (From BS Levy, DH Wegman. The occupational history in medical practice: What questions to ask and when to ask them. Postgrad Med 1986; 79:301.)

patient's problem; work in confined spaces (Fig. 3-2); and new substances or changed processes at work.

Many workplace chemicals and other substances are referred to only by brand names, slang terms, or coded numbers. It should be possible, however, for a physician to obtain the ingredients of most chemicals and to determine the nature of any hazard (see Appendix A). The federal Hazard Communication Standard (see Chap. 9) and, in many states and localities, Right-to-Know laws facilitate the process whereby workers and their physicians (and other health care workers), with only limited information, can determine the toxic effects of these substances.

It is important to quantify these exposures as accurately as possible. Clinicians can estimate the degree of exposure by determining the duration of

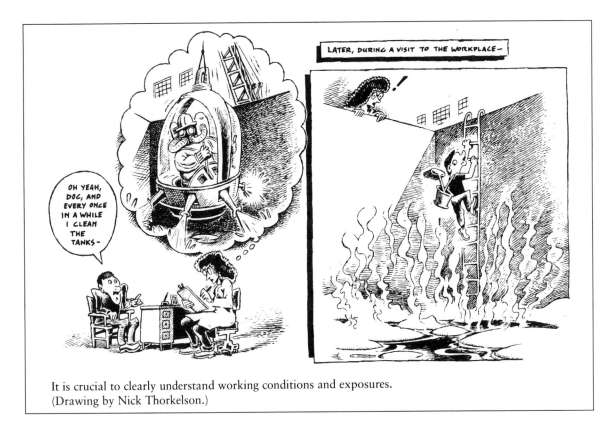

It is crucial to clearly understand working conditions and exposures. (Drawing by Nick Thorkelson.)

exposure and route of entry. Large amounts of volatile substances, such as solvents, can be inhaled unknowingly, especially if they do not irritate the upper respiratory tract or if they do not have a strong odor. Large amounts of certain substances—again, solvents are a good example—can be absorbed through the skin with the worker unaware of the degree of this exposure. The patient should be asked to describe the amount of a potentially hazardous material that contacts skin or clothes, or is inhaled, on a typical workday. The patient should also provide information on eating, drinking, and smoking in the workplace (contamination of hands can lead to inadvertent ingestion of toxic materials) (Fig. 3-3); handwashing and showering at work; changing workclothes; and who cleans workclothes.

It should be determined if personal protective equipment (PPE, such as gloves, workclothes, masks, respirators, and hearing protectors) has been provided, and if, when, and how often the worker has used this equipment. If PPE is not being used, it is important to determine the reasons. Masks and respirators are frequently not worn because of poor fit, discomfort in hot weather, and difficulty in communicating. In addition, masks and respirators that are not properly maintained are ineffective. If PPE is being used, one should determine if it appears to fit and work properly. One should ask whether protective engineering systems and devices, such as ventilation systems, are present in the workplace and whether they seem to function adequately.

*Timing of Symptoms.* Information on the time course of the patient's symptoms is often vital in determining if a given disease or syndrome is work-related or not. The following questions are

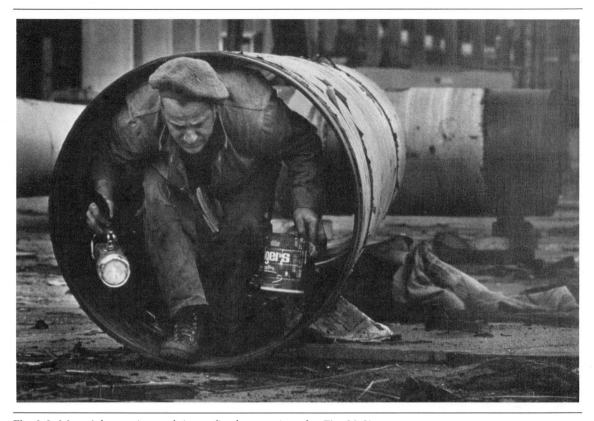

**Fig. 3-2.** Many jobs require work in confined spaces (see also Fig. 30-2).

often useful: "Do the symptoms begin shortly after the start of the workday? Do they disappear shortly after leaving work? Are they present during weekends or vacation periods? Are they time-related to certain processes, work tasks, or work exposures? Have you recently begun a new job, worked with a new process, or been exposed to a new chemical in the workplace?"

Questions on recent changes at work are often critical in suspecting or proving that a disease is work-related. On the basis of the responses to these and related questions, the physician can determine if the period from the start of exposure to the onset of symptoms and the time course of the patient's symptoms are consistent with those of the suspected illness. For example, certain irritants with low water solubility will produce severe pul-

monary damage and even fatal pulmonary edema with onset about 12 to 18 hours after work ceases. Symptoms of byssinosis ("brown lung") are characteristically worse on returning to work on Monday morning. Nitroglycerin workers, whose blood vessels have dilated due to work exposure to nitrates, may suffer "withdrawal" angina while away from work. Thus, since latent periods vary, occupational etiologies should not be ruled out because timing of symptoms does not initially correlate with time at work.

*Epidemiology of Symptoms or Illness Among Other Workers.* The patient's knowledge of other workers at the same workplace or in similar jobs elsewhere who are suffering from the same symptoms or illness may be the most important clue to

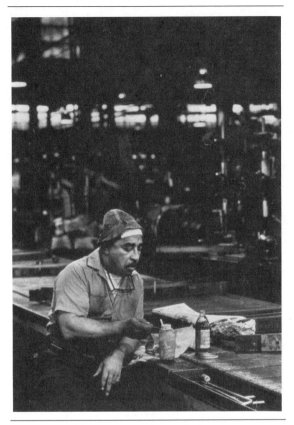

**Fig. 3-3.** Workers eating in the workplace may ingest toxic substances. (Photograph by Earl Dotter.)

recognizing work-related disease. The physician should inquire further what the affected workers share in common such as similar job, exposure, physical location in the workplace, age, or gender. One should ask about birth defects among offspring, fertility problems, cancer incidence, and high turnover of workers or their early retirement for health reasons. Workers and then their physicians linked the pesticide dibromochloropropane (DBCP) to male sterility and the catalyst dimethylaminopropionitrile (DMAPN) to bladder neuropathy by recognizing that similarly exposed workers had the same medical problems. Unfortunately,

workers may not always be aware of symptoms present in coworkers.

*Non-Work Exposures and Other Factors.* Sometimes there is a synergistic relationship between occupational and nonoccupational factors in causing disease. The physician should ask if the patient smokes cigarettes or drinks alcohol; if so, amount and duration should be quantified. For skin problems, questions should be asked regarding recent exposure to new soaps, cosmetics, and clothes. The physician should also ask: Does the patient have hobbies (such as woodworking or gardening) or other non-work activities that involve potentially hazardous chemical, physical, biologic, or psychological exposures that may account for the symptoms? Does the patient live near any factories, waste dump sites, or contaminated sources of water? Does the patient live with someone who brings hazardous workplace substances home on workclothes, shoes, or hair? The same suggestions noted in the Work Exposures section apply here: repeated questioning, quantification of exposure to the degree possible, and obtaining generic names of substances. Questioning should be aimed at determining both current and past exposures.

Other information the physician obtains may supplement the occupational history. It is useful to know whether the patient has had preplacement or periodic physical and laboratory examinations at work. For example, preplacement audiograms or pulmonary function test results may be helpful in determining if hearing impairment or respiratory symptoms are work-related or not. Since Occupational Safety and Health Administration (OSHA) regulations mandate periodic screening of workers with certain exposures (such as asbestos and coke oven emissions), and since many employers are voluntarily providing health screening in the workplace, it is increasingly likely that such information may be available to a physician, if the worker approves of its release. Finally, it is often useful to ask the patient whether there is some reason to suspect that the symptoms may be work-related.

## When to Take a Complete Occupational History

A work history should always contain information on past and present jobs of the patient to provide a good understanding of how he or she spends the workday and what potential health hazards may exist. It is impossible to obtain a detailed, 20-minute or longer occupational history on every patient seen; every medical history, however, should include the individual's two major previous jobs and his or her current job.

In the following situations the physician should have a strong suspicion of occupational factors or influences on the development of the problem and take a detailed, complete occupational history. Many symptoms appear to be nonspecific, but have their origin in occupational exposures.

*Respiratory Disease.* Virtually any respiratory symptoms can be work-related. It is all too easy to diagnose acute respiratory symptoms as acute tracheobronchitis or viral infection when the actual diagnosis may be occupational asthma, or chronic respiratory symptoms as chronic obstructive pulmonary disease (COPD) when the actual diagnosis may be asbestosis. Viruses and cigarettes are too often assumed to be the sole agents responsible for respiratory disease. Adult-onset asthma is frequently work-related but often not recognized as such. In addition, patients with preexisting asthma may have exacerbations of their otherwise quiescent condition when exposed to workplace sensitizers. Less commonly, pulmonary edema can be caused by workplace chemicals such as phosgene or oxides of nitrogen; a detailed work history should therefore be obtained for anyone with acute pulmonary edema when no likely nonoccupational cause can be identified (see Chap. 22).

*Skin Disorders.* Many skin disorders are nonspecific in nature, bothersome but not life-threatening, and self-limited. Diagnoses are often nonspecific, and all too often a brief occupational history is not taken that might identify the offending irritant, sensitizer, or other factor. Contact dermatitis, which accounts for about 90 percent of all work-related skin disease, does not have a characteristic appearance. Determination of the etiologic agent and work-relatedness depends on a carefully obtained work history (see Chap. 24).

*Hearing Impairment.* Many cases of hearing impairment are falsely attributed to aging (presbycusis) or other nonoccupational causes. Millions of American workers were exposed to hazardous noise at work; thus, a detailed occupational history should be obtained from anyone with hearing impairment. Recommendations for the prevention of future hearing loss should also be made (see Chap. 16).

*Back and Joint Symptoms.* Much back pain is at least partially work-related in etiology, but there are no tests or other procedures that can differentiate work-related from non–work-related back problems; the determination of likelihood depends on the occupational history. A surprising number of cases of arthritis and tenosynovitis are caused by unnatural repetitive movements associated with work tasks. Ergonomics, the study of interactions between worker and machine, helps prevent some of these problems (see Chaps. 8 and 23).

*Cancer.* A significant percentage of cancer cases is known to be caused by work exposures, and each year more occupational carcinogens are discovered. Initial evidence that a workplace substance is carcinogenic has come more often from individual clinicians' reports than from large-scale epidemiologic studies. This effort can be facilitated if occupational histories are obtained on all patients with cancer. Of importance in considering occupational cancer is that exposure to the carcinogen may have begun 20 or more years before diagnosis of the disease and that the exposure need not have been continued over the entire time interval (see Chap. 14).

*Exacerbation of Coronary Artery Disease Symptoms.* Exposure to stress and to carbon monoxide and other chemicals in the workplace may increase the frequency or severity of the symptoms of coronary artery disease (see Chap. 28).

*Liver Disease.* As with respiratory disease, it is all too easy to give liver ailments common diagnoses, such as viral hepatitis or alcoholic cirrhosis, rather than less common diagnoses of work-related toxic problems. It is always important to take a good occupational history with liver disease. Hepatotoxins encountered in the workplace are discussed in Chapter 30.

*Neuropsychiatric Problems.* The possibility of relating neuropsychiatric problems to the workplace is often overlooked. Peripheral neuropathies are more frequently attributed to diabetes, alcohol abuse, or "unknown etiology"; central nervous system depression to substance abuse or psychiatric problems; and behavioral abnormalities (which may, in fact, be the first sign of work-related stress or less frequently a neurotoxic problem) to psychosis or personality disorder. More than 100 chemicals (including virtually all solvents) can cause central nervous system depression, and several neurotoxins (including arsenic, lead, mercury, and methyl *n*-butyl ketone) can produce peripheral neuropathy. Carbon disulfide exposure can cause symptoms that mimic a psychosis (see Chap. 26).

*Illnesses of Unknown Cause.* A detailed complete occupational history is an essential part of all cases in which the cause of illness is unknown or not certain, or the diagnosis is obscure. The need to search carefully for a work-related source in such illnesses results from the increasing concern with low-level environmental exposures as a cause of symptoms or disease. While this concern has been raised forcefully by groups concerned about hazardous waste disposal sites and indoor air quality (see Chap. 21), increasingly medical authorities have found reason to look more closely at this complex topic.

A key principle in toxicology—and occupational health—is that the biologic response to a chemical or physical agent is primarily a function of exposure dose. While health effects from high levels of exposure will be more frequent and/or more severe than those from lower levels, more people are exposed to lower than higher levels of exposure, in the workplace and in the general environment. It is important, therefore, that health professionals who are approached by workers with symptoms they think are related to low levels of exposure to chemical substances develop a caring and careful approach to addressing these concerns.

Symptoms associated with low-level exposures are often difficult to evaluate since the exposure may be hard to document and the symptom pattern much less specific than that of a well-established disorder. Health professionals may, therefore, be skeptical and wish to dismiss the complaints or direct these patients to other specialists. This attitude is supported when there is the impression that complaints are being driven by psychosocial aspects of the job or other non–health-related factors.

As the complex nature of human physiology and its response to toxic materials evolves, however, there are compelling reasons why such cases should be examined systematically before they are set aside. These include the fact that indirect toxic responses, such as allergic responses, may well not have a clear "threshold" dose below which effects do not occur; human variability is such that even a normal distribution of responses includes a few individuals who will respond at the low dose extremes; and increasing experience with confusing problems, such as the sick building syndrome, makes clear that some patterns of response are environmentally related in the absence of readily identified causal factors.

While the laboratory investigation of the syndromes represented in these workers may predominate, the history is still central in the final determination of how to care for such individuals.

1. If the problem is related to classic allergy, it may be possible to identify patterns of response of those who are severely atopic that effectively explain the nonspecific stimuli associated with lower symptom severity between actual allergic attacks.
2. Anxiety disorders may be associated with chemical or other environmental stimuli resulting in symptoms interpreted as caused by the environment. A careful medical history should identify the need to have such individuals evaluated by a specialist, particularly since relevant diagnoses may be ones of exclusion.
3. Sick building syndrome, a newly described disorder due to poor ventilation, is discussed further in Chap. 21. Characteristic symptoms of fatigue as well as respiratory, dermal, and central nervous system complaints are reported in association with a specific environment. Here the history should identify similar illnesses in coworkers and the isolation of difficulties to a single environment with improvement in others.
4. Most recently attention has been drawn to a syndrome referred to as multiple chemical sensitivities (MCS) [1, 2]. This syndrome is reported to affect multiple systems and occur in multiple, unrelated environments. Stimulants are reported to include such seemingly unrelated low-level chemical exposures as perfumes, petroleum derivatives, and smoke. While there is often a willingness to attribute these symptoms to a primary anxiety disorder, it is important to note that few of the MCS cases meet the established criteria for this psychiatric diagnosis. It is hoped that careful and well-documented medical and environmental histories will shed light on MCS as more knowledge develops.

In concluding this section on the diagnosis of symptomatic workers, it is surprising how current the following advice still is [3]:

If the recording intern would only treat the poison from which the man is suffering with as much interest as he gives to the coffee the patient has drunk and tobacco he has smoked, if he would ask as carefully about the length of time he was exposed to the poison as about the age at which he had measles, the task of the searcher for the truth about industrial poisons would be made so very much easier.

## Screening for Occupational Disease

Screening for occupational disease is the search for previously unrecognized diseases or physiologic conditions that are caused or influenced by work-associated factors. It may be part of an individual physician's evaluation of a patient's health or of a large-scale prevention effort by an employer, union, or some other organization. Screening methods can include questionnaires seeking suggestive symptoms or exposures, examinations and laboratory tests, or other procedures. To be widely used, the methods should be simple, noninvasive, safe, rapid, and usually relatively inexpensive. Screening is one technique in a continuum for the prevention of occupational disease. Other techniques include eliminating hazards from the workplace, containing hazards with engineering controls, protecting workers with personal protective devices such as gloves and respirators, measuring intoxicants in the environment (environmental monitoring) or in biologic samples (biologic monitoring), and detecting and treating occupational disease at early stages when it is reversible or more easily treatable [4]. As with screening for nonoccupational diseases, screening for work-related diseases only *presumptively* identifies those individuals who are likely (and those who are unlikely) to have a particular disease. Further diagnostic tests are almost always necessary to confirm the diagnosis and assess the severity of the individual's condition.

Although screening data may eventually lead to more effective primary prevention measures, the purpose of screening is the identification of conditions already in existence at a stage when their progression can be slowed, halted, or even reversed. Screening is therefore a secondary prevention measure. Primary prevention measures that reduce workers' exposure to occupational hazards are, in general, more likely to improve health and prevent disease (see Chaps. 4 and 6).

While the main goal of screening is the early detection and treatment of disease, other goals include the evaluation of the adequacy of exposure control and other means of primary prevention, the detection of previously unrecognized health effects suspected on the basis of toxicologic and other studies, and suitable job placement. Clearly screening data, in addition to their clinical use for the protection of the individual screened, may be useful in a surveillance system to be analyzed epidemiologically for the protection of the community of similarly exposed workers [5].

The employees at a particular workplace are a logical target for screening for occupational disease because they have some risk factors in common (their workplace exposures) and a clear opportunity for prevention in common (reduction or elimination of those exposures). In addition, a workplace may provide excellent opportunities for screening for treatable nonoccupational diseases such as hypertension. To be effective, screening programs for occupational disease must meet the following five criteria:

1. *Screening must be selective*—applying only the appropriate tests to the population at risk of developing specific diseases, given its exposures, demographic features, and other factors. A "shotgun" approach, which involves a battery of tests (such as a "chemistry profile") applied indiscrimi-

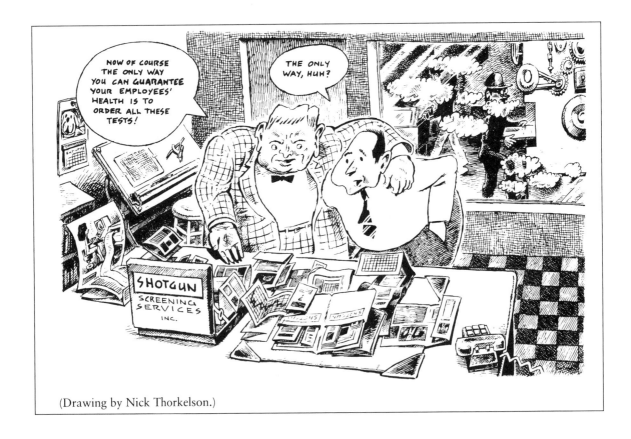

(Drawing by Nick Thorkelson.)

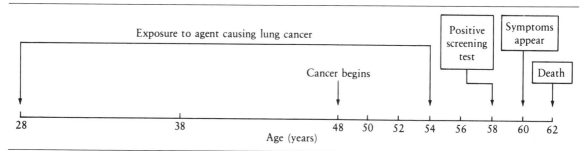

**Fig. 3-4.** Phases of cancer development. If the course of the disease cannot be positively influenced by early detection and effective treatment, there is no advantage to screening an individual for early detection of the disease. Current screening tests for lung cancer have yet to be proved effective. Screening may detect cancer earlier than would occur without screening, but the eventual time of death is not significantly changed.

nately without regard to the diseases for which the population is at risk, is generally not effective. The natural history of the exposure-disease relationship should be considered in application of screening tests. For example, screening workers exposed to asbestos in the first few years after the start of exposure may lead to a false sense of security, since the disease process will not have had time to be manifest on screening examination.

2. *Identifying the disease in its latent stage as opposed to identifying it when symptoms appear must lead to treatment that impedes the progression of the disease* in a given individual or to measures that prevent additional cases (Fig. 3-4). The major justification for screening for disease for which there is no therapy is to allow an opportunity to control exposure and prevent disease in others similarly exposed.

3. *Adequate follow-up is critical and further diagnostic tests and effective management of the disease must be available, accessible, and acceptable* both to examiner and worker. Lack of follow-up is a frequent deficiency in screening programs for occupational disease. Workers who have been screened should receive test reports along with interpretation of test results and summary data for the entire group tested.[2] Follow-up also entails

that action will be taken to reduce or totally eliminate the hazard. Some follow-up actions are job transfer for the ill worker and improving the ventilation systems of the plant; job transfer without controlling the underlying problem may mean that another worker will be exposed to the same hazard.

4. *The screening test must have good reliability and validity.* Reliability reflects the reproducibility of the test. Validity reflects the ability of the test to identify correctly which individuals have the disease and which do not. Validity is evaluated by examining sensitivity and specificity. *Sensitivity is* the proportion of those with the disease that the test identifies correctly; *specificity is* the proportion of those without the disease that the test identifies correctly. Another measure of a screening test is *predictive value positive,* which is often more useful clinically than sensitivity or specificity; it indicates the proportion of those found with a positive screening test who actually have the disease (Table 3-1).

5. *The benefits of the screening program should outweigh the costs.* Benefits consist primarily of improved quality and length of life—that is, reduced morbidity, disability, and mortality. Costs include economic costs (the expenses of performing the screening tests and further diagnostic tests and of managing those with the disease) and human costs (the risks, inconvenience, discomfort,

_____
[2]OSHA requires that records of medical surveillance be made available to the affected employee. They can be transmitted to third parties only with the written consent of the worker.

**Table 3-1.** Hypothetical data: Screening of 100,000 workers for colon cancer*

| Test outcome | Colon cancer present | | |
| --- | --- | --- | --- |
| | Yes | No | Total |
| Positive | 150 | 300 | 450 |
| Negative | 50 | 99,500 | 99,550 |
| Total | 200 | 99,800 | 100,000 |

*Sensitivity* = 150/200 = 75%. The test was (correctly) positive for 75% of actual cancer cases, but 25% of the actual cases were not detected.
*Specificity* = 99,500/99,800 = 99%. The test was (correctly) negative for 99% of those who actually did not have colon cancer.
*Predictive value positive* = 150/450 = 33%. Of those with a positive test, 33% actually had colon cancer.

and anxiety of screening and the diagnostic work-ups of "false positives"). Screening tests in the community must be inexpensive since they compete with other public health resources such as immunization. It should not be assumed that effective screening tests for occupational disease must be inexpensive as they do not compete for the same resources. The cost-benefit equation is often difficult to determine and relies on tenuous assumptions. Therefore, such analysis should not be allowed to obscure the primary objective of screening: early identification of work-related disease. Advocates of screening should be cautious that increased survival in those detected with disease, as compared with individuals detected when their symptoms occur, is not a result of lead-time bias or length bias. In lead-time bias, the added survival of individuals with detected disease results from adding part of the preclinical detection period to postdiagnosis survival, not from altering the actual time that individuals die. In length bias, an apparent increased survival results from the greater probability of detecting indolent, more benign disease, rather than quickly developing disease that is less likely to be detected because it is present for a shorter period of time.

There must be mutual trust among the individuals who have requested or authorized the screening program, the health professionals who are administering it, and the workers being screened. Without such trust, workers may be reluctant to be screened. This trust is developed, in part, by management personnel and health professionals assuring workers that screening data will be kept strictly confidential, will be used only for the stated purpose of the screening program, and will not adversely affect the worker's salary or other benefits. In addition, for any screening program to be effective, it cannot be used as a tool to discriminate—sexually, racially, or otherwise—against a specific group of workers.

### Screening Approaches

Reviewed below are current screening approaches to five major categories of work-related disease: nonmalignant respiratory disease, hearing impairment, toxic effects, cancer, and back problems. As we review these categories, you will note that few current screening approaches for occupational disease meet all five criteria for effective screening.

### Nonmalignant Respiratory Disease.
Screening for acute work-related respiratory diseases such as irritant pneumonitis is generally not possible. Pathologic changes due to exposure to irritant or toxic gases and fumes develop so quickly that there is no opportunity to screen for these disorders during a latent stage.

Many chronic work-related respiratory diseases, however, are amenable to screening. These diseases usually have very long periods from initial exposure to first appearance of symptoms—often years. Early identification of workers with asymptomatic pulmonary disease and reduction or elimination of their hazardous exposure may reverse the disease process or at least halt or slow its progression. Once well established, however, most of these diseases are not reversible by currently available treatment, and they account for much morbidity, disability, and mortality (see Chap. 22).

Screening approaches for occupational respiratory diseases range from simple questions to sophisticated tests of pulmonary function. The four basic approaches are history of respiratory symptoms, physical examination, chest x-rays, and pulmonary function tests. Usually two or more of these approaches are used in combination. Each approach, of course, has its strengths and weaknesses.

HISTORY. By means of direct questioning or use of a standardized questionnaire,[3] one can elicit information on the presence of respiratory symptoms, including cough, sputum production, wheezing, and dyspnea. The worker is questioned about the presence of these symptoms, their time course, and their relationship to airborne substance exposure, exertion, and work habits. The worker is also questioned about work history and in detail about cigarette smoking history. Although this approach is simple, inexpensive, without risk, usually acceptable to the worker, and capable of being performed by paramedical personnel or the worker, it suffers from major weaknesses. With some diseases such as asbestosis, cough, dyspnea on exertion, and other symptoms often do not appear until the disease is moderately advanced. The worker with lung disease may fail to report certain symptoms such as "smoker's cough" that may be considered acceptable or unimportant to smokers. The worker may choose not to report certain symptoms for fear of losing a job or being labeled an unhealthy person. Finally, respiratory symptoms are often due to causes other than chronic lung disease. (The first three of these weaknesses have to do with low sensitivity, the last with low specificity.)

PHYSICAL EXAMINATION. Performing a physical examination is generally a less helpful screening approach than obtaining a history of previously unrecognized respiratory symptoms. It, too, is simple, inexpensive, without risk, acceptable to the worker, and capable of being done by paramedical personnel, but it, too, has low sensitivity and specificity, and is rarely helpful in screening for work-related pulmonary disease. For example, by the time basilar rales are heard in an individual with asbestosis, significant fibrosis has already occurred, and such physical signs as clubbing and cyanosis are usually associated with far-advanced disease.

CHEST X-RAYS. Chest x-rays also have significant limitations in the early detection of chronic respiratory disease. This screening approach is more expensive and requires special equipment. In addition, with periodic x-rays a given worker may face some cumulative radiation hazard. Moreover, chest films are usually not very sensitive or very specific, the presence or absence of abnormalities does not always correlate with the intensity of symptoms, early physiologic abnormalities, and actual pathology. Chest films also fail to reveal early changes of COPD, and they are subject to much variation in technique and interpretation. Despite these limitations, chest films can play an important role in the early diagnosis and assessment of work-related restrictive diseases, especially if chest x-ray abnormalities begin to appear relatively early in the course of chronic disease. Chest x-rays are discussed again later in this chapter in the context of lung cancer screening.

PULMONARY FUNCTION TESTING. Although it requires special equipment and therefore is more costly than performing histories or physical examinations, pulmonary function testing is a reasonably sensitive screening approach for work-related respiratory diseases, and it generally provides more useful screening information than the other approaches (Fig. 3-5). Pulmonary function tests

[3]An excellent questionnaire, developed by the American Thoracic Society, was published in BG Ferris. Epidemiology standardization project. Am Rev Respir Dis 1978; 118:7–54. It is also available from the National Heart, Lung, and Blood Institute, Bethesda, MD 20892.

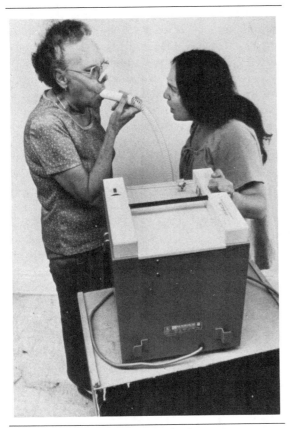

Fig. 3-5. Pulmonary function testing. (Photograph by Earl Dotter.)

used for screening are relatively easy to perform, and, if properly done, the results are reproducible.

Pulmonary function testing suffers from two general limitations: the range of normal is wide, and if the worker being tested does not cooperate fully, artifacts can appear, especially in tests requiring maximal effort. The first limitation can be countered by periodic testing of the same individual; test results in a given worker can be followed over time and abnormalities identified when greater than expected decreases in function occur. The second limitation can be addressed by applying standardized rules for acceptable tests (see Chap. 22).

The two most frequently used screening tests of pulmonary function are forced vital capacity (FVC) and forced expiratory volume in the first second of expiration ($FEV_1$). FVC is the maximal volume of air that can be exhaled forcefully after maximal inspiration. For most people it closely approximates the vital capacity without a forced effort. FVC is reduced relatively early in restrictive diseases such as asbestosis. $FEV_1$ is the volume of air that can be forcefully expelled during the first second of expiration with a maximal effort after the lungs have been filled completely. It is reduced in both restrictive and obstructive disease but relatively more so than FVC in obstructive disease. In the early course of asthma, it returns toward normal when the attack ends spontaneously or with bronchodilators. Advances in assessing pulmonary dysfunction are occurring but generally require validation before they are ready for routine use [6]. For further discussion, see Chapter 22.

Evaluation of workers for nonoccupational risk factors that may predispose them to occupational pulmonary disease is another, although controversial, approach. This is actually a method of primary prevention rather than screening. For example, some employers identify smokers, who may be at increased risk of acquiring a variety of occupational pulmonary diseases, and restrict them from certain jobs. This approach is sometimes opposed by workers who feel that it is unfair discrimination. One large asbestos company has prohibited workers from smoking in the workplace—even at its corporate offices—and has refused to hire new workers who smoke. This approach is controversial also because it can encourage employers to avoid eliminating hazardous conditions and instead find workers with "iron constitutions" who can withstand these conditions. The status of such programs in the U.S., since the passage of the Americans with Disabilities Act, is unclear. Decisions on this subject obviously involve both scientific assessments and public policy considerations of equity.

Screening for $\alpha_1$-antitrypsin deficiency is an example of a similar approach to risk factor identification. Individuals with a severe deficiency of this protein (1 in 5,000 of the general population) are at very high risk of developing emphysema and chronic bronchitis and should not work in a dusty workplace. It has not been established, however, if those individuals with lesser degrees of this deficiency are at increased risk of developing respiratory diseases.

Although there are many opportunities to screen for occupational respiratory disease, it is difficult to detect such disease before significant loss of lung function has occurred. Therefore, more reliance should be placed on methods of primary prevention, such as ventilation systems, changed work practices, and substitution of hazardous substances with nonhazardous ones.

*Hearing Impairment.* Several million Americans suffer chronic work-related hearing impairment, and several million American workers are exposed to loud noise at work that poses a threat to hearing (see Chap. 16). Even at the current OSHA standard of 90 decibels of sound pressure (dBA) for eight hours of workplace noise exposure, it is estimated that 10 percent of those exposed for a lifetime will have significant hearing impairment. By the time a worker notices hearing impairment, irreversible sensorineural damage affecting the sound frequencies of human conversation has usually occurred. However, long before a worker notices any hearing impairment, significant changes can be seen in the audiogram. Screening for hearing impairment is therefore important in workers exposed to loud noise.

The first sign of hearing impairment is a dip in the audiogram, usually at 3,000 to 6,000 Hz (cycles per second). If hearing impairment progresses, the audiologic abnormality becomes more severe and covers a broader range of frequencies. Discovery of an abnormal audiogram can point to the need to prevent hearing impairment by reduction of noise at the source, modification of the work procedures creating the noise, use of personal protective equipment (earmuffs or earplugs),

or removal of the worker from a noisy work environment.

Audiograms should be performed as part of the preplacement examination of workers who will be exposed to loud noise at work so that a baseline will be available for comparison with later audiograms. They should be repeated on exposed workers every year. Audiograms should not be performed within 14 hours of any significant noise exposure; if done sooner, a temporary threshold shift may be mistakenly identified as a permanent one. As with other screening tests, it is usually best to compare test results repeated on an individual over time rather than with "normal limits." It is particularly important to note that deterioration of hearing due to loud noise exposure is fairly rapid for the first years of exposure. Therefore, the effectiveness of a screening program is maximal during this initial work period.[4]

Audiometry is generally accepted as a useful screening approach and is widely performed in industry in the United States. However, its value can be undermined by poor technique, such as inadequate calibration of equipment, excess noise in the testing room, headphone position variations, headset pressure against the external ears, examiner and tester biases, improved performance of the subject after familiarization with the testing procedure, obstruction of the ear canal, tinnitus, simulation or malingering, and fluctuation of the subject's criterion for threshold identification of the test tone. A National Institute for Occupational Safety and Health (NIOSH) study several years ago indicated that 80 percent of industries surveyed used inadequate audiometric equipment. However, most of these problems can be minimized with appropriately trained technicians and adequate equipment.

---

[4]It is useful to remember as a rule of thumb that the maximum temporary threshold shift (i.e., the asymptomatic level of threshold shift) determined by several measurements taken consecutively over 8 to 24 hours is considered a possible indicator of future permanent hearing impairment due to continued work in the same noise environment. (Personal communication from R Hamernik to B Levy.)

*Toxic Effects.* Three components are involved in the prevention of the toxic effects of workplace chemicals: evaluating the toxicity of the chemical itself (preferably before it is introduced, as the Toxic Substances Control Act mandates) by animal studies and short-term in vitro assays, environmental monitoring of levels of the chemical in workplace air to determine if it is controlled in accordance with recommended or mandated standards, and biologic monitoring (see also Chap. 13).

Biologic monitoring is the testing of blood, urine, or exhaled air of individuals to determine either the body's level of a hazardous chemical and metabolites (evidence of exposure) or reasonably specific biochemical changes that are associated with cellular damage (screening for early health effects). For the screening to be effective, it must detect early ("sentinel") biologic effects before serious health effects occur. As with other evaluation approaches, once biologic monitoring of any kind indicates that workers have excessive exposure or early toxic effects, measures must be taken to reduce their exposure to the responsible agents. Following are three examples of biologic monitoring:

Several volatile organic compounds, including benzene and toluene, if inhaled or absorbed through the skin, produce metabolites that can be measured in urine.

Organophosphate pesticides, before exerting any known health effects, begin to inhibit both plasma and red blood cell cholinesterase. The activity of plasma cholinesterase (pseudocholinesterase) reflects absorption of the organophosphate, and the activity of the red cell cholinesterase correlates well with the degree of adverse effect.

Various tests have been used to evaluate lead exposure or body burden and the biologic effects of lead (Table 3-2). Biologic monitoring for lead is particularly useful because the early effects of lead poisoning are reversible and because symptoms of early toxicity, such

as headache and fatigue, are nonspecific, or the patient is asymptomatic (see Chaps. 13, 26, 27, and 31).

Biologic monitoring has a different use from environmental monitoring because it takes into consideration host differences in, for example, susceptibility to toxic effects and absorption, distribution, and biotransformation of the substance. It also considers possible multiple exposures (both occupational and nonoccupational) and multiple routes of absorption. A crucial issue is the relationship of environmental monitoring and biologic monitoring. Since environmental monitoring leads to control of exposure before absorption of the hazardous chemical, it is preferable. Biologic monitoring, however, should not be considered a substitute for environmental monitoring. Given the potential for multiple routes of exposure that are not well assessed by environmental monitoring (for example, percutaneous absorption), biologic monitoring should be used as a valuable adjunctive technique.

Biologic monitoring is still in an early stage of development and has several limitations. There is no health effect parameter for many substances; as each new parameter is developed, its relation must be established, on the one hand, to the amount of exposure and, on the other, to the disease. The biologic half-lives of many toxins are not known. Screening may erroneously be done at the wrong time and therefore fail to identify acute intoxication or transient effects. For many known biologic parameters, the range of normal is wide, so it is necessary to base the interpretation of testing on a series of tests on the same individual over time. This fact demonstrates the importance of performing baseline biologic monitoring specific to known or anticipated hazards during the preplacement examination. Quality control in laboratories varies; it is essential that laboratories performing biologic monitoring ensure accurate results.

These potential problems make it crucial to plan biologic monitoring carefully. Workers who may

**Table 3-2.** Evaluation of the various tests that have been used to monitor workers with lead exposure

| Exposure monitoring tests (evaluation of lead exposure or lead body burden) | Screening tests (evaluation of biologic action of lead) |
|---|---|
| Lead in blood<br>  Evaluates amount of lead absorption, therefore reflects intensity of lead exposure<br>  As absorption increases it reaches a plateau, so it is not an accurate measure of body burden<br>  Laboratory technique must be very good<br>Lead in urine<br>  Ease of obtaining specimens<br>  Disadvantages of fluctuating kidney function and fluid intake affecting test results<br>Lead in urine after administration of a chelating agent<br>  Reflects fraction of lead in body that can be mobilized, therefore probably indicates amount that is metabolically active<br>  Too complex and dangerous for screening test<br>Lead in hair<br>  Indicates past exposure, so of limited use in occupational disease | Hemoglobin/hematocrit<br>  Easy to obtain<br>  Do not correlate with blood lead below 70 μg/dl<br>Coproporphyrins in urine<br>  Low specificity<br>  Do not increase until the blood level is about 50 μg/dl<br>Free erythrocyte protoporphyrins (including measurement of zinc protoporphyrin [ZPP])<br>  Useful, but reflect bone marrow lead 3 months before<br>  Some false positives, including iron deficiency<br>Porphobilinogen in urine<br>  Not useful because increase occurs after toxic symptoms present<br>Delta-aminolevulinic acid (ALA) in urine<br>  Very useful, reflects amount of metabolically active lead in body<br>  Very sensitive, very specific but returns slowly toward normal after exposure ceases<br>Activity of delta-aminolevulinic acid dehydratase (ALA-D) in erythrocytes<br>  This enzyme inhibited by lead<br>  Very sensitive and specific<br>  But must keep specimen at 0°C |

Source: R Lauwerys. Biological criteria for selected industrial toxic chemicals: A review. Scand J Work Environ Health 1975;1:139.

be exposed must be identified. The appropriate parameter to monitor them must be chosen. Baseline measurements made before exposure and measurements after exposure must be appropriately timed. There is also much room for error in the choice of specimen, the storage and handling of specimens, and the interpretation of results. However, biologic monitoring holds much promise, and with the increase of toxic substances in the workplace and greater recognition of toxic hazards, it can play an important preventive role.

*Cancer.* Screening has a limited role in occupational cancer control. National Cancer Institute data support the concept that early detection of cancer followed by appropriate treatment can increase survival of some patients with certain cancers. Approaches that have been used to screen for different cancers include examination of exfoliated cells by the Papanicolaou technique (Pap smear), x-rays, proctosigmoidoscopy, identification of a substance in the blood or other body fluid that may be a specific marker for a given malignancy, breast self-examination, measures of organ function, and tests to detect colon cancer by identifying occult blood in the stool. These approaches widely vary in effectiveness (see Chap. 14).

Few screening approaches of any kind, however, have been proved to reduce mortality from cancer. As with screening for most chronic diseases, discussion of the effectiveness of cancer screening has been greatly confused by studies that do not differentiate between true mortality reduction and merely earlier identification.

A dramatic increase in lung cancer mortality has taken place in the past 50 years. Attempts to detect lung cancer early have recently focused on periodic chest x-rays and cytologic examinations of sputum, which tend to complement one another; chest x-rays are more useful for detecting peripherally situated cancers while sputum cytology can identify early squamous cell carcinoma involving major airways. Relatively few cases of lung cancer give a positive result on both tests at the same time. Although these tests are often used to screen for lung cancer, neither has been convincingly shown to be effective. Usually, by the time either of these tests presumptively identifies a lung cancer, it has metastasized and is incurable. Well-controlled studies have demonstrated that addition of sputum cytology to chest x-ray screening does not significantly reduce mortality from all types of lung cancer but suggests that mortality from squamous cell carcinoma is reduced [7]. A report of three randomized trials of screening for early lung cancer suggests that sputum cytology detects 15 to 20 percent of all lung cancer, mostly squamous cell carcinoma, with a relatively good prognosis, and that chest x-ray alone may be a more effective test for early-stage lung cancer than previous reports have suggested. However, a randomized clinical trial at the Mayo Clinic has shown that both procedures offered every 4 months had no advantage in survival over standard medical practices [8].

The status of attempts to screen for bladder cancer is much the same as that for lung cancer. The approaches used most frequently in recent years have been a search for occult blood and cytologic examination of exfoliated cells in urine. These approaches have been successfully used to identify asymptomatic individuals with early bladder cancer in a population at high risk of bladder cancer because of exposure to aromatic amines [9]. However, whether screening in this or similar high-risk groups will lead to prolongation of life or decreased morbidity has not been evaluated in a controlled clinical trial.

Given the continued high incidence of cancer (and the substantial incidence of occupational cancer), its severity, and frequent lack of effective treatment, attempts will no doubt continue to develop better screening tests. In the meantime, health professionals should not raise false hopes of workers, since most currently available screening tests are of unproved effectiveness, and instead should concentrate on measures of primary prevention. These measures include testing workplace substances for carcinogenicity, limiting exposure to proved or suspected carcinogens, and encouraging smoking cessation, since smoking is associated with lung, bladder, and other cancers.

*Back Problems.* When the term *screening* is used in relation to back problems in the workplace, it usually refers to preplacement identification of preexisting back problems, both work-related and not, or of a predilection to back problems. Three methods have been traditionally used to try to identify workers at high risk of work-related back problems: history, physical examination, and x-rays of the lumbosacral spine. None of these methods has been effective in controlling low back injuries. X-rays have been used on the basis of a hypothesis, now shown to be false, that developmental abnormalities of the spine predispose to low back injury. The persistent use of back x-rays to detect such abnormalities not only is without benefit but also discriminates unnecessarily against prospective workers with x-ray abnormalities. X-rays do not necessarily predict future back injury risk and create unnecessary x-ray exposure. Although the only effective control for back problems today seems to be the ergonomic approach of designing the job to fit the worker, some evidence indicates that measurements of strength and fitness before the start of work can predict back injuries (see Chaps. 8 and 23). In addition, strength measurements can be used to match a worker's strength to job requirements.

*Possibilities for Improved Screening*
Opportunities for effective screening for occupational diseases at present are relatively limited, and most available screening approaches do not meet the criteria outlined earlier in this chapter. Unless screening approaches are improved, much time, effort, and limited resources may be wasted; workers may face unnecessary risks and experience unnecessary anxiety and inconvenience; and workers and employers may become disillusioned with preventive approaches in general.

The general industry standards for specific hazardous exposures, published by OSHA, specify re-quirements for medical surveillance of exposed workers [10]. They may include preplacement and periodic screening histories, examinations, and tests. Table 3-3 illustrates some of the specific screening tests required by OSHA. OSHA also requires employers to keep records of this surveillance and to make these records available to affected employees. The records can also be made available to physicians or other third parties on specific written request.

Suggested principles for screening and biologic monitoring of the effects of exposure in the workplace and many related articles were the subject of an intensive national conference held in Cincinnati in July 1984 and published as the August and October 1986 issues of the *Journal of Occupational Medicine*. Extensive discussions of various aspects of screening are included in these issues. A central theme expressed in these discussions is the following: "Screening and monitoring, in and of themselves, prevent nothing; only the appropriate intervention, in response to results of these tests, can prevent" [11].

Table 3-3. Selected OSHA standards for medical surveillance

| Exposure | History | Physical examination | Other tests/procedures |
|---|---|---|---|
| Airborne asbestos | Especially respiratory symptoms | Especially chest examination | Chest x-ray FVC and $FEV_1$ |
| Vinyl chloride | Especially alcohol use, history of hepatitis, transfusions | Especially liver, spleen, and kidneys | Liver function tests |
| Inorganic arsenic | Yes | Especially nasal and skin examinations | Chest x-ray Sputum cytology |
| Benzene | Including alcohol use and medications | Yes | Complete blood count Reticulocyte count Serum bilirubin |
| Dibromochloropropane (DBCP) | Including reproductive history | Especially genitourinary system | FSH, LH Males: also sperm count Females: also total estrogen |

Key: FSH = follicle-stimulating hormone; LH = luteinizing hormone.
Source: Occupational Safety and Health Administration, U.S. Department of Labor. Code of Federal Regulations (CFR), Title 29: General industry (Revised July 1, 1993). Washington, D.C.: U.S. Government Printing Office, 1984.

# Occupational Surveillance for Disease Control

*Occupational surveillance* is the systematic and ongoing collection, analysis, and dissemination of information on disease, injury, or hazard for the prevention of morbidity or mortality. Surveillance as it applies to populations should be differentiated from the *medical surveillance* of individuals. Medical surveillance, also known as medical monitoring and sometimes as periodic medical screening, is focused on the interview and examination of the individual. *Public health surveillance*, of which occupational surveillance is a subset, is focused on populations. While the overriding goal of medical surveillance and public health surveillance is the same—prevention, the specific goals are different.

There are five goals of public health surveillance as applied to occupational disease:

1. To identify illnesses, injuries, and hazards that represent new opportunities for prevention. New opportunities can be new problems, as might occur with the introduction of a new hazardous machine, or the belated identification of a long-standing, but ignored, problem or the recurrence of a problem controlled previously.
2. To define the magnitude and distribution of the problem in the workforce. Information on magnitude and distribution is useful for planning intervention programs. While no hazard is acceptable, the more common and severe problems deserve more immediate attention.
3. To track trends in the magnitude of the problem as a rudimentary method of assessing the effectiveness, or lack thereof, of prevention efforts—whether the problem is getting better or worse. Epidemics can be tracked on their rise or their decline.
4. Targeting, the identification of categories of occupations, industries, and specific worksites that require attention—either in the form of consultation, educational efforts, or inspection for compliance with established regulations.

5. The public dissemination of information so that wise personal and societal decisions can be made.

There is a *continuum of outcomes* that could be the subject for surveillance. The continuum may range from the presence of an exposure or hazard, to early and subclinical health effects of that hazard, to morbidity and associated medical care and disability, and finally mortality. Choice of an appropriate exposure or health outcome for surveillance should depend on the goal of surveillance that is sought. Other considerations should include an assessment of whether the proposed reporting entity, such as the physician or the employer, will report the occurrence; the accuracy of the system in detecting real problems and minimizing false-positive leads; the timeliness of the system in producing useful information; and the cost of the system in relationship to other systems that could be supported instead.

There are two kinds of surveillance. One is based on the intensive investigation of cases (case-based); the other is more embedded in epidemiologic methods, especially the determination of the distribution or rate of disease, injury, or hazard in the population (rate-based). An underlying philosophy for case-based surveillance has been called the sentinel health event (occupational) [SHE(O)] method [12]. An SHE(O) has been defined as a case of disease, injury, or exposure that represents a failure of the system for prevention. While a list of SHE(O)s has been published, it should not inhibit one from focusing on other adverse entities that are more germane to a local situation.

Rate-based surveillance is embedded in epidemiology in that it seeks to establish the rate of occurrence of the disease, injury, or exposure and to track that rate over time or compare it to the rate in some other population. Surveillance differs from epidemiologic research, however, in that surveillance is an ongoing activity with goals directly related to the functioning of the public health system, while epidemiologic research is concerned about assessing the association between effect and etiologic agent. Epidemiologic research also involves an intensive collection of data during a limited period of time, rather than being an ongoing collection and assessment of data as is part of surveillance. While it is valuable to discern the differences between surveillance and research in their pure forms, in reality, these distinctions often blur.

Surveillance can be used to monitor either the occurrence of diseases (or physiologic abnormalities) or the presence of hazardous substances and worker exposures to them. This section focuses on its use in monitoring the occurrence of injury and disease. For chronic diseases caused by workplace exposures, monitoring of *exposures,* however, may be more useful. This possibility exists because a number of exposure-effect relationships are sufficiently well described that long-term exposure to known levels of a material can be said to predictably result in the chronic illness. Furthermore, the long latency period between exposure and onset of chronic work-related disease makes it difficult to associate the exposure with the disease in an individual case. For diseases of shorter latency, direct disease surveillance may be very useful.

In contrast to communicable disease surveillance, which is largely based on physician reporting, there are a variety of models for occupational disease surveillance. Some of these are broadly based while others can be done on a plant-specific or job-specific basis.

### Broad-Based Occupational Surveillance Programs

***Surveillance Based on Death Certificates.*** The National Occupational Mortality System (NOMS) of NIOSH collects and codes mortality and occupational information from about 500,000 death certificates a year from 23 states in the U.S. This allows analysis of differential mortality patterns among occupations and industries, as well as comparison of distribution of industries and occupations among diseases. This is one of the few systems capable of providing information about women and minorities in the workforce. NIOSH also conducts surveillance for fatalities from injuries through the National Traumatic Occupational Fatalities (NTOF) system, which collects from all states death certificates in which the cause of death is an injury at work.

***Surveillance Based on Employer Records.*** An annual survey of a large sample of employers is performed by the Bureau of Labor Statistics (BLS) of the U.S. Department of Labor. Using information from the required "OSHA 200" log of injuries and illnesses, these data provide broad estimates of work-related disease and injury. However, the survey is limited by the absence of specific criteria for determining the occupational relationship of disease, the limited sensitivity of the "OSHA 200" log for detecting cases, and assurance of confidentiality, which limits the usefulness of the survey for identifying cases or plants for in-depth follow-up investigations.

***Surveillance Based on Workers' Compensation.*** Although readily available in most states, workers' compensation data are limited by nature because they include only those who file (generally those with the more severe injuries and illnesses), they exclude most cases of chronic work-related *disease,* and they are limited by adjudication procedures and diagnostic criteria that vary from state to state (see Chap. 10). However, these data have been very useful in identifying new problems such as violence toward women workers, and in providing estimates of the magnitude of newly identified problems such as disability from knee disease in carpet installers. In Ohio, workers' compensation readily identified companies with excessive dermatitis, as well as the offending agent [13].

***Cancer Registries.*** Hospital-based, regional, or statewide cancer incidence registries can be useful sources of surveillance data on cancer, but often have only limited, if any, information on occupation.

*Physician Reporting.* In some locations, such as Alberta (Canada), Great Britain, West Germany, and selected states in the U.S., the law requires physicians to report all work-related diseases and injuries or certain specified ("scheduled") conditions. Where this is effectively enforced, the scheduled diseases can be tracked and epidemics identified early.

*Laboratory-Based Reporting.* A state-based national system, Adult Blood Lead Epidemiology and Surveillance (ABLES), collects information from the 26 U.S. states that require laboratories to report to them cases of individuals with excessive lead levels. This information has proved useful in making national estimates of lead poisoning, tracking trends, identifying underserved occupations and industries, and targeting specific worksites with excessive cases. The limitations in laboratory-based reporting include the limited number of conditions for which laboratories can be involved; an irony is that workers with the most inadequate resources available are the least likely to even be monitored for lead.

*Sentinel Event Approaches.* Examples of sentinel event approaches are present in both Great Britain and the U.S. In Great Britain, the SWORD system was developed to identify new and survey known types of occupational respiratory disease, using reports from thoracic and occupational physicians [14]. Preliminary success has led to efforts to replicate the model for occupational dermatitis. In the U.S., NIOSH is working with 36 states to develop state-based systems for surveillance of occupational disease and injury. A central element of this effort is the Sentinel Event Notification System for Occupational Risks (SENSOR), which includes silicosis, occupational asthma, amputations, cadmium poisoning, carpal tunnel syndrome, child-labor injuries and illnesses, noise-induced hearing loss, pesticide poisoning, spinal cord injuries, and tuberculosis [15]. New conditions are also being explored for inclusion in SENSOR. For example,

three states are now utilizing workers' compensation reports and networks of dermatologists to report occupational dermatitis, and two states are testing surveillance of severe occupational burns, using reports from hospital burn units.

### Focused Occupational Surveillance Programs

*Surveying Workers.* Interviews and examinations of workers represent an effective surveillance approach, especially for estimating the magnitude and distribution of occupational problems in the workforce. In addition to focused efforts at specific work locations, large interview surveys addressing the prevalence of cumulative trauma disorders, dermatitis, and other conditions have been conducted by the National Center for Health Statistics (NCHS). NCHS conducts other large examination surveys that contain limited information relevant to occupation, such as blood lead.

*Union Records.* Unions may have morbidity or mortality data, often related to medical or death benefit programs, which can be used for surveillance. Even without this information, union records can define the exposed, or at-risk, population in order to look for adverse health outcomes in state vital registry records or cancer registries.

*Employer Records.* Employer records can be helpful for finding morbidity data, although such data are likely to be underestimates of the actual incidence of disease; such records may also provide valuable information on exposure.

*Disability Records.* Disability records can be examined as a potentially useful source of surveillance data (see Chap. 11).

### Conclusion

With time, it is likely that improved surveillance of occupational disease will yield additional useful information. In evaluating occupational surveillance, it is most important to be clear on the goal(s) for the specific surveillance system and recognize that not every system will meet every goal.

More information on surveillance of occupational disease can be obtained from (1) the Surveillance Coordinating Activity at NIOSH (4676 Columbia Parkway, Cincinnati, OH 45226); (2) workers' compensation system agencies in most states; (3) the Bureau of Labor Statistics of the U.S. Department of Labor in Washington, D.C.; and (4) the occupational disease and injury epidemiologists in most state health or labor departments.

## References

1. Ashford NA, Miller CS. Chemical exposures: Low levels and high stakes. New York: Van Nostrand Reinhold, 1991.
2. Cullen MR. Low level chemical exposure. In L Rosenstock, MR Cullen. eds. Textbook of clinical occupational and environmental medicine. Philadelphia: Saunders, 1994.
3. Hamilton A. Industrial poisons in the U.S. 1925.
4. Halperin WE, Frazier TM. Surveillance for the effects of workplace exposure. Annu Rev Public Health 1985; 6:419–32.
5. Halperin WE, et al. Medical screening in the workplace: Proposed principles. J Occup Med 1986; 28:547–52.
6. Kreiss K. Approaches to assessing pulmonary dysfunction and susceptibility in workers. J Occup Med 1986; 28:664–9.
7. Frost JK, et al. Sputum cytopathology: Use and potential in monitoring the workplace environment by screening for biological effects of exposure. J Occup Med 1986; 28:692–703.
8. Fontana RS. Lung cancer screening: The Mayo program. J Occup Med 1986; 28:746–50.
9. Schulte P, Ringen K, Hemstreet G. Optimal management of asymptomatic workers at high risk of bladder cancer. J Occup Med 1986; 28:13–7.
10. OSHA, U.S. Department of Labor. General industry: OSHA safety and health standards (29 CFR 1910). Washington, D.C.: U.S. Government Printing Office, 1978.
11. Millar JD. Screening and monitoring: Tools for prevention. J Occup Med 1986; 28:544–6.
12. Rutstein D, et al. The sentinel health event (occupational): A framework for occupational health surveillance and education. Am J Public Health 1983; 73:1054–62.
13. O'Malley M, et al. Surveillance of occupational skin disease using the supplementary data system. Am J Ind Med 1988; 13:291–300.
14. Meredith SK, Taylor VM, McDonald JC. Occupational respiratory disease in the United Kingdom 1989: A report to the British Thoracic Society and the Society of Occupational Medicine by the SWORD project group. B J Ind Med 1991; 48:292–8.
15. Baker EL. Sentinel Event Notification System for Occupational Risks (SENSOR): The concept. Am J Public Health 1989; 79 (suppl.):18–20.

## Bibliography

### Recognition

Bureau of Labor Statistics, U.S. Department of Labor. Towards improved measurement and reporting of occupational illness and disease. (Symposium proceedings, Albuquerque, NM, 1985.) Washington, D.C.: U.S. Department of Labor, 1987.
*State-of-the-art review of practical issues in occupational disease surveillance and proposals for the future.*

Froines JR, Dellenbaugh CA, Wegman DH. Occupational health surveillance: A means to identify work-related risk. Am J Public Health 1986; 76:1089.
*Introduction to the concept of hazard surveillance.*

Goldman RH, Peters JM. The occupational and environmental health history. JAMA 1981; 246:2831.
*An excellent article with more detail on the occupational history.*

### Screening

Halperin WE, Schulte PA, Greathouse DG. eds. (Part I) and Mason TJ, Prorok PC, Costlow RD eds. (Part II). Conference on medical screening and biological monitoring for the effects of exposure in the workplace. J Occup Med 1986; 28:543–788, 901–1126.
*An in-depth, up-to-date, comprehensive review on screening in the workplace.*

Halperin WE, et al. Medical screening in the workplace: Proposed principles. J Occup Med 1986; 28:547–52.
*Questions the adequacy of current recommendations on screening in the workplace and proposes a revised set of principles for such screening.*

Hathaway GJ, et al. eds. Chemical hazards in the workplace. 3rd ed. Philadelphia: Lippincott, 1991.

*Includes recommended screening examinations and tests for workers exposed to any of almost 400 substances.*

Lauwerys RR. Industrial chemical exposure: Guidelines for biological monitoring. 2nd ed. Davis, CA: Biomedical Publications, 1993.

*Presents concepts of biologic monitoring and reviews current knowledge on numerous specific agents.*

Morrison AS. Screening in chronic disease. Monographs in epidemiology and biostatistics, vol 7. 2nd ed. New York and Oxford: Oxford University Press, 1992.

*An excellent text on the epidemiology of screening.*

Silverstein MA. Analysis of medical screening and surveillance in 21 OSHA standards: Support of a generic medical surveillance standard. Am J Ind Med 1994; 26(3).

*An excellent review article.*

World Health Organization. Early detection of occupational diseases. Geneva: WHO, 1986.

*An excellent guide on the principles of and approaches to early detection and control of various occupational diseases.*

## Surveillance

Ashford NA, et al. Monitoring the worker for exposure and disease: Scientific, legal, and ethical considerations in the use of biomarkers. Baltimore: Johns Hopkins Press, 1990.

*This monograph covers issues related both to screening and surveillance. The considerations given to the issues raise a number of important questions about what are the objectives of efforts to evaluate biologic materials from workers, how these are used effec-tively, as well as how the measurements can be of little or no use for the objectives identified.*

Bureau of Labor Statistics, U.S. Department of Labor. Towards improved measurement and reporting of occupational illness and disease. (Symposium proceedings, Albuquerque, NM, 1985.) Washington, D.C.: U.S. Department of Labor, 1987.

*State-of-the-art review of practical issues in occupational disease surveillance and proposals for the future.*

Halperin WE, Frazier TM. Surveillance and the effects of workplace exposure. Ann Rev Public Health 1985;6:419.

*A systematic review that provides a careful integration of the range of issues related to surveillance in work settings.*

Halperin W, Baker EL, Monson RR. eds. Public health surveillance. New York: Van Nostrand Reinhold, 1992.

*This book covers basic principles of public health surveillance and provides discussions of specific subject areas particularly relevant to the occupational setting including occupational disease, hazard surveillance, AIDS, chronic disease, and injury.*

Mullan RJ, Murthy LI. Occupational sentinel health events: An updated list for physician recognition and public health surveillance. Am J Ind Med 1991; 19:775–99.

*Adaptation of the general concept of sentinel health events to occupational disease.*

Wegman DH. Hazard surveillance. In W Halperin, EL Baker, RR Monson. eds. Public health surveillance. New York: Van Nostrand Reinhold, 1992.

*Provides conceptual framework for the surveillance of hazards. This is a primary prevention approach especially relevant for long latency diseases.*

# 4

# Preventing Occupational Disease

David H. Wegman and Barry S. Levy

Occupational diseases and injuries are, in principle, preventable. Among the approaches to preventing occupational diseases are developing awareness of occupational health hazards among workers and employers, assessing the nature and extent of hazards, and introducing and maintaining effective control measures. Sometimes these approaches are successfully undertaken solely by employers and workers within a specific workplace. Other times there is also the need for external involvement, ranging from encouragement by appropriate individuals or agencies outside the specific workplace to promulgation and rigorous enforcement of occupational health and safety regulations.

Although specific circumstances will require a variety of different approaches, it is important for physicians and other health professionals to recognize the vital role they can play in preventing work-related disease. This role requires going beyond treating individual patients both to help prevent recurrence of disease and to prevent initial occurrence of disease in other similarly exposed workers.

The opportunities for prevention of work-related disease or injury that are available to the health professional are different depending upon whether his or her role is related solely to *individual* patients or whether it extends also to *groups* of workers in companies or unions. This chapter covers opportunities and responsibilities that present themselves to health care providers in caring for individual patients with newly identified work-related diseases or injuries, and a summary of prevention measures that are possible when the health professional also has a formal relationship with, and responsibility to, an employer.

## Methods of Prevention

Measures to prevent occupational disease and injury can be considered as either (1) applied to the process or workplace, or (2) applied to the individual worker. These are further described below as well as illustrated in many places in this text (see particularly Chap. 6).

### Measures Applied to the Process or Workplace

*Substitution of a Nonhazardous Substance for a Hazardous One.* An example is the frequent substitution of synthetic vitreous fibers, such as fibrous glass, for asbestos. Substitution carries with it, however, certain risks because substitute materials have often not been adequately tested for health effects and may, in fact, be hazardous. For example, years ago fire protection was enhanced by replacing flammable cleaning solvents with carbon tetrachloride. Increased use of carbon tetrachloride, however, led to identification of its hepatotoxicity and its subsequent replacement by less toxic chlorinated hydrocarbons. Even now, there is concern that use of chlorinated hydrocarbons should be reduced to better protect the general environment. The lesson in this evolution is

## TOXICS USE REDUCTION AND OCCUPATIONAL HEALTH PROMOTION
Kenneth Geiser

Conventional approaches to protecting workers from dangerous levels of exposure to toxic chemicals in the workplace are based on two assumptions: (1) There are thresholds of exposure below which no ill effect will occur, and (2) engineering and management controls can maintain exposures below those thresholds. Such regulations limit, but do not stop, toxic chemical exposure. What if these assumptions proved wrong and even small amounts of toxic chemical exposure over long periods could lead to illness? This is not an unreasonable possibility. For example, it is commonly accepted that there are no safe threshold levels for occupational exposure to carcinogens. Yet, many workers are daily exposed to low levels of carcinogens, because it is argued that certain carcinogens are so indispensable or cost-effective, that it is worth risking the health of some workers to continue to use these chemicals at the workplace.

A different example is provided by considering lead in the manufacture of automobile batteries. The largest American manufacturer of auto batteries has argued that lead, which is a confirmed reproductive hazard, is essential to battery production. The management of the firm was even willing to go to court to defend its exclusion of women from certain battery production areas due to the reproductive hazards of lead. Most reviewers of this case including the courts accepted the firm's own research that concluded that there were no feasible alternatives to lead in automobile battery manufacture. Yet, just a decade ago, when the solar-powered car was undergoing rapid technological development, a host of alternatives to lead batteries emerged because lead was simply too heavy a material for solar cars. In other words, when the conditions are right, industry can rapidly move to replace toxic materials in production processes. Yet, such solutions are little considered when firms seek to alter workplaces to meet exposure threshold standards.

Environmentalists, too, have been faced with increasing evidence that years of government pollution control regulations have not produced an acceptably safe or clean environment. Such conclusions have pushed environmental advocates to search for new approaches to toxic chemical management that would more fundamentally reduce the accumulation of highly persistent toxins in the environment.

One such approach is called toxics use reduction (TUR), which shifts the focus of engineering and management activities from complying with pollution emission threshold standards to changing production processes so as to reduce or eliminate the use of toxic chemicals in production. By reducing the use or release of toxic chemicals in production processes, firms may prevent, rather than merely control, the generation of dangerous pollutants.

Toxics use reduction is no pipe dream. From 1990 to 1993, 10 states passed some kind of TUR law. Typically, these laws require firms to report publicly a list of targeted toxic chemicals and to prepare plans on how they will change production processes to reduce or eliminate the use of these chemicals. States that promote TUR often provide free technical assistance to firms to assist managers in finding ways to reduce the use of toxic chemicals.

Firms may change production processes by, for example:

- Substituting chemicals in the raw material inputs
- Reformulating the product so as to reduce the use of a toxic chemical
- Redesigning the production processes
- Modernizing or upgrading the production technologies
- Improving operations and maintenance programs

- Recycling toxic chemicals back into the processes in closed systems

Industrial firms have begun to adopt TUR programs in order to meet environmental regulations. Some illustrative examples include the following:

At a Massachusetts company that produces folded and printed cartons for commercial clients, the conventional operations used large quantities of isopropyl alcohol (IPA) in the fountain solutions for the offset printing presses. The IPA solution was mixed by hand into tap water, resulting in variable quality solutions, worker inhalation of alcohol fumes, and costly releases of volatile organic compounds to the environment. By redesigning the processes, management was able to install a centralized, closed-loop recycling system for the fountain solutions and reverse osmosis equipment to filter incoming water. With better management of the fountain solution system, the company was able to find and use a substitute for the IPA. Thus, environmental emissions, vapor exposure for workers, flammability hazards, use of raw material quantities, and costs were all reduced along with the elimination of permits for IPA use.

Another company was able to eliminate its use of chlorofluorocarbon metal cleaners in the manufacture of its communication equipment through a process of substituting aqueous-based cleaners and eliminating unnecessary cleaning steps. A third company was able to reduce its discharge of mercury to the sewer system by redesigning its camera battery pack to fully replace the mercury battery. The U.S. Department of Defense developed a process in which small plastic beads are air blasted at the surface of airplanes to remove old paint, eliminating the need for methylene chloride–based paint strippers and cutting the time of removing paint by 80 percent.

In each of these cases, production managers have gone beyond the conventional approaches to regulatory compliance. Instead of simply meeting the minimal standards of the regulations, they have sought to reconsider the production system itself in order to prevent the use of hazardous chemicals.

Many of these projects have been initiated by managers attempting to cut hazardous waste treatment costs or attempting to avoid the need for complying with environmental regulations. Occupational health protection is less often cited as a motivation. Yet, TUR programs may be equally valuable for reducing the risks at the workplace. There are many opportunities for complying with chemical exposure regulations by applying TUR principles to redesign production processes and substitute chemicals, thereby reducing or eliminating the use of dangerous toxic chemicals.

## Bibliography

Rossi M, Ellenbecker M, Geiser K. Techniques in toxics use reduction. New Solutions 1991;1:25–32.

---

not that substitution is hopeless, but that the introduction of a substituted material should be considered only a first step and that the impact of the substitution must always be followed to determine whether initially unrecognized problems develop after increased use of the new material.

*Installation of Engineering Controls and Devices.* These approaches are more often available than substitution and cover a wide range of effective options to reduce both chemical and ergonomic hazards. Some examples of common approaches are:

- The installation of ventilation exhaust systems that remove hazardous dusts (Fig. 4-1)
- The use of jigs or fixtures to reduce static muscle contractions in holding parts or tools
- The application of appropriately designed soundproofing materials to reduce loud noises that cannot be engineered out of a work process
- Installing tools on overhead balancers to eliminate torque and vibration transmitted to the hand
- The construction of enclosures to isolate hazardous processes

**Fig. 4-1.** Local exhaust ventilation used to protect a worker from asbestos dust generated in working with clutch plates. (Photograph by Earl Dotter.)

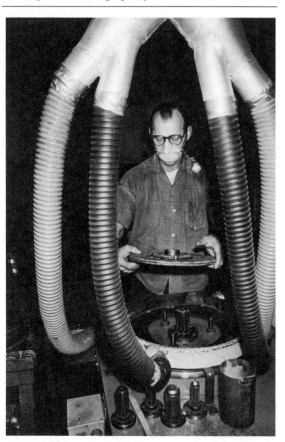

- Installing hoists to eliminate manual lifting of containers or parts
- The careful maintenance of process equipment to reduce or eliminate fugitive emissions from processes designed as closed systems or the development of unwanted vibrations as equipment ages

Although the installation of these engineering controls can be substantial initial capital expenditures, these controls often save money by reducing materials use, toxic and other material wastes, and costs of disease, injury, and absenteeism. Often, the reasons such approaches are not considered or implemented is the lack of awareness that such solutions are available.

*Job Redesign, Work Organization Changes and Work Practice Alternatives.* There are a number of changes that can be introduced which take advantage of methods designed to directly improve work processes so that several different types of risks can be reduced or eliminated. These include job redesign, changes in work organization, and alternative work practices. Job redesign, which often combines engineering and administrative aspects, typically seeks several related objectives: to increase job content, to make the physical work less redundant or repetitive, and to improve workers' opportunity to exercise individual or collective autonomy in decision-making. (See further discussion in Chap. 19.)

Changes in work organization, often closely integrated with individual job redesign, are directed to eliminating undesirable features in the structure of work processes. For example, a change from piece-rate work (with incentive wages) to hourly-rate work removes inappropriate pressure and tension—both physical and mental—on affected workers. Piece-rate work has been associated with higher rates of musculoskeletal problems in a variety of work settings. Machine pacing has the unfortunate consequence of enforcing repetitive and mind-numbing work; another example of a change in work organization is elimination of this kind of work pacing.

Work practice alternatives can, through relatively limited change, lead to important improvements in the work environment. For example, dust exposures in a variety of settings can be significantly reduced by introducing vacuum cleaning in place of compressed air to clean dusty surfaces and utilizing wet mopping in place of dry sweeping wherever possible.

As a rule, these preventive measures tend to be more effective than the following methods that primarily impact the worker. The four measures that follow potentially reduce the damage that may result from workplace hazards without actually removing the source of the problem.

### Measures Primarily Directed Toward the Worker

*Education and Advice. Education and advice* concerning specific work hazards are essential. Workers should always be given full information about workplace hazards and means of reducing their risk (Fig. 4-2). Many safety measures necessitate changed behavior by workers, which also requires education or training. Workers who are not aware of job hazards will not take the health and safety precautions necessary for protecting themselves and their coworkers. (See box on education of workers and information on the Hazard Communication Standard in Chap. 9.)

*Personal Protective Equipment. Use of personal protective equipment,* such as respirators, earplugs, gloves, and protective clothing (Fig. 4-3) will continue to be necessary in a number of settings where it is the only available protective measure. However, this approach to controlling a hazard often has important limitations; for example, workers will often resist wearing such protection because it is cumbersome or causes other difficulties. It is important that the effectiveness of personal protective equipment be evaluated in actual use where the experimentally determined effective-

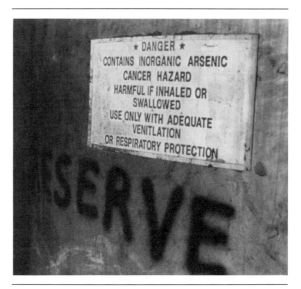

Fig. 4-2. Hazardous labeling regulations require that labels such as this one be improved to gain attention readily and in appropriate languages.

ness claimed by its manufacturer may not apply. In the U.S., the Occupational Safety and Health Administration (OSHA) has developed lists of acceptable personal protective equipment that can be helpful in proper selection and use of these devices. OSHA and other authorities have also emphasized the need for and importance of developing a complete *program* for personal protective equipment, not only a requirement for its *use.* Adequate programs will include requirements for proper fitting of the equipment (especially with respirators), education about proper use, and a plan for maintenance, cleaning, and replacement of equipment or parts. The costs of an effective personal protective equipment program are significant, making it particularly important to recognize that use of such equipment should only be accepted when no alternative controls are present.

*Organizational Measures. Organizational measures,* taken by the employer, may offer some protection. For example, exposure can be reduced somewhat by implementing work schedules such

## EFFECTIVELY EDUCATING WORKERS
Margaret Quinn and Nancy Lessin

A prerequisite to effective health and safety programs is education. The most effective approach to teaching health and safety acknowledges that the worker is the one most familiar with his or her job. Workers can thus identify hazards, both apparent and hidden, that may be associated with their work. Worker involvement in prioritizing educational needs and in the design and content of training are major determinants of meaningful and useful programs. Workers also should be included in the development and implementation of the solutions to health and safety problems. Education regarding solutions should include a discussion of the traditional occupational hygiene hierarchy of hazard controls (see Chap. 6) that emphasizes hazard elimination, and not be limited to training on the use of personal protective equipment. In addition to worker involvement with needs assessment and program design, additional guidelines for successful educational programs include the following:

1. *Develop an educational program in the trainee's literal and technical language.* The educator should also understand the social context and psychosocial factors of a workplace that may affect a worker's ability to participate in an educational program or to perform certain work practices in response to a potential hazard.

2. *Define specific and clearly stated goals for each session* based on a needs assessment that has involved representatives of the workers to be trained. Begin each program with a concise overview and reinforce the key issues that come up during the session.

3. *Build an evaluation mechanism that can be easily adapted to each program.* The evaluation process should be designed to judge the effectiveness of the educational program in attaining goals set by both the trainer and trainees.

4. *Use participatory teaching methods, which draw on the experience that workers already have, in place of a traditional lecture approach.* Participatory or learner-centered teaching methods are designed to foster maximum worker participation and interaction. They constitute an approach to labor education based on the understanding that adults bring an enormous amount of experience to the classroom that should be used in the training program. In addition, adults learn more effectively by doing rather than listening passively. Learners' experiences are incorporated into the course material and are used to expand their grasp of new concepts and skills. Basing new knowledge on prior practical experience will help the learner solve problems and develop safe solutions to unforeseen hazards. Instructors offer specialized knowledge; workers have direct experience. This combination leads to effective, long-lasting solutions to health and safety problems.

Participatory learning generally requires more trainer-trainee interaction than lecture-style presentations. Large groups should be limited to approximately 20 participants, and these groups may break down into groups of 3 to 6 for small group exercises. Participatory teaching methods can include the use of:

1. *Large group discussion or "speakouts."* The participants share their experiences relative to a particular hazard or situation.
2. *"Brainstorming sessions."* The instructor throws out a particular question or problem; the participants call out their ideas. The ideas are recorded on a flipchart so that they become a collective work. In this activity, the trainer elicits information from the participants rather than presenting it in a didactic manner.
3. *"Buzz groups."* This is a small group discussion or exercise. Groups of three to six participants are formed. Each group discusses a particular problem, situation, or question

and records the answers or views of the group.

4. *"Case studies."* This is a particular form of small group exercise in which participants get to apply new knowledge and skills in the exploration of solutions to a particular problem or situation.

5. *"Discovery exercises."* Participants go back into the workplace to obtain certain items such as OSHA 200 logs or they may perform activities such as interviewing coworkers on a particular hazard. This information is brought back into the classroom for discussion.

6. *"Hands-on training."* The participants practice skills, such as testing respirator fit, simulating asbestos removal or hazardous waste cleanup (Fig. 4-4), calculating lost workday injury rates from OSHA 200 logs, or handling and learning the uses and limitations of industrial hygiene monitoring equipment.

7. *"Report-back sessions."* Following the "buzz groups," the class reconvenes as a larger group. A spokesperson for each buzz group reports on the group's answers or views. Similarities and differences are noted between groups, and patterns may be discovered.

Participatory learning techniques are well-established methods practiced in labor education programs, schools of education, labor unions, and committees or coalitions for occupational safety and health (COSH groups). These groups have demonstrated that it is possible to use participatory methods even for educational programs that require that specific, technical knowledge be conveyed. For example, the OSHA Hazard Communication Standard has worker training requirements for using material safety data sheets (MSDSs), forms that contain brief information regarding chemical and physical hazards, health effects, proper handling, storage, and personal protection for a particular substance. Training on MSDSs should cover how to obtain the data sheets, how to interpret them, and their uses and limitations, and give the participants practice in each of these areas. Rather than presenting the MSDS in a lecture-style format, the information can be taught more effectively with a participatory exercise such as the one that follows:

The first part has workers going back into their work areas, finding a labeled chemical container, and seeking an MSDS for that substance. During this part of the exercise, workers become familiar with where MSDSs are located in their particular workplaces and the processes required to find them. It also serves to identify problems in the system that can be corrected, for example, missing MSDSs or locked file cabinets for which no one on that shift had the key.

A second part of the exercise divides the class into small groups who review sample MSDSs and collectively answer questions such as: "Is the substance flammable?" "What are the health effects associated with it?" "Does it require wearing gloves?" and "What ventilation is required?" During the "report-back session," the instructor asks for the answers from all of the groups and reviews how to read and interpret MSDSs in general. A final part of the exercise has participants looking up the chemicals covered in the sample MSDSs in other sources such as the NIOSH *Pocket Guide to Chemical Hazards.* In some situations, more hazards, especially health hazards, are discovered when other sources are consulted. Thus, students learn about the uses and limitations of MSDSs and get practice in using additional sources.

A goal of all health and safety educational programs should be the promotion of hazard recognition and hazard elimination. The use of participatory teaching and learning methods will assist in achieving this goal.

# Bibliography

Clement D. The Hazards of Work: Occupational safety and health training manual. New Market, TN: Highlander Research and Education Center, 1980.

The Labor Institute. Sexual harassment at work: A training workbook for working people. New York: The Labor Institute, 1994.

Massachusetts Coalition for Occupational Safety and Health (MassCOSH) Women's Committee. Occupational safety and health course for working women. Boston: MassCOSH, 1981.

Massachusetts Coalition for Occupational Safety and Health (MassCOSH). English as a second language health and safety curriculum for working people. Boston: MassCOSH, 1993.

*The National Institute of Environmental Health Sciences (NIEHS) established regional training centers to develop materials and training for Hazardous Waste Site Workers. The materials from all regions are available from the National Clearing-house, the George Meany Center for Labor Studies, 10000 New Hampshire Avenue, Silver Spring MD 20903; 301-431-5425. Two examples of educational manuals are:* Hazardous waste site workers basic health and safety course, The New England Consortium, Department of Work Environment. Lowell, MA: University of Massachusetts Lowell, 1990.

Chemical and radioactive hazardous material workbook. New York: Oil, Chemical and Atomic Workers/Labor Institute, 1993.

Wallerstein N, Weinger M. eds. Special issue on empowerment education. Am J Indus Med, 1992; vol 22.

Wallerstein N, Rubenstein H. Teaching about job hazards: A guide for workers and their health providers. Washington, D.C.: American Public Health Association, 1993.

Wallerstein N, Pillar C, Baker R. Labor educator's health and safety manual. Berkeley, CA: Labor Occupational Health Program, Center for Labor Research and Education, Institute of Industrial Relations, University of California, 1981.

that workers spend carefully limited amounts of time in areas with potential exposure. Such measures require good environmental monitoring data in order to develop appropriate schedules, and care must be taken to make certain that the result is not simply to distribute more widely the exposure to substances that can be controlled by engineering approaches. Another preventive administrative measure is a preplacement examination to avoid placing individuals on jobs in which individual risk factors place the worker at higher risk for specific disease(s) or injury from that job. The requirements of the U.S. Americans with Disabilities Act place a special responsibility on those carrying out preplacement examinations (see box in Chap. 11, p. 229).

*Screening and Surveillance. Screening and surveillance for early detection of disease* separately or together may lead to the identification of need for control measures to prevent further hazardous exposure to workers (see Chap. 3). Unlike the methods described above, which are designed to prevent occurrence of occupational disease by *primary* prevention, screening and surveillance activities are part of *secondary prevention*. Both screening and surveillance are directed toward identifying health events or documenting early evidence for adverse health effects that have already occurred. However, both screening and surveillance can lead to primary prevention measures; early detection of disease or abnormality can identify inadequate control measures, allowing them to be corrected so that other workers can be protected.

By recognizing potential or existing work-related disease, health professionals can initiate activities leading to one or more of these methods of prevention. They can play an active role in education by informing workers and employers about potentially hazardous workplace exposures and ways of minimizing them. They can advise appropriate use of respirators or other personal protective equipment. They can also screen workers and

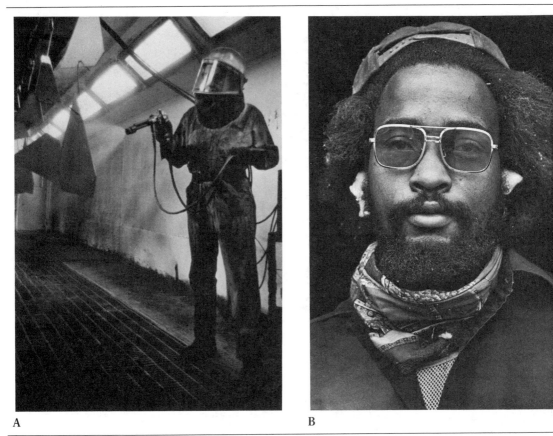

**Fig. 4-3.** A. Spray painter with respiratory protection. B. Makeshift personal protective equipment. Cotton plugs are not effective as personal protective equipment. Only adequately fitting earplugs or earmuffs are effective. (Photographs by Earl Dotter.)

facilitate screening of coworkers who may be at high risk for certain diseases. Consultation with specialists in occupational medicine, occupational hygiene, or occupational safety may be necessary to facilitate these activities.

## Initiating Preventive Action

Once a health professional identifies a probable case of work-related disease or injury, it is crucial to take preventive action while also providing ap-

propriate treatment and rehabilitation services as necessary. Failure to consider the prevention opportunities along with the necessary therapeutic measures may lead to recurrence or worsening of the disease in the affected worker—and the continuation or new occurrence of similar cases among workers in similar jobs, either at the same workplace or at other workplaces. A health professional has at least the following five opportunities for preventive action after identifying a case of work-related disease: advise the patient, contact the patient's union or other labor organization, contact

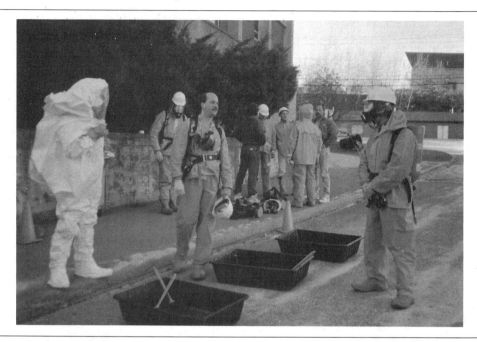

**Fig. 4-4.** Hands-on field training for hazardous waste workers.

the patient's employer, inform the appropriate government authority, and contact an appropriate research or expert group. Often some combination of these possible approaches is undertaken.

*Advise the Patient*

The health professional should always advise the worker concerning the nature and prognosis of his or her condition, and the possibility that there are appropriate engineering controls to remove the relevant hazards; that there may be a need, even if only temporarily, for personal protective equipment at work; or, in extreme circumstances, that there is the necessity to change jobs. The health professional should alert the patient to the need to file a workers' compensation report to protect his or her rights to income replacement as well as medical and rehabilitation services (see Chap. 10). These reports will also trigger the employer to consider listing the health event as a reportable injury or illness and possibly lead the insurance carrier to

provide consultative services to the employer to assess the problem area and consider appropriate control measures.

At times, the health professional may be called upon to provide advice to the patient concerning legal remedies should a health problem result in a contested workers' compensation claim or the need for registering a complaint with an appropriate government agency, as discussed below. It is important to remember that a worker's options may be limited; the worker may not wish to file a claim for workers' compensation or register a complaint with a government agency, fearing job loss or other punitive action. However, it is essential to inform a worker of potential hazards. It is not appropriate to withhold this information because of the possibility of upsetting the patient. A health professional cannot assume that even a large and relatively sophisticated employer will have adequately educated its workers about workplace hazards. (It should be noted that once a patient is informed of the work-relatedness of a disease in writing, this may start the "time clock" on the notification procedures and statute of limitations for workers' compensation; see Chap. 10.)

### Contact the Patient's Union or Other Labor Organization

If it is agreeable to the affected worker, the health professional should inform the appropriate union or other labor organization of the potential health hazards suspected to exist in the workplace. The provision of this information may help to alert other workers to a potential workplace hazard, facilitate investigation of the problem, possibly identify additional similar cases, and eventually facilitate the implementation of any necessary control measures. (Keep in mind, however, that only about 15 percent of workers in the United States belong to a union.)

### Contact the Patient's Employer

The health professional, again only with the patient's consent, may choose to report the problem to the employer. This can be effective in initiating preventive action. Many employers do not have the staff to deal with reported problems adequately, but they can obtain assistance from insurance carriers, government agencies, academic institutions, or private firms in order to gain the necessary assistance to provide a safe workplace. In addition to triggering workplace-based prevention activity, discussions with the employer may lead to obtaining useful information concerning exposures and the possibility of similar cases among other workers. Depending on the circumstance, it can be particularly helpful to the health professional to arrange with an employer to visit a patient's work area. This presents the opportunity to observe firsthand the possible hazardous environment as well as to establish the necessary rapport with managers to involve them in preventive measures.

While the law prohibits employers from firing workers for making complaints to OSHA, it does not prohibit them from firing workers who have a potentially work-related diagnosis. In the U.S., only the federal lead and cotton dust standards *mandate* the removal of workers from jobs that are making them sick. The medical removal protection section of the federal lead standard provides temporary medical removal for workers at risk of health impairment from continued lead exposure, as well as temporary economic protection for workers so removed (see Chaps. 13, 26, 27, 29, 31 for more information on lead). It states, "During the period of removal, the employer must maintain the worker's earnings, seniority and other employment rights and benefits as though the worker had not been removed." The cotton dust standard, however, does not offer such protection.

### Inform the Appropriate Governmental Regulatory Agency

If a case of occupational disease appears to be serious or may be affecting others in the same workplace, it is wise for the worker or the health professional to consider filing a complaint with the appropriate governmental agency. He or she can notify the federal OSHA or the appropriate state occupational safety and health agency. OSHA establishes and enforces standards for hazardous exposures in the workplace and undertakes inspections, both routinely and in response to complaints from workers, physicians, and others (see Chap. 9). In about half of the states in the United States, the program is implemented directly by federal OSHA, which is part of the U.S. Department of Labor; in the other states, a state agency—often the state department of labor—implements the program. Both federal OSHA and the state agency may investigate a workplace in response to a complaint. Most state agencies will make recommendations to improve the situation, but only those states with OSHA-delegated authority can order changes to improve health and safety in the workplace and impose fines if these changes are not made.

LABOR-MANAGEMENT HEALTH
AND SAFETY COMMITTEES

The benefits from seeking the participation of labor unions and workers in the development and implementation of occupational health and safety programs and research can be substantial. As a consequence of the experience and intimate knowledge of the actual work processes, workers and their unions often can add significantly to the understanding of a health or safety problem and determine the best approach to prevention of risks. Their participation also aids in both understanding and explaining the nature and importance of programs and research efforts as well as interpreting the impact and meaning of these to individual workers (Fig. 4-5).

One effective means for including workers and their labor unions in the development and improvement of approaches to prevention is through joint labor-management health and safety committees in the workplace. These committees are groups of representatives of workers and managers that meet periodically to systematically review workplace health and safety hazards and their control, and to respond to specific complaints concerning workplace health and safety. For these committees to function effectively, labor representatives need to be truly representative of workers and not simply appointed by management.

These committees have been legally authorized and are more generally active in some countries, such as Canada, while in the United States they are less common, usually the result of collectively bargained agreements. Proposed OSHA reform legislation in the U.S. would require health and safety committees to be operating in many more workplaces than at present.

Recent studies in Canada, where joint health and safety committees have been mandated, suggest that this particular form of involvement can be unusually effective. Documented reduction in work injuries and resolution of health and safety problems have been shown in the absence of governmental intervention. Effective committees tend to have cochairs and equal representation, readily available training and information, and well-established procedures. An important feature of successful committees is sufficient authority for action either as a committee or on the part of the management representatives.

Typically, labor-management health and safety committees meet on a monthly basis for 1 to 2 hours. They review, evaluate, and respond to worker and manager complaints and concerns about working conditions and workplace hazards. They periodically walk through the workplace to observe and assess working conditions as well as possible health and safety hazards. Also, they often systematically evaluate work practices and procedures as well as materials used in the workplace regarding their impact on workplace health and safety.

As effective as labor-management health and safety committees can be, they are most effective when seen as one component of a more general prevention program that also relies on the development and enforcement of government regulations.

The health professional should always inform the patient in advance of notifying federal or state agencies. Although OSHA and the Mine Safety and Health Administration (MSHA) regulations protect U.S. workers who file health and safety complaints against resultant discrimination by the employer—that is, against loss of job, earnings, or benefits—this protection is difficult to enforce, and workers' fears are not unfounded. Health professionals should familiarize themselves with pertinent laws and regulations. For example, if the worker does not file an "11-C" (antidiscrimination) complaint within 30 days of a discriminatory act, his or her rights are lost. In the U.S., health

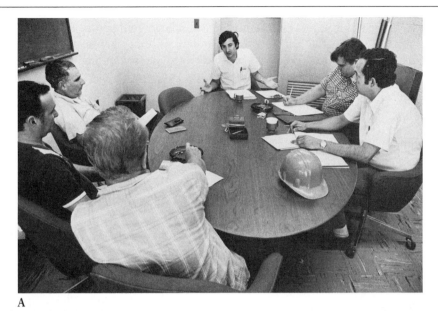

A

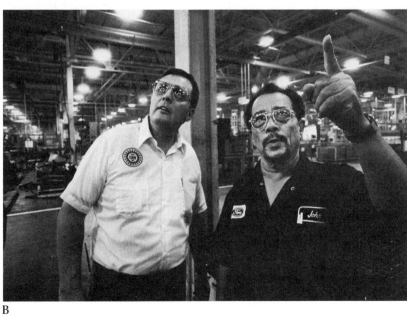

B

**Fig. 4-5.** Joint labor-management health and safety committees are increasingly important in ongoing workplace prevention activity. A. Medical surveillance, screening programs, and a wide variety of other occupational health issues are discussed by committee. B. A worker points out a faulty oil line in a grinder to the union health and safety representative (man in white shirt).

professionals and workers (or their union, if one exists) have the right, guaranteed by the Freedom of Information Act, to obtain the results of an OSHA inspection.

### Contact an Appropriate Research or Expert Group

The health professional may choose to refer the patient for an additional review to an occupational health academic center or to report the identified situation to an agency or other organization conducting research on occupational safety and health such as:

- The National Institute for Occupational Safety and Health, or NIOSH (see Chapter Appendix) especially the hazard evaluation group at NIOSH, which responds to complaints of possibly serious occupational health or safety hazards
- An appropriate state agency, usually within the state departments of labor or public health
- A medical school or school of public health (several of these schools have NIOSH-sponsored occupational health and safety Educational Resource Centers; see Chapter Appendix)
- Some other group with expertise, experience, and interest in research concerning work-related medical problems

Occasionally, the health professional who is reporting a work-related medical problem may undertake or assist in a research investigation of the problem. No matter who conducts the research, identifying additional cases and investigating these cases and the workplace will often lead to new information. Publishing epidemiologic studies or even case reports alerts others to newly discovered hazards and ways of controlling them.

## The Consulting Physician's Role

Most employed persons in the United States work in plants that do not have formal workplace health and safety programs. While there are publications available to guide those employed to provide such programs, there is little guidance to give to health care providers who might have the opportunity to offer components of such programs on a consultant basis or from a community-based practice. Today, an increasing number of physicians are being asked to advise, consult with, or provide a full range of services to an industry or a union on a part-time basis. Initial invitations may be focused on very limited activities, such as preplacement physical examinations, return-to-work evaluations, and reviews of cases in which there have been workers' compensation claims. A physician consulting on a part-time basis to an employer or a union, however, can and should insist on being permitted to undertake preventive measures; in any such relationship, the physician should have the authority to obtain data; to share data with those who need to have this information, including the workers; and to take preventive and corrective action.

The following are reasons that can be introduced to encourage an employer to adopt components of a comprehensive program:

- *Government regulations.* With the incentive of government regulations, small employers need to consider some basic in-plant health and safety program of high priority.
- *Pressure from organized labor.* In workplaces where workers are represented by a union, health and safety concerns are often given higher priority and may be dealt with through collective bargaining. Such programs are most effective when health care providers are involved in efforts for which both the union and the employer have developed common objectives.
- *Enlightened self-interest.* Effective workplace safety and health programs should reduce workers' compensation and medical care costs and increase productivity.

Opportunities should be actively sought to become involved as a consultant to a workplace-based health and safety program. While special knowledge is required for the most comprehensive aspects of such a program, a well-educated health professional should be able to establish the basic components of this program. There are a variety of types of consulting activities that may be requested. However, every effort should be made to provide services not simply as requested, but to follow a prevention-based order of priorities. The following is a recommended priority for program activities:

1. *Programs designed to identify and control both new and old risks.* The identification and control of risks depends on a series of activities designed to build an effective ongoing program. The critical first action should be to undertake a

Advice to employees and employers should be practical.
(Drawing by Nick Thorkelson.)

comprehensive baseline hazard survey documenting major chemical, physical, and biologic hazards along with the important sources of psychosocial, ergonomic, and safety risks. The results of this survey should be organized in terms of priorities for improvement and frequency of follow-up evaluation. The results should be maintained in an easily accessible form, preferably an electronic database system, facilitating review and additions. The baseline survey of risks should be followed by implementation of a hazard-based surveillance program designed to update the status of risks and to document successful reduction in risks that have not previously been appropriately controlled. When possible, objective measurements should be collected and maintained; however, regular observations alone can be an important surveillance tool. Close cooperation with workplace safety managers and with other consultants, if any, is important, particularly when introducing new control strategies. The importance of systematic and periodic evaluation of the effectiveness of controls cannot be overemphasized.

2. *Programs designed to properly match jobs to employees.* A basic principle of occupational health and safety is that jobs should be designed to fit the worker. Unfortunately, too often the reverse has been the case. A consultant should set high priority on the need to evaluate every job and determine how the job design or equipment can be altered or replaced in order to best fit human capacities (see Chaps. 8, 9, 19, and 23). Although cost may be used as an argument against such alterations, the development of a program to implement changes over time as the opportunity permits is essential.

A consultant should carefully examine any limitations listed for job eligibility and determine that these are essential, rather than items of convenience or simply common practice. With the passage of the Americans with Disabilities Act, a much greater effort will likely be placed on designs to fit the worker.

Two circumstances exist where attention should focus on the worker and not the job: (1) *Following return to work after an absence due to illness or injury.* Too often this reentry is either inappropriately accelerated or characterized by an overly cautious approach. The proper middle course can be achieved if careful estimates are made both of the requirements for the job and the temporary or permanent limitations of the returning worker. Directives such as "light work" are too nonspecific and are likely to impede successful reentry to active work, unless they are more specific. (2) *Where there is an appropriately justified job limitation,* such as high-frequency hearing ability or ability to meet high physical demands on short notice. Only when the consultant is convinced that the worker characteristics are essential, should he or she be involved in accepting such limitations on job eligibility and determining that a worker meets the stated conditions.

Health care providers should be asked to play an important role in a comprehensive personal protective equipment (PPE) program concerning issues about fitting and dispensing of any and all types of PPE. While care should be taken to determine that the proper equipment has been selected and is being used appropriately, the question should always be asked regarding why such equipment is required and what alternative engineering solutions can be used or planned.

3. *Programs designed to identify early evidence of work-related health effects while they are still reversible.* Medical monitoring or screening data are designed to identify early evidence of control failures at the workplace. Generally, results are applied to the individual to guard against future damage. However, all such data should also be used in a prevention context. Collection and analysis of data on screening or monitoring results, along with any data on disease or injury morbidity, disability, or mortality of workers, must be routinely compared with information concerning hazards experienced in the workplace along with the nature and levels of exposure to these hazards (see #1, above) in order to seek unrecognized opportunities for intervention and risk reduction.

4. *Programs designed for treatment and rehabilitation of occupational illnesses and injuries.* Generally, workers' compensation regulations of various states in the U.S. require employers to provide treatment and appropriate rehabilitative measures for work-related illnesses and injuries. This requirement may cause employers to seek consulting arrangements with health care providers. Although the determination of work-relatedness may be difficult in some cases, it is important that prompt and appropriate treatment and rehabilitative measures be initiated irrespective of the determination of work-relatedness. Numerous studies have documented the importance of early, effective medical intervention in leading to successful return to work at full capacity. While it may be possible to plan to have treatment services provided at a workplace medical department, many times appropriate arrangements can be made for prompt and efficient care in a nearby physician's office or in a community outpatient medical facility or hospital. Underlying this activity is the principle that the best possible treatment is the most effective and least expensive in the long run.

5. *Programs designed for hazard communication.* All members of a workforce should understand the nature of work risks, the actions taken by the management to control these risks, and the importance of engineering controls as a primary prevention priority. Those unavoidable circumstances in which individual worker responsibility is an important component of control need to be explained in a way that encourages and supports cooperation. The need to use personal protective equipment (when it is the only recourse) or the role of administrative rules (for example, cleaning spills or maintaining clear aisles) should be understood as components of a control program without promoting the idea that workers are to "blame" when failures occur.

Any risk communication effort directed at specific hazard incidents needs to begin by ascertaining what the affected workers perceive to be a health or exposure concern. It should explain also what is generally known about these hazards, what is known about the possibility of risk related to the work setting, what efforts (present and future) are being undertaken to determine whether the risk is work-related, and the nature of the chemical control effort at the location. Experts in risk communication should be consulted in planning and carrying out this effort.

Most health professionals are reluctant to go beyond treating or advising their patients when they suspect work-related medical problems. While it is understandable that they might not want to get involved in legal proceedings or other complex situations that may require siding with either employer or employee, it is really a failure in the responsibility of a health professional if he or she does not go beyond providing treatment of an occupational condition. While only a few health professionals may have gained the medical and medicolegal expertise to provide the full range of needs for patients with work-related medical problems, participating in the active efforts at prevention related to each occupational disease or injury is essential. Since each event is, in principle, preventable, there is an obligation to seek to prevent the next occurrence.

Preventing these problems requires the active participation of almost *all* health professionals, not only those who have a particular interest or expertise in the field. All health professionals should be willing to take appropriate action to ensure that workplace hazards are correctly identified, investigated, and controlled. To do this effectively, health professionals need to develop appropriate methods for advice, consultation, and referral. They also must recognize that persistence—sometimes extraordinary persistence—is necessary to solve complex problems. Nevertheless, there are few other areas of medicine where the health professional has such a vast opportunity to practice prevention and to make such a difference.

## APPENDIX
# Summary of Information Concerning NIOSH

Although the National Institute for Occupational Safety and Health (NIOSH) and the Occupational Safety and Health Administration (OSHA) were both created by the Occupational Safety and Health Act of 1970, they are two distinct agencies with separate responsibilities. OSHA is in the Department of Labor and is responsible for creating and enforcing workplace safety and health regulations. NIOSH, which is part of the Centers for Disease Control and Prevention in the Department of Health and Human Services, is responsible for conducting research, training, and field studies, and making recommendations for the prevention of work-related illnesses and injuries.

The main responsibilities of NIOSH include investigating potentially hazardous working conditions, as requested by employers or employees; evaluating hazards in the workplace, ranging from chemicals and repetitive trauma to machinery and radiation; creating and disseminating methods for preventing disease, injury, and disability; conducting research and providing scientifically valid recommendations for exposure limits to hazardous chemicals, physical agents, and processes; and providing education and training to individuals preparing for careers in the field of occupational safety and health.

NIOSH responds to requests for investigations of workplace hazards through the Health Hazard Evaluation (HHE) program. An HHE is a work-site study designed to evaluate potential workplace health hazards. HHEs can be requested by a management official, a current employee (provided that two other current employees sign the request), or any officer of a labor union representing the employee. If a hazard is detected, NIOSH notifies the workers, the employer, and the Department of Labor and makes recommendations for reduction or removal of the hazard. The HHE program serves as a useful surveillance tool, keeping NIOSH abreast of emerging workplace concerns.

NIOSH conducts a wide range of surveillance activities in order to determine the number of workers exposed to specific hazards and what industries and occupations are at risk (see Chap. 3). Ongoing surveillance allows NIOSH to address the most critical problems in occupational safety and health.

In order to set program objectives, NIOSH has developed a list of the 10 leading categories of work-related diseases and injuries in the U.S. and proposed strategies for prevention in each category. The 10 categories are occupational lung disease, musculoskeletal injuries, occupational cancers, severe traumatic injuries, occupational cardiovascular diseases, disorders of reproduction, neurotoxic disorders, noise-induced hearing loss, dermatologic conditions, and psychological disorders.

Because the nature of work is constantly evolving, NIOSH is examining additional areas of safety and health related to risks associated with work in new work environments and with new technologies. In addition, NIOSH is now prioritizing areas that have received inadequate attention in the past, such as agriculture and construction, indoor environmental quality, occupational infectious disease, and occupational safety and health for minorities and women. At the same time, NIOSH is devoting extra effort to identifying improved approaches to control of such long-standing occupational disease problems as lead poisoning and silica-related diseases.

To disseminate research findings, NIOSH publishes a variety of reports and other materials. NIOSH publications are designed to inform workers, employers, and occupational safety and health professionals of hazards and how to avoid them. Additionally, NIOSH develops documents to forward its scientific recommendations to OSHA and Mine Safety and Health Administration (MSHA) for consideration in the standard-setting processes.

Finally, in order to improve and maintain competence of the occupational safety and health professionals, NIOSH provides a wide variety of training programs, which focus on occupational medicine, occupational nursing, industrial hygiene, and occupational safety.

NIOSH is headquartered in Washington, D.C. with administrative offices in Atlanta, Georgia and with seven working divisions located in Morgantown, West Virginia, and Cincinnati, Ohio. These are:

*Division of Biomedical and Behavioral Science (DBBS).* It conducts research in toxicology, neurologic and behavioral science, and ergonomics. Responsibilities include laboratory and field studies of biomechanical, psychological, neurobehavioral, and physiologic effects of physical, psychological, biomechanical, and selected chemical stressors. It also develops biologic monitoring and diagnostic procedures to improve worker health.

*Division of Physical Sciences and Engineering (DPSE).* It conducts research to develop procedures and equipment for the measurement of occupational safety and health hazards and for the development of effective engineering controls and work practices. It also maintains a quality control reference program for industrial hygiene laboratories.

*Division of Respiratory Disease Studies (DRDS).* It conducts epidemiologic, environmental, clinical, and laboratory research focused on all aspects of occupational respiratory disease. It also has specific responsibilities from the Mine Safety and Health Act (the National Coal Workers X-Ray Surveillance and the National Coal Workers Autopsy Study, certification of x-ray facilities, mine plan approvals, and B-reader examinations).

*Division of Safety Research (DSR).* It conducts research on occupational injury prevention through studies of risk factors and the effectiveness of prevention efforts. It also has responsibility for the federal respirator and coal mine dust personal sampler unit testing and certification program. It conducts research to provide criteria for improving respirators and other personal protective equipment and devices.

*Division of Standards Development and Technology Transfer (DSDTT).* It has responsibility for development of NIOSH policy and recommendations, with special attention to new occupational health and safety standards. It publishes *Current Intelligence Bulletins* to disseminate new scientific information, and *Alerts* to identify opportunities for preventive interventions. It also undertakes quantitative risk assessment efforts to prioritize issues for regulatory attention. It coordinates NIOSH testimony for U.S. Department of Labor hearings, and maintains databases such as NIOSHTIC, RTECS, library services, technical information services, the Institute Archives, and the toll-free telephone number (see Appendix A).

*Division of Surveillance, Hazard Evaluations and Field Studies (DSHEFS).* It has responsibility for surveillance of the extent of hazards and occupational illnesses. It conducts legis-latively mandated health hazard evaluations at the request of employees or employers. It also conducts a broad range of industry-wide epidemiologic and industrial hygiene research programs, with wide responsibility for occupational illnesses not included in DBBS or DRDS. It is also responsible for energy-related health research related to workers at U.S. Department of Energy facilities.

*Division of Training and Manpower Development (DTMD).* It develops programs to increase the numbers and competence of occupational safety and health professionals. Its responsibilities include the development of curriculum programs and courses, the presentation of a broad continuing education program, and the administration of a major training grant program to foster development of academically based training programs.

To further assist professionals and the public, NIOSH provides a *toll-free information system.* To access it telephone 1-800-35-NIOSH or 1-800-356-4674. NIOSH specialists provide technical advice and information on subjects in occupational safety and health.

# 5
# Epidemiology

Ellen A. Eisen and David H. Wegman

All health care providers need to be aware of the importance of epidemiologic concepts in evaluating occupational risks. A woman may ask her gynecologist if the difficulty she and her husband are having in conceiving a child could be due to work exposure to a chemical. A nurse practitioner may be requested to judge the work-relatedness of a bladder cancer in a 60-year-old patient who has worked for 40 years in a textile dye plant. A workplace physician may be required to determine if the use of a chemical recently shown to cause cancer in mice has increased the incidence of lung cancer among production workers. A company occupational hygienist may be asked whether the recent introduction of a new chemical is causing acute respiratory irritation in a small group of exposed employees. The director of a state health department may recommend ongoing disease surveillance for occupational groups exposed to known and suspected toxic materials. Clearly, these judgments require differing levels of epidemiologic expertise, ranging from a familiarity with the literature to the ability to design a health study. The objective of this chapter is to assist occupational health professionals in reading the relevant epidemiologic literature critically and in considering the potential value of the full range of epidemiologic approaches available for the identification and prevention of specific work-related health problems.

The relationship between any group of workers and their work environment is dynamic rather than static, constantly changing over time. For example, workers are hired and others leave the workforce, exposures vary over time because of job transfers or changes in technology or the production process, the workforce ages, and individuals alter personal habits, such as cigarette smoking. The epidemiologist uses analytic tools to examine this complex mix of variables in an attempt to develop new understandings of the effects of workplace exposures on disease, disability, or death. The analytic methods used to examine epidemiologic data have become more sophisticated over the past two decades as the focus of occupational epidemiology has shifted to the detection of early health effects associated with lower-level exposures.

The approaches of clinical medicine and epidemiology work together particularly well in addressing occupational health problems. The clinical approach focuses on the individual and is concerned with diagnosis, treatment, and education of the individual regarding risk factors and preventive behavior. In contrast, the epidemiologic approach focuses on groups and is concerned with identifying subgroups of the population at high risk for particular diseases, providing evidence for new causal associations, estimating dose-response relationships, and determining the effectiveness of exposure control measures. Although these two approaches employ different techniques, they share the same ultimate goal of preventing occupational disease or injury and resulting disability or death.

Several applications of epidemiology are relevant to occupational settings: the surveillance of already recognized occupational disease or injury (see Chap. 3), the systematic study of relations between health effects and known or suspected workplace hazards, and the evaluation of the effectiveness of a control intervention in the reduction of disease or injury. In epidemiology, the health "response" may be a discrete endpoint, such as disease diagnosis, or the measurement of a biologic parameter, such as pulmonary function. The measure of "exposure" may be as crude as membership in an occupational group, such as shipbuilders, or as refined as the average daily time-weighted average exposure to a particular substance.

Much greater emphasis has been placed on the measure of response than on the measure of exposure because traditionally epidemiologists were trained as clinicians and, therefore, were more oriented toward measuring health outcomes. More recently, however, the development of environmental and occupational epidemiology has involved a closer relationship to the environmental and quantitative sciences. Consequently, epidemiologists have begun to collaborate more effectively with toxicologists, ergonomists, environmental scientists, and statisticians to improve the collection of exposure data and to develop more precise methods for estimating exposures that account for uptake, metabolism, and excretion of toxic materials.

## Measuring Exposure

In occupational settings, a distinction should be made between exposure (what we can measure) and dose (what we would like to measure). Dose is the amount of a substance that is delivered to the organs or tissues where the effect is manifested. Although the epidemiologist would like to study the health effects associated with actual dose levels, studies are generally based on exposure as measured in the external environment. Exposure is characterized by intensity (e.g., parts per million) and the duration over which it occurs. Cumulative

exposure is therefore a product of intensity and duration and is an approximation of dose (to an organ or tissue). A review of the possible degrees of refinement for approximating dose should place this aspect of the epidemiologic study in perspective.

### Potential Exposure

The most common measure of exposure in epidemiologic studies is a crude indicator of potential exposure, that is, the history of ever having been employed in a specific industry or specific job. Here, the information is in categorical form, such as presence or absence of employment in a particular industry or job. It is important to realize that the estimate of exposure to a specific causative agent may be greatly diluted by such a surrogate measure. For example, in a study of diesel exposure among railroad workers, only 7 percent of workers were found to be exposed to diesel fumes. The title "railroad worker," therefore, was a very crude measure of exposure since 93 percent of railroad workers would be misclassified as exposed. If, however, the association between exposure and response is very strong, the effect of such dilution is not too damaging. For example, lung cancer has been associated with asbestos in studies in which exposure was no more specific than past employment in a shipyard, where fewer than half of the workers have asbestos exposure [1].

### Quantity of Exposure

Ideally, the measure of exposure would reflect both intensity and duration. Because data on duration of employment may be more easily and accurately determined than intensity of exposure, duration is frequently used as the dose surrogate. Although it may sometimes appear that no data on length of employment are available, indirect data sources can often provide the required information. Pension plan eligibility, for example, may provide at least a dichotomous measure of duration, such as less than or greater than 10 years of employment. Documentation of the actual number of years employed is preferred and frequently is available from payroll records or from union seniority records.

A more refined surrogate for exposure can be created if a complete work history is available for each subject, including documentation of specific jobs, years in those jobs, and potential exposure to specific materials. Information about job-specific potential exposures permits the aggregation of jobs with common exposures [2]. A thorough history would include information on the gaps during time employed, such as time away from work due to prolonged sick leave, periods of layoffs, or military leave.

### Estimates of Exposure Levels

Occupational hygiene measurements of work environments permit an estimation of exposure levels. Variation in exposure occurs as a result of changes in daily work assignments both between days and often within any given day, differences in work habits, seasonal changes in ventilation patterns, and use of personal protective equipment. Current exposure estimates are most relevant for acute effects. Current exposure can only be used to estimate past exposure in environments with well-documented stability in the production process.

### Estimates of Cumulative Historic Exposure

In occupational studies of disease with long induction periods, that is, the so-called chronic diseases, the exposure variable of interest is often the total exposure history. Although this has rarely been measured directly, it is often possible to reconstruct cumulative exposure during past employment. The approach is to estimate job-specific exposures and their variation in level over time. Exposure reconstruction may require compilation of current and historical industrial hygiene data and interviews of plant personnel about the history of process and exposure changes. Information on production rates and exposure control methods over time is also extremely valuable. To compute cumulative exposure, these estimated exposure levels are then weighted by the number of years in successive jobs and summed over all jobs held by each worker. Further refinements are also possible. For example, in studies of respiratory disease in the Vermont granite industry, it was learned that an exhaust ventilation system had been installed throughout the industry in the late 1930s in an effort to eliminate silicosis. However, no occupational hygiene measurements were available before the introduction of these controls. To estimate these early exposures there was an unusual opportunity to reopen an old granite shed and operate it without environmental controls.

The assumptions implicit in the arithmetic computation of cumulative exposure should be noted. First, one year of exposure to 20 fibers/cc of asbestos is treated as equivalent to 10 years of exposure to a tenth of that level (2 fibers/cc). Second, exposure that occurred 20 years ago is assumed equivalent to the exposure last year. More complex weighting schemes are possible but should be based on specific biologic hypotheses about the relative importance of different exposure patterns. For example, suppose one hypothesizes a 10-year latency interval between the initiation of a cancer and its clinical manifestation. One could then "lag" exposure by 10 years so that a subject's cumulative exposure at any point is always accumulated up to 10 years before that point.

### Biologic Monitoring

Evaluation of workers for toxic agents (or their metabolites) in blood, urine, or exhaled air sometimes permits improved estimation of real dose. When a biologic index of exposure exists, its advantage over environmental measurements is that it accounts for exposures from multiple routes, including inhalation, skin absorption, and ingestion. For example, the use of urinary hippuric acid levels is an estimate of the total current dose of toluene to an exposed worker via both lung and skin absorption. Blood lead is another familiar and commonly used biomarker. Many of the available biomarkers, however, measure only active or current levels, not total body burden, and so are most appropriately used in the assessment of health effects associated with current exposures. Unfortunately, no biologic monitoring tests currently exist for a substantial number of hazardous workplace substances. However, biologic monitoring is deservedly receiving much more attention today and useful measures of the body burden of toxic agents can be expected. For example, recent evidence suggests that x-ray fluorescence of bone can effectively estimate total body burden of lead [3].

In summary, there are a wide variety of ways to estimate both current and past exposures. Each has advantages and disadvantages in terms of efficiency and precision. It is important to recognize the range of methods available as well as the assumptions and limitations inherent in each method. An accurate measure of exposure is equally as important as the measurement of health outcome in arriving at an unbiased and precise estimate of an exposure-response relationship.

# Common Measures of Disease Frequency

The significance of a number of individuals with a diagnosed disease or an abnormal test result, in general, cannot be interpreted without knowing the size of the population from which the individuals come. An exception to this rule is the occurrence of a disease that is so rare that detection of even a single case indicates a hazard. Three cases of angiosarcoma diagnosed during a three-year period among a group of workers exposed to vinyl chloride was sufficient to make a plant physician suspect that the chemical was a carcinogen [4]. In contrast, the problem with a simple case count is illustrated by the example of a study of workers in a coated fabrics plant where 68 individuals were found to have a peripheral neuropathy [5]. Even though this endpoint is uncommon in the general population, it is not sufficiently rare that the expected number of case values can be treated as zero. A case count by itself has little or no meaning without a standard of reference, that is, expressing incidence in terms of the size of the population at

risk. There are several different ways to measure disease frequency in an exposed group and to express it in relation to the frequency in a reference (nonexposed) group. Such measures are called rates and relative risks.

## Rates

A rate is the frequency of a disease per unit size of the group (or population) being studied. The simplest quantity, known as point prevalence, is based on the number of cases present at a single point in time.

$$\text{Prevalence rate} = \frac{\substack{\text{number of cases present} \\ \text{at a given time}}}{\substack{\text{total population} \\ \text{at that given time}}}$$

To improve our understanding of the 68 cases of peripheral neuropathy in the coated fabrics plant, we need a denominator. The total plant population was 1,157, which results in a plant prevalence rate of 68/1,157 = 5.9 percent. To determine if it is excessive, this rate can then be compared with the rate in the general population or other appropriate comparison group. A limitation of a prevalence rate, however, is that it counts all cases of the disease, without differentiating between old and new cases.

A rate that removes the previously diagnosed or existing cases and focuses more clearly on new or recent events is the incidence rate, which is based on the number of *new* cases occurring during a specified period of time.

$$\text{Incidence rate} = \frac{\substack{\text{number of new cases} \\ \text{during a specified time period}}}{\substack{\text{total population} \\ \text{at risk during that time period}}}$$

In the coated fabrics plant, of the 68 prevalent cases, 50 had occurred in the past year. Since the onset of 18 cases had occurred before this year, the population at risk of developing a new case was regarded as 1,139 (1,157 − 18). Using these numbers we arrive at the plant-wide annual incidence rate of 50/1,139 = 4.4 percent for the preceding year.

In order to understand whether this incidence rate reflects an underlying hazard, it is necessary to have an estimate of an appropriate comparison rate. One possibility would be the annual incidence rate of peripheral neuropathy in another workplace. Occasionally population data are available from national surveys. In this case, however, it was possible to identify the subpopulation of workers (the print department) that was exposed to a suspect neurotoxic agent. Thus, comparison rates can be estimated *within* the plant population based on subgroups of the workers defined according to exposure status. In this case, 970 employees worked outside the print department. Among them, there were 16 new cases, resulting in an annual incidence rate of 16/970 = 1.6 percent. By contrast, 34 of the 169 employees in the print department had onset of peripheral neuropathy in the past year, an annual incidence rate of 34/169 = 20.0 percent. A difference of more than 10-fold is observed when these two rates are compared.

### Person-Time

When members of the study group are followed for varying lengths of time, in contrast to the pre-vious example in which everyone was observed for one year, the appropriate denominator is person-time, usually expressed in units of person-years. This denominator takes into account not only the number of individuals but also the time period over which they were at risk of developing the disease. It therefore permits the inclusion of individuals newly hired or recently terminated. An example of how to calculate one individual's contri-bution to a person-years denominator is illustrated in Fig. 5-1.

The rates discussed above, calculated without consideration of factors such as age or calendar year, are known as *crude* rates. Crude rates can be misleading. For example, suppose the crude disease rate is high for an exposed group of workers when compared with a nonexposed group. If the exposed group also has a higher proportion of elderly individuals, and disease incidence increases with age, the differences observed in their crude disease rates may only reflect differences in age.

Rates estimated for homogeneous subgroups of the population defined by specific levels of a factor such as age, for example, are called age-specific rates. Sometimes an elevated disease risk will only exist in one subgroup, for example, younger workers. In the first published report of the relationship between lung cancer and exposure to bischloro-methyl ether (BCME), the average age of death for

**Fig. 5-1.** Person-years experienced by a person entering a follow-up at age 23½ in mid-1952 and leaving in mid-1962. (Adapted from RR Monson. Occupational epidemiology, 2nd ed. Boca Raton, FL: CRC Press, 1989.)

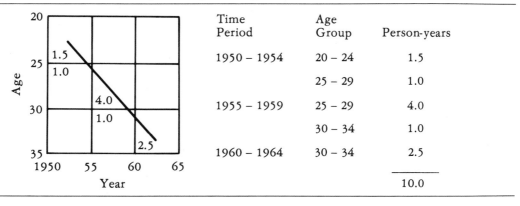

| Time Period | Age Group | Person-years |
|---|---|---|
| 1950 – 1954 | 20 – 24 | 1.5 |
| | 25 – 29 | 1.0 |
| 1955 – 1959 | 25 – 29 | 4.0 |
| | 30 – 34 | 1.0 |
| 1960 – 1964 | 30 – 34 | 2.5 |
| | | ————— |
| | | 10.0 |

**Table 5-1.** Age effect on incidence of myocardial infarction[a]

| Location | Cases | Population at risk | Age-specific incidence rate | |
|---|---|---|---|---|
| FACTORY 1 | | | | |
| Workers < 45 yrs | 4 | 400 | 10.0 | |
| Workers ≥ 45 yrs | 18 | 600 | 30.0 | |
| FACTORY 2 | | | | |
| Workers < 45 yrs | 10 | 800 | 12.5 | |
| Workers ≥ 45 yrs | 10 | 200 | 50.0 | |
| | | | CRUDE INCIDENCE RATE | AGE-ADJUSTED INCIDENCE RATE[b] |
| ALL WORKERS | | | | |
| Factory 1 | 22 | 1,000 | 22.0 | 18.0 |
| Factory 2 | 20 | 1,000 | 20.0 | 27.5 |

[a]The incidence rate is expressed as new myocardial infarctions occurring in a 10-year period of observation per 1,000 population
[a]Based on age distribution summed for Factory 1 and Factory 2

the affected men was 46 years, well below the average for the general population [6]. Risk in this specific age subgroup might not have been detected had only a crude lung cancer rate been calculated.

### Standardization (Adjustment) of Rates

Although specific rates can provide valuable information, it is cumbersome to compare many specific rates, for example, rates in five-year age categories over several decades. For this reason, methods have been developed for estimating a single summary rate, which takes account of differences in the distribution of population characteristics such as age. These rates are known as *adjusted* or *standardized* rates. Two types of adjustment are commonly used: direct and indirect adjustment. These methods can be illustrated with examples of adjustment for age.

*Direct.* The rates of disease in each of the specific age categories in the two (or more) study groups being compared are multiplied by the number of person-years within each age category in a standard population with a fixed distribution of subjects. The resulting total number of cases computed for each of the two groups is then divided

by the total number of subjects in the standard population to form summary rates that are *directly* comparable.

*Indirect.* The age-specific rates of disease in a reference population (typically, the national population) are applied to the number of subjects in each of the age categories of a study group to produce an expected number. This expected number is then compared with the total number observed in each category, summed across all age categories in the study group. The comparison usually takes the form of a standardized ratio of observed/expected outcomes. *Indirectly* standardized rates in two study populations cannot be compared unless the distributions of the categories, such as age groups, are approximately the same in the two study groups.

Table 5-1 provides an example of the use of adjusted rates. For a more detailed description of these types of adjustment, see the appendix at the end of the chapter.

## Comparisons of Rates

Independent of whether rates are presented by homogeneous subgroups or adjusted for appropriate

**Table 5-2.** Derivation of relative and attributable risk

| Disease | Exposure Present | Absent | Total |
|---|---|---|---|
| Present | a | c | a + c |
| Absent | b | d | b + d |
| Total | a + b | c + d | a + b + c + d |

Exposed disease rate = a/(a + b)
Nonexposed disease rate = c/(c + d)
Relative risk = a/(a + b) ÷ c/(c + d)
Attributable risk = a/(a + b) − c/(c + d)

variables in the entire group, the rates must be compared between groups to evaluate the effects of exposure. The two most common comparisons (estimates of risk) are the ratio of rates (relative risk) and the difference between rates (attributable risk).

### Relative Risk

The relative risk, or rate ratio, is designed to communicate the relative importance of an exposure by comparing rates from an exposed population to a nonexposed or normal population. In its simplest form, it is the ratio of two rates (Table 5-2). Referring again to neuropathy in the coated fabrics plant, the relative risk (or *incidence rate ratio*)

is 0.20/0.016 = 12.5. When examining different diseases or the effects of different hazards, relative risks can be compared directly. For example, the relative risk of lung cancer in smokers compared to nonsmokers (Table 5-3) is very large (32.4), whereas that for cardiovascular disease is small (1.4). This suggests that smoking is a more potent lung carcinogen than cardiotoxic agent.

### Attributable Risk

Whereas the relative risk is a measure of the potency of the hazard, the attributable risk measures the magnitude of the disease burden in the population ascribed to the exposure under study. This concept is particularly useful in occupational disease studies because occupational exposures are generally only one of several possible causes of any specific disease. The attributable risk is calculated by subtracting the rate of the particular disease in the nonexposed population from that in the exposed population (see Table 5-2). This risk difference is attributed to the exposure.

In the example of the impact of cigarette smoking on health, Table 5-3 shows that the smoking-attributable risk for lung cancer (2.20) is smaller than the smoking-attributable risk for cardiovascular disease (2.61). The attributable risk takes account of both potency and magnitude of disease in the population. Despite the lower relative risk of

**Table 5-3.** Relative and attributable risks of death from selected causes associated with heavy cigarette smoking by British male physicians, 1951–1961

| Cause of death | Death rate[a] among nonsmokers | Death rate[a] among heavy smokers[b] | Relative risk | Attributable risk[a] |
|---|---|---|---|---|
| Lung cancer | 0.07 | 2.27 | 32.4 | 2.20 |
| Other cancers | 1.91 | 2.59 | 1.4 | 0.68 |
| Chronic bronchitis | 0.05 | 1.06 | 21.2 | 1.01 |
| Cardiovascular disease | 7.32 | 9.93 | 1.4 | 2.61 |
| All causes | 12.06 | 19.67 | 1.6 | 7.61 |

[a]Annual death rates per 1,000.
[b]Heavy smokers are defined as smokers of 25 or more cigarettes per day.
Source: R Doll, AB Hill. Mortality in relation to smoking: Ten years' observations of British doctors. Br Med J 1964; 1:1399.

smoking for cardiovascular disease, the elimination of smoking would produce a larger absolute reduction of cardiovascular disease than for lung cancer.

Relative risks are commonly presented in epidemiologic studies as the measure of association between an exposure and a disease outcome. In contrast, attributable risks are useful in setting priorities for public health interventions or control.

## Types of Epidemiologic Study Designs

Epidemiologic studies can be categorized into three general types: cross-sectional, cohort, and case-control. The cross-sectional design is characterized by the collection of both exposure and health information at one point in time, typically on a study population of current employees. By contrast, cohort studies measure the incidence of disease over time. As in cross-sectional studies, the cohort is defined on the basis of exposure and disease outcomes are compared between subjects with and without exposure. Cohorts are, generally, a complete enumeration of either current employees or past workers. In either case, the cohort is followed through time and the incidence of disease or death is observed. Unlike both the cross-sectional and cohort study designs, the study group in a case-control study is defined on the basis of disease status (Fig. 5-2). In this design, exposures are compared between subjects with and without disease.

### Cross-Sectional Studies

The cross-sectional study is a common approach used in field investigations when an immediate evaluation of a perceived hazard is necessary. In this type of study design, either the frequency of existing (prevalent) disease is compared between

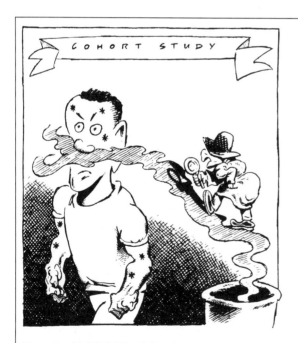
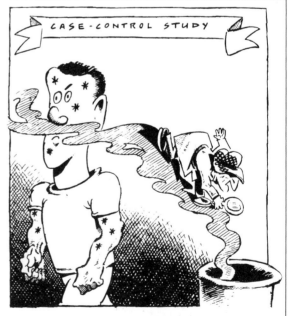

(Drawing by Nick Thorkelson.)

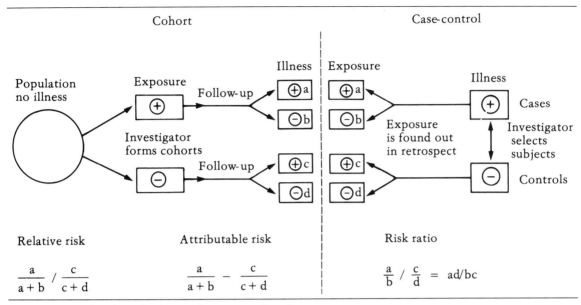

**Fig. 5-2.** General outline of cohort and case-control studies.

groups defined by exposure status, or the prevalence of exposure is compared between disease groups. The exposure categories can be defined as exposed versus nonexposed, or according to an exposure gradient (for example, high, medium, low). Exposure classification can be based on either current exposure or lifetime exposure as estimated by historical records.

*Example (Cross-Sectional Study—Exposure Based)*
A pathology resident died of an acute heart attack at the age of 28. In discussing this incident, a number of other pathology residents noted that they had been experiencing abnormal heart rhythms (palpitations). It was discovered that those with palpitations appeared to have worked with fluorocarbon propellants. This led to a study of all employees in the pathology department (the exposed group) where these propellants were used to prepare frozen sections of pathology tissue and to clean instruments or specimen slides. A radiology department (the nonexposed group) of similar size and distribution of staff and physicians was selected as a nonexposed comparison group. Each

individual was asked about the occurrence of palpitations and the current use of fluorocarbon propellants. Those exposed had twice the prevalence of palpitations of the nonexposed group [7].

*Example (Cross-Sectional Study—Disease Based)*
In the study just described, the investigators wanted to further explore their hypothesis that exposure to fluorocarbon propellants accounted for the elevated risk of palpitations in the pathology department. Accordingly, a follow-up analysis was designed in which groups were defined on the basis of disease. The pathology department staff was divided into those with palpitations (cases) and those without palpitations at the end of follow-up (controls). Among the cases, 40 percent had exposure, while among those without palpitations only 20 percent had exposure, for an odds ratio of 2.7 [7].

### Cohort Studies
Another common type of study in work settings is the retrospective cohort study. In this study design,

a group known to be exposed (either currently or in the past) is identified and followed to disease or death. The experience of mortality or disease incidence observed in the study group is compared to that of a nonexposed reference group.

Some retrospective cohort studies compare mortality (or incidence) in exposed and unexposed cohorts to estimate relative risks. For example, mortality in a cohort of workers exposed to asbestos in textile manufacturing might be compared with that of an unexposed cohort of silk textile workers. When a nonexposed group is not available, which is typically the case, the cause-specific mortality of the exposed cohort can be compared to that of the general population (assumed to be nonexposed). This results in an approximation of a relative risk, known as the standardized mortality ratio or standardized morbidity ratio (SMR). If the number of deaths observed in the exposed cohort is equal to the number expected based on death rates in the standard population, the SMR = 1.0, which indicates neither an excess nor a deficit of risk. If the SMR is greater than 1.0, the data suggest an increased risk in the exposed population.

To compute an SMR, the cause-specific death rates of the general population are applied to the exposed cohort's age distribution, resulting in an indirectly standardized measure (see Chapter appendix). Therefore, SMRs for different exposed cohorts should not be compared unless the age distributions of each are similar.

To conduct an SMR study, the following information must be obtained for each member of the cohort: date of birth, date of entry into cohort, date of leaving cohort, vital status, and cause of death for those who died. With these data, person-years of risk can be determined that take into consideration times when workers entered or left during the study period. This permits a calculation of years at risk, adjusting for different lengths of time since entry into the study. This type of study, however, requires personnel records with accurate employment data. When such data on the total population at risk are lacking, as is often the case, the

mortality experience can be evaluated by proportional mortality analysis.

Cause-specific proportional mortality ratios (PMRs) are calculated as the proportion of all deaths represented by each specific cause of death. These ratios in the study population are compared to the cause-specific ratios from the general population and are adjusted for age, sex, race, and year of death (again, indirect standardization).

In contrast to the SMR, however, an excess or deficit of deaths in causes other than the one under scrutiny can affect the proportional distributions. Therefore, the PMR results are less valid than SMR results. For example, an excess of accidental deaths will lead to a reduced proportion of all other causes. Consequently, when the proportions of other causes of death are compared to the proportions in the general population, deaths from a specific nonaccidental cause may appear to be lower than expected, although they are actually equal or higher. Despite the greater difficulty in interpreting PMR results, they have often provided the first clue that an occupational factor is associated with a specific cause of death.

***Example (Retrospective Cohort Mortality Study, SMR).*** A study of mortality in steelworkers was planned in 1962 [8]. The workers were selected for study if they were employed in 1953 and were followed to the end of 1962 for vital status. Over 59,000 workers were followed and 4,716 deaths recorded. When the number of deaths from specific causes were compared to the number expected, based on deaths in the study country, there appeared to be no excess (SMR for all cancer = 0.92). The study population was large enough, however, to examine a subgroup and to compare the observed deaths to those expected had the mortality experience of the rest of the workers (documented as nonexposed) prevailed.

This in-depth evaluation led to the discovery that lung cancer risk was higher among the coke plant workers and that the excess was much greater for the nonwhite employees. Further analysis showed that the workers employed on the top of coke ovens (the most heavily exposed job assignment) had the highest risk for lung cancer (Table 5-4). The large size of the study population permitted detailed examination of a number of subgroups. As a result, the very high risk of lung cancer in coke oven workers was extracted from the overall "normal" results.

*Example (Retrospective Cohort Mortality Study, PMR).* In 1949 British researchers determined that nickel was an occupational carcinogen. Since this finding was based primarily on case reports, an epidemiologic investigation was undertaken to examine the magnitude and duration of risk. Over 15,000 deaths from the region were grouped according to occupation reported on the death certificates and were examined for the proportional distribution of lung cancer [9]. Occupations were divided into those using nickel, other occupations with suspected cancer risks, and those with no known cancer risks ("all others"). This permitted use of the last category as a locally generated comparison group.

Based on the age distribution of the nickel workers, roughly 10 lung cancers would have been expected if the "all other" occupation proportions applied. However, a total of 48 lung cancer deaths were observed, almost five times the number expected (PMR = 4.86). Three explanations for this finding were considered: (1) the "all other" occu-

pations might have had an unusually low number of lung cancer deaths, (2) the nickel workers might have had an unusually low number of "other causes" of death, or (3) the lung cancer excess could be real. The proportion of lung cancer in the "all other" occupations was very close to that for the country as a whole, which eliminated the likelihood of the first explanation. The second explanation was eliminated because it would have required deaths from all other causes in nickel workers to be one-fifth of the national experience, a highly unlikely event. The conclusion that the lung cancer excess was real still leaves open the question of whether the cause of the excess was likely to be nickel exposure or whether it was due to confounding by cigarette smoking. The association between lung cancer and nickel was accepted as probable and was later corroborated by an SMR study.

*Example (Prospective Cohort Mortality Study).* In 1970 Finnish researchers published the results of a retrospective cohort study that provided the first clear evidence of an association between carbon disulfide exposures and both incidence and death from cardiovascular disease. The investigators continued to follow the study populations prospectively. Five years later results for carbon disulfide–exposed workers showed a 4.7-fold excess mortality for ischemic and other heart diseases compared with a reference cohort of paper mill workers. These disturbing results led to the introduction of a prevention program, which included transfer of symptomatic workers and increased efforts at exposure control.

Continued prospective examination of mortality in these populations documented a striking reduction in cardiovascular disease risk (Fig. 5-3). In the two years immediately following the interventions, the risk of cardiovascular disease mortality decreased to 3.2. Over the course of the next eight years, the rate ratio fell to 1.0, indicating no excess risk relative to the nonexposed comparison group [10].

Table 5-4. Standardized mortality ratios for lung cancer among nonwhite men according to employment in coke ovens for five years or more

| Work area | Observed | Expected | SMR |
|---|---|---|---|
| Side oven | 19 | 9.5 | 200 |
| Part-time topside | 9 | 2.3 | 391 |
| Full-time topside | 23 | 1.9 | 1210 |
| Total coke oven | 51 | 19.0 | 268 |

Source: Adapted from CK Redmond, et. al. Long term mortality study of steelworkers. Department of Health and Human Services (NIOSH) publication no. 81-120, 1981.

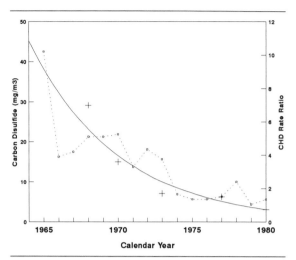

**Fig. 5-3.** Decrease in coronary heart disease (CHD) following decrease in exposure to carbon disulfide among viscose rayon manufacturing workers. Dotted line (····) shows change in exposure levels following introduction of controls in 1965 and in 1972. Solid line (—) shows smoothed curve of change in CHD mortality.

*Example (Retrospective Cohort Morbidity Study).* Reproductive outcomes were of interest in a study of the use of sterilizing agents in a cohort of approximately 1,000 hospital nurses [11]. The objective was to examine the reproductive experience of nurses with respect to sterilizing activities. Questionnaires and medical records were used to collect information retrospectively about both exposure and pregnancy history as far back as 30 years.

The frequency of spontaneous abortion was only slightly higher when comparing total spontaneous abortions among current sterilizing nurses to that for currently nonexposed nurses. A more striking difference was observed, however, when examining results stratified according to whether exposure to sterilizing agents had occurred during a past pregnancy. Among the exposed the rate was 16 percent compared to the nonexposed, whose rate was only 6 percent. Of the three specific sterilizing agents considered, ethylene oxide showed the strongest association with spontaneous abortions.

*Example (Prospective Cohort Morbidity Study).* A study was designed to characterize adverse respiratory effects associated with exposure to toluene diisocyanate (TDI). Since TDI was already known as a cause of asthma, the study was designed to measure other types of acute and chronic respiratory effects. Pulmonary function tests, including forced expiratory volume in the first second of expiration ($FEV_1$), were administered to all workers at a polyurethane foam manufacturing firm on the first shift on a Monday morning. The workers were divided into three exposure groups, and were retested at the end of the workday (a one-day prospective study design).

Generally, $FEV_1$ changes only slightly over the course of a workday. These workers, however, were, on average, losing lung function over the shift, and the amount of loss increased with exposure (Table 5-5). To examine whether this acute response (presumably due to bronchospasm) reflected a more persistent (chronic) effect, those still employed were retested four years later. Annual decline in $FEV_1$ was estimated in the same three exposure groups [12]. Again, an exposure-related response was observed (Table 5-5), with the highest exposed group losing lung function at the greatest annual rate. Cigarette smoking habits did not explain the effects noted in either the one-day or the four-year prospective study.

**Case-Control Studies**

Another common type of epidemiologic study for identifying occupational hazards is the case-control, or case-referent, study. In this study design, the investigator compares the frequency of exposure between groups with and without the disease of interest (see Fig. 5-2). The case-control design is particularly well suited to study diseases that occur with low incidence since a cohort study would have to be prohibitively large to generate enough cases. Furthermore, since the study population in

Table 5-5. Acute and chronic change in FEV₁ by exposure group in polyurethane foam manufacturing workers

|  | FEV$_1$ differences (in ml) | |
| --- | --- | --- |
| Exposure group | Cross-shift change | Annual change |
| Low | −78* | 0.5 |
| Medium | −108 | −33.25 |
| High | −180 | −60.5 |

*Negative change means loss over day or year.
Source: Adapted from DH Wegman, et. al. Accelerated loss of FEV-1 in polyurethane production workers: A four year prospective study. Am J Ind Med 1982; 3:209–15.

a case-control study is defined by disease status rather than exposure status, such studies allow the risks associated with several different exposures to be evaluated within the same study population. (If the study population in a cohort study is defined broadly enough, for example, workers in an automobile manufacturing plant, several different specific exposures may also be assessed within a single cohort. However, the assessment of multiple exposures is not a typical feature of cohort studies.)

There are two types of case-control studies: (1) studies nested within cohort studies and (2) registry-based case-control studies. In nested case-control studies, all cases of the selected disease are identified from the cohort and controls are sampled from among those without the disease. Disease status may be determined at death from a particular disease in a mortality study, or disease incidence based on diagnosis while alive. In registry-based case-control studies, all cases of disease that occur in the registry are identified during a defined time period, and controls can be selected in one of two ways. If the registry is known to include all cases from a defined population (a population-based registry), then controls can be sampled from that same defined population. On the other hand, if the registry is not population-based, such as a registry of cases collected from a single hospital, then patients with other diseases from the same hospital can be used for comparison.

The measure of risk in a case-control study is the *odds ratio*, which differs from the rate ratio

in that it is a ratio of the odds of exposure (exposed : nonexposed) among the cases compared with the odds of exposure among the controls. From Table 5-2, it can be seen that a/b is the odds of exposure among the cases, and c/d is the odds of exposure among the controls. Odds ratios are used as approximations of rate ratios that are obtained in cohort studies. Their interpretations are similar: OR = 1 means no excess or deficit of risk.

A case-control study does not have to include all the cases within a defined population. Valid results may still be obtained in situations in which the case group includes only a sample of all cases. The major requirement for a valid case-control study is that both cases and controls are selected *without* prior knowledge of past exposure history.

*Example (Registry Case-Control Study).* A team of investigators wanted to examine the effect of environmental arsenic exposure on several different disease risks (lung and blood cancers, heart disease, and cirrhosis of the liver) [13]. A parish in Sweden surrounding a copper smelter was selected for study. Deaths from the above causes were classified into four case groups. Controls included deaths from all other well-defined causes. In this study it was assumed that the control group was representative of the general population, and that the cases were a representative sample of all cases. The results for lung cancer are presented in Table 5-6. This study clearly was more feasible than a cohort study would have been.

Table 5-6. Arsenic exposure and lung cancer mortality

| Lung cancer | Arsenic exposure | | Total |
|---|---|---|---|
| | Present | Absent | |
| Cases | 18 | 11 | 29 |
| Controls | 18 | 56 | 74 |
| Total | 36 | 67 | 103 |

$$\text{Relative odds} = \frac{18 \times 56}{18 \times 11} = 5.1$$

Source: Adapted from O Axelson, et. al. Arsenic exposure and mortality, a case referent study from a Swedish copper smelter. Br J Ind Med 1978; 35:8–15.

*Example (Nested Case-Control Study).* A case-control study of larynx cancer was conducted within a cohort of automobile workers exposed to several different types of metal working fluids, commonly referred to as machining fluids [14]. Results were based on 108 cases of larynx cancer, including both incident and deceased cases, and five controls matched to each case. Methods for retrospective exposure assessment were used to calculate lifetime exposures to specific types of machining fluids (straight, soluble, and synthetic), as well as to specific components of the fluids. Risks were then estimated according to the different machining fluid types.

Results suggested that straight mineral oils were associated with almost a two-fold excess in larynx cancer risk. Because extensive data had been collected on these complex mixtures, the investigators were then able to examine specific components of straight machining fluids. Evidence was found of an association with elemental sulfur, commonly added to straight machining fluids to improve the integrity of the materials under extreme pressure and heat. Sulfur was required for high stress applications, which in turn were more likely to produce polyaromatic hydrocarbons (PAHs) during the process. Thus, the importance of the association with sulfur in the machining fluid may be due to an association with exposures to PAHs as well as straight machining fluids.

# Selection of Type of Study

The study designs described in the previous section have relative strengths and weaknesses. The selection of which design to use is based on a variety of factors.

## Cross-Sectional Studies

Cross-sectional cohort studies have several advantages over longitudinal studies. First cross-sectional studies permit the examination of disease morbidity or measures of physiologic function. Second, since the subjects are alive at the time of the study it is often possible to collect information directly on nonoccupational risk factors such as cigarette smoking or diet (potential confounders). Finally, since both disease prevalence and exposure data are collected at one time they generally require less time to complete than cohort or case-control studies.

These studies also have important limitations. They are regarded as less appropriate for investigating causal relationships because they are based on prevalent, rather than incident, cases of disease. A second limitation derives from the fact that they are based on actively employed workers, and do not include employees who have terminated or retired prior to the study. Because, in the presence of an occupational hazard, workers whose health has been affected are more likely to leave that workforce, the absence of those workers may result in an underestimate of the association of interest.

## Longitudinal Cohort Studies

These studies focus on exposure and look ahead to outcome or disease incidence. Thus several outcomes can be studied in the same population. Longitudinal cohort studies can occur completely in the past (retrospective) or in both the past and future (prospective). Data collected on exposure retrospectively are dependent on the quality of past records, in contrast to data collected prospectively according to a specific study plan. If questionnaires or interviews about past exposures are used, selective recall can be a source of bias. Furthermore, since retrospective studies typically rely on outcomes recorded for other purposes, the endpoint is likely to be cause of death or disease diagnosis. Both types of cohort studies have the advantage over cross-sectional studies of including the entire population of interest. Both types of cohort studies suffer from the fact that long-term follow-up is difficult and some subjects will inevitably be "lost to follow-up."

### Case-Control Studies

In contrast to cross-sectional and cohort studies, case-control studies start by identifying disease and seek information about exposures. The case-control design is especially efficient when the disease is rare because a cohort study is unlikely to produce a sufficient number of cases. Case-control studies are also valuable when multiple possible exposures are being explored in the etiology of a specific disease. For example, if the investigator wishes to examine a spectrum of diseases associated with an exposure (for example, lead), a cohort study is desirable, but if the interest is in studying the causes of a specific disease (for example, bladder cancer), then the case-control study is more suitable.

The principal advantage of the case-control study is its relative simplicity and reduced cost. In addition this type of study is well suited to the assessment of several different exposures. On the other hand, these studies are regarded as slightly more susceptible to biases (see below). For example, exposure information may be recalled differently by subjects with and without disease. Moreover, it is necessary to identify a control group that estimates the exposure history of the population that generated the cases.

## Problems Related to Validity

Careful consideration needs to be given to a study's validity, that is, the lack of bias. Bias is defined as a distortion of the measure of association between exposure and health outcome. The degree to which the inferences drawn from a study are warranted is determined largely by the absence of bias. Because epidemiologic studies are observational studies rather than planned experiments, they are prone to biases, some of which are unavoidable. Epidemiologists should provide sufficient information for the reader to understand what potential sources of bias are present and how those biases are addressed. There are three sources of bias: selection bias, misclassification, and confounding.

### Selection Bias

Selection bias results from the inappropriate inclusion or exclusion of subjects in the study population. For example, it was customary in studies of pulmonary function to exclude subjects who did not perform reproducible pulmonary function tests. It was subsequently discovered that subjects who had difficulty performing a reproducible forced expiratory maneuver had compromised respiratory health [15]. Thus the exclusion of such subjects may result in an overestimation of the health status of a working population, and possibly the underestimation of a dose-response association if one exists.

Most types of selection bias, such as excluding short-term workers from the study population, cannot be corrected or controlled for; they can only be prevented. To prevent selection bias in a cohort study, the investigators should be kept unaware ("blinded") of cohort members' outcome status. Similarly, in case-control studies, investigators should be blinded as to the exposure status of those with cases and of controls. Furthermore, selection of subjects should not be influenced by prior knowledge or suspicion of health outcome in a cohort study or of exposure status in a case-control study.

The most common type of selection bias seen in occupational epidemiologic studies is the "healthy worker effect" (HWE). The bias results from employers or workers themselves selecting out of the study groups rather than resulting from an investigator's error or oversight. For example, as described earlier, cross-sectional studies may result in an underestimate of the dose-response association if the occupational exposure produces disease that in turn causes workers to leave the workforce. Another example of HWE, common to cohort mortality studies, occurs because employed people are healthier than the general population, which includes the aged, the chronically ill, and those who are otherwise unfit to gain and maintain employment. The disparity in health between the employed and unemployed is likely to be greatest at the time of hire and gradually to decrease over the period of employment. The HWE has generally been found to be more pronounced among nonwhites.

As a result of the HWE, studies of illness or death among work populations often show lower rates of some chronic diseases (for example, cardiovascular diseases) when compared to the general population. In the steelworkers mortality study described previously, the overall SMR, expected to be 1.00, was only 0.82 for steelworkers when the surrounding county mortality rates were used for a comparison. Unfortunately, appropriate alternative comparison groups of sufficient size are rarely available. When possible, HWE bias is minimized by using a nonexposed comparison group drawn from within the study population. The HWE will be reduced, although not necessarily eliminated, when analyses are based on this sort of "internal" comparison between exposed and nonexposed workers. Even when comparisons are made between workers, job transfers and temporary time off work may result in reduced exposure for workers with slight impairment. Recent progress has been made in developing analytic methods for adjusting for this source of bias. However, studies of worker populations must always be interpreted with this problem in mind.

## Misclassification

Misclassification (information bias) refers to an investigator's inappropriate placement of an individual into a specific category or group. Either disease or exposure can be misclassified. However, for purposes of illustration, we will focus on exposure misclassification because it is more relevant for occupational epidemiology. There are two types of misclassification: nondifferential and differential.

Exposure misclassification that is nondifferential is the random misassignment of exposure that occurs *regardless* of disease status. Nondifferential misclassification is common in occupational studies, where there is often little information on subjects' exposure and subjects cannot be well classified into exposure categories. The net effect is a reduced ability to detect exposure-disease associations when such associations truly exist. The problem is generally worse in retrospective studies where adequate documentation of historical exposures is more difficult. Although many epidemiologists are comforted by the fact that nondifferential misclassification only reduces the apparent difference in disease rates between exposed and nonexposed groups, it is virtually impossible to demonstrate that the observed effect is actually an underestimate of the true effect. Thus, nondifferential misclassification may result in an existing occupational hazard going unrecognized.

Bias of a different sort is presented by misclassification that is "differential," that is, where the likelihood of misassignment of exposure *is* related to disease status. This type of bias can result in either a stronger or a weaker association than *truly* exists. Although differential misclassification is less common in occupational epidemiology, there are situations in which it may be anticipated, such as with biologic monitoring, where greater exposure estimation and health outcome detection occur simultaneously. In cohort studies, differential misclassification is commonly prevented by keeping the investigator "blind" about exposure status when collecting outcome information. In this manner, any errors in collection should be randomly distributed among both exposed and nonexposed groups. In case-control studies, controlling such bias is much more complicated; it is difficult for the investigator, and generally impossible for the subject, to be unaware of the disease status when exposure information is being obtained. Prevention of differential misclassification depends on trying to collect data as objectively as possible.

### Confounding

Confounding is present when two study groups (for example, exposed and nonexposed) are not comparable with respect to a characteristic that is also a risk factor for the disease. For example, in a study comparing stomach cancer in coal and iron miners, chewing tobacco was considered as a potential confounder. Tobacco chewing is more common among coal miners because tobacco smoking is prohibited in a coal mine and, furthermore, it may be an independent risk factor for stomach cancer.

Confounding can be controlled either in the design of the study or in the analysis of the epidemiologic data. In case-control studies, matching study subjects on potential confounders in the design phase can facilitate its control in the analysis. To control confounding in the previous example of stomach cancer, subjects could be matched on tobacco-chewing habits so that the proportion of tobacco chewers is the same among cases and controls.

Stratification is the major approach to the control of confounding in the analysis phase of cross-sectional, cohort, or case-control studies. A confounder, such as age, is used to define strata (for example, 10-year age groups). The independent effect of the primary exposure of interest can be examined in each stratum. Stratification, however, presents problems in that the more potential confounders considered, and the more refined the strata become, the larger the study group necessary to estimate stable measures of risk.

As the number of strata increases, there are likely to be some strata that contain few or no subjects at all. For example, if age, smoking, race, and gender must be controlled for simultaneously, there may be no nonsmoking 40- to 45-year-old white women in the study population. In this case, stratification becomes an inadequate method of controlling confounding, and one must turn to mathematical modeling methods to control confounding statistically.

Multivariate models impose particular mathematical forms on the dose-response relationships, such as a linear or exponential form. By restricting the data to a specific structure, one can interpolate between sparse strata. Mathematical modeling generally involves "smoothing" the data to equalize the distributions of confounders across exposure categories.

## Interpretation of Epidemiologic Studies

The interpretation of epidemiologic studies depends on the strength of the association, the validity of the observed association, and supporting evidence for causality. In studies of discrete health outcomes (for example, cancer), the strength of an association is usually measured by the size of the relative risk estimate for the exposed compared to that for the nonexposed. The magnitude of the difference in physiologic parameters (for example, $FEV_1$) is a measure of the strength of the association in other types of studies. Further evidence of an effect is provided by dose-response relations in which the effect estimate increases over strata defined by increasing exposure. Although spurious risk estimates can occur, it is unlikely they will occur in an exposure-related manner.

Statistical tests of significance and confidence intervals are generally presented along with estimates of the relative risk. Statistical tests, however, do not measure the strength of the association or provide evidence of causality. Statistical tests evaluate only the likelihood that the observed association could have occurred by chance alone, assuming that one expects no effect *a priori*. For example, "probability (p) < 0.05" indicates that the likelihood of observing an effect at least as large as the one observed is less than 5 percent, given that no effect actually exists. Some investigators will not interpret an effect as significant unless p is less than 0.01; others will require only that p be less than 0.10. In any event, the significance level is merely a guide to numerical stability, particularly when the available number of subjects is small, and can be used as supporting evidence for exposure-related associations. Confidence intervals provide more information than "p" values alone because they also indicate a range of plausible effect estimates of risk consistent with the data from the study.

The statistical power of a study to detect a true effect depends on the background prevalence of the disease or exposure, the size of the cohort, the length of follow-up, and the level of statistical significance required. For example, a small cohort followed for a brief time can result in a falsely negative result. For this reason, it is important, when interpreting a negative study, to examine whether the design itself precluded a positive finding. For example, in a recent retrospective cohort study of formaldehyde exposure, despite having 600,000 person-years of observation, the study had only 80 percent power to detect a fourfold risk in nasal cancer mortality [16]. The power was low because nasal cancer has such a low background prevalence that even if the true relative risk were 3.5, the absolute difference in rates would be so small that a much larger study would have been needed

---

## GUIDE FOR EVALUATING EPIDEMIOLOGIC STUDIES

To assist health professionals in reading, understanding, and critically evaluating epidemiologic studies, the following questions (adapted from Monson's *Occupational Epidemiology*) should serve as a useful guide.

### Collection of Data

1. What were the *objectives* of the study? What was the association of interest?
2. What was the primary *outcome* of interest? Was this accurately measured?
3. What was the primary *exposure* of interest? Was this accurately measured?
4. What *type of study* was conducted?
5. What was the *study base*? (process of subject selection, sample size, etc.)
6. *Selection.* Was subject selection based on the outcome or the exposure of interest? Could the selection have differed with respect to other factors of interest? Were these likely to have introduced a substantial bias?
7. *Misclassification.* Was subject assignment to exposure or disease categories accurate? Were possible misassignments equally likely for all groups? Were these likely to have introduced a substantial bias?

8. *Confounding.* What provisions (study design, subject restrictions, etc.) were made to minimize the influence of external factors before the analysis of the data?

### Analysis of the Data

9. What *methods* were used to control for confounding bias?
10. What *measure of association* was reported in the study? Was this appropriate?
11. How was the *stability* of the measure of association reported in the study?

### Interpretation of Data

12. What was the *major result* of the study?
13. How would the interpretation of this result be affected by the previously noted *biases*?
14. How would the interpretation be affected by any nondifferential *misclassification*?
15. To what larger population may the results of this study be *generalized*?
16. Did the *discussion* section adequately address the limitations of the study? Was the final conclusion of the paper a balanced summary of the study findings?

to find the association significant. Formulas for calculating the statistical power associated with a given sample size, as well as the converse, are available in standard biostatistics and epidemiology texts.

When an association appears to be present, the validity of the association still must be evaluated. This can be done in studies that provide sufficient detail on design and results. The internal validity should be evaluated by examining for selection bias, misclassification bias, and particularly confounding. Since all studies will suffer to some degree from problems with validity, a judgment must be made concerning the importance of the biases. Any systematic errors should be evaluated for both the direction and magnitude of their effect.

Finally, the consistency of the association—that is, the repeated demonstration of a particular association in different populations and by different investigators—is valuable supporting evidence of an association. Toxicology data and reasonable consistency with a postulated biologic mechanism may also assist in determining causal associations. It should be recognized that, unlike experimental sciences, epidemiology cannot "replicate" studies. Therefore, circumstances of worker populations and their environments, including confounders, are never identical from one study to the next. This means that findings from several different studies of the same exposure, for example, require both an interpretation within the specific context of each study as well as more generally within the context of the other related research.

# References

1. Blot WJ, et al. Lung cancer after employment in shipyards during World War II. N Engl J Med 1978; 299:620–24.
2. Corn M, Esmen NA. Workplace exposure zones for classification of employee exposures to physical and chemical agents. Am Ind Hyg Assoc J 1979; 40: 47–60.
3. Hu H, Pepper L, Goldman R. Effect of repeated occupational exposure to lead, cessation of exposure, and chelation on levels of lead in bone. 1991; Am J Ind Med 20:723–35.
4. Creech JL, Johnson MN. Angiosarcoma of liver in the manufacture of polyvinyl chloride. J Occup Med 1974; 16:150–51.
5. Billmaier D, et al. Peripheral neuropathy in a coated fabrics plant. J Occup Med 1974; 16:668–71.
6. Figueroa WG, Raszkowski R, Weiss W. Lung cancer in chloromethyl methyl ether workers. N Engl J Med 1973; 288:1096–97.
7. Speizer FE, Wegman DH, Ramirez A. Palpitation rates associated with fluorocarbon exposure in a hospital setting. N Engl J Med 1975; 292:624.
8. Redmond CK, et al. Long term mortality experience of steelworkers. Department of Health and Human Services (NIOSH) publications no. 81–120, 1981.
9. Doll R. Cancer of the lung and nose in nickel workers. Br J Ind Med 1958; 15:217–23.
10. Nurminen M, Hernberg S. Effects of intervention on the cardiovascular mortality of workers exposed to carbon disulfide: 15 years follow up. Br J Ind Med 1985;42:32–35.
11. Hemminki K, et al. Spontaneous abortions in hospital staff engaged in sterilizing instruments with chemical agents. Br Med J 1982; 285:1461–63.
12. Wegman DH, et al. Accelerated loss of FEV-1 in polyurethane production workers: A four year prospective study. Am J Ind Med 1982; 3:209–15.
13. Axelson O, et al. Arsenic exposure and mortality, a case referent study from a Swedish copper smelter. Br J Ind Med 1978; 35:8–15.
14. Eisen EA, et al. Mortality studies of machining fluid exposure in the automobile industry III: A case-control study of larynx cancer. Am J Ind Med 1994; 26(2).
15. Eisen EA, Robins JM, Greaves IA, Wegman DH. Selection effects of repeatability criteria applied to lung spirometry. Am J Epidemiol 1984; 120:734–42.
16. Blair A, et al. Mortality among industrial workers exposed to formaldehyde. J Natl Cancer Institute 1986; 76:1071–84.

# Bibliography

Ahlbom A, Norell S. Introduction to modern epidemiology. 2nd ed. Chestnut Hill, MA: Epidemiology Resources, 1990.
Beaglehole R, Bonita R, Kjellström. Basic epidemiology. Geneva: World Health Organization, 1993.
*Two introductory texts on the core ideas underlying epidemiologic research are useful starting points for*

*more advanced reading. The second book is available worldwide (through WHO) and a teacher's guide can be obtained for use with the text.*

Checkoway H, Pearce NE, Crawford-Brown DJ. Research methods in occupational epidemiology. New York: Oxford University Press, 1989.

*Very readable full text on epidemiologic approaches specific to occupational studies. Numerous examples are provided to guide the reader in understanding both the simple and complex issues that need to be addressed.*

Colton T. Statistics in medicine. Boston: Little, Brown, 1974.

*Basic statistics text written in a reasonable fashion with a functional index. Good general reference for statistics.*

Hernberg S. Introduction to occupational epidemiology. Chelsea, MI: Lewis, 1992.

*An excellent introductory text that is well written and illustrated. Aimed at the reader who is new to occupational epidemiology although somewhat familiar with principles of epidemiology.*

Kleinbaum DG, Kupper LL, Morgenstern H. Epidemiologic research: principles and quantitative methods. Belmont CA: Lifetime Learning Publications, 1982.

*The basic text in epidemiology that provides principles of epidemiology in substantial detail as well as the quantitative basis for the research methods. Particularly useful as a reference.*

Monson RR. Occupational epidemiology. 2nd ed. Boca Raton, FL: CRC Press, 1989.

*A systematic review of methods as applied specifically to occupational settings. A practical textbook for those doing occupational studies.*

Olsen J, Merletti R, Snashall D, Vuylsteek K. Searching for causes of work-related diseases: An introduction to epidemiology at the work site. Oxford: Oxford Medical Publications, 1991.

*A practical introduction to epidemiology for health professionals with no formal training in the discipline. It is written to assist professionals to better plan and carry out investigation of worksite health problems.*

Rothman KJ. Modern epidemiology. Boston: Little, Brown, 1986.

*Probably the best general text on epidemiologic methods designed both for the novice and the expert. Organized in a way that makes it useful to read through or to use as a general reference.*

Steenland K. Case studies in occupational epidemiology. New York: Oxford University Press, 1993.

*Provides the reader the opportunity to explore further many of the questions discussed in the chapter by practical and detailed presentation of case studies of different types of epidemiologic studies.*

# Adjustment of Rates

For the purposes of illustration, adjusting for the differences in age will be examined in detail. Table 5-1 presents a hypothetical problem involving the myocardial infarction (MI) experience in two viscose rayon factories. To compare the incidence of MI in Factory 1 and Factory 2, a summary rate is calculated in each factory. If crude rates are calculated, it would appear that workers in Factory 2 have a slightly greater risk. A comparison of these rates, however, ignores the rather striking difference in age distribution of the populations in the two factories. These can be taken into account by adjusting for the differences by either the direct method or the indirect method.

## Direct Adjustment

The principle of direct adjustment is to apply the age-specific rates determined in the study groups to a set of common age weights, such as a standard age distribution. The selection of the standard is somewhat arbitrary but often is chosen as the sum of the specific age groups for the two or more study groups. Thus, in Table 5-1, the standard population would be: less than 45 years = 1,200, 45 years or older = 800. The specific rates are applied to this set of weights and then added to create an adjusted rate.

$$\text{Factory 1} = \frac{0.010 \times 1,200 + 0.030 \times 800}{2,000}$$

$$= \frac{12 + 24}{2,000} = 0.018$$

$$\text{Factory 2} = \frac{0.0125 \times 1,200 + 0.050 \times 800}{2,000}$$

$$= \frac{15 + 40}{2,000} = 0.0275$$

Not only is the magnitude of the MI rate affected by the adjustment procedure, but also the rank order is reversed. Note that if another age distribution had been selected as the standard (for example, $<45 = 1,500$, $\geq45 = 500$), the standardized rates would change and the rate for Factory 1 would become 0.015 while that for Factory 2 would become 0.022. Thus, the magnitude of the two adjusted rates has no inherent meaning. However, they can be compared, and although the size of the ratio will change slightly it will be closely duplicated regardless of the weights; in these two examples of weighting, the ratios of the adjusted rates are 1.53 and 1.47.

## Indirect Adjustment

In indirect adjustment standard rates are applied to the observed weights or the distribution of specific characteristics (for example, age, sex, or race) in the study populations. This provides a value for the number of cases (events) that would be expected if the standard rates were operating. These expected cases can be compared to those actually observed for each study group in the form of a ratio. In Table 5-1, assume a national standard rate for MI of 1/1,000 (0.001) for those under 45 and 2/1,000 (0.002) for those 45 years or older. The expected cases in the two factories would be

Factory 1 $= 0.001 \times 400 + 0.002 \times 600$
$$= 0.4 + 1.2 = 1.6$$

Factory 2 $= 0.001 \times 800 + 0.002 \times 200$
$$= 0.8 + 0.4 = 1.2$$

These expected values are, in turn, compared to the observed values to calculate a standardized morbidity ratio.

$$\text{Factory 1 } SMR = \frac{22}{1.6} = 13.8$$

$$\text{Factory 2 } SMR = \frac{20}{1.2} = 16.7$$

It is tempting to compare the two SMRs and calculate a ratio similar to that calculated for the directly standardized rates. However, this is one of the drawbacks of indirect standardization. Since the age distributions and age-specific rates are significantly different for the two factories, the resulting comparison of the two SMRs would not distinguish differences due to disease incidence rate from differences due to a different age distribution.

It is reasonable then to ask why indirectly standardized rates are used. One reason is that often only one population is being studied, so comparison to the general population experience is convenient and possibly the only reasonable comparison available. Probably of greater importance is the instability of observed rates. In the example presented here, if five rather than two age groups were used and it was also necessary to adjust for both race and sex, then the total number of subdivisions necessary would be $5 \times 2 \times 2 = 20$. With a maximum of 22 cases in either factory, several of the subdivisions would contain no cases and therefore have no reliable rate estimate. Even in the illustration provided, one case more in Factor 1 workers under 45 years of age would have changed the age-specific incidence rate to 12.5, and one case less, to 7.5, a very large relative difference.

# 6
# Occupational Hygiene

Thomas J. Smith and Thomas Schneider

Occupational hygiene is the environmental science of anticipating, recognizing, evaluating, and controlling health hazards in the working environment with the objectives of protecting workers' health and well-being and safeguarding the community at large. It encompasses the study of chronic and acute conditions emanating from hazards posed by physical agents, chemical agents, biologic agents, and stress in the occupational environment, as well as concern for the outdoor environment. As an example, an occupational hygienist would be asked to determine the composition and concentrations of air contaminants in a workplace where there have been complaints of eye, nose, and throat irritation. The hygienist in this situation would also determine if the contaminant exposures exceeded the permissible exposure limits required by the Occupational Safety and Health Administration (OSHA) or other national limits. If the problem was the result of airborne materials (a conclusion that might be reached in consultation with a physician or epidemiologist), then the hygienist would be responsible for selecting the techniques used to reduce or eliminate the exposure such as installing exhaust ventilation around the source of the air contaminants and isolating it from the general work area, and follow-up sampling to verify that the controls were effective. Most occupational hygienists have earned either a bachelor's degree in science or engineering or a master of science degree in industrial hygiene. Occupational hygienists tend to specialize in specific technical areas because the scope of the field has so greatly expanded.

Occupational hygienists must work with physicians to develop comprehensive occupational health programs and with epidemiologists to perform research on health effects. It has been traditional to separate occupational hygiene and safety, but the trend has been to broaden the training for each to include the other. This has led to the specialty of risk management for evaluating and controlling all types of hazards in the workplace. At present occupational hygienists generally do not deal with mechanical hazards or job activities that can cause physical injuries; these are the responsibility of the safety specialists (see Chap. 7). However, it is not uncommon for private companies to have a single individual responsible for both occupational hygiene and safety who has no formal training in either area.

Most occupational hygienists work for large companies or governmental agencies. A small but growing number work for labor unions. For whomever they work, occupational hygienists unfortunately are often located in organizational units where they have little organizational power to force necessary changes. Hygienists who work for labor unions may be restricted in their access to the workplace for sampling and exposure measurements, which can limit their ability to assess and control hazards.

The closeness of working relationships between occupational hygienists and occupational physicians varies. Some have close collaborative activities with extensive exchange of information, while others operate with nearly complete independence and have little more than formal contact. A physician who is familiar with the workplace, job activities, and health status of workers in all parts of the process may be very helpful in guiding the occupational hygienist in assessing environmental hazards and vice versa. Within a framework of multidisciplinary approaches, occupational hygienists and physicians should collaborate with safety specialists, production units, personnel departments, worker representatives, and delegates of the health and safety committees. Where contact among these groups is minimal, many opportunities are lost for improving the effectiveness of health hazard control and the prevention of adverse effects.

## Anticipation, Recognition, Evaluation, and Control of Hazards

Anticipation of hazards has become an important responsibility of the occupational hygienist. *Anticipation* refers to the application of and mastery of knowledge that permits the occupational hygienist to foresee the potential for disease and injury. The occupational hygienist should thus be involved at an early stage in planning of technology, process development, and workplace design.

An electronics company was developing a new process for making microcomputer chips. The process involved dissolving a photographic masking agent in toluene and then spraying the mask on a large surface covered with chips. The company's hygienist noted that this would expose the workers to potentially high airborne levels of toluene. She suggested they substitute xylene, which has a lower vapor pressure, and modify the process to use smaller amounts of solvent, which would reduce the amount of hazardous waste generated by the process. It is common that process engineers or industrial researchers will propose using hazardous materials or will not consider the interaction of the worker and the process or machine. Consequently, hygienists can prevent many problems that will be expensive to fix after installation by reviewing early plans and findings of pilot plant experiments.

An overview of the production process may be most easily obtained by describing the complete flow from raw material to final product. Production can be subdivided into its component unit processes. In this stepwise fashion the processes with hazards can be recognized, the worker exposures evaluated, and the exposures in nearby areas assessed. Examples of some common unit processes and their hazards are given in Table 6-1. This general approach, and the hazards of a wide range of common industrial processes, are discussed in more detail in Burgess' *Recognition of Health Hazards in Industry: A Review of Materials and Processes* (see Bibliography).

The approach can be illustrated by considering a small company that manufactures tool boxes from sheets of steel by a six-step process: (1) Sheets of steel are cut into the specified shape; (2) sharp edges and burrs are removed by grinding; (3) sheets are formed into boxes with a sheet metal bender; (4) box joints are spot welded; (5) boxes are cleaned in a vapor degreaser in preparation for painting; and (6) boxes are painted in a spray booth. Production steps 2, 4, 5, and 6 use unit processes with known sources of airborne emissions; their hazards are given in Table 6-1 and should be evaluated. It may also be necessary to evaluate the exposures of workers involved with steps 1 and 3 because they may be located near enough to the operations with hazards to have significant exposure.

The design of job tasks and an individual's work habits can both have an important influence on exposures. For example, a furnace tender's exposure to metal fumes will depend on the length of tools used to scrape slag away from the tapping hole in the furnace and on the instructions for performing the task. Lack of adequate tools or sufficient operating instructions may cause excessive exposure to fumes emitted by molten materials. Similarly, the furnace tender who is positioned close to the slag as it runs out of the furnace may receive a much higher exposure to fume than a co-worker who stands farther away from the slag.

**Table 6-1.** Common unit processes and associated hazards by route of entry*

| Unit process | Route of entry and hazard |
|---|---|
| Abrasive blasting (surface treatment with high-velocity sand, steel shot, pecan shells, glass, aluminum oxide, etc.) | Inhalation: silica, metal, and paint dust<br>Noise |
| Acid/alkali treatments (dipping metal parts in open baths to remove oxides, grease, oil, and dirt) | |
| Acid pickling (with HCl, $HNO_3$, $H_2SO_4$, $H_2CrO_4$, $HNO_3$/HF | Inhalation: acid mist with dissolved metals<br>Skin contact: burns and corrosion, HF toxicity |
| Acid bright dips (with $HNO_3$/$H_2SO_4$) | Inhalation: $NO_2$, acid mists |
| Molten caustic descaling | Inhalation: smoke and vapors |
| Bath (high temperature) | Skin contact: burns |
| Blending and mixing (powders and/or liquid are mixed to form products, undergo reactions, etc.) | Inhalation: dusts and mists of toxic materials<br>Skin contact: toxic materials |
| Cleaning (application of cleansers, solvents, and strong detergents to clean surfaces and articles; and operation of devices to aid cleaning, such as floor washers, waxers, polishers, and vacuums) | Inhalation: dust, vapors<br>Skin contact: defatting agents, solvents, strong bases |
| Crushing and sizing (mechanically reducing the particle size of solids and sorting larger from smaller with screens or cyclones | Inhalation: dusts and mists of toxic materials<br>Noise |
| Degreasing (removing grease, oil, and dirt from metal and plastic with solvents and cleaners) | |
| Cold solvent washing (clean parts with ketones, cellosolves, and aliphatic, aromatic, and stoddard solvents) | Inhalation: vapors<br>Skin contact: dermatitis and absorption<br>Fire and explosion (if flammable)<br>Metabolic: carbon monoxide formed from methylene chloride |
| Vapor degreasers (with trichloroethylene, methyl chloroform, ethylene dichloride, and certain fluorocarbon compounds) | Inhalation: vapors; thermal degradation may form phosgene, hydrogen chloride, and chlorine gases<br>Skin contact: dermatitis and absorption |
| Electroplating (coating metals, plastics, and rubber with thin layers of metals) | Inhalation: acid mists, HCN, alkali mists, chromium, nickel, cadmium mists<br>Skin contact: acids, alkalis<br>Ingestion: cyanide compounds |
| Copper, chromium, cadmium, gold, silver | |
| Forging (deforming hot or cold metal by presses or hammering) | Inhalation: hydrocarbons in smokes (hot processes), including polyaromatic hydrocarbons, $SO_2$, CO, $NO_x$, and other metals sprayed on dies (e.g., lead and molybdenum)<br>Heat stress<br>Noise |

(continued)

127

**Table 6-1.** (continued)

| Unit process | Route of entry and hazard |
|---|---|
| Furnace operations<br>(melting and refining metals; boilers for steam generation) | Inhalation: metal fumes, combustion gases, for example, $SO_2$ and CO<br>Noise from burners<br>Heat stress<br>Infrared radiation, cataracts in eyes |
| Grinding, polishing, and buffing<br>(an abrasive is used to remove or shape metal or other material) | Inhalation: toxic dusts from both metals and abrasives<br>Vibration from hand tools<br>Noise |
| Industrial radiography<br>(x-ray or gamma ray sources used to examine parts of equipment) | Radiation exposure |
| Machining<br>(metals, plastics, or wood are worked or shaped with lathes, drills, planers, or milling machines) | Inhalation: airborne particles, cutting oil mists, toxic metals, nitrosamines formed in some water-based cutting oils, endotoxin<br>Skin contact: cutting oils, solvents, sharp chips<br>Noise |
| Materials handling and storage<br>(conveyors, forklift trucks are used to move materials to/from storage) | Inhalation: CO, exhaust particulate, dusts from conveyors, emissions from spills or broken containers |
| Mining<br>(drilling, blasting, mucking to remove loose material, and material transport) | Inhalation: silica dust, $NO_2$ from blasting, gases from the mine<br>Vibration stress<br>Heat stress<br>Noise |
| Painting and spraying<br>(applications of liquids to surfaces, for example, paints, pesticides, coatings) | Inhalation: solvents as mists and vapors, toxic materials<br>Skin contact: solvents, toxic materials |
| Repair and maintenance<br>(servicing malfunctioning equipment; cleaning production equipment and control systems) | Inhalation: dust, vapors, and gases from the operation<br>Skin contact: grease, oil, solvents |
| Quality control<br>(collection of production samples, performance of test procedures that produce emissions) | Inhalation: dusts, vapors, and gases<br>Skin contact: solvents |
| Soldering<br>(joining metals with molten lead or silver alloys) | Inhalation: lead or cadmium particulate (*fumes*) and flux fumes |
| Welding and metal cutting<br>(joining or cutting metals by heating them to molten or semi-molten state)<br>Arc or resistance welding<br>Flame cutting and welding<br>Brazing | Inhalation: metal fumes, toxic gases and materials, flux particulate, etc.<br>Noise: from burner<br>Eye and skin damage from infrared and ultraviolet radiation |

*The health hazards may also depend on the toxicity and physical form(s) (gas, liquid, solid, powder, etc.) of the materials used. For further information see WA Burgess. Recognition of health hazards in industry: A review of materials and processes. (2nd ed.) New York: Wiley, 1994.

Therefore, an important part of an evaluation is the observation of work practices used in hazardous unit processes.

*Recognition* of problems in a new or unfamiliar workplace generally requires that the occupational hygienist engage in the following activities:

Collection of background information on production layout, processes, and raw materials.

Visits to the workplace to become familiar with the production processes and their hazards. Their visits are crucial for detecting unique aspects of the workplace that may strongly affect exposures. Information is collected on

- Type, composition, and quantities of substances and materials, including raw materials, intermediate products, and additives
- Design of work processes and tasks
- Emission sources
- Design and capacity of ventilation systems or other control measures. Flow visualization with smoke tubes can give information on effectiveness of local exhausts or process ventilation

Recording of work practices, worker position relative to sources, and task duration. Cleaning routines and performance, and tidiness, are important determinants of exposure.

If this initial appraisal cannot for certain rule out a hazard, a basic survey has to be made to provide quantitative information about exposure of workers. Particular account has to be taken of tasks with high exposure. Sources of information are: earlier measurements, measurements from comparable installations or work processes, reliable calibrations or modeling based on relevant quantitative data, and air sampling to determine range of exposures. Sampling, which may show that sensory impressions under- or overestimate exposures; for example, the odor threshold for most solvents is well below the level at which they present a toxic exposure hazard. If this information is insufficient to enable valid comparisons to be made with the limit values, a full-scale survey has to be undertaken. The full-scale survey will examine all phases of workplace activities—both normal activities and abnormal or infrequent ones, such as maintenance, reactor cleaning, or simulation of malfunctions. The survey activities may take several weeks or months in a complex manufacturing or chemical plant.

Farm workers were experiencing episodes of depressed blood cholinesterase levels from organophosphate exposure despite the fact that they were observing the required waiting times before re-entry into sprayed fields and wearing long-sleeved shirts and gloves to prevent skin contact. The pesticide had a very low vapor pressure so there was no significant inhalation exposure. However, it was known that environmental moisture decomposes this type of pesticide. Since the weather was very dry during these episodes there was concern that the pesticide was not decomposing as rapidly as expected. Consequently, despite the skin protection, there could still be sufficient skin absorption of the pesticide to affect cholinesterase levels. Skin sampling with patches showed that fine dust was sifting through the cloth of the shirt sleeves and depositing pesticide on the workers' arms in substantial quantities. The problem was solved by extending the standard re-entry times.

The *evaluation* of recognized or suspected hazards by the hygienist uses techniques based on the nature of the hazards, emission sources, and routes of environmental contact with the worker. For example, *air sampling* can show the concentration of toxic particulates, gases, and vapors that workers may inhale; *skin wipes* can be used to measure the degree of skin contact with toxic materials that may penetrate the skin; biological samples (blood or urine) can provide data where there are multiple routes of entry; and *noise dosimeters* record and electronically integrate workplace noise levels to determine total daily exposure. Both acute and chronic exposures should be considered in the evaluation because they may be associated with different types of adverse health effects. The workplace is not a static environment: Exposures may change by orders of magnitude over short distances from exposure sources, such as welding, and over short time intervals because of intermittent source output or incomplete mixing of air contaminants. It is also common that operations and materials used or produced may change, as do job titles and definitions. The nature of these changes and their possible effects must be recognized and taken into consideration by the occupational hygienist.

In the 1940s a company that produced cadmium pigment and other products decided to operate a long-term monitoring program for cadmium exposures because of their concern about the chronic effects of cadmium. This program was very thoughtfully designed around existing sampling and analysis methodologies. They collected routine fixed location air sampling with chemical analysis of cadmium in the dust. All of the work areas where cadmium dust might be present were sampled at the same locations on a regular schedule so that the time profile of exposure could be determined. Later, when more sophisticated methods for personal sampling were developed, they used both methods for several years so that the relationship between the personal exposures in each area could be correlated with the fixed location data. As a result, it was possible to develop a clear picture of the inhalation exposures of the workers and to estimate their personal doses of cadmium over a substantial period of time. These chronic exposure estimates were critical for studies of exposure-response relationships for pulmonary and renal effects of the cadmium exposures. The point is to structure all monitoring programs (long-term and acute problems) with a clear focus on the individual's sources of exposures and the ultimate objective to estimate dose. Monitoring organized completely around compliance with today's standards will probably be unable to answer tomorrow's questions about hazards associated with personal exposures.

The effects of environmental controls such as ventilation and personal protective equipment that intervene between the emission source and the worker must also be considered.

The hygienist's decision on whether a hazard is present is based on three sources of information: (1) scientific literature and various exposure limit guides such as the threshold limit values (TLVs) of the American Conference of Governmental Industrial Hygienists[1] (ACGIH), a set of consensus standards developed by occupational hygienists, toxicologists, and physicians from governmental agencies and academic institutions, or the World Health Organization (WHO) recommendation[2]; (2) the legal requirements of OSHA (in some cases these are less stringent than the TLVs because the TLVs have been updated) or legal requirements of other countries; and (3) interactions with other health professionals who have examined the exposed workers and evaluated their health status. In cases in which health effects are present but exposures do not exceed the TLVs, WHO recommendations, or OSHA or other national requirements, the prudent hygienist will assume a relationship if it is consistent with the facts. Exposure limits of either type are designed to prevent adverse effects in most exposed workers but are not absolute levels below which effects could not occur. The supporting data for many of these exposure limits are sometimes viewed as insufficient, out-of-date, or based too much on evidence of toxic effects and not enough on recent evidence of carcinogenicity, mutagenicity, or teratogenicity.

Once a hazard is identified and the extent of the problem evaluated, the hygienist's next step is to design a control strategy or plan to reduce exposure to an acceptable level. Such controls may include (1) changing the industrial process or the materials used to eliminate the source of the hazard, for example, changing to clean technologies; (2) isolating the source and installing engineering controls such as ventilation systems; and (3) using administrative directives to limit the amount of exposure a worker receives, or, as a final resort, re-

---

[1]Can be obtained from ACGIH, 6500 Glenway Avenue, Bldg. D-5, Cincinnati, OH 45211.
[2]Can be obtained from WHO, CH-1211, Geneva 22, Switzerland.

quiring the use of personal protective equipment. The approaches in (3) are less reliable because they depend on enforcement by management and conscientious application by the workers, both of which can fail. Usually the control strategy will include a combination of these approaches, particularly where there may be delays in installing engineering controls. In designing control strategies, account should also be taken of the environmental impact (for example, emissions, waste, accidents, storage, spills, leaks). Action can be taken at the process, materials, component, systems, and strategic level. Education of both workers and supervisors is an important part of any control strategy; both must understand the nature of the hazards and support the efforts taken to control or eliminate them. Implementation of control measures should be supervised and their efficiency evaluated.

Automobile manufacturers have been very concerned about the hazards of coolants used on machining and grinding operations. Workers complain of skin and inhalation problems associated with exposure to liquids splashed on their skin and mists in the air. In the recent past controls were installed based on hypotheses about the causal factors, but without an investigation of the specific causes for exposures. As is often the case, some hypotheses were later found to be incorrect and it was determined that incomplete control had been achieved despite substantial expenditures. It was shown that inhalation exposures had been only partially controlled by local exhaust ventilation and enclosure of processes, but a relationship was still found between symptoms and reduced pulmonary function associated with exposures at levels below the current allowable exposure. Analysis of the coolants also revealed that material safety data sheets (MSDSs) were inaccurate and more hazardous materials were being used than were known to the machining department. Investigations are now being planned to determine what engineering controls will be needed to further reduce the exposures. Substitution of alternate types of coolant components and better control of microbial contaminants are part of the planned investigations. This example points out that controlling hazards in large, complex manufacturing operations is

very frequently a stepwise process and that control strategies are most effective when based on complete knowledge of the nature of problems.

After hazards are controlled, the hygienist may recommend a routine hazard surveillance program to ensure that controls remain adequate. This type of surveillance is most effective when done in close association with a medical surveillance program designed to detect subtle effects that may occur at low levels of exposure.

The following sections indicate how assessment and control techniques are utilized. The approach for toxic materials is used as a paradigm, which can be employed for other environmental hazards: noise, vibration, ionizing and nonionizing radiation, heat, cold, poor lighting, and infectious agents.

### Exposure Pathways

The hazard of a given exposure to a toxic material depends on the toxicity of the substance and on the duration and intensity of contact with the substance. Thus, adverse effects can result from chronic low-level exposure to a substance or from a short-term exposure to a dangerously high concentration of it. However, the pharmacologic mechanisms by which effects are caused differ for acute and chronic effects. Occupational hygienists are concerned with both long-term, low-level exposures and brief acute exposures and strive to characterize both.

In assessing a given hazardous material, the hygienist determines the route of exposure by which workers contact it and by which it may enter their bodies. There are four major routes of exposure: (1) direct contact with skin or eyes, (2) inhalation with deposition in the respiratory tract, (3) inhalation with deposition in the upper respiratory tract and subsequent transport to the throat and ingestion, and (4) direct ingestion of contaminated food or drink. In the workplace, several concurrent routes of exposure may occur for a single toxic substance.

Inhalation of airborne particulates, vapors, or gases is by far the most common route of exposure and therefore occupies much of a hygienist's efforts at assessment and control. Skin absorption may be important if the substance is lipid soluble or the skin's barrier is damaged or otherwise compromised. Ingestion of contaminated food and drink is a problem, especially for particulate and liquid materials, whose degree of risk may depend on the worker's level of awareness of the hazard and personal hygiene habits and on the availability of adequate facilities for washing and eating at the workplace. Contamination of cigarettes with toxic materials and their subsequent inhalation is also a problem for some substances. For example, workers handling lead ingots are exposed to a low-level hazard from small amounts of lead by eating contaminated food or by inhaling small amounts of lead fumes from contaminated cigarettes. However, workers refining lead at temperatures above 800°F are exposed to a serious hazard from inhaling large amounts of lead fume if they work close to unventilated refining kettles for several hours a day. Workers handling liquid nitric acid are exposed to the hazard of direct contact with the liquid on their skin, but they may also be exposed to a respiratory hazard from inhaling acid mist generated by an electroplating process using the nitric acid. In these examples the toxic materials cause different types and magnitudes of hazards because their physical forms vary: solid material versus small-diameter airborne particulates, and liquid material versus airborne droplets.

*Anticipation and Recognition.* The first problem the hygienist faces in evaluating an unfamiliar workplace for toxic hazards is the identification of toxic materials. In many cases, such as a lead smelter or pesticide manufacturing process, the emission sources for toxic materials are clearly evident. Even in these examples, however, some hazards may not be evident without a careful examination of an inventory of the chemicals to be used or in use in the facility, including raw materials, by-products, products, wastes, solvents, cleaners,

and special-use materials. Lead smelter workers are also exposed to carbon monoxide and sometimes to arsenic and cadmium; pesticide workers are subject to solvent exposures. Relatively nontoxic chemicals may be contaminated with highly toxic ones; for example, low-toxicity chlorinated hydrocarbons used in weed killers (2,4-T) may contain dioxin, which is highly toxic, and technical-grade toluene may contain significant amounts of highly toxic benzene. In some cases, toxic materials may not be hazards because there are no emissions into the work areas and only small amounts are handled, such as in a chemical laboratory.

Material safety data sheets, which list the composition of commercial products, are available from manufacturers and can be useful, but they are sometimes too general or out-of-date. Toxicity data on specific substances can be obtained by literature searches—either manually or by computer—or by searches of databases for toxic materials (see Appendix A).

As noted earlier, exposure to toxic substances can also occur by contamination of food, drink, or cigarettes. Therefore, the hygienist determines if facilities for eating and drinking are physically separated from the work area, if facilities for washing are close to eating areas, and if sufficient time is permitted workers to use both of these facilities. Protective clothing and facilities for showering after a work shift should also be provided. Workers' understanding of hazards from toxic materials they are using must also be assessed. Finally, the hygienist determines the existence and enforcement of rules prohibiting eating, drinking, and smoking in areas with toxic substances.

*Measurement Techniques.* Two types of environmental sampling techniques are available.

*Direct reading instruments* have sensors that detect the instantaneous air concentration and may produce a reading on a dial or store a complete eight-hour time profile in a small datalogger for later retrieval. Some are expensive and all require careful calibration and maintenance to obtain accurate data. The detector tube is another type of direct reading instrument of considerable use in determining approximate concentrations of air contaminants. This simple device uses a small hand pump to draw air through a bed of reagent in a glass tube that changes color or develops a length of stain that is proportional to the concentration of a given gaseous air contaminant. The conventional tube is suitable for short-term sampling, but tubes are available that are capable of measuring time-weighted average exposure levels. This is an advantage since a few short-term samples can misrepresent long-term average exposures. Tubes are available that have been manufactured under strict quality control and their uncertainty is specified. Consideration must always be given to interference from other substances (cross-sensitivity), which usually is specified on the data sheets.

*Sample collectors* that remove substances from the air for analysis in a laboratory may be a less expensive alternative to direct reading instruments. *Personal sampling is* a common approach used by the occupational hygienist to obtain accurate and precise measurements of workers' exposures to particulate and gaseous air contaminants; the worker wears the sampler like a radiation dosimeter. Particulate contaminants are collected with filters, and gases and vapors are collected by solid adsorbents or liquid bubblers. The sampling apparatus is generally quite simple, consisting of a small air pump usually worn on a worker's belt, connected by tubing to the collector, and attached to the worker's lapel. (Some gas and vapor collectors are passive—they use diffusion instead of an air pump to move the contaminant into the sampler.) With the appropriate selection of a gas or particulate collector or both combined in a sampling train, it is possible to measure the average concentration of an air contaminant in the worker's breathing zone during an eight-hour work shift.

Collection devices for toxic particulates may capture either total dust—that is, all particle sizes that can enter the collector—or only the respirable dust—that is, only particles that can penetrate the terminal airways and alveolar spaces (less than 5 micrometers [$\mu$]). Total particulate samples are collected if the toxic substance causes systemic health problems, as lead and pesticides do. Respirable dust samples are collected if the particulate causes chronic pulmonary disease such as pneumoconiosis. There is some controversy about the size of particles that cause chronic bronchitis and, therefore, which type of sample to collect. However, the type of sampler should be matched to the route of entry, type of effect, and target tissue (Fig. 6-1).

Charcoal and other sorbent packed into tubes have been the most common adsorption collectors for gases and vapors; a small amount of charcoal inside a small glass tube acts as an activated surface that will retain nonpolar materials such as benzene. These collectors are commonly used to measure inhalation exposures to solvents such as vapor exposures of printers. Collectors such as impingers or bubblers will collect gases and vapors into liquid from air drawn through them. Bubblers are less convenient to use than charcoal tubes but may be required for some compounds such as sulfur dioxide. New adsorbent types and use of chemosorption (for example, in impregnated filters) has greatly extended the range of substances that can be sampled and these have largely replaced the use of bubblers to collect reactive gases. The specific methods are discussed in detail in the OSHA *Analytical Methods Manual* (see Bibliography).

The passive or badge-type samplers are much more convenient to use for gas and vapor sampling than the collectors that require air pumps, and they have better worker acceptance because many workers do not like the weight of the pumps. After the sampling period is completed, the cover is replaced on the badge and it is sent to a laboratory for analysis. They are convenient and relatively inexpensive. Several passive samplers have well-documented sampling rates. They may surpass active samplers in accuracy, if contamination from liquid splashes during use can be avoided.

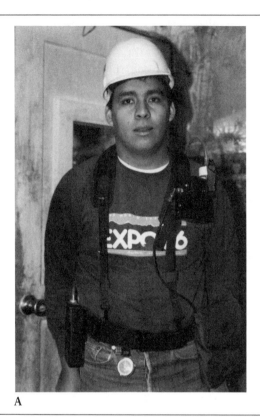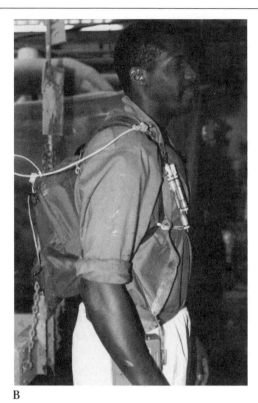

A                                        B

**Fig. 6-1.** Monitoring equipment can be used to collect samples to measure personal exposures on the job. A. Particulate sampler (*arrow*) is connected to portable pump located on worker's right hip. Here more sophisticated sampling is being accomplished by adding a real-time direct reading aerosol sampler and logging device (black box on chest and package on left hip). B. Vapor sampling tubes on worker's chest usually collect a time-weighted sample to measure chemical exposure. Here a direct reading aerosol measurement system has been added (in the backpack) to permit collection of real time data in a logging device. (Photograph by Susan Woskie.)

*Sampling Strategy.* The hygienist must design a sampling strategy that takes into account the types of hazards, variations in exposure, and routes of exposure and the uses for the data, for example, risk assessment or source of control and evaluation. The approach should enable most efficient use of resources. The use of personal measurement in the strategy is designed to reflect the accumulation of exposure from a variety of sources that a worker may encounter in the course of a work shift. In some cases exposure may only occur dur-

ing certain operations. When it is clear that high emissions from certain activities/sources will occur and it is decided that sampling will only be done during the period of highest exposure, this approach is called worst-case sampling. It is frequently found that workers in adjacent areas, not directly involved with the air contaminant of interest, may also have significant exposures because the air contaminant drifts into their work areas.

Variability in exposure levels can be large due to day-to-day variation in work pattern, production rate, and differences in the process. Differences in personal work habits, and wind velocity and direction, also cause variation. The exposed populations should be subdivided into smaller, well-defined groups of workers performing identical or similar tasks. Properly selected subgroups reduce within-group variability, which has the advantage that resources can be concentrated on the highest exposed groups, although these may be difficult to identify a priori. Single samples are generally avoided wherever possible because it is difficult to know whether the sample value is representative. Additionally, because workers have different work habits and techniques, there may be differences in average exposures among workers [1]. Several replicate samples on workers may indicate how important these differences are and how much the assumption of uniform mean exposure within groups is violated.

In addition to personal sampling, the occupational hygienist also uses fixed location sampling in the sampling strategy. In this approach the sampler is set at a given location that has some useful relationship to a source of exposure. This type of sampling is advantageous because it can allow determination of features of the exposure that would be difficult with personal samples. For example, a large sampler can be used to determine the particle size distribution of airborne dust in a work area or to collect a large quantity of airborne material for detailed chemical analysis if the composition of the contaminants is not known. These samplers can be very useful for identifying and characterizing sources of exposure and assessing the effectiveness of engineering controls. As with personal sampling, to get the most out of the effort, it is very important to select carefully the sampling location and strategy for fixed location sampling. In some cases a combination of personal and fixed location samples is used to describe a given problem completely; for example, personal samples are used to describe the highly variable exposures of steelworkers tending a blast furnace while stationary samples measure exposures to the uniform,

well-mixed air levels they experience while waiting in the lunchroom for their next job assignment (2 to 4 hours per work shift). In some cases, such as cotton dust exposures, only fixed location sampling techniques are available.

In general, the principal applications of fixed location sampling are to identify and characterize sources within a work area and to evaluate the effectiveness of emission control systems such as local exhaust ventilation. Many large plants use continuous multipoint sampling of gases and vapors with central analysis. Instant action can be taken if concentrations go out of control, that is, exceed specified limits. Continuous monitoring at stationary sites should be part of the total quality management process.

In some occupational settings the most important route of exposure is skin contact. Skin contact is difficult to evaluate with environmental sampling because even if the amount of skin contamination can be determined, it is not possible to know how much of the contaminant has already penetrated into the body or would penetrate given sufficient time. Two principal sampling approaches are employed. First, cloth patches can be used to cover given locations of skin, such as the forehead, back of the neck, back of the hands, and forearms, to measure the amount of contamination per unit area that resulted during a period of exposure. The second approach is to use wipe sampling, in which an area of skin is washed with an appropriate, nontoxic solvent to determine the quantity of contamination. Both of these techniques have been used to estimate pesticide exposures of agricultural workers. Addition of a fluorescent whitening agent to the pesticide as a tracer allows visualization of contamination. Additionally, wipe sampling on surfaces can be used as a method to detect and control the indiscriminate distribution of toxic materials throughout the workplace environment with which workers may come in contact. This type of sampling is also useful in estimating the risk of one person relative to another or of one area relative to another. It is, however, difficult to know in absolute terms the quantity of contaminant that may actually penetrate the skin and become a health problem. Biologic monitoring is probably the best method for determining the intensity of skin exposures to a substance for which such a monitoring test is available (see Chaps. 3 and 13).

Some nonpolar substances such as pesticides and solvents may enter the body both via the respiratory tract and through skin contact. In these cases both skin contact and air exposure must be evaluated to completely assess the risk. Biologic sampling that integrates these two routes of intake may be a practical necessity. However, two important theoretical problems are associated with biologic monitoring. Some types of tests may represent detection of adverse effects, such as monitoring red blood cell cholinesterase in pesticide-exposed workers. As a result they detect excessive exposures only after the effects have occurred. Tissue levels of environmental contaminants represent a dynamic interaction because the exposure is rarely constant. As a result, there is a complex relationship between exposures and levels of compounds and metabolites in blood, urine, exhaled breath, and other biologic media. This relationship is controlled by toxicokinetics of the particular agents [2]. Consequently, proper interpretation of findings from biologic monitoring for a given worker requires some knowledge of the temporal variations in the worker's exposure. In many situations, biologic monitoring should only be used to verify that exposures have been controlled. Its use in detecting high exposures should be limited (for example, when absorption is primarily through the skin).

It is almost never possible to evaluate ingestion as a route of exposure with sampling. Occasionally, samples of food and drink may be collected to assess the level of contamination; however, this sort of exposure is likely to be extremely variable and episodic in nature, so that environmental sampling is usually an ineffective way of assessing exposure. Again, biologic monitoring is the method of choice to monitor this route of exposure.

*Controls.* SUBSTITUTION. Substances and materials that pose health risks or impair health and safety should not be used if they can be substituted. Substitution is part of the toxics use reduction and waste management concept. Potential benefits to health and safety have to be balanced against technological and economic consequences. This balance should include product properties, production process, environment, and reliability of supply, since substitution is the method of choice, whenever possible. For example, less-toxic toluene may be an adequate replacement for benzene. Regular auditing of use of substances and materials provides inspiration for substitution and keeps the substitution process active.

LIMITATION OF RELEASE AND OF BUILDUP OF CONTAMINATION. If substitution is not possible, then the next step is to attempt to control or limit releases and prevent the buildup of toxic materials in the worker's environment. Local exhaust ventilation combined with source isolation will control process emissions. General room ventilation is used to prevent the buildup of hazardous concentrations in the work area from contaminants escaping local exhaust, fugitive emissions (from seals, valves, pumps), spills, and so forth. An example of these two ventilation approaches is shown in Fig. 6-2.

Local exhaust systems surround the point of emission with a partial or complete enclosure and attempt to capture and remove the emissions before they are released into the worker's breathing zone. Figures 6-3 through 6-5 show several examples of local ventilation systems; a wide variety of types are available with differing degrees of effectiveness. Unfortunately, it is not possible before installation to determine precisely the effectiveness of a particular system, although this is an area of active research. As a result it is important to measure exposures and evaluate how much control has been achieved after a system is installed. Unless contaminant sources are totally enclosed, collection will only capture a percentage of the total emission. Release of smoke from smoke tubes at

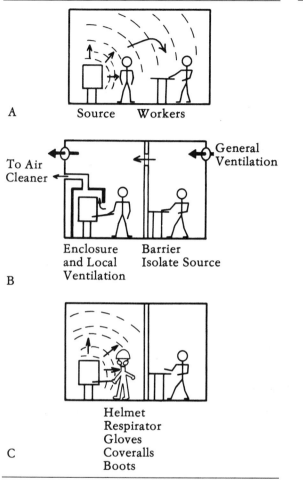

A    Source    Workers

To Air Cleaner ←

General Ventilation

Enclosure and Local Ventilation

Barrier Isolate Source

B

Helmet
Respirator
Gloves
Coveralls
Boots

C

**Fig. 6-2.** Examples of controls for airborne exposures. A. Workers with primary and secondary exposure to source emissions. B. Ventilation and source isolation to control exposures. C. Personal protection and source isolation to control exposures. (From Harvard Occupational Health Program.)

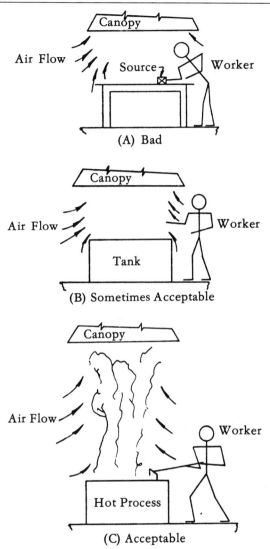

Canopy

Air Flow    Source    Worker

(A) Bad

Canopy

Air Flow    Worker

Tank

(B) Sometimes Acceptable

Canopy

Air Flow    Worker

Hot Process

(C) Acceptable

**Fig. 6-3.** The proper use of a canopy hood, which will not draw the air contaminants through the worker's breathing zone. The worker's location is crucial. (From National Institute for Occupational Safety and Health. *The Industrial Environment—Its Evaluation and Control.* Washington, D.C.: NIOSH, 1973, p. 599.)

the point of contaminant generation is a useful technique for visualizing the flow of air toward the exhaust. It may reveal if the distance to the exhaust is too large, if there are cross-drafts or strong air disturbances, or if the worker creates wakes, all of which greatly reduce the collection efficiency. A good system may collect 80 to 99 percent, but a

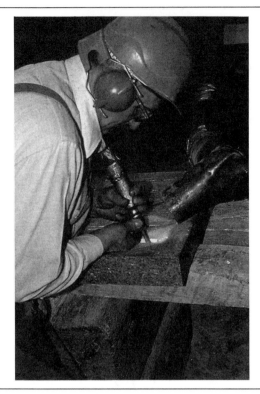

Fig. 6-4. Local exhaust ventilation successfully captures dust produced by stone cutting. (From Harvard Occupational Health Program.)

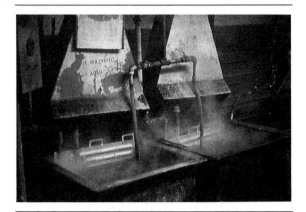

Fig. 6-5. Electroplating protected by local slot exhaust ventilation. (From Harvard Occupational Health Program.)

poor system may capture only 50 percent or less. Careful maintenance must be performed on the system to maintain efficiency. Poor maintenance is probably most responsible for system failures.

The increasing cost of energy has made the practice of ventilating work areas with outside fresh air an increasingly expensive process. Considerable effort is being directed to the design of systems that can recirculate decontaminated air or use heat exchangers so the heat value is not lost.

LIMITATION OF CONTACT. The third important approach to controlling exposures to toxic materials is to limit worker contact either by automation, by isolating processes using toxic materials from the remainder of the work area so that the potential for contact with these materials is limited (Fig. 6-6), or by furnishing workers with personal protective equipment such as dust or gas masks (respirators) or hoods or suits with externally supplied air for controlling inhalation of toxic materials (Fig. 6-7). Many people mistakenly think that the use of respirators is a simple and inexpensive way to control exposure to toxic airborne materials. However, there is discomfort in wearing these masks, poor worker acceptance, and variable levels of protection achieved. There are extensive OSHA requirements for an adequate respirator program to ensure that the quality of the devices is maintained and that workers are receiving adequate protection. It should be noted that the cost of a good respirator program for lead dust exposures is reported to be $1,000 per worker per year or more. The fitting of respirators is an extremely important aspect that is commonly neglected; a poorly fitting respirator provides substantially less protection than expected because, even if the filters are highly efficient, air leaks around the edges of the face mask.

The use of rubber gloves and protective clothing does not automatically ensure that workers are

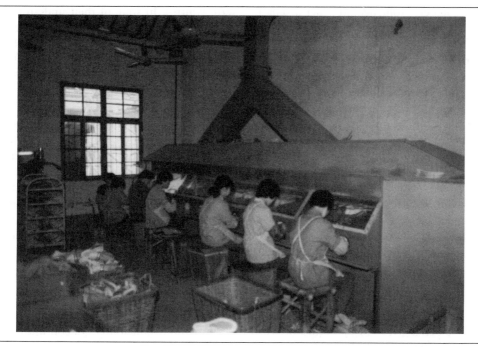

**Fig. 6-6.** A glovebox enclosure system prevents solvent exposure to workers gluing shoes. (Photograph by Barry Levy.)

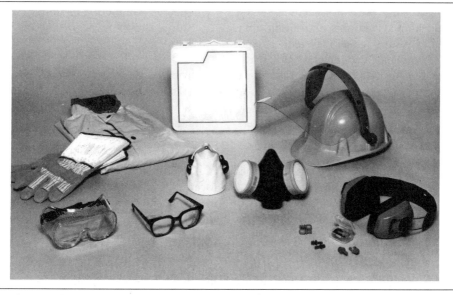

**Fig. 6-7.** Several types of personal protective equipment. (Courtesy of James Schaepe, M.D.)

protected adequately. Toluene and other aromatic solvents readily penetrate rubber gloves; thus, glove composition must be matched to the chemical nature of the substance. Similarly, long-sleeved shirts or coveralls may not prevent skin contact with toxic dusts because small dust particles can sift through the openings between threads in woven cloth. A study of orchard workers showed the effects of pesticide exposures even though they had been wearing dust masks to prevent inhalation of the dust and long-sleeved shirts to prevent skin exposure. Special testing indicated that, despite wearing the shirts, their arms were covered with dust that contained pesticide. Tests with fluorescent dusts showed similar findings, which indicated that even impermeable protective suits are difficult to seal to prevent migration of dust past cuffs and the neck opening.

An important part of limiting contact with hazardous substances is the requirement that protective clothing be changed each day and not worn outside the work area. This effort is also facilitated by the requirement for showers after the work shift.

Some reduction in exposure can be obtained by administrative controls such as schedules where workers spend limited amounts of time in areas with potential exposure, which may reduce exposure below recommended guidelines. While this approach may be effective in certain situations, it requires good exposure data to demonstrate its effectiveness and the careful attention of supervisory personnel, may be an inefficient use of workers, and may be inappropriate for controlling exposures to carcinogens.

Ideally, all the control approaches described should be used together to develop an overall control strategy that will deal with all aspects of toxic material exposure in a particular workplace. Short-term measures such as extensive use of personal protective equipment may be adopted immediately after a problem is recognized to allow time for developing engineering controls or process modifications that will provide more long-

term control. In spite of their undesirable aspects (OSHA's previous policy was to use them only as a last resort), respirators may be the only effective control device for some exposures such as those faced by maintenance or cleanup workers.

### Noise Problems

Occupational exposure to excessive noise is an important problem that is evaluated and controlled in part by occupational hygienists (see also Chap. 16). Hygienists are trained to measure the intensity and quality of noise, assess its potential for producing damage, and devise means to control noise exposures. Two principal types of workplace noise have somewhat different techniques of evaluation and control:

Continuous noise is produced by high-velocity air flow in compressors, fans, gas burners, and motors. Crushing, drilling, and grinding are important sources of continuous noise because a large amount of energy is used in a small space.

Impact noise results from sharp or explosive inputs of energy into some object or process, such as hammering or pounding on metal or stone, dropping heavy objects, or materials handling.

During the evaluation of a workplace, a hygienist looks for sources of excessive noise, determines which workers are exposed, and then selects an evaluation strategy to clarify the nature and extent of the exposures. If the noise is continuous or almost continuous, a hand-held noise survey meter is used to determine the noise levels at the worker's location. If the exposure involves impact noises, an electronic instrument that records and averages the high-intensity but short-duration pulses is used to characterize the source and exposures.

Typically, workers spend variable amounts of time exposed to noise sources, and they may work at different distances from the sources, which will alter their exposures. Exposures may also vary because the output of noise sources may change over time. Therefore, the average (time-weighted) exposure may not be easy to estimate, even though the sources may present clear potential for overexposure. This problem has been solved by the use of small noise dosimeters worn by the workers that electronically record sound levels and indicate average noise levels during the work shifts. Dosimeters are very useful for describing average exposures. Some dosimeters store eight-hour time traces in a datalogger, which can be displayed and linked to records of worker activities. A typical noise evaluation will include both source noise level and dosimeter measurements.

National requirements and TLV guidelines are used by the hygienist to evaluate noise data and decide if a hazard is present. In addition to the hazard to hearing, noise also affects verbal communication, which may create a hazard by interfering with warnings and worker detection of safety hazards such as moving equipment. The current OSHA standard for continuous noise for eight hours is 90 dBA.[3] Higher levels are permitted for shorter periods of time [3]. The OSHA standard allows levels of noise exposure that will protect some but not all workers from the adverse effects of workplace noise. The TLV for an eight-hour exposure to noise (1993) is 85 dBA, which is significantly lower than the 90-dBA OSHA standard for (continuous) noise.

Although techniques exist to obtain an overall time-weighted average of noise exposures received in several different work settings, no techniques exist for assessing the hearing risks of combined exposure to both continuous and impulse noise. Workers exposed to both continuous and impulse noise are numerous; they include brass foundry workers who are exposed to continuous noise from gas burners and to impulse noise from brass ingots dropping into a metal bin from a conveyor.

The strategies for controlling noise are similar to those used for toxic material control:

*Substitution.* Use another process or piece of equipment; electrically heated pots for melting metal can be used instead of gas-heated pots to eliminate burner noise.

*Prevent or reduce release of noise.* Modify the source to reduce its output, enclose and soundproof the operation, or install mufflers or baffles; noisy air compressors can be fitted with mufflers and placed in soundproofed rooms to control their noise; impact-absorbing materials can be installed to eliminate impulse noise from ingots dropping into a metal bin.

*Prevent excessive worker contact.* Provide personal protective equipment such as earplugs or earmuffs, or provide a control booth.

As with toxic materials, the overall strategy to control exposures usually involves separate approaches for various aspects of the problem. It may be necessary to consult an acoustical engineer with advanced evaluation and engineering expertise for dealing with complex noise problems. If engineering controls are not completely effective or are impractical, ear protectors may be required; however, the effectiveness of these devices is limited because sound may also reach the ear by bone conduction. A full shift exposure above 120 dBA cannot be controlled adequately using earplugs or muffs (see Chap. 16).

### Radiation Problems

Radiation hazards are commonly first identified by occupational hygienists, but the responsibility for their evaluation and control overlaps among the occupational hygienist, the health physicist, and the radiation protection officer (see Chaps. 15 and 17).

Exposure to ionizing radiation can be external (from x-ray machines or radioactive materials) or internal (from radioactive substances in the body).

---

[3]dBA means decibels on the "A" scale, which is related to the human ear's response to sound.

External exposures can be monitored instrumentally by several methods; the type of detector system chosen for a given problem depends on the nature of the ionizing radiation. Personal monitoring is commonly performed with badges of photographic emulsions, thermal luminescent materials, or induced radiation materials that will indicate the cumulative dose during the period worn. Data from these measurement systems can be used to construct relatively accurate estimates of tissue exposure. If there are also detailed supporting data on worker activities, sources of exposure and points of intervention can also be identified.

Nonionizing radiation is also an external exposure problem. This type of radiation includes a variety of electromagnetic waves ranging from short-wavelength ultraviolet, through visible and infrared, to long-wavelength microwaves and radiowaves. Exposures to ultraviolet, visible, and infrared radiation are measured with photometers of various types. Microwaves and radiowaves can also be measured by several standardized techniques, but there is some controversy over the exposure intensities required to produce adverse effects.

Exposures to radioactive materials can be evaluated with similar methodology to that used for toxic substances. Personal air sampling, surface sampling, and skin contamination measurements can be used to quantify exposures by their route of contact or entry into the body. For example, personal air sampling in uranium mines can measure the miners' exposure to respirable radioactive particles that will be deposited in their respiratory tracts. Internal levels of some radionuclides can be detected outside the body and measured directly if they emit sufficient penetrating radiation, such as gamma rays emitted from radioactive cobalt. However, most cannot be detected externally; the quantities of radioactive substances reaching sensitive tissues usually must be estimated by determining the worker's external exposures and making assumptions about the amount entering the body and being transported to the site(s) of adverse effects.

The Nuclear Regulatory Commission has set standards for allowable ionizing radiation exposures for both external and internal sources. These exposure limits, based on the work of an earlier governmental agency, the National Council on Radiation Protection and Measurements, can be used, like TLVs, to decide if a given exposure presents a health risk. They also have many of the same problems associated with TLVs: They were based on limited data obtained at high-dose levels and include many assumptions and extrapolations that have not been verified. They are especially controversial because they contain an inherent assumption of a threshold below which there is no cancer risk. Radiation protection programs have strict requirements about techniques for handling radioactive materials and working with radiation sources and also require extensive routine exposure monitoring and medical monitoring.

Exposure limits for nonionizing radiation have been set by OSHA based on published scientific data, the TLVs developed by the ACGIH, and standards developed by the American National Standards Institute. Equivalent limits have been developed by WHO and a number of countries (see Bibliography). The eyes and the skin are the critical organs to be protected, and the standards are set for the most susceptible areas. There is concern about reproductive hazards for these agents. Standards also have been developed for lasers based on ophthalmoscopic data and irreversible functional changes in visual responses. As with other types of standards, the numerical limits cannot be treated as absolute, and the margin of safety for many is uncertain.

Control of external ionizing and nonionizing radiation exposures is achieved by minimizing the amounts of radiation used, isolating the processes, shielding the sources, using warning devices and interlocking door and trigger mechanisms to prevent accidental exposures, educating workers and supervisors about the hazards, and, if necessary, requiring use of personal protective equipment. For example, an industrial x-ray machine used to check castings for flaws is placed in a separate room with extensive lead shielding, and the x-ray machine cannot be triggered when the door is open. The room also has signs warning of the hazard. A red warning light inside the room is lit for 30 seconds before the x-rays are released so that a worker inside the room when the door is closed could activate an emergency override switch to prevent operation of the x-ray machine. All personnel working around the x-ray operation are required to wear film badges to monitor their accumulated x-ray exposure.

Control of internal radiation exposures from radioactive materials is very similar to controls for toxic materials. The objectives are to use minimal amounts of radioactive materials; isolate the work areas; enclose any operations likely to produce airborne emissions; use work procedures that prevent or minimize worker contact with contaminated air or materials; have workers wear personal protective equipment to prevent skin contact, eye exposure, or inhalation of materials; monitor environmental contamination levels; and educate workers about the hazards. Some or all of these measures will be used in a typical radiation control problem. Careful supervision of work activities and monitoring of program implementation are required to provide adequate protection.

Traditional work environments, such as factories and heavy industry, have been long-term concerns of hygienists. These are now a growing concern in developing countries that seek to balance the economic benefits of industry against the health costs of sufficient worker protection. In some developed countries there has been a growing concern about the office environment and the health effects associated with energy-efficient, tightly sealed buildings. These buildings are now recognized as a possible source of hazardous exposure to emissions from building materials, such as formaldehyde, and to viable agents and their toxins (Chap. 21). All of these problems are of interest to the occupational hygienist.

## References

1. Rappaport SM. Assessment of long-term exposures to toxic substances in air (review). Ann Occup Hyg 1991; 35:61–121.
2. Fiserova-Bergerova V. Modeling of inhalation exposure to vapors: Uptake, distribution, and elimination. Boca Raton, FL: CRC Press, 1983.
3. Occupational Safety and Health Administration, U.S. Department of Labor. General industry: OSHA safety and health standards (29 CFR 1910). Washington, D.C.: U.S. Government Printing Office, 1993.

## Bibliography

Clayton GD, Clayton FE, eds. Patty's industrial hygiene and toxicology. New York: Wiley; vols. 1A and IB, 4th ed., 1991; vols. 2A–2F, 4th ed., 1993–1994; 3A and 3B, 3rd ed., 1993–1994.

National Institute for Occupational Safety and Health. The industrial environment—its evaluation and control. Washington, D.C.: NIOSH, 1973.

*Two useful and comprehensive general references on industrial hygiene. Patty's works (now edited by the Claytons), although somewhat unwieldy, are the professional's reference work. The NIOSH volume has the advantage of being reasonably priced, but can be difficult to use for specific problems because of the poor quality of its index.*

American Conference of Governmental Industrial Hygienists. Industrial ventilation. 20th ed. Cincinnati: ACGIH, 1988.

Colton CB, Birkner LR, Brosseau L. Respiratory protection—a manual and guideline. Akron, OH: AIHA, 1991.

Schwope AD, Costas PP, Jackson JO. Guidelines for selection of chemical protective clothing. Cincinnati: ACGIH, 1987.

*Manuals containing recommendations for the design and operation of ventilation systems to control air contaminants, along with other protective approaches.*

Burgess WA. Recognition of health hazards in industry: A review of materials and processes. (2nd ed.) New York: Wiley, 1994.

*The source of much of the data in Table 6-1. A highly recommended reference.*

Considine DM. Chemical and process technology encyclopedia. New York: McGraw-Hill, 1974.
*A technical source for gathering background information.*

Hawkins NC, Norwood SK, Rock JC. A strategy for occupational exposure assessment. Akron, OH: AIHA, 1991.

Rappaport SM. Assessment of long-term exposures to toxic substances in air (review). Ann Occup Hyg. 1991; 35:61–121.
*While these two works contain much useful information they are difficult to follow in places and require a strong background in statistics. They are important because they lay out the rationale for sampling strategies to determine compliance with OSHA's permissible exposure limits.*

OSHA analytical methods manual. Washington, D.C.: OSHA, U.S. Department of Labor; Part I–Organic Substances, vols. 1–3, 1990; Part 2–Inorganic Substances, vols. 1–2, 1991.
*Designed for the laboratory chemist and industrial hygienist.*

World Health Organization. Occupational hygiene in Europe. Development of the profession. European occupational health series no. 3. Copenhagen: WHO Regional Office for Europe, 1992.

Draft European Standard prEN 689. Workplace atmospheres–guidance for the assessment of exposure to chemical agents for comparison with limit values and measurement strategy. Draft version, 1992.

Harvey B, Crockford G, Silk S. eds. Handbook of occupational hygiene, vols. 1–3. London: Crone Publications, 1992.
*These references contain all the relevant material about standards in Europe and a number of other countries.*

The way things work. Vols. I and II. New York: Simon & Schuster, 1967 and 1971.
*A practical encyclopedia on industrial processes and other technological items that can be used to obtain basic background information to guide a hazard evaluation.*

NIOSH criteria for a recommended standard: Occupational exposure to hand-arm vibration. National Institute for Occupational Safety and Health, DHHS (NIOSH) publication no. 89-106, 1989.

Pelmear PL, Taylor W, Wasserman DE, eds. Hand-arm vibration: A comprehensive guide for occupational health professionals. New York: Van Nostrand Reinhold, 1992.

Griffin MJ. Handbook of human vibration. London: Academic, 1990.

# 7
# Occupational Safety: Prevention of Accidents and Overt Trauma

W. Monroe Keyserling

An *accident* is an unanticipated, sudden event that may cause an undesired outcome such as property damage, bodily injury, or death. *Injury* is physical damage to body tissues caused by an accident or by exposure to environmental stressors. Many work injuries result from accidents, such as a heavy object falling and crushing bones in a worker's foot. Some work injuries, however, are not associated with accident, but are caused by normal work activities, such as tendinitis on a repetitive assembly-line or data entry job. The occupational basis of these nonacute injuries may not always be recognized due to the lack of a well-defined causative event.

Each year, work accidents produce staggering costs in terms of loss of life, pain and suffering, lost wages for the injured, damage to facilities and equipment, and lost production opportunity. Based on estimates released by the National Safety Council in 1990, the annual toll of workplace accidents in the United States included 10,400 deaths (9 per 100,000 workers), 1,700,000 disabling injuries, and more than 75 million lost workdays. The estimated cost, including lost wages, medical and rehabilitation payments, insurance administrative costs, property losses, and other indirect costs was approximately $49 billion [1]. The above figures underestimate both the count and cost of all work accidents and injuries, however, because of the underreporting of certain non-acute injuries and the omission of certain indirect costs. For example, carpal tunnel syndrome, tendinitis, and related upper-extremity cumulative trauma disorders are classified as occupational *dis-*

*eases* and do not show up in the above statistics. Furthermore, the dollar costs reported above do not include governmental payments (such as welfare and social security) to the families of deceased or permanently disabled workers.

As a result of the aggressive implementation of industrial safety programs following World War II and the passage of the Occupational Safety and Health Act in 1970, the annual rate of accidental industrial fatalities in the U.S. declined from about 33 per 100,000 workers in 1945 to 9 at the beginning of this decade. Certain industries, such as mining, agriculture, and construction, however, have continued to experience high rates of fatal accidents. Death rates for these industries ranged between 30 and 40 per 100,000 workers in 1989 [1]. The safest U.S. industries in 1989 were retail trade (such as apparel and furniture stores) and service (finance, insurance, real estate, and education), where death rates ranged between 4 and 6 per 100,000 workers [1]. While nonfatal accidents have generally declined during the last four decades, the construction, agriculture, manufacturing, transportation, and mining sectors continue to experience high rates of disabling injuries.

In certain instances, the consequences of a workplace accident can affect people outside the confines of a plant, sometimes with catastrophic results. Such was the case in Bhopal, India, where over 2,000 people died following the release of a toxic gas from a chemical plant.

The principal responsibility of the safety professional is to reduce the risk of injuries and disorders by preventing accidents and controlling hazardous

**Table 7-1.** Selected examples of occupational injuries and affected workers

| | Overt trauma | |
| --- | --- | --- |
| Cause | Injury or disorder | Affected occupations |
| Mechanical energy | Lacerations | Sheet metal workers, press operators, meat/poultry processors, woodworkers, carpenters, forestry workers, fabric cutters, glass workers |
| | Fractures | Construction workers, miners, materials handlers |
| | Contusions | Any worker exposed to low energy impacts |
| | Amputations | Press operations, meat/poultry processors, saw operators, machine operators and repairers |
| | Crushing injuries | Materials handlers, construction workers, press operators, calender operators, maintenance workers, miners |
| | Eye injuries (struck by foreign objects) | Miners, grinders, machine tool operators, carpenters, roofers |
| | Strains/sprains (overt) | Materials handlers, miners, baggage handlers, mail handlers, construction workers |
| Thermal extremes | Burns | Foundry workers, smelter workers, cooks, welders, roofers, glass workers, mechanics |
| | Heat strain | Firefighters, smelter workers, steelworkers, hazardous waste cleanup workers, cooks |
| | Cold strain | Utility workers, forestry workers, meat/poultry processors, firefighters |
| Chemical reactivity | Burns | Masons and cement workers, hazardous waste workers, chemical plant workers |
| | Toxicity (including asphyxiation) | Firefighters, hazardous waste workers, confined space workers |
| Electrical energy | Electrocution, shocks, burns | Utility workers, construction workers, operators of electrical equipment and tools, electricians |
| Radiation | Burns, radiation illness | Hospital workers, industrial radiographers, nuclear workers |

| | Cumulative trauma | |
| --- | --- | --- |
| Cause | Injury or disorder | Affected occupations |
| Heavy lifting, prolonged sitting, awkward posture | Back pain | Materials handlers, nurses, truck drivers, sewers, assemblers, mechanics, construction workers, miners, maintenance workers |
| Repetitive motions, prolonged postures, awkward postures, forceful exertions | Upper-extremity cumulative trauma disorders (e.g., tendinitis, carpal tunnel syndrome) | Assemblers, data entry operators, word processors, clerical workers, journalists, meat/poultry processors, packers, sewing machine operators, press operators, musicians |
| Vibration | Raynaud's syndrome | Forestry workers (power saw operators), grinders, air-hammer operators |

exposures in the work environment. Common examples of these hazards and affected occupational groups are listed in Table 7-1. Traditionally, safety professionals have concentrated their efforts on the prevention of accidents and *acute trauma* injuries such as amputations, fractures, lacerations, burns, and electrocution. These injuries typically are immediately apparent to the victim and can be directly linked to a well-defined event or exposure. In recent years, safety professionals have also become concerned with the prevention of *cumulative trauma* disorders such as chronic back pain, tendinitis, and carpal tunnel syndrome. Unlike the general downward trend in the rates of fatalities and acute injuries, cumulative trauma problems increased dramatically throughout the 1980s, particularly in the manufacturing and service sectors.

The remainder of this chapter emphasizes topics related to the prevention of acute trauma. For additional discussion of cumulative trauma disorders and injuries, see Chaps. 8 and 23.

**Table 7-2.** Major causes of work injury classified by accident type

Struck by
Caught in, under, or between (CIUB)
Fall from elevation
Fall on same level
Overexertion (see Chap. 8)
Motor vehicle accident
Other
    Contact with electric current
    Struck against
    Contact with temperature extremes (see Chap. 17)
    Rubbed or abraded
    Bodily reaction
    Contact with radiation, caustics, toxic and noxious substances (see Chaps. 13, 15, and 17)
    Public transportation accident
Unknown

Source: American National Standards Institute. Method of recording basic facts relating to the nature and occurrence of work injuries. (std. #Z16.2). New York: American National Standards Institute, 1962.

## Safety Hazards in the Work Environment

Safety hazards and the injuries they cause can be categorized in many different ways. The American National Standards Institute (ANSI, see Appendix B) uses a system for classifying the cause of work injuries according to *accident type*. This approach, summarized in Table 7-2, considers the conditions and events that caused the accident and has been adopted by workers' compensation boards in many states. The ANSI classification system is used in the following discussion of the causes and prevention of common work accidents.

### Struck By

The classification "struck by" applies to a broad variety of cases in which a worker is hit by a moving object or particle. Typical accident scenarios include: a construction worker who suffers a concussion when hit by a hammer that is accidentally kicked off a scaffold, a warehouse worker who fractures a leg when hit by a moving fork truck, and a grinding machine operator who is permanently blinded when struck in the eyes and face by the fragments of an exploding grinding wheel.

Falling objects cause approximately one-third of these accidents. Items dropped from overhead (such as hand tools, construction materials, and equipment being hoisted to an upper floor of a building) can cause severe head, neck, and shoulder injuries, such as fractures, concussions, and lacerations. In some instances, these injuries are fatal. Effective methods for preventing these events include:

1. Installing covers or side rails to enclose or contain materials carried on overhead conveyor systems (Fig. 7-1)
2. Placing toe boards on all overhead work platforms to prevent materials or tools from being kicked off
3. Installing nets or gratings above workers assigned to hazardous areas

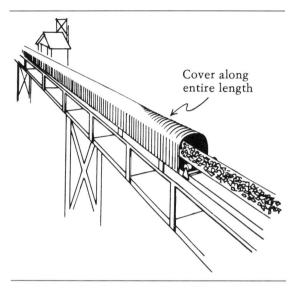

Fig. 7-1. Overhead conveyors should be enclosed to prevent loose materials from falling on people walking or working below. (Reprinted with permission. National Safety Council. Accident prevention manual for industrial operations: Engineering and technology. 9th ed. Chicago: National Safety Council, 1988, p. 118.)

4. Providing and requiring the use of safety helmets
5. Training workers to follow safe rigging practices when hoisting materials overhead
6. Painting safety warnings on floors to indicate work zones where overhead hazards are present

Objects dropped during materials handling tasks, such as lifting and carrying, can cause severe "struck by" injuries to the feet and toes; crush injuries, fractures, and contusions are quite common. Objects that are manually carried should be equipped with handles that allow workers to maintain a firm grasp and should not exceed safe weight-lifting limits. (See discussion of manual materials handling in Chaps. 8 and 23.) Finally, foot protection (safety shoes and metatarsal guards) must be provided and worn whenever these hazards exist.

Flying objects are another cause of "struck by" injuries. Small airborne particles released during operations such as grinding, chipping, and machining can cause severe eye injuries and blindness. These operations should be fully enclosed whenever possible. The use of compressed air for cleaning dust and chips may also be hazardous as small particles can rapidly accelerate to very high velocities. Occupational Safety and Health Administration (OSHA) regulations require that the pressure of cleaning air be limited to 30 pounds per square inch (PSI) to minimize this hazard. Eye and face protection is a critical factor in the prevention of eye injuries. All workers exposed to operations that can release flying particles and fragments must be provided with and *constantly* wear the appropriate personal protective equipment, such as safety glasses, safety goggles, and face shields (see Chap. 25).

The remainder of "struck by" injuries are caused by a variety of factors. In-plant vehicles, such as fork lifts and other industrial trucks, can strike workers, causing fractures and severe trauma to internal organs. Construction tools, such as nail guns used by roofers, use high-pressure air or ex-

Fig. 7-2. The belt drive in this power transmission system is completely enclosed by a barrier guard. (From Occupational Safety and Health Administration. Concepts and techniques of machine guarding. OSHA pub. no. 3067. Washington, D.C.: Occupational Safety and Health Administration, 1980: 13.)

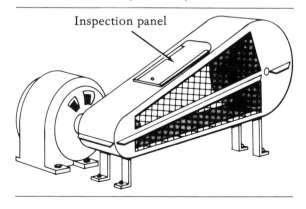

plosive charges to drive nails and other fasteners into wood and concrete. Because of design defects or improper use, or both, these tools are capable of shooting high-velocity projectiles that can cause serious injuries. Machines with moving parts that can strike a worker, such as the rotating blades of a lawnmower, are common hazards. All moving parts of machines and power transmission systems that can either strike or ensnare a person should be fully enclosed within a barrier guard (Fig. 7-2).

Programmable robots, which are becoming common in many manufacturing and assembly operations, present a special hazard. They have very limited sensory capabilities, such as vision, hearing, or touch, to detect the presence of a worker. If a person enters the work zone of a robot without taking the necessary precautions to deactivate and lock out all sources of energy, he/she may be struck or entrapped during subsequent movements of the system. Research is currently under way to im-

---

## A ROBOT-RELATED FATALITY

A 34-year-old operator of an automated die-cast system went into cardiorespiratory arrest and died after being pinned between the back-end of an industrial robot and a steel safety pole (Fig. 7-3). The robot had been installed in an existing production line to remove and transfer parts. The victim had 15 years' experience in die-casting and had completed a one-week course in robotics three weeks before the accident.

The victim entered the work zone of the operating robot before the accident, presumably to clean up scrap that had accumulated on the floor. Despite training and warnings to avoid this practice, he apparently climbed over or walked around the safety rail that surrounded two sides of the robot's work envelope. The gate in the safety rail was interlocked. (Had the worker used the gate, power to the robot should have been shut off.) No other presence-sensing devices (for example, electric eyes, pressure-sensitive floor mats, etc.) were installed.

This case demonstrates both the failure of a worker to recognize all of the hazards associated with robots and serious defects in the design of a robotic system. While workers may readily recognize hazards associated with movement of the "working-end" of a robotic arm, they may not recognize dangers associated with the movement of other parts of the system. In this case, the victim was trapped between a

fixed steel pole and the back-end of the robot. Because he was not standing in the movement envelope of the robot's working arm, he apparently presumed that he was not in danger. Furthermore, the existing safety rail and interlock gate failed to block access to the robot's work zone while the system was powered and in motion.

To prevent a recurrence of this accident, several actions must be taken. Several design changes are needed. The enclosure rail must be modified so that workers cannot walk around or step over the barrier. The robot control system must be enhanced to assure that hardware is placed in a nonpowered, safe condition whenever the barrier rail is opened or crossed. Inside the barrier, floors should be painted to indicate zones of movement for all parts of the robot system. Administrative changes are also needed. Workers must be trained to recognize *all* hazards associated with the specific robot installation. This training must be enhanced periodically with refresher courses to prevent complacency and overconfidence. Finally, supervisors must assure that no worker is ever permitted to enter the operational area of a robot without first putting the system into safe condition.

Adapted from NIOSH publication no. 85-103, Request for assistance in preventing the injury of workers by robots. Cincinnati: National Institute for Occupational Safety and Health, December 1984.

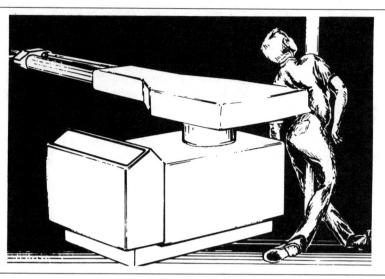

**Fig. 7-3.** Die-cast operator crushed between "back-end" of robot and post. (From National Institute for Occupational Safety and Health. Request for assistance in preventing the injury of workers by robots. Pub. no. 85-103. Cincinnati: National Institute for Occupational Safety and Health, 1984.)

prove the sensory abilities of robots in order to prevent this type of accident. In the meantime, however, all workers assigned to robot installations should receive special training in robot safety. For a case report of a robot-related fatality, see the box on page 149.

### Caught In, Under, or Between

Accidents classified as "caught in, under, or between" (frequently abbreviated as CIUB) include those where the injury is caused by the crushing, squeezing, or pinching of a body part between a moving object and a stationary object, or between two moving objects. Frequently, these accidents are associated with operations that involve the use of mechanized equipment, such as power presses and calenders. A power press is a machine used to cut and shape contoured sheet metal products, such as automobile body panels, household appliances, and metal furniture. When a power press is operated, unprocessed stock material (typically a flat piece of sheet metal) is loaded to the machine and placed on the lower die. The machine is then activated, causing the upper die to close down on the sheet metal with tremendous force (up to several tons). If any part of the body is between the dies during this action, it can be severely crushed or amputated (Fig. 7-4).

Calenders are large heavy rolls used to compress raw materials, such as slabs of steel or rubber, into sheets of precise thickness. It is possible for a limb to become caught in the "in-running pinch point" between these rollers and to be crushed or amputated (Fig. 7-5). When working with large presses or calenders, the entire body may be drawn into the dies or rollers, killing the worker.

When power presses and calenders are in use, the most hazardous operations involve the feeding and removal of stock, since these tasks place workers' hands near moving machine parts. Effective systems for preventing accidents during these activities include *barrier guards,* devices that enclose the dangerous zone before the machine can be activated; *two-handed "safety" buttons,* devices that are positioned in a safe location and require simultaneous activation in order to start the ma-

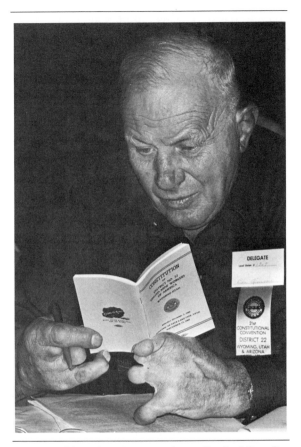

Fig. 7-4. Although not necessarily totally disabling, finger amputations are disfiguring and may reduce job opportunities. (Photograph by Earl Dotter.)

chine (Fig.7-6); and *presence-sensing systems* such as electric eyes that prevent the operation of a machine while any part of the body is in the danger zone. In addition, all machines that can catch clothing or body parts in a "pinch point" should be equipped with emergency stop buttons that can be easily reached by the operator with either hand. Because all of the above systems are quite sophisticated, they must be designed and installed by qualified personnel.

Maintenance activities, such as setup, cleanup, the unjamming of parts, and repair, are also asso-

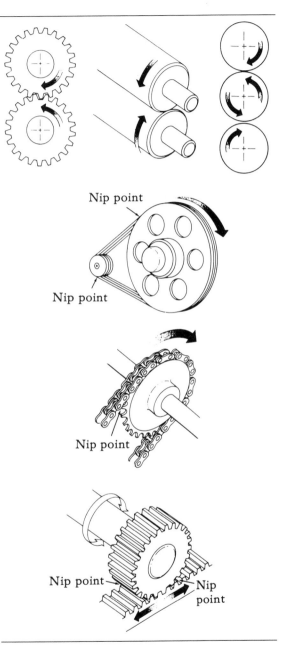

Fig. 7-5. Common examples of in-running pinch points. (From Occupational Safety and Health Administration. Concepts and techniques of machine guarding. OSHA pub. no. 3067. Washington, D.C.: Occupational Safety and Health Administration, 1980: 3–4.)

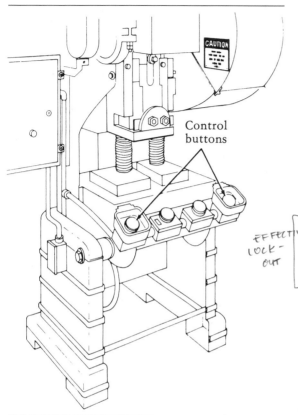

Control buttons

**Fig. 7-6.** Two-handed safety buttons assure that both hands are out of the danger zone before the machine cycle starts. (From Occupational Safety and Health Administration. Concepts and techniques of machine guarding. OSHA pub. no. 3067. Washington, D.C.: Occupational Safety and Health Administration, 1980: 38.)

ciated with CIUB accidents. These operations are particularly hazardous because of the necessity to remove or bypass guards in order to reach locations that require maintenance. (Such was the case in the robot-related fatality case study presented in the box.) Maintenance workers require special training in safe procedures for working with powered machines and equipment that are temporarily unguarded.

Maintenance activities should only be performed when the machine has been put into a nonpowered state. This can be done using "lock-out" procedures that prevent the machine from being started during servicing (Fig. 7-7). Lock-out is now required by OSHA and provides a simple but reliable procedure for protecting workers during maintenance. Before a worker services a piece of equipment, the power switch is placed in the "off" position. The switch is then secured in the "off" position using the personal padlocks of each maintenance worker assigned to the job. Because each worker carries the key to his/her padlock, it is practically impossible to restart the machine until all workers have left the danger zone and removed their locks. Effective lock-out programs require the support and active participation of both management and workers. Policies that prohibit any maintenance activities prior to placing machines in a safe, locked-out state must be developed and rigorously adhered to by all personnel.

As a result of the Occupational Safety and Health Act of 1970 and increasing product liability lawsuits settled in favor of injured workers, employers and machine tool manufacturers in the U.S. have been under increasing legal and economic pressure to upgrade guarding systems on presses, calenders, and other machines. This has resulted in a decrease in the frequency of CIUB and struck-by incidents in the U.S. over the last two decades. Unfortunately, the older machines that have been rendered obsolete because of inadequate guarding and other safety deficiencies are sometimes exported to manufacturers in developing countries. Workers who use these machines are not afforded the protection provided by contemporary guarding technology. In addition, workers in developing countries often lack the necessary training and personal protective equipment needed to operate these machines safely.

*Fall from Elevation*
This category covers incidents in which a worker falls to a lower level and is injured on impact against an object or the ground. Typical injuries include fractures, sprains, strains, contusions,

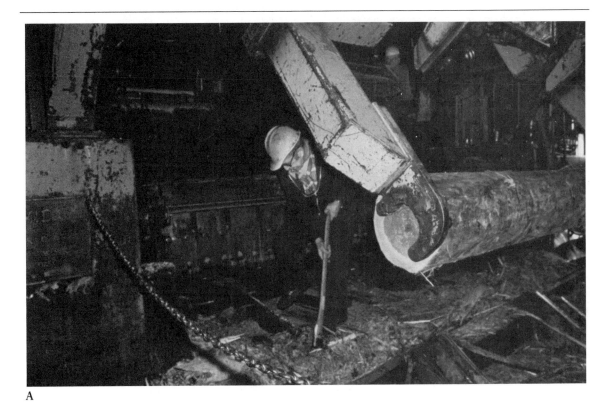

A

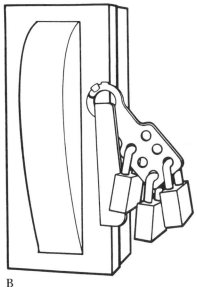

B

**Fig. 7-7.** Lock-out is a control measure used to prevent premature accidental activation of a power switch. A. Maintenance worker has locked operating switch in the "off" position with a personal key. Without lock-out, he could be caught in this machine when the operator restarts it. (Photograph by Earl Dotter.) B. In this diagram, three workers' locks are in place, preventing accidental activation of the power switch. (From Occupational Safety and Health Administration. Concepts and techniques of machine guarding. OSHA pub. no. 3067. Washington, D.C.: Occupational Safety and Health Administration, 1980: 60.)

damage to internal organs, and death. The nature and severity of the injury is primarily determined by the velocity and orientation of the body at the time of impact. Over 40 percent of these falls occur in the construction industry, where work activities are frequently performed on temporary, elevated structures that are exposed to rain, snow, and ice (Fig. 7-8). Maintenance workers in manufacturing plants frequently fall while performing repairs from ladders and other temporary work surfaces. Falls from elevated scaffolds, walkways, and work platforms are usually due to insufficient or nonexistent guardrails. The American National Standards Institute (see Appendix B) has developed standards for the design and safe use of scaffolds and elevated work platforms. Many of these standards have been adopted by OSHA.

Falls from ladders account for over 20 percent of work injuries in the "fall from elevation" category. In a common fall scenario, the accident is initiated by a slippage of the worker's shoe on a ladder rung, which is followed by a loss of grip at the hands. For fixed vertical ladders, this type of accident is sometimes caused by insufficient toe space between the ladder and the structure to which it is mounted. In other cases (particularly outdoor locations where the ladder is slippery), the slip may be caused by insufficient friction between the shoe and the ladder rung. Other falls are caused by slippage or breakage of the ladder itself. These can be prevented in many cases by close compliance with safety standards developed by OSHA and ANSI.

Personal protective devices have been developed to reduce the risk of severe injuries and fatalities that result from falls from elevations, including safety belts, harnesses, lanyards, and lifelines. In spite of the protection offered by these devices, contusions, fractures, strains, and severe deceleration injuries to internal organs can occur when fall protection devices are used.

**Fig. 7-8.** Construction workers have high rates of occupational injuries, many of which are caused by falls. (Photograph by Ken Light.)

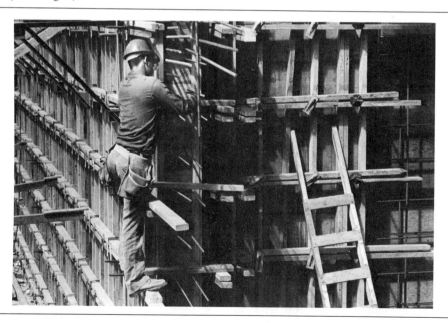

### Fall on the Same Level

Although rarely fatal, serious injuries such as fractures, sprains, strains, and contusions occur when workers lose their footing or balance and fall to the surface supporting them. Slipping, a loss of traction between the shoes and the floor, accounts for about half of all "same level" falls in industry. Most slips are caused by an unanticipated reduction in shoe-floor friction, such as when walking from a dry surface to a wet or oily surface, or from a nonskid surface to a highly polished one. These accidents can be controlled by using similar floor surfaces throughout a work area and by preventing and quickly cleaning up liquid spills. Many slips occur on floor surfaces where friction is relatively uniform, but low, such as in slaughterhouses and food processing plants, and on floors where oil spills are common. In these environments, floor surfaces and shoe soles must be carefully selected to provide adequate friction.

Trips and missteps, usually because of unseen objects on a floor or unexpected changes in floor elevation, are another frequent cause of "same level" falls. These accidents can be prevented through good housekeeping (keeping floors and aisles clear), good maintenance (repairing cracks and uneven surfaces), and good lighting. Finally, warning devices, such as caution signs, are useful in situations where a hazardous floor condition is temporary (such as during mopping and other maintenance) and is being corrected. However, warning signs should never be used on a permanent basis. Instead, the underlying problem must be eliminated.

### Overexertion and Repetitive Trauma

Overexertion and repetitive trauma injuries, such as low back pain, strains, sprains, and tendinitis, are caused by jobs that involve excessive physical effort or highly repetitive patterns of usage of localized muscles and joints. Awkward work posture is frequently a confounding or aggravating factor in these injuries. In recent years, overexertion and repetitive trauma injuries have accounted for over one-fourth of workers' compensation costs in the U.S. In some facilities, these injuries now account for well over one-half of workers' compensation costs. These injuries frequently occur on jobs that involve manual materials handling—this is, where human power is used to lift, push, pull, or carry an object—or highly repetitive hand motions, such as working on an assembly line, operating a sewing machine, or performing high-speed keyboard operations. For a detailed discussion of the recognition and prevention of these injuries, see Chaps. 8 and 23.

### Motor Vehicle Accidents

Motor vehicle accidents are frequently overlooked as a serious occupational hazard. While they account for fewer than 10 percent of workers' compensation payments, they are responsible for almost one-third of work-related deaths. Controlling injuries and deaths due to vehicle accidents is a complex problem. Driver selection (including screening for substance abuse) and training may help reduce the frequency and seriousness of accidents. Daily limits on driving time may reduce operator fatigue as a cause of accidents. Vehicle inspection programs, routine preventive maintenance, and regular use of seat belts also help. Investigations to determine the causes of motor vehicle accidents can lead to measures that prevent recurrence. Details on these and other loss control programs for motor vehicles are available from the National Safety Council, the Insurance Institute for Highway Safety, and the National Highway Traffic Safety Administration (see Appendix B).

### Other Causes of Physical Trauma

About one-fourth of work accidents do not fall into any of the categories discussed thus far. "Contact with electric current" results in shocks and electrical burns, which are sometimes fatal. The critical factor that determines the seriousness of electric shock is the amount of current that flows through the victim, particularly through the chest cavity. Studies have shown that an alternating current of only 100 mamp at the commercial frequency of 60 Hz (standard in the U.S.) may cause ventricular fibrillation or cardiac arrest, or both, if the current passes through the chest cavity. Power supplies commonly found at construction sites, in manufacturing facilities, and even in households are sufficiently high to drive fatal currents through the body.

Construction workers are frequently the victims of electrical accidents because they use electrically powered tools and equipment in wet outdoor locations. Control programs for construction sites should include effective grounding of all electrical equipment, double insulation of all electrical hand tools, and/or ground fault circuit interrupters. Regular inspections of all equipment and power cords should be performed to assure that insulation is intact. Personal protective devices, such as insulated gloves, boots, and clothing, must be worn. Metal ladders and heavy equipment, such as cranes and "cherry pickers," present a special problem at construction sites since they can accidentally become energized on contact with "live" overhead wires. Special precautions must be taken when working below or near overhead lines, such as substituting with wood ladders and de-energizing power sources.

The classification "struck against" is used to describe cases in which a worker collides with a stationary object. Typical injuries include contusions, abrasions, lacerations, and fractures. Head injuries are common and are associated with low ceilings and working in confined spaces. Hand and finger injuries are also common and are frequently caused by forceful exertions with poorly designed or improperly selected tools. The severity of "struck against" injuries can sometimes be controlled by using personal protective equipment, such as safety helmets and gloves, and through improved design of workstations and tools.

"Contact with temperature extremes" refers to incidents in which tissue damage (either burning or freezing) results from exposure to hot or cold solids, liquids, or gases. Control measures include insulation, using robots and other automation in extreme thermal environments, and personal pro-

tection such as heat-resistant clothing and gloves. (For additional information on thermal extremes, see Chap. 17.)

The category "rubbed, abraded, or scratched" refers to relatively minor tissue damage resulting from prolonged contact with rough or sharp objects. Common sites of these injuries are the hands (using abrasives for cleaning or polishing) and the knees (prolonged kneeling on a rough surface). In most instances, these incidents can be controlled by covering the objects with padded materials or handholds, or by wearing protective clothing.

## Elements of a Safety Program

### Organization and Responsibilities

An effective safety program results from a multidisciplinary effort involving interactions among many groups within an organization. To develop a program, it is necessary to establish a plant-level safety committee with overall authority and responsibility for administering the program. This "steering" committee includes upper-level managers (typically the plant manager or designate, and heads of production departments), the plant physician and/or nurse, the safety manager, staff managers (from the engineering, purchasing, maintenance, and industrial relations departments), and labor representatives (the president and/or safety steward in plants with union representation, employee representative(s) in plants without unions). This committee establishes policy, sets goals, and oversees the activities of departmental safety committees that run the day-to-day safety program and solve problems on the plant floor. For the safety program to be effective, the departmental committees must encourage active participation by foremen and hourly workers.

*Upper-level managers* establish a safety policy, develop the policy into a program, and assure that the program is effectively executed. Although safety policies vary from one organization to another, most include the following items:

1. A commitment to provide the greatest possible safety to all employees and to ensure that all facilities and processes are designed with this objective. Similarly, purchasing policies must provide that all equipment, machines, and tools meet the highest safety standards.
2. A requirement that all occupational injuries and accidents be reported, and corrective action taken to assure that similar incidents do not occur.
3. Clear explanations to all employees of their exposures to safety and health hazards, and the establishment of training programs to inform employees of how to minimize their risk of being affected.
4. Regularly scheduled systems safety analyses of all processes and workstations to identify potential safety hazards so that corrective actions can be taken before accidents occur. (Systems safety is discussed later in this chapter.)
5. Disciplinary procedures for employees who engage in unsafe behavior and for supervisors who encourage or permit unsafe activities.

While the chief executive officer is ultimately responsible for the safety of all employees, this responsibility should be delegated throughout all levels of management.

*Floor supervisors* play a key role in the execution of safety programs because of their direct contact with employees. Supervisors must ensure that all equipment comply with applicable safety standards and regulations, and that employees use safe work practices. In addition, the supervisor must make certain that all injuries are promptly reported and treated. Some organizations use "safety competitions," in which supervisors compete to achieve the best safety record. These contests yield beneficial results when supervisors are encouraged to bring their departments into compliance with applicable safety standards and regulations. Unfortunately, however, such competitions sometimes discourage the accurate reporting of accidents or appropriate medical care for injuries. For

this reason, safety competitions may lead to unintended and counterproductive results, and should be undertaken with caution. Care should also be taken to avoid giving supervisors incompatible goals, such as unreasonably high production standards, when lower rates are necessary to assure safety.

Larger worksites usually have a full-time *safety director,* a manager responsible for the day-to-day administration of the safety program. Typical responsibilities include developing and presenting safety training, inspecting facilities and operations for unsafe conditions and practices, conducting accident investigations, maintaining accident records and performing analyses to identify causal factors, and developing programs for hazard control. The safety director must work with the *engineering* and *purchasing* departments to assure that equipment and facilities are designed and purchased in compliance with all applicable safety standards. The safety director also works closely with the plant's medical staff to assure that all injuries and illnesses are properly recorded and investigated. A full-time safety director should be certified by the Board of Certified Safety Professionals (BCSP). For smaller worksites that do not employ a full-time safety director, the duties described above should be assigned to managerial personnel on a part-time basis or obtained from a qualified safety consultant.

Regardless of the size and structure of the plant's medical services, *physicians and nurses* play an essential role in the plant safety program through primary treatment of injured workers and by helping to identify workplace hazards. While the causes of overt trauma injuries are usually obvious, causes of cumulative trauma are often subtle and difficult to identify. By evaluating patterns of employee injuries, disorders, and complaints, the physician or nurse can provide early detection of potentially hazardous operations and processes. Whenever disorders or complaints are suspected of being work-related, this information should be reported to the plant safety director and the responsible supervisor. The physician or nurse, or both, should participate in the subsequent worksite investigations to identify specific hazards or stresses that could be causing the observed injuries, and in planning the subsequent hazard control programs. Finally, physicians and nurses must work closely and cooperatively with supervisors to assure the prompt reporting and treatment of all work-related health and safety problems.

The *maintenance department* and *skilled trades* (electricians, millwrights, and others) play a critical role in the success of the safety program by routinely inspecting facilities, equipment, and tools, and servicing them when necessary. Individuals in these groups should receive special training to enhance their knowledge of safety hazards and control technology.

Finally, *workers* play an essential role in the successful execution of a safety program. Before a new assignment, a worker must be educated regarding specific hazards associated with the new job. Training should include both hazard recognition and control techniques. If personal protective equipment is required to assure safety, training must cover how to inspect, maintain, and wear such equipment. Training must emphasize the responsibility of each worker to maintain a safe workstation and to comply with safe work practices. Part of this responsibility includes reporting unsafe conditions to foremen and employee safety representatives so that corrective action can be taken.

*Employee participation* is an important component of the total safety program. Each worker is an expert in his or her job, and should be actively involved in inspections and systems safety analyses. If modifications are deemed necessary to reduce hazards, worker acceptance of new equipment, tools, and work methods is an essential ingredient in the successful implementation of change. For this reason, workers should actively participate in the design of equipment and process safety features and the selection of personal protective equipment.

### Hazard Discovery and Identification

A completely successful safety program would identify and eliminate all hazards *before* any accidents occur. Systems safety analysis is a subdiscipline of safety engineering concerned with the discovery and evaluation of hazards so that actions can be taken to prevent or substantially reduce the likelihood of an accident. Over 30 different systems safety methodologies have been developed for specific applications, such as aircraft design and consumer product safety. One of these methodologies, job safety analysis (JSA), has been found to be particularly useful for identifying hazards in the work environment.

Job safety analysis is performed by an interdisciplinary team composed of the worker, supervisor, and safety/health specialist. If the analyzed job or process is technically complex, the responsible engineers and skilled trades workers should also participate. The first step in JSA is to break the job down into a sequence of work elements. The next step is to scrutinize each element to identify existing or potential hazards. To do this effectively, the worker must simulate or "walk through" each element, explaining the details of the element to the team and describing previous accidents or "near misses" and the associated causes. Team members rely on experience and expertise in their specialty areas to identify any additional hazards. The results of this analysis are used to recommend changes to the workstation, process, or methods in order to eliminate or effectively control all identified hazards.

Certain operations pose special hazards to both workers and the surrounding community because of the storage, use, or production of materials that are either highly toxic or reactive (i.e., having the potential to cause major explosions or fires). These types of operations are usually associated with the chemical and petroleum industries, but can also be found in the pharmaceutical, food processing, paper, automotive, and electronic industries. Because these operations have the potential for a catastrophic accident with multiple deaths and widespread property damage, OSHA issued a process safety standard in 1992. The standard is performance based and addresses 12 major points, including:

- Developing a written description of potential hazards
- Performing comprehensive analyses to evaluate hazards and to establish priorities for implementing changes to enhance safety
- Formalizing and enforcing safe operating procedures to reduce the likelihood of an accident
- Emergency response planning (for example, evacuation procedures, coordination with community law enforcement and firefighting agencies, etc.)

Job safety analysis and the process safety standard are widely regarded as useful techniques for the identification and control of hazards *prior to* accidents, injuries, or illnesses. To maximize their effectiveness, these techniques must be formally incorporated into the safety program and practiced on a regular basis.

## Reference

1. National Safety Council. Accident facts. 1990 ed. Chicago: National Safety Council, 1990.

## Bibliography

Brauer RL. Safety and health for engineers. New York: Van Nostrand Reinhold, 1990.
*A comprehensive text that is significantly more quantitative and engineering oriented than most contemporary books on safety and health. This book covers a broad range of topics and problems faced by engineers and other safety and health professionals. Numerous illustrations, sample problems, and reference citations enhance the presentation of technical topics.*

Clemens PL. A compendium of hazard identification and evaluation techniques for systems safety application. Hazard Prevention, March 1982.
*Provides a brief summary of 25 frequently used systems safety techniques. An excellent bibliography directs the reader to detailed descriptions of each approach.*

Fullman JB. Construction safety, security, and loss prevention. New York: Wiley-Interscience, 1984.
*Discusses management and engineering aspects of construction safety. Covers hazards unique to the construction environment such as scaffolding and excavations.*

Hammer W. Occupational safety management and engineering. 4th ed. Englewood Cliffs, NJ: Prentice Hall, 1989.
*A useful reference or instructional text that covers both engineering and management aspects of occupational safety and industrial hygiene. Engineering chapters are organized by generic hazard types and include topics not found in many current safety texts (for example, vibration, thermal stress, explosive materials). Management chapters provide broad topical coverage of many issues, including employee training, workers' compensation, safety legislation, accident investigation, and data management.*

National Safety Council. Power press safety manual. 3rd ed. Chicago: National Safety Council, 1979.
*Covers basic safety issues related to the design, setup, operation, and guarding of mechanical power presses.*

National Safety Council. Accident prevention manual for business and industry: Engineering and technology. 10th ed. Chicago: National Safety Council, 1992.
*Reference manual for identification and control of generic safety topics such as machine guarding, fire, electricity, materials handling, and building maintenance. Well illustrated with topical chapters that summarize relevant safety standards and established control technology.*

Winburn DC. Practical electrical safety. New York: Marcel Dekker, 1988.
*Covers basic issues related to effects of electrical current on the human body and controlling exposures to electrical hazards in residential, occupational, and construction settings. Summarizes major points of the National Electrical Code and relevant federal standards.*

# 8

# Occupational Ergonomics: Promoting Safety and Health Through Work Design

W. Monroe Keyserling

*Ergonomics* is the study of humans at work to understand the complex interrelationships among people, their work environment (such as facilities, equipment, and tools), job demands, and work methods. A basic principle of ergonomics is that all work activities cause some level of physical and mental stress. If these stresses are kept within reasonable limits, work performance should be satisfactory and the worker's health and well-being should be maintained. If stresses are excessive, however, undesirable outcomes may occur in the form of errors, accidents, injuries, or a decrement in physical or mental health.[1]

Ergonomists evaluate stresses that occur in the work environment and the corresponding abilities of people to cope with stress. The goal of an occupational ergonomics program is to create a safe work environment by designing facilities, furniture, machines, tools, and job demands to be compatible with workers' attributes (such as size, strength, aerobic capacity, and information processing capacity) and expectations. A successful ergonomics program should simultaneously improve health and enhance productivity.

The following examples call attention to ergonomic issues that are relevant to the prevention and control of health and safety problems in the contemporary workplace:

---

[1]An *accident* is defined as an unanticipated, sudden event that results in an undesired outcome, such as property damage, injuries, or death. An *injury* is defined as damage to body tissues. Injuries can be associated with accidents, but can also result from normal stresses in the environment.

## Prevention of Accidents

Designing a machine guard that allows a worker to operate equipment with smooth, nonawkward, time-efficient motions. This minimizes inconveniences introduced by the guard and decreases the likelihood that it will be bypassed or removed.

Studying the biomechanics of human gait to determine forces and torques acting between the floor surface and the sole of the shoe. This information can be used to improve the friction characteristics of floor surfaces and shoe soles to reduce the risk of a slip or fall.

Designing warning signs for hazardous equipment and work locations so that workers take appropriate actions to avoid accidents (for example, de-energizing powered equipment before maintenance and donning appropriate personal protective equipment). Warnings are particularly important for inexperienced workers or if the hazards are hidden or subtle.

## Prevention of Excessive Fatigue and Discomfort

Designing a computer workstation (equipment and furniture) and associated tasks so that an operator can use a video display terminal (VDT) and keyboard for an extended period without experiencing visual fatigue or musculoskeletal discomfort. Discomfort may be a precursor of serious problems such as tendinitis or carpal tunnel syndrome.

Evaluating the metabolic demands of a job performed in a hot, humid environment to develop a work-rest regimen that prevents heat stress.

Establishing maximum work times for transportation workers (for example, truck drivers, airline pilots) to reduce the risk of drowsiness due to sleep deprivation.

### Prevention of Musculoskeletal Disorders

Evaluating lifting tasks to determine stresses acting at the lower back and designing lifting tasks to prevent back injuries.

Evaluating workstation layouts to discover causes of postural stress and designing changes to eliminate or reduce awkward work postures that cause cumulative trauma disorders. Eliminating awkward postures can also reduce fatigue.

Evaluating highly repetitive manual assembly operations and developing alternative hand tools and work methods to reduce the risk of cumulative trauma disorders such as tendinitis, epicondylitis, tenosynovitis, and carpal tunnel syndrome.

The remainder of this chapter describes several subdisciplines of ergonomics concerned with occupational safety and health.

## Human Factors Engineering

Human factors engineering, sometimes called engineering psychology, is concerned with perceptual, cognitive, and psychomotor aspects of work. Human factors engineers design procedures, equipment, and the work environment to minimize the likelihood of an accident caused by human error. Common causes of work accidents due to human error include:

1. *Failure to perceive or recognize a hazardous condition or situation.* In order to react to a dangerous situation, a worker must perceive that danger exists. Many workplace hazards, such as excessive pressure inside a boiler that could cause an explosion, a fork truck approaching from behind in a noisy factory, unguarded machinery in a poorly lit room, or the sudden release of an odorless, colorless toxic gas, are not easily perceived through human sensory channels. These situations require special informational displays, such as a pressure gauge with "redlines" to indicate a dangerous condition inside the boiler, a horn or beeper that sounds automatically when the fork truck moves, a warning sign at the entrance to the equipment room or better lighting within the room, or an automatic alarm system that signals the release of toxic gases.

2. *Failures in the information processing or decision-making processes.* Decision making involves combining new information with existing knowledge to provide a basis for action. Errors can occur at this stage if the information processing load is excessive. For example, during the Three Mile Island nuclear power plant accident, operators were required to react to an overwhelming number of simultaneous alarms. Decision-making errors can also occur if previous training was incorrect or inappropriate for handling a specific situation.

3. *Failures in motor actions following correct decisions.* Following a decision, it is frequently necessary for a worker to perform a motor action such as flipping a switch or adjusting a knob to control the status of a system or machine. Problems can occur if required actions exceed motor abilities. For example, the force required to adjust a control valve in a chemical plant should not exceed a worker's strength. Errors can occur if controls are not clearly labeled or if manipulation of the control causes an unexpected response. Switches that start potentially dangerous machinery or equipment should be guarded to prevent accidental activation. This is accomplished by covering the switch, locking it in the "off" position, or placing it in a location where it cannot be accidentally touched.

Effective human factors engineering is essential for workplace safety, even when the simplest machines and equipment are involved.

## Work Physiology

Work physiology is concerned with stresses that occur during the metabolic conversion of stored biochemical energy sources to mechanical work. If these stresses are excessive, the worker will experience fatigue. Fatigue may be localized to a relatively small number of muscles or may affect the entire body.

### Static Work and Local Muscle Fatigue

Static work occurs when a muscle or muscle group remains in a contracted state for an extended period. High levels of static work can be caused by sustained awkward posture, such as that of a mechanic who must continuously flex the trunk while repairing an automobile engine, or by high strength demands associated with a specific task, such as using a tire iron to unfreeze a badly rusted wheelnut when changing a tire.

When a muscle contracts, its blood vessels are compressed by the adjacent contractile tissue. Vascular resistance increases with the level of muscle tension and the blood supply to the working muscle decreases. If the muscle cannot relax periodically, the demand for metabolic nutrients exceeds the supply and metabolic wastes accumulate. The short-term effects of this condition include ischemic pain, tremor, and/or a reduced capacity to produce tension. Any of these effects can severely inhibit work performance [1].

Figure 8-1 shows the relationship between the intensity and duration of a static exertion. A contraction of maximum intensity can be held for only about six seconds. At 50 percent of maximum intensity, the limit is approximately one minute. To sustain a static contraction indefinitely, muscle tension must be kept below 15 percent of maximum strength.

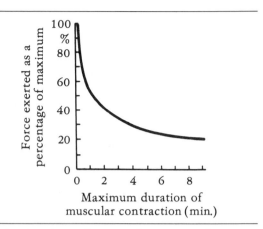

**Fig. 8-1.** Maximum duration of a static muscle contraction for various levels of muscular contraction. (From WM Keyserling, TJ Armstrong. Ergonomics. In JM Last. ed. Maxcy-Rosenau public health and preventive medicine. 12th ed. Norwalk, CT: Appleton-Century-Crofts, 1986.)

Static work also causes a temporary increase in the peripheral resistance of the cardiovascular system. Significant increases in heart rate and mean arterial blood pressure have been observed in conjunction with short-duration static contractions [2]. Caution should be exercised when placing a person with a history of cardiovascular disease on a job that requires moderate or heavy static exertions. If feasible, the job should be modified to reduce the intensity and duration of these exertions.

Dynamic activities involving cyclical contraction and relaxation of working muscle are generally preferable to static work. If, however, the job requires highly repetitive or forceful exertions, a variety of localized cumulative trauma disorders may occur to musculoskeletal tissue or peripheral nerves, or both (see below and Chap. 23).

### Dynamic Work and Whole-Body Fatigue

Whole-body dynamic work occurs when large skeletal muscle groups repeatedly contract and relax while a task is being performed. Common examples of dynamic work activities include walking on a level surface, pedaling a bicycle, climbing stairs, and carrying a load.

The intensity of whole-body dynamic work is limited by the capacity of the pulmonary and cardiovascular systems to deliver adequate supplies of oxygen and glucose to the working muscles and to remove the products of metabolism. Whole-body fatigue occurs when the collective metabolic demands of working muscles throughout the body exceed this capacity. Symptoms of whole-body fatigue include shortness of breath, weakness in working muscles, and a general feeling of tiredness. These symptoms continue and may increase until the work activity is stopped or decreased in intensity.

For extremely short durations of whole-body dynamic activity (typically four minutes or less), a person can work at an intensity equal to his or her aerobic capacity. As the duration of the work period increases, the work intensity must decrease. If a task continues for one hour, the average energy expenditure for this period should not exceed 50 percent of the worker's aerobic capacity. For a job that is performed for an eight-hour shift, the average energy expenditure should not exceed 33 percent of the worker's aerobic capacity.

Aerobic capacity varies considerably within the population. Table 8-1 presents mean aerobic capacities for untrained (i.e., nonathletes) men and women of various ages. Aerobic capacity peaks in

the third decade (20–29 years) for both men and women. At age 50, average aerobic capacity decreases to about 90 percent of the peak value; by age 65 it falls to about 70 percent of the peak [3]. Note that these are average values for each age-sex stratum and do not reflect the full range of variability among the adult population. This variability is an important consideration in evaluating ergonomic stress; a job that is relatively easy for a person with high aerobic capacity can be extremely fatiguing for a person with low capacity. In particular, some older workers may have difficulty performing jobs with high energy expenditure requirements.

The prevention of whole-body fatigue is accomplished through good work design. The energy demands of a job should be sufficiently low to accommodate the adult working population, including persons with limited aerobic capacity. This can be accomplished by designing the workplace to minimize unnecessary body movements (excessive walking or climbing) and providing mechanical assists (such as hoists or conveyors) for handling heavy materials. If these approaches prove infeasible, it may be necessary to provide additional rest allowances to prevent excessive fatigue. This is particularly true in hot, humid work environments due to the metabolic contribution to heat stress (see Chap. 17).

In establishing metabolic criteria for jobs that involve repetitive manual lifting, the National Institute for Occupational Safety and Health (NIOSH) [4] recommends that the average energy expenditure during an eight-hour work shift should not exceed 3.5 kcal/min. Applying the "33 percent" rule to the values in Table 8-1, the NIOSH rate would be acceptable to most of the adult population. Caution should be practiced when placing persons with low levels of physical fitness on metabolically strenuous jobs.[2]

Table 8-1. Average aerobic capacities (kcal/min) of untrained men and women for various ages

| Age | Men | Women |
|-----|------|-------|
| 20 | 15.0 | 11.0 |
| 30 | 15.0 | 9.5 |
| 40 | 13.0 | 8.5 |
| 50 | 12.0 | 8.0 |
| 60 | 10.5 | 7.5 |
| 70 | 9.0 | 6.5 |

Source: J Stegemann. Exercise physiology: Physiologic bases of work and sport. Chicago: Year Book, 1981.

[2]Aerobic capacity can be determined by measuring oxygen uptake and carbon dioxide production during a stress test. For additional information on measuring or estimating aerobic capacity, see [1].

To assess the potential for whole-body fatigue, it is necessary to determine the energy expenditure rate for a specific job. This is usually done in one of three ways:

1. *Table reference.* Extensive tables of the energy costs of various work activities have been developed and can be looked up (see Bibliography for references).
2. *Indirect calorimetry.* Energy expenditure can be estimated for a specific job by measuring a worker's oxygen uptake while performing the job.
3. *Modeling.* The job is analyzed and broken down into fundamental tasks such as walking, carrying, and lifting. Parameters describing each task are inserted into equations to predict energy expenditure.

There is no "best" method for determining energy expenditure. The selection of a method is often a trade-off between the availability of published tables or prediction equations for the specific work activities of interest versus the time and expenses associated with data collection for indirect calorimetry.

## Biomechanics

Biomechanics is concerned with the mechanical properties of human tissue and the response of tissue to mechanical stresses. Some injury-causing mechanical stresses in the work environment are associated with overt accidents, such as crushed bones in the feet caused by the impact of a dropped object. The hazards that produce these injuries can usually be controlled through safety engineering techniques (see Chap. 7). Other injurious mechanical stresses are more subtle and can cause cumulative trauma injuries. These stresses can be external, such as a vibrating chain saw that causes Raynaud's syndrome, or internal, such as

compression on spinal discs during strenuous lifting.

Work-related overexertion disorders (also called cumulative trauma disorders, or CTDs) often result from excessive biomechanical stress. These disorders are frequently seen in the lower back, neck, shoulders, or upper extremities and include a variety of injury and disease entities such as sprains, strains, tendinitis, bursitis, and carpal tunnel syndrome [4–6]. Because these disorders impair mobility, strength, tactile capabilities, and/or motor control, affected workers may be unable to perform their jobs. In many industries, overexertion is the leading cause of workers' compensation expenditures. At companies whose operations include a large amount of manual materials handling or repetitive assembly, overexertion disorders may account for well over one-half of all occupational health and safety expenditures. For additional information on musculoskeletal disorders and related overexertion syndromes, refer to Chap. 23.

Ergonomists and other health professionals are often called on to perform job analyses to identify and control exposures to biomechanical risk factors that cause overexertion injuries and disorders. These risk factors can be grouped into the following six categories [7]:

1. Forceful exertions
2. Awkward postures
3. Localized contact stresses
4. Vibration
5. Temperature extremes
6. Repetitive/prolonged motions or activities

In addition to identifying the presence of these risk factors, job analysis determines specific aspects of the job (for example, workstation layout, production standards, work organization and work methods) that cause or contribute to worker exposures. This information must be obtained in order to effectively design and implement job modifications.

The following sections present a brief discussion of each risk factor.

### Forceful Exertions

"Whole-body" exertions, such as strenuous lifting, pushing, and pulling can cause back pain and other injuries and disorders (Fig. 8-2). Because the lifting and handling of heavy weights are the most commonly cited activities associated with occupational low back pain, NIOSH [4] has issued guidelines for the evaluation and design of jobs that require manual lifting. These guidelines consider task factors, such as lift frequency, workplace ge-

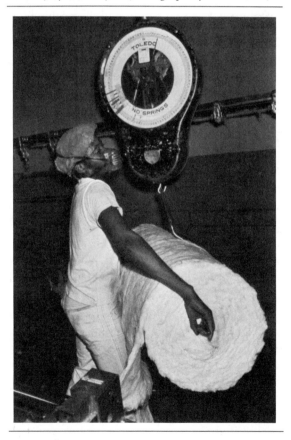

**Fig. 8-2.** Lift assists are necessary to prevent the risk of back injury on this job. (Photograph by Earl Dotter.)

ometry, and posture to establish the amount of weight that a person can safely lift. Factors other than object weight play a significant role in the amount of force that workers can safely exert during lifting and other manual transfer tasks. Because of the effect of long moment arms, handling relatively light loads can stress muscles in the back and shoulder if the load is held at a long horizontal distance in front or to the side of the body.

One or more of the following approaches may prove useful in reducing the magnitude of forces exerted during whole-body exertions:

1. Reduce the weight of the lifted object by decreasing the size of a unit load (for example, placing fewer parts in a tote bin, purchasing smaller bags of powdered or granular materials)
2. Reduce extended reach posture by removing obstructions (for example, rails on storage bins) that prevent the worker from getting close to the lifted object
3. Use gravity or mechanical aids (for example, conveyors, hoists, articulating arms, etc.) to assist the worker or eliminate the manual exertion (Fig. 8-3)

Forceful exertions of the hands (e.g., cutting with knives or scissors, tightening screws, "snapping" together electrical connectors, using the hands/fingers to sand or buff parts) can cause upper-extremity disorders such as tendinitis or carpal tunnel syndrome. Pinch grips, heavy tools, poorly balanced tools, poorly maintained tools (for example, dull knives or scissors), or low friction between the hand and tool increase the forces exerted in the finger flexor muscles and tendons. Gloves may increase force requirements of some jobs because of reduced tactile feedback, reduced friction, or resistance of the glove itself to stretching or compression. Environmental conditions may also increase force requirements as some rubber and plastic materials lose their flexibility when cold and become more difficult to shape or manipulate. One or more of the following approaches

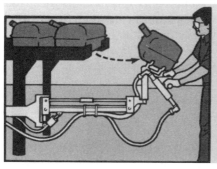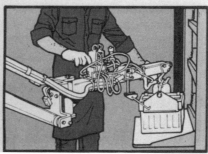

Fig. 8-3. Mechanical assist devices can reduce or eliminate forceful exertions during manual materials handling activities such as lifting or carrying. (Courtesy of the University of Michigan and the UAW/Ford Joint National Committee on Health Safety. From University of Michigan Center for Ergonomics. Fitting jobs to people: An ergonomics process. Ann Arbor, MI: The Regents of the University of Michigan, 1991.)

may prove useful in reducing the forcefulness of hand exertions:

1. Substitute power tools (electric or pneumatic) for manual tools. If a power tool is infeasible, redesign the manual tool to increase mechanical advantage or otherwise decrease required hand forces.
2. Suspend heavy tools with "zero-gravity" balance devices.
3. Treat slippery handles on tools and other objects with friction enhancement devices or treatments to minimize slippage within the hands.
4. Move the handle of an off-balance tool closer to the center of gravity or suspend the tool in a way that minimizes off-balance characteristics.
5. Use torque control devices (reaction arms, automatic shut-off) on power tools such as air wrenches, nut runners, or screwdrivers (Fig. 8-4). Investigate if torque can be reduced without adversely affecting product quality.
6. If high force is required to assemble poorly fitting parts, consider the following: (a) improve quality control to achieve better fit or (b) use a lubricant to facilitate the assembly of tightly fitting parts.

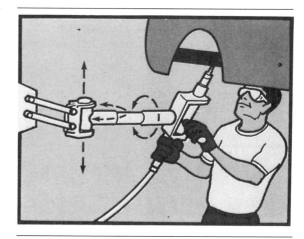

Fig. 8-4. Torque control devices can substantially reduce the amount of force exerted when air wrenches and similar tools are used. Note that the weight of the tool is also borne by the device, further reducing the force exerted by the worker. (Courtesy of the University of Michigan and the UAW/Ford Joint National Committee on Health Safety. From University of Michigan Center for Ergonomics. Fitting jobs to people: An ergonomics process. Ann Arbor, MI: The Regents of the University of Michigan, 1991.)

7. Prewarm rubber and plastic components if these become cold and unmalleable during storage.

### Awkward Posture

Awkward posture at any joint may cause transient discomfort and fatigue. Prolonged awkward postures may contribute to disabling injuries and disorders of musculoskeletal tissue or peripheral nerves, or both. Awkward trunk postures such as those shown in Fig. 8-5 increase the risk of back injuries [8]. Raising the elbow above shoulder height or reaching behind the torso can increase the likelihood of musculoskeletal problems in the neck and shoulders. The worker shown in Fig. 8-6 must position his arms in an extended forward reach because of poor workstation layout.

Most awkward postures of the trunk and shoulder result from excessive reach distances (for example, bending into bins or reaching behind the body to place or retrieve parts, reaching overhead to high shelves and conveyors, reaching overhead or in front of the body to activate machine controls) and can be eliminated through improved workstation layout. In general, workers should not reach below knee height or above shoulder height. Routine forward reaches should be performed with the trunk upright and the upper arms nearly parallel to the trunk. Where possible, workstations and equipment should offer adjustability to accommodate workers of different body sizes.

Allowing workers to sit while working reduces fatigue and discomfort in the legs and feet and can increase stability of the upper body. (Note: A high level of body stability is essential for precision manual tasks.) However, prolonged sitting may be a factor in the development of back pain. A well-designed workseat (for example, one with good lumbar support and adjustability of the seat pan and backrest) enhances comfort and can reduce the risk of health problems. Layouts that allow

**Fig. 8-5.** A method for classifying nonneutral trunk postures. (From WM Keyserling. Postural analysis of the trunk and shoulders in simulated real time. Ergonomics 1986; 29:569–83.)

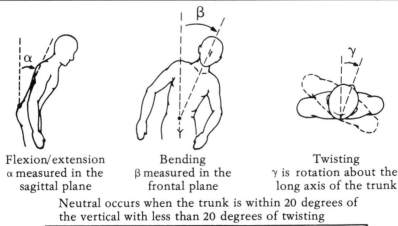

Flexion/extension
$\alpha$ measured in the
sagittal plane

Bending
$\beta$ measured in the
frontal plane

Twisting
$\gamma$ is rotation about the
long axis of the trunk

Neutral occurs when the trunk is within 20 degrees of
the vertical with less than 20 degrees of twisting

| STANDARD TRUNK POSTURES | |
|---|---|
| 1. Stand-extension ($\alpha < -20°$) | 6. Lie-on back or side |
| 2. Stand-neutral | 7. Sit-neutral |
| 3. Stand-mild flexion ($20° < \alpha \le 45°$) | 8. Sit-mild flexion |
| 4. Stand-severe flexion ($\alpha > 45°$) | 9. Sit-twisted/bent |
| 5. Stand-twisted/bent ($\beta$ or $\gamma > 20°$) | |

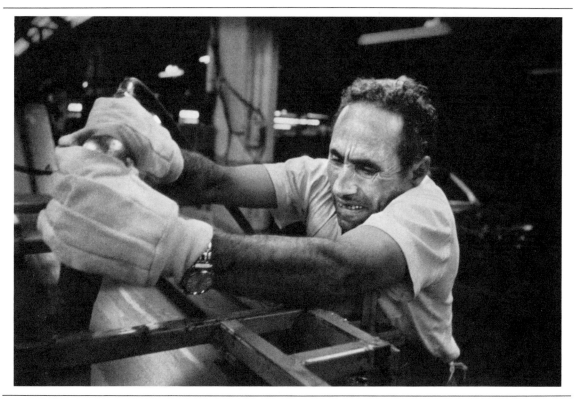

**Fig. 8-6.** This job involves exposure to several risk factors associated with the development of upper-extremity cumulative trauma disorders. (Photograph by Earl Dotter.)

workers to alternate between standing and sitting postures are also desirable.

Awkward upper-extremity postures can occur at the shoulder (discussed above), elbow, or wrist. It is important to avoid frequent or prolonged activities that require a worker to bend the wrist. Hand tool features, such as the shape and orientation of handles, in combination with workstation layout (location and orientation of work surfaces), play an important role in determining wrist postures. See Fig. 8-7 for examples of how tool selection and workstation layout affect upper-extremity posture.

### Localized Contact Stresses
Local mechanical stresses result from concentrated pressure during contact between body tissues and

an object or tool. "Hand hammering" (i.e., using the palm as a striking tool) is used in some manufacturing operations as a method of getting two parts to fit together. This activity, which can irritate nerves and other tissues in the palm, can be avoided by using a mallet. Hand tools with hard, sharp, or small-diameter handles (for example, knives, pliers, scissors) can irritate nerves and tendons in the palm or fingers. This problem can be controlled by either padding or increasing the radius-of-curvature of tool handles. In some bench assembly activities and office jobs, contact stresses result from resting the forearms or wrists against a sharp, unpadded workbench edge. This problem can usually be controlled by either rounding or padding the edge, or by providing a support for the forearm and wrist.

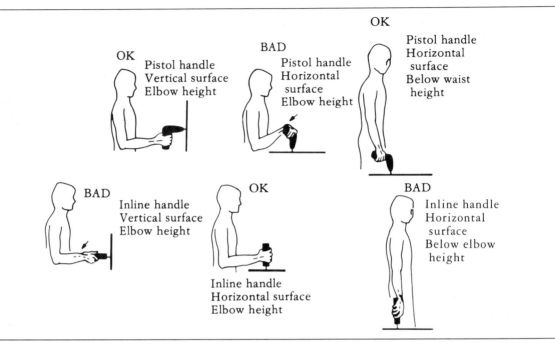

**Fig. 8-7.** Examples of neutral and nonneutral wrist postures associated with various combinations of tool selection and work station layout. (From T Armstrong. An ergonomics guide to carpal tunnel syndrome. Akron, OH: American Industrial Hygiene Association, 1983. Reprinted with permission by American Industrial Hygiene Association.)

Seated workstations that produce localized pressure on the posterior knee and thigh can impair circulation to the lower extremities, causing swelling and discomfort in the lower legs, ankles, or feet. A common cause of this condition in both factories and offices is a work seat that is too high, allowing the lower legs to dangle free. Because the full weight of the lower extremities hangs from the work seat, concentrated compressive forces can squeeze tissues in the area where the thighs contact the front edge of the seatpan. A solution to this problem is to provide adjustable seats. Another solution is to provide a foot rest to support some of the weight of the lower extremities.

*Vibration*

Exposure to whole-body vibration that occurs while driving or riding in motor vehicles (including fork trucks and off-road vehicles) may be a factor that increases the risk of back pain. Because driving tasks are usually performed in a seated posture, most drivers are exposed to two back pain risk factors. Driving over rough surfaces for prolonged periods and/or vehicle seats with poor suspension systems increase vibration exposure. Standing on vibrating floors (e.g., near power presses in a stamping plant or near shakeout equipment in a foundry) may also result in exposure to whole-body vibration.

Localized vibration of the upper extremity (also called segmental vibration) can occur when using powered handtools such as screwdrivers, nutrunners, grinders, jackhammers and chippers. Other exposures include holding parts against grinding wheels or prolonged gripping of a vibrating steering wheel. Localized vibration may contribute to the development of carpal tunnel syndrome and vibration-induced Raynaud's syndrome. Proper tool selection can help in reducing exposure. For example, a torquing tool that uses an automatic shut-off system produces less vibration exposure than a slip-clutch mechanism. Many manufacturers offer a variety of low-vibration hand tools.

### Temperature Extremes

Exposure to unusually hot or cold ambient temperatures can produce a variety of adverse health effects, as discussed in Chap. 17. In addition to considering the general thermal characteristics of the workroom (for example, air temperature, air movement, relative humidity), it is also necessary to look at temperature extremes that affect the hands. For example, handling extremely hot or cold parts may require the use of special gloves that increase the force requirements of the job (see above). In jobs that involve the use of pneumatic tools, air from high-pressure lines and tool exhaust ports may be directed onto the hands causing local chilling and reduced manual dexterity and tactile sensitivity. This exposure can be controlled by eliminating leaks and/or directing exhausted air away from the hands.

---

## OCCUPATIONAL VIBRATION EXPOSURE
Robert G. Radwin
### Sources of Vibration Exposure

Workers are exposed to vibration from a variety of sources. *Whole-body* vibration (WBV)—vibration transmitted to the entire body via the seat or the feet, or both—often originates from vehicular motion in construction, transportation, and shipping. *Hand and arm vibration* (HAV), by contrast, is limited to the extremities and results from exposures commonly generated by use of power hand tools and vehicle controls. The nature of the adverse effects of vibration exposure depends on the particular vibration characteristics of the source. For example, the effects of sea sickness from ship motion are quite different from the effects of helicopter vibration on the pilot's vision, or the effects of the vibration from a power grinder on tactile sensitivity of the operator.

Although standards for WBV exposure are internationally recognized, there is less universal agreement about the standards for HAV exposures. For many years, problems associated with the effects of HAV vibration on the vascular system, such as vibration white finger, autonomic disturbances, perception, discomfort, and other abnormalities, have received attention. More recently, however, efforts have been directed to determining the degree to which HAV vibration is important for musculoskeletal and peripheral nerve disorders.

With this effort has come a set of problems associated with developing an improved understanding of the natural history of the pathologic processes involved. For example, neurologic disorders, such as carpal tunnel syndrome (CTS), and vascular disorders, such as Raynaud's disorder, have been difficult to separate since several early symptoms for both disorders are similar. Hence the effects of CTS and the early stages of hand-arm vibration syndrome are sometimes confounded. Studying the relative effects of hand transmitted vibration in the context of other ergonomic stress factors is complicated by the fact that many jobs that use vibrating hand tools also involve considerable repetitive or awkward motions of the upper limb to manage tools that also provide HAV. Highly repetitive work can affect vibration exposure through accumulated doses of repeated vibration exposures. These interactions have certainly complicated the study of ergonomic stress factors and their effects combined with hand-transmitted vibration.

### Exposure Assessment

Primary among the factors considered important in human vibration exposure are vibration:

*Magnitude* (measured as acceleration in units of gravity or often reported in dB from a reference accelerator)

*Frequency* (measured in cycles per second as hertz)

*Duration of exposure* (measured in time intervals appropriate to tasks)

The magnitude and frequency of vibration exposure are commonly measured using continuous recording devices attached to small accelerometers—electronic sensors containing piezoelectric or piezoresistive materials that measure the time course and magnitude of acceleration. Measurements are made at the point where the body comes into contact with the vibrating source. While the accelerometers can be clamped directly to handles of power hand tools for measuring HAV, special accelerometers have been developed for placement between the seat and a vehicle operator's buttocks for WBV measurements. By recording continuous vibration measurements, spectral analyzers can be used to study vibration frequency in detail.

The closer the tool or equipment vibration frequency is to the natural or resonant vibration frequency of the body part affected, the more damaging the vibration. Therefore, frequency is particularly relevant in understanding how to redesign tools or equipment, or in determining the appropriate vibration isolation systems. Exposure duration is also important both for determining relevant exposure variables in population studies and in understanding the limits that must be placed on duration of exposure when vibration cannot be eliminated. Sufficiently detailed measurements of duration often require using time studies or work sampling.

The effective measurement of HAV exposure is more difficult than for WBV. A variety of factors determine the nature and amount of HAV exposure. One of the more important ones is the nature of the coupling between the hands and the vibrating source. A forceful grip will result in increased vibration transfer to the hand and arm because of better coupling between the vibrating handle and the hand. While factors such as handle location, tool weight, and position of the work can affect the force of the grip required, force is also affected by the vibrating handle. Vibration can introduce disturbances in muscular control via a reflex mediated through the response of muscle spindles to the vibration stimulus. This reflex, known as the tonic vibration reflex, appears as a gradual increase in muscle activity. Consequently, hand tool vibration alone can result in excessive grip exertions when a vibrating handle is held. Factors associated with the dynamic coupling between hand and tool are usually not accounted for in HAV measurements when accelerometers are attached directly to the vibrating source. Vibration measurements taken directly off the hands, however, are more difficult to obtain and are usually not performed.

Work standards and individual work methods are another aspect of worker vibration exposure. One study found that the prevalence of hand-arm vibration syndrome was greater among incentive workers than among hourly workers. It suggested that the intensity of incentive work resulted in increased vibration transmission and therefore exposure, presumably due to increased grip exertions and the resulting improved coupling between the hand and the power tool. Handle location and the type of tool also can have a dramatic effect on the level of vibration transmitted to the operator. Vibration measurements, taken at points where workers normally grip these tools, made from a large chipping hammer running at full throttle, indicated that the acceleration was attenuated substantially; between the chisel end and the rear handle, the magnitude had a ratio of approximately $78 : 1$ ($23,400$ m/s$^2$ at the chisel and $299$ m/s$^2$ at the rear handle).

## Control of Vibration

WBV levels can often be reduced through use of vibration isolation and suspension systems imposed between the operator and the vibrating source.

HAV is more difficult to control and requires consideration of a variety of features of the vibration source. Vibration is an intrinsic property of power hand tool operation and may even be the desired action of a particular tool. Vibration levels associated with power hand tools depend on tool properties, including size, weight, method of propulsion, and the tool drive mechanism. For example, continuous vibration is inherent in reciprocating and rotary power tools, while impulsive vibration is produced by tools operating by shock and impact action, such as impact wrenches or chippers. The tool power source, such as air power, electricity, or hydraulics, can also determine the nature and amount of vibration. Accessory attachments may become a source of vibration if they fit improperly or cause a tool to become unbalanced. An example is a loosely fitting extension shaft on a nutrunner, causing a hand tool that is usually considered to have a low vibration magnitude to produce considerable vibration as a result of the wobbling action of the rotating spindle. Tools that require maintenance, or tools that become unbalanced, are also potential sources of vibration. Vibration is also generated at the tool-material interface by cutting, grinding, drilling, or other actions. Vibration levels are affected by work piece material properties including hardness and surface characteristics such as roughness or shape. Other features of importance include characteristics of abrasive discs and their contact with areas of surfaces as well as the type of fastener being used.

Modifications in work methods can be used to reduce both the patterns and levels of vibration exposure produced. Examples of modifications in work methods are redesigning production processes in order to reduce or eliminate vibrating hand tools, redistributing the work among workers, and introducing external tool support devices in order to reduce grip force or eliminate the need to hold tools when they are not in use. Care must be taken to determine that a change in work method or material does not, in turn, create an unanticipated new problem. For example, reducing a sanding pad grit abrasiveness may decrease the overall vibration *level*. However, it is important to be sure that the consequence of the reduced abrasiveness is not simply to increase the time interval necessary to complete the sanding task, leading to increased *duration* of vibration exposure time as well as prolongation of the duration of repetitive work.

Some tool manufacturers are now offering tools designed to produce less vibration. However, add-on accessories for standard tool handles have met with only mixed success. One partially successful new design feature has been use of rubber handle coverings. While some studies have shown that these did not significantly reduce vibration level, researchers have found that their use resulted in lower grip exertions and, hence, a change in the coupling of hand and tool. It is thought that this reduction in grip exertion may be due to improved frictional characteristics between the hand and tool handle. Personal protection devices, such as antivibration gloves, are another method of providing vibration isolation to the hands and arms. A problem with some antivibration gloves is the large amount of absorbing material necessary, making grasp difficult and interfering with hand motions. This calls attention to the fact that even if gloves or other antivibration apparel can prevent vibration transmission to the hands, they should be used cautiously since they may increase grip exertions, especially when gloves fit poorly.

## Repetitive and Prolonged Activities

The biomechanical and physiologic strain experienced by a worker is related to the cumulative exposure to all the risk factors discussed previously. Because ergonomic risk factors are often related to specific work activities, jobs that involve high repetition or prolonged activities (e.g., driving 5,000 screws per day on an assembly line or continuous word processing in an office) typically involve higher exposures than nonrepetitive jobs (for example, rework/repair in a factory, a supervisory position in an office). Studies have shown that jobs with a basic cycle time of 30 seconds or less (i.e., a production rate of two or more parts per minute) have an elevated rate of carpal tunnel syndrome and related disorders. Longer cycle times do not necessarily result in lower risk of injury if basic hand motions are repeated within the cycle. Workers in jobs in which over 50 percent of the work cycle involves similar motion patterns have also shown elevated rates of upper-extremity disorders [9].

Repetitiveness as a risk factor is not limited to upper-extremity problems. Frequent lifting and other manual materials handling activities increase the risk of back pain [4].

Repetitiveness can often be measured or estimated using industrial engineering records and other work standards. For example, on an assembly line, repetitiveness is a function of the line speed or the time allowed to complete one unit of work. For a clerk in a bank or insurance office, repetitiveness can be a function of the number of forms processed per day. For a supermarket checker, repetitiveness is a function of the number of items scanned over the course of a work shift (Fig. 8-8). Where work standards do not exist, repetitiveness can sometimes be estimated as the percentage of time spent in certain postures or performing certain activities.

Resolving problems of repetition can be a major challenge. Two possible approaches are job enrichment and job rotation. The premise behind these approaches is to increase the overall variety of activities performed by a worker to reduce the repet-

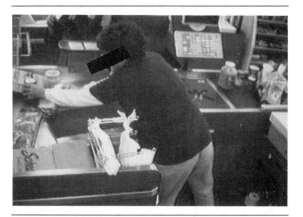

**Fig. 8-8.** Supermarket checkout persons using bar-code readers can be at risk for carpal tunnel syndrome.

itiveness of any specific stressful activity. While good in theory, these approaches may be very difficult to implement. Job enrichment and job rotation will not prove feasible in work locations where there are no "low-repetition" jobs to combine with the "high-repetition" jobs. Even in situations in which a good mix of low- and high-repetition jobs exists, there may be other barriers (for example, increased learning time, seniority practices) that present significant barriers. In these instances, it may be necessary to establish a participatory ergonomics program and to educate management and workers before attempting these interventions.

## Components of an Ergonomics Program

An effective program for controlling overexertion injuries and disorders starts with the commitment and involvement of management to provide the organizational resources and motivation to control ergonomic hazards in the workplace. Management must also perform regular reviews and evaluations of the program to assure that program goals are met in a deliberate and timely manner. Because ergonomic programs focus on improving the complex interrelationships among workers and their jobs, employee involvement is essential to assuring the success of the program [5].

An effective program should include the following components:

- Surveillance of health and safety records to identify patterns of overexertion injuries and illnesses
- Job analysis to identify worker exposures to risk factors that cause overexertion injuries and illnesses
- Job design (and redesign if necessary) to reduce or eliminate ergonomic risk factors
- Training of managers, engineers, and workers in the recognition and control of ergonomic risk factors
- Medical management of injured workers to improve the chances for a speedy return to work

Limited resources must be directed at those jobs with the greatest ergonomic problems. One approach for identifying high-hazard jobs is to analyze available medical, insurance (workers' compensation insurance, in particular), and safety records (such as the OSHA 200 log) for evidence of high rates of cumulative trauma disorders in certain departments, job classifications, or workstations. This approach is called *passive surveillance* because it relies on previously collected information. Passive surveillance may underestimate the true level of cumulative trauma problems. (For example, at small plants that do not have in-plant medical services, a worker may seek treatment from his or her personal physician. Unless the worker requests coverage under the workers' compensation system, the complaint and associated treatment may not appear in any company records.) *Active surveillance* involves a more aggressive approach to identifying potential problems. Active surveillance may include employee surveys to identify jobs associated with elevated rates of discomfort in the back, neck, shoulders, and upper extremities. Active surveillance may also include interviews with supervisors and personnel managers to identify jobs with high turnover. If other

employment opportunities are available, workers often seek relief by leaving jobs with unusually high physical stresses before a cumulative trauma injury develops.

Once the high-risk jobs have been identified, the next step is to determine the specific causes of exposure so that corrective actions can be taken. This activity involves job analysis to identify the various risk factors discussed previously and the development of engineering or administrative controls to reduce or eliminate exposures. The appropriateness of an intervention to reduce ergonomic stress will vary among and within facilities. Changes that are practical at one workstation may not be appropriate for other workstations. Alternatives must be evaluated to determine the best strategy for resolving each ergonomic problem. It is also important to recognize that most solutions will require some degree of "fine tuning" to assure that they are acceptable to workers and accomplish the intended reductions in ergonomic stress. Follow-up job analyses should be performed to assure that the solution is working effectively and that no new stresses have been introduced. Follow-up health surveillance is also recommended to detect any changes in the pattern of injuries, illnesses, or employee complaints.

# References

1. Rodahl K. The physiology of work. London: Taylor and Francis, 1989.
2. Armstrong TJ, et al. Static work elements and selected circulatory responses. Am Ind Hyg Assoc J 1980; 41:254–60.
3. Stegemann J. Exercise physiology: Physiologic bases of work and sport. Chicago: Year Book, 1981.
4. Waters TR, Putz-Anderson V, Garg A, Fine LJ. Revised NIOSH equation for the design and evaluation of manual lifting tasks. Ergonomics 1993; 36:749–76.
5. Occupational Safety and Health Administration (OSHA). Ergonomics program management guidelines for meatpacking plants. Publication no. OSHA-3121. Washington, D.C.: U.S. Department of Labor, 1990.
6. Putz-Anderson V. ed. Cumulative trauma disor-

ders—a manual for musculoskeletal diseases of the upper limbs. London: Taylor and Francis, 1988.

7. Keyserling WM, Armstrong TJ, Punnett L. Ergonomic job analysis: A structured approach for identifying risk factors associated with overexertion injuries and disorders. Appl Occup Environ Hyg 1991; 6:353–63.

8. Punnett L, et al. A case-referent study of back disorders in automobile assembly workers: The health effects of nonneutral trunk postures. Scand J Work Environ Health 1991; 17:337–46.

9. Silverstein BA, Fine LJ, Armstrong TJ. Occupational factors and carpal tunnel syndrome. Am J Ind Med, 1987; 11:343–58.

# Bibliography

Chaffin DB, Andersson GBJ. Occupational ergonomics. 2nd ed. New York: Wiley-Interscience, 1991.
*This text discusses in detail the biomechanical basis of many occupational injuries and disorders, with special emphasis on the lower back. Quantitative methods of job analysis are presented, with numerous examples of ergonomic approaches to equipment, tool, and workstation design.*

Durnin JVGA, Passmore R. Energy, work, and leisure. London: Heineman Educational Books, 1967.
*Presents numerous tables of the metabolic cost of common occupational, household, and recreational activities. A useful reference text.*

Garg A, Chaffin DB, Herrin GD. Prediction of metabolic rates for manual materials handling jobs. Am Ind Hyg Assoc J 1978; 39:661–74.
*Describes the development and validation of a modeling approach to estimate energy expenditure rates associated with common materials handling tasks. Equations for predicting energy expenditure are included in an appendix to this paper.*

Grandjean E. Fitting the task to the man—an ergonomic approach. London: Taylor and Francis, 1985.
*A well-written survey text that covers all aspects of ergonomics. Chapters on fatigue and work physiology provide an excellent introduction to these topics.*

Keyserling WM, Armstrong TJ. Ergonomics. In WN Rom. ed. Environmental and occupational medicine. 2nd ed. Boston: Little, Brown, 1992, pp. 1179–96.
*A general review of occupational ergonomics with emphasis on anthropometry, work physiology, and biomechanics. A total of 96 references include many recent journal articles on ergonomic topics.*

Occupational Safety and Health Administration (OSHA). Ergonomics program management guidelines for meat-packing plants. Publication no. OSHA-3121. Washington, D.C.: U.S. Department of Labor, 1990.
*Although written specifically for the red-meat industry, this document presents general guidelines for establishing and managing effective ergonomics programs at worksites. A section on the medical management of injured workers is included along with employee surveillance instruments for assessing discomfort and other symptoms.*

Putz-Anderson V. ed. Cumulative trauma disorders—a manual for musculoskeletal diseases of the upper limbs. London: Taylor and Francis, 1988.
*Discusses etiology and prevention of upper-extremity cumulative trauma disorders. Covers a broad range of topics, including biomechanics of upper-extremity cumulative trauma disorders, analysis of health records, and design of workstations, tools, and work methods to control exposure risk factors.*

Sanders MS, McCormick EJ. Human factors in engineering and design. 6th ed. New York: McGraw-Hill, 1987.
*A useful reference text for many topics in human factors engineering, including lighting, displays, controls, and information processing. Well illustrated with numerous examples.*

Waters TR, Putz-Anderson V, Garg A, Fine LJ. Revised NIOSH equation for the design and evaluation of manual lifting tasks. Ergonomics 1993; 36:749–76.
*This article presents a methodology developed by NIOSH for identifying potentially hazardous lifting activities. Biomechanical, physiologic, and psychophysical criteria are used to establish an equation for predicting safe weight-lifting limits based on task characteristics, such as workplace geometry, lifting frequency, and characteristics of the lifted object. This equation is based on recent research findings and replaces an earlier version released by NIOSH in 1981. Extensive references to relevant research are cited throughout the article.*

# 9

# Government Regulation of Occupational Health and Safety

Nicholas A. Ashford

The use of chemicals, materials, tools, machinery, and equipment in industrial, mining, and agricultural workplaces is often accompanied by health and safety hazards or risks (Fig. 9-1). These hazards cause occupational disease and injury that place heavy economic and social burdens on both workers and employers. Because voluntary efforts in the free market have not succeeded historically in reducing the incidence of these diseases and injuries, government intervention into the activities of the private sector has been demanded by workers. This intervention takes the form of the regulation of health and safety hazards through standard-setting, enforcement, and the transfer of information.

In the United States, toxic substances in the workplace are regulated primarily through three federal laws: the Mine Safety and Health Act of 1969 (see box on p. 179), the Occupational Safety and Health Act (OSHAct) of 1970, and the Toxic Substances Control Act (TSCA) of 1976. The federal legislation has remained essentially unchanged since its passage, and serious attempts at reauthorization are being planned.

The OSHAct established the Occupational Safety and Health Administration (OSHA) in the Department of Labor to enforce compliance with the act, and the National Institute for Occupational Safety and Health (NIOSH) in the Department of Health and Human Services (under the Centers for Disease Control) to perform research and conduct health hazard evaluations. The Office of Pollution Prevention and Toxic Substances in the Environmental Protection Agency (EPA) administers TSCA.

The evolution of regulatory law under the OSHAct has profoundly influenced other environmental legislation and especially the evolution of TSCA. This chapter addresses federal regulation, focusing on standard-setting, enforcement mechanisms, and Right-to-Know provisions.

The OSHAct requires OSHA to (1) encourage employers and employees to reduce hazards in the workplace and to implement new or improved safety and health programs; (2) develop mandatory job safety and health standards and enforce them effectively; (3) establish "separate but dependent responsibilities and rights" for employers and employees for the achievement of better safety and health conditions; (4) establish reporting and recordkeeping procedures to monitor job-related injuries and illnesses; and (5) encourage states to assume the fullest responsibility for establishing and administering their own occupational safety and health programs, which must be at least as effective as the federal program.

As a result of these responsibilities, OSHA inspects workplaces for violations of existing health and safety standards; establishes advisory committees; holds hearings; sets new or revised standards for control of specific substances, conditions, or use of equipment; enforces standards by assessing fines or by other legal means; and provides for consultative services for management and for employer and employee training and education. In all of its procedures, from the development of standards through their implementation and enforcement, OSHA guarantees employers and employees the right to be fully informed, to participate ac-

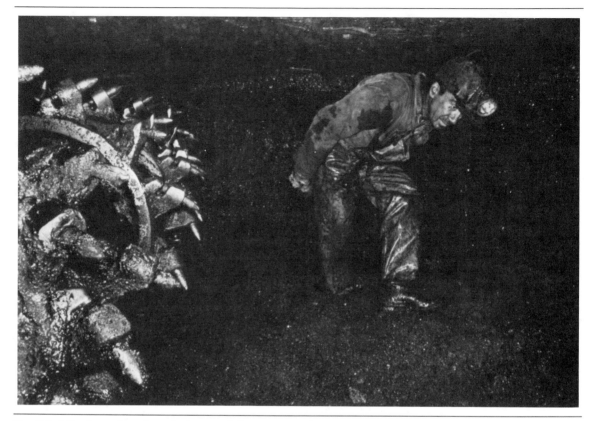

**Fig. 9-1.** Mine hazards such as the increased dust exposure from continuous mining machines are regulated by the Mine Safety and Health Administration (MSHA). (Photograph by Earl Dotter)

tively, and to appeal its decisions (although employees are limited somewhat in the latter activity).

The coverage of the OSHAct initially extended to all employers and their employees, except self-employed people; family-owned and -operated farms; state, county, and municipal workers; and workplaces already protected by other federal agencies or other federal statutes (Fig. 9-2). In 1979, however, Congress exempted from routine OSHA safety inspections approximately 1.5 million businesses with 10 or fewer employees. (Exceptions to this are allowed if workers claim there are safety violations.) Since federal agencies, such as the U.S. Postal Service, are not subject to OSHA regula-

tions and enforcement provisions, each agency is required to establish and maintain its own effective and comprehensive job safety and health program. OSHA provisions do not apply to state and local governments in their role as employers. OSHA requires, however, that any state desiring to gain OSHA support or funding for its own occupational safety and health program must provide a program to cover its state and local government workers that is at least as effective as the OSHA program for private employees.

OSHA can begin standard-setting procedures either on its own or on petitions from other parties, including the Secretary of Health and Human Services, NIOSH, state and local governments,

WHAT YOU NEED TO KNOW
ABOUT THE MINE SAFETY AND
HEALTH ADMINISTRATION
—James L. Weeks

The Mine Safety and Health Administration (MSHA) is designed to protect the approximately 350,000 miners engaged in the most dangerous industrial occupation in the United States. Historically, federal government intervention in mine safety and health was the responsibility of the U.S. Bureau of Mines in the Department of the Interior. The bureau was organized in 1910 for the purpose of conducting research into mine disasters and thereafter acquired increasing authority and responsibility to promote mine safety. This role culminated in the federal Coal Mine Health and Safety Act of 1969, which created the Mining Enforcement Safety Administration (MESA). This act was amended in 1977, at which time MESA's name was changed to the Mine Safety and Health Administration (MSHA), it was moved to the Department of Labor, and all mines (not only coal mines) were included under its jurisdiction.

MSHA's structure and function are similar to those of OSHA. In general, it is required to write and enforce regulations and employs a corps of inspectors to inspect mines. Citations carry penalties that mine operators may appeal in court, including the U.S. Supreme Court. Mine operators may request variances from standards and may receive technical assistance from MSHA or the Bureau of Mines. Miners have the right to request inspections and to participate in most aspects of rule-making and enforcement. They are promised protection from discrimination for engaging in activities protected by the act.

MSHA differs from OSHA in some important ways. Its enforcement powers are significantly greater, and it is part of a comprehensive and reasonably successful plan to prevent occupational lung diseases among coal miners.

With respect to enforcement, MSHA must inspect every mine on a regular basis. MSHA must inspect underground mines at least four times each year and surface mines twice each year. Inspectors have the authority on their own to close all or parts of mines if there is an imminent danger. Mine operators must submit for approval a mine plan, showing how they will control the principal hazards—methane, respirable coal mine dust, and danger from roof falls. All injuries and some accidents that do not produce injuries (such as fires, floods, and unplanned roof falls) must be reported to MSHA, not merely recorded and posted annually as under OSHA. Mine-specific data on injuries, accidents, and dust measurements are available. Mine operators must train miners in health and safety for 40 hours for new miners, and 8 hours annually thereafter. Mine operators must inspect and log the results of certain inspections for each work shift. Such regulations have resulted in a significant decline in underground and surface coal mine fatality rates from when the Coal Mine Act was passed in 1969 to the present (Fig. 9-3).

MSHA is also part of a comprehensive effort to control occupational lung diseases, such as coal workers' pneumoconiosis (commonly known as "black lung"). Mine operators as well as MSHA inspectors conduct surveillance of exposure to respirable dust and crystalline silica. For purposes of determining compliance with the exposure limit, underground mine operators must take five dust samples every 2 months at high-risk jobs and surface operators must take one sample every 2 months. MSHA is required to take samples annually.

Medical surveillance is also required. New miners must have a chest x-ray when first starting work as a miner; after this, operators must offer follow-up chest x-rays approximately every 5 years. Miners with positive films may exercise rights to medical removal, with a transfer to a less dusty job (see Chap. 22).

NIOSH is conducting a long-range prospective study of the occurrence and progression of black lung in relation to exposure to dust. The Bureau of Mines conducts research and development activities on control technologies for occupational health and safety hazards, such as respirable dust, methane, diesel exhaust, noise, fires and explosions and unsafe roofs. These efforts have resulted in a significant decline in exposure to respirable dust and in the occurrence of coal workers' pneumoconiosis.

The 1969 act created a novel federal government program to compensate miners who were totally disabled by pneumoconiosis. Largely because of difficulty in establishing a precise etiology for miners' respiratory disease, the black lung program is complex and controversial. By the mid-1980s approximately $1.6 billion in payments was being sent annually to recipients and their families. Initially, payments were made out of the general treasury and the program was administered by the Social Security Administration. Several amendments to the act moved the program to the Department of Labor, and payments are currently made by the miner's last mining employer or, if that employer cannot be found, out of a disability trust fund.

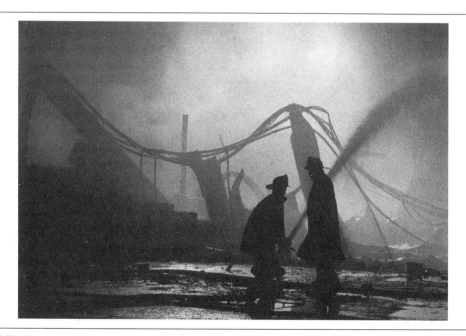

**Fig. 9-2.** OSHA's positive impact on general industry health and safety in the U.S. unfortunately does not extend to municipal workers such as firefighters. (Photograph by Marvin Lewiton)

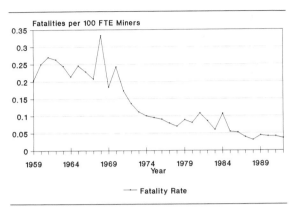

Fig. 9-3. Underground bituminous coal mine fatality rates, 1959 to 1991. FTE = full-time equivalent miners. (Source: Mine Safety and Health Administration)

any nationally recognized standards-producing organization, employer or labor representatives, or any other interested person. The standard-setting process involves input from advisory committees and from NIOSH. When OSHA develops plans to propose, amend, or delete a standard, it publishes these intentions in the *Federal Register*. Subsequently, interested parties have opportunities to present arguments and pertinent evidence in writing or at public hearings. Under certain conditions OSHA is authorized to set emergency temporary standards, which take effect immediately but expire within six months. OSHA must first determine that workers are in grave danger from exposure to toxic substances or new hazards and are not adequately protected by existing standards. Standards can be appealed through the federal courts, but filing an appeals petition will not delay the enforcement of the standard unless a court of appeals specifically orders it. Employers may make application to OSHA for a variance from a standard or regulation if they lack the means to comply readily with it or if they can prove that their facilities or methods of operation provide employee protection that is at least as effective as that required by OSHA.

OSHA requires employers of more than 10 employees to maintain records of occupational injuries and illnesses as they occur. All occupational injuries and diseases must be recorded if they result in death, one or more lost workdays, restriction of work or motion, loss of consciousness, transfer to another job, or medical treatment (other than first aid).

## Standard-setting and Obligations of the Employer and the Manufacturer or User of Toxic Substances

### Legal Background for OSHA Obligations

The OSHAct provides two general means of protection for workers: (1) a statutory general duty to provide a safe and healthful workplace, and (2) adherence to specific standards by employers. The act imposes on virtually every employer in the private sector a general duty "to furnish to each of his employees employment and a place of employment which are free from *recognized hazards* that are causing or are likely to cause death or serious physical harm. . . ." A recognized hazard may be a substance for which the likelihood of harm has been the subject of research, giving rise to reasonable suspicion, or a substance for which an OSHA standard may or may not have yet been promulgated. The burden of proving that a particular substance is a recognized hazard and that industrial exposure to it results in a significant degree of exposure is placed on OSHA. Since standard-setting is a slow process, protection of workers through the employer's general duty obligation is especially important, but it is crucially dependent on the existence of reliable health effects data.

The OSHAct addresses specifically the subject of toxic materials. It states, under Section 6(b)(5) of the act, that the Secretary of Labor (through OSHA), in promulgating standards dealing with toxic materials or harmful physical agents, shall set the standard that "most adequately assures, to the extent *feasible*, on the basis of the *best available evidence* that *no* employee will suffer material

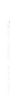

impairment of health or functional capacity, even if such employee has a regular exposure to the hazard dealt with by such standard for the period of his working life." By these words, one can see that the issue of exposure to toxic chemicals or carcinogens that have long latency periods, as well as to reproductive hazards, is covered by the act in specific terms.

Under Section 6(a) of the act, without critical review, OSHA initially adopted as standards, called permissible exposure limits (PELs), the 450 threshold limit values (TLVs) recommended by the American Conference of Governmental Industrial Hygienists (ACGIH) as guidelines for protection against the toxic effects of these materials. In the 1970s, under Section 6(b), OSHA set formal standards for asbestos, vinyl chloride, arsenic, dibromochloropropane (DBCP), coke oven emissions, acrylonitrile, lead, cotton dust, and a group of 14 carcinogens. In the 1980s OSHA regulated benzene, ethylene oxide, and formaldehyde as carcinogens and asbestos more rigidly as a carcinogen at 0.2 fibers per cubic centimeter. In the 1990s OSHA regulated cadmium, bloodborne pathogens, glycol ethers, and confined spaces. OSHA also lowered the PEL for formaldehyde from 1 ppm to 0.75 ppm (over an 8-hour period) and issued a process safety management rule. Under consideration are standards for methylenedianiline, hexavalent chromium, and silica. Also imminent are new reporting requirements.

The burden of proving the hazardous nature of a substance is placed on OSHA, as is the requirement that the proposed controls are technologically feasible. The necessarily slow and arduous task of setting standards substance by substance makes it impossible to realistically deal with 13,000 toxic substances or 2,000 suspect carcinogens on NIOSH lists. Efforts have been made to streamline the process by proposing generic standards for carcinogens.

The inadequacy of the 450 TLVs adopted under Section 6(a) of the act is widely known. The TLVs originated as guidelines recommended by the ACGIH to protect the *average* worker from either recognized acute effects or easily recognized chronic effects. The standards are based on animal toxicity data or the limited epidemiologic evidence available at the time of the establishment of the TLVs. They do not address the sensitive populations within the workforce or those with prior exposure or existing disease, nor do they address the issues of carcinogenicity, mutagenicity, and teratogenicity. These standards were adopted en masse in 1971 as a part of the consensus standards that OSHA adopted along with those dealing primarily with safety.

As an example of the inadequacy of protection offered by the TLVs, the 1971 TLV for vinyl chloride was set at 250 ppm, whereas the later protective standard (see below) recommended no greater exposure than 1 ppm (as an average over 8 hours)—a level still recognized as unsafe but the limit that the technology could detect. Another example is the TLV for lead, which was established at 200 $\mu$g per cubic meter, whereas the later lead standard was established at 50 $\mu$g per cubic meter, also recognizing that that level was not safe for all populations, such as pregnant women or those with prior lead exposure. The ACGIH has updated its TLV list every two years. While useful, an updated list would have little legal significance unless formally adopted by OSHA. OSHA did try, unsuccessfully, to adopt an updated and new list of PELs in its Air Contaminants Standard in 1989. (See discussion below.)

Under Section 6(b) of the OSHAct, new health standards dealing with toxic substances were to be established utilizing the mechanism of an open hearing and subject to review by the U.S. Circuit Courts of Appeals. The evolution of case law associated with the handful of standards that OSHA promulgated through this section is worth considering in detail. The courts addressed the difficult issue of what is adequate scientific information necessary to sustain the requirement that the standards be supported by "substantial evidence on the record as a whole." The cases also addressed the extent to which economic factors were permitted or required to be considered in the setting of the standards, the meaning of "feasibility," the question of whether a cost-benefit analysis was required or permitted, and, finally, the extent of the jurisdiction of OSHAct in addressing different degrees of risk.

### The Carcinogens Standard

In an early case challenging OSHA's authority to regulate 14 carcinogens, the District of Columbia Circuit Court of Appeals first addressed the issue of substantial evidence. For 8 of the 14 carcinogens, there were no human (epidemiologic) data. Industry challenged OSHA's ability to impose controls on employers in the absence of human data. Here the court expressed its view that some facts, such as the establishment of human carcinogenic risk from animal data, were on the "frontiers of scientific knowledge" and that the requirement for standards to be supported by substantial evidence in these kinds of social policy decisions could not be subjected to the rigors of other kinds of factual determinations. Thus, OSHA was permitted to require protective action against substances known to produce cancer in animals but with no evidence of producing cancer in humans. It was not until 1980 that the U.S. Supreme Court in the benzene case (see below) placed limits on the extent of OSHA's policy determination on carcinogenic risk.

### The Asbestos Standard

In the challenge to OSHA's original asbestos standard—in which asbestos was regulated as a classic lung toxin and not as a carcinogen—the Industrial Union Department of AFL-CIO unsuccessfully challenged the laxity of the standard, claiming that OSHA improperly weighed economic considerations in its determination of feasibility. OSHA indeed was permitted to consider economic factors in establishing feasibility. The District of Columbia Circuit Court of Appeals went on to state, however, that a standard might be feasible even if some employers were forced out of business, as

long as the entire asbestos-using industry was not disrupted. In 1986, OSHA revised the standard from 2 fibers per cubic centimeter to 0.2 fibers per cubic centimeter, thus finally acknowledging it as a carcinogen.

### The Vinyl Chloride Standard

In the industry challenge to OSHA's regulation of vinyl chloride at 1 ppm, the Second Circuit Court of Appeals reiterated OSHA's ability to make policy judgments with regard to matters "on the frontiers of scientific knowledge" when it declared that there could be no safe level for a carcinogen. In addition, the court said that since 1 ppm was the lowest feasible level, OSHA was permitted to force employers to comply even though it had performed no formal risk assessment or knew how many tumors would be prevented by the adoption of this protective level. Another noteworthy aspect of the case was the recognition that OSHA could act as a "technology forcer" and require controls not yet fully developed at the time of the setting of the standard.

### The Lead Standard

Protection from lead exposure had been provided through the TLV of 200 µg per cubic meter. This level was long recognized as inadequate for workers who accumulated lead in their body tissues and for women (and possibly men) who intended to have children. As a result, based on the limits of technological feasibility, OSHA promulgated a new standard that permitted no exposure greater than 50 µg per cubic meter, averaged over an 8-hour period. In addition, because this was still unsafe for many workers, OSHA also provided that workers be removed with pay and employment security if their blood lead levels exceeded 50 µg per deciliter of blood *or* if there were grounds to remove them based on risks to their reproductive system. The legality and necessity of this additional provision, known as Medical Removal Protection (MRP), was unsuccessfully challenged by the Lead Industries Association. (MRP has since been required in a limited way in the cotton dust and benzene standards.) OSHA specifically provided that workers in workplaces with air-lead levels over an "action level" of 30 μg per cubic meter have the benefit of a continuing medical surveillance program, including periodic sampling of blood-lead levels and removal from exposure above the action level after finding of blood levels in an individual worker above 50 μg per deciliter, with job return when the worker's level fell below 40 μg per deciliter.

Removal could also be triggered by other medical conditions deemed to create an unusual risk for lead exposure (for example, pregnancy). OSHA provided that workers' pay and seniority be maintained by the employer during any periods of medical removal (up to 18 months), even if such removal entailed sending the worker home. In actual practice, many employers have reduced the ambient air-lead level well below 50 μg per cubic meter, which results in the removal of fewer workers.

### The Benzene Standard

Following the first serious successful industry challenge of an OSHA benzene standard in the Fifth Circuit Court of Appeals, the U.S. Supreme Court, in a controversial and divided majority opinion, chided OSHA for not attempting to evaluate the benefits of changing the permissible exposure level for benzene from 10 ppm (the former TLV) to 1 ppm. The Court argued that OSHA is obligated to regulate only "significant risks" and that without a risk assessment of some kind OSHA could not know whether the proposed control addressed a significant risk. The Court was careful to state that it was not attempting to "statistically straitjacket" the agency, but that at a minimum the benefits of regulation needed to be addressed to meet the substantial evidence test. The Court did not give useful guidance concerning what constituted a significant risk. It stated that a risk of death of 1 in 1,000 was clearly unacceptable, while a risk of 1 in 1 billion might be tolerated. This three-orders-of-magnitude range, of

course, represents the area on which the arguments have always been centered.

The implications of the benzene decision for future standards will depend on the nature of the particular OSHA administration. There is little question that had OSHA performed a risk assessment for benzene at the time, it could have argued that the risk it was attempting to address was actually significant. The precise requirement and nature of a risk assessment sufficient to meet the substantial evidence test remains quite unclear. In late 1985, OSHA again proposed to lower the permissible exposure limit from 10 ppm to 1 ppm, and in 1987, the standard was set at that level. OSHA, however, after intervention by the Office of Management and Budget (OMB), declined to establish a short-term exposure limit.

The petroleum industry argued in the benzene case that not only must a risk assessment be performed, but a cost-benefit analysis must also be done in which the risks of exposure must be balanced against the benefits of the chemical. The question, however, was not decided in the benzene case but was addressed in a later case challenging OSHA's cotton dust standard. The Supreme Court not only acknowledged that cotton dust did represent a significant risk but also indicated that a cost-benefit balancing was neither required nor permitted by the OSHAct since Congress had already struck the balance heavily in favor of worker health and safety.

### The Generic Carcinogen Standard

In 1980 OSHA promulgated a generic carcinogen standard by which questions of science policy, already settled as law in cases dealing with other standards, were codified in a set of principles. During the process of developing the generic carcinogen standard, OSHA and NIOSH developed lists of chemical substances that would probably be classified as suspect carcinogens. Each agency composed a list of approximately 250 substances. Thus far, OSHA has declined to formally list any substance under the carcinogen standard.

In setting or revising standards for formaldehyde, ethylene oxide, asbestos, and benzene, the agency has proceeded to act as if the generic carcinogen standard did not exist, thus following the historically arduous and slow path to standard-setting.

### Emergency Temporary Standards (ETS)

In Section 6(c), the OSHAct authorizes OSHA to set emergency temporary (6 month) standards for toxic exposures constituting a "grave danger" on publication in the *Federal Register* and without recourse to a formal hearing.

Before OSHA lowered its permanent standard for asbestos from 2 to 0.2 fibers per cubic centimeter, it attempted to protect workers by promulgating an ETS at 0.5 fibers per cubic centimeter. In 1984 the Fifth Circuit Court of Appeals denied OSHA the ETS, arguing that the cost involved defeated the requirement that the ETS be "necessary" to protect workers.

### Short-Term Exposure Limits

Short-term exposures to higher levels of carcinogens are generally considered more hazardous than longer exposures to lower levels. OSHA issued a new standard for exposure to ethylene oxide (EtO) in 1984, but excluded a short-term exposure limit (STEL) that had originally been prepared, in deference to objections from the Office of Management and Budget. Ralph Nader's Health Research Group sued the Secretary of Labor in 1986 over OSHA's continuing failure to issue the STEL. In 1987 the District of Columbia Circuit Court of Appeals ordered OSHA to establish a STEL for ethylene oxide by March 1988. OSHA complied by setting a STEL of 5 ppm over a 15-minute period.

### The Air Contaminants Standard

It is obvious that the slow arduous process of promulgating individual health standards under Section 6(b)(5) of the OSHAct could never catch up with advances in scientific knowledge concerning the toxicity of chemicals. The ACGIH has updated their TLV list every 2 years, and while not as protective as workers and their unions would have liked, the recent updated lists did advance protection over the 1969 list that OSHA adopted into law in 1971. In 1989 OSHA decided to update the original list in a single rule-making effort through the 6(b) standard revision route. The agency issued more protective limits for 212 substances and established limits for 164 chemicals that were previously unregulated. Neither industry nor labor was satisfied with the standards. Industry, while giving general support, objected to the stringency of some of the PELs. Labor objected to their laxity, citing NIOSH recommendations not adopted, and generally objected to the rush-it-through process. The Eleventh Circuit Court of Appeals vacated the standard on July 7, 1992, ruling that OSHA failed to establish that a significant risk of material health impairment existed for each regulated substance [required by the benzene decision], and that the new exposure limit for each substance was feasible for the affected industry. OSHA decided not to appeal the decision to what it perceived as a conservative Supreme Court. Thus, the original and inadequate TLV list remains in effect and 164 new substances remain unregulated. OSHA, however, could argue that those 164 substances are "recognized hazards" and enforceable through OSHA's general duty clause (see below).

### The Consumer Product Safety Act

The implementation of the OSHAct, with burden of proof placed on the government, cannot keep pace with the proliferation of chemicals in the work environment, and it is certainly no safeguard against general environmental contamination or consumer product hazards. The burden of proving "unreasonable risk" in consumer products is placed on the Consumer Product Safety Commission, which has taken action on only a few chemical problems, including fluorocarbons, vinyl chloride, and formaldehyde in foam insulation.

*The Toxic Substances Control Act*

TSCA enables the EPA to require data *from industry* on the production, use, and health and environmental effects of chemicals. The EPA may regulate by requiring labeling, setting tolerances, or banning completely and requiring repurchase or recall. The EPA may also order a specific change in chemical process technology. In addition, TSCA gives aggrieved parties, including consumers and workers, specific rights to sue for damages under the act, with the possibility of awards for attorneys' fees. (This feature was missing in the OSHAct.)

Under TSCA, the EPA must regulate "unreasonable risks of injury to human health or the environment." EPA has issued a regulation for worker protection from asbestos at the new OSHA limit of 0.2 fibers per cubic centimeter, which applies to state and local government asbestos abatement workers not covered by OSHA. The EPA has declared formaldehyde a "probable carcinogen" and will proceed to regulate it to supplement OSHA's actions. Although the potential for regulating workplace chemicals is there, the EPA has not been aggressive in this area. Between 1977 and 1990, of the 22 regulatory actions taken on existing chemicals, 15 addressed polychlorinated biphenyls (PCBs). Only regulations pertaining to asbestos, hexavalent chromium, and metal-working fluids had a strong occupational exposure component.

One strength of TSCA is its ability to shift onto the producer the requirement to prove that a substance is safe to the extent that exposure to it does not present an "unreasonable risk of injury to human health or the environment." Used together, the OSHAct and TSCA provide potentially comprehensive and effective information-generation and standard-setting authority to protect workers. In particular, the information-generation activities under TSCA can provide the necessary data to have a substance qualify as a "recognized hazard," which, even in the absence of specific OSHA standards, must be controlled in some way by the employer to meet the general duty obligation under the OSHAct to provide a safe and healthful workplace.

The potentially powerful role of TSCA regulation was seriously challenged by the Fifth Circuit Court of Appeals in October 1991, when it overturned the EPA's omnibus asbestos phase-out rule issued in July 1989. The Court, which is generally unfriendly to environmental, occupational health, and consumer product regulation, argued that under TSCA, the EPA should have considered alternatives to a ban that would have been less burdensome to industry. The case was not appealed to the Supreme Court and the EPA is considering what steps to take next to resurrect the regulatory authority of TSCA. Pressure is mounting for reauthorization of the act.

## Enforcement Activities

Standard-setting, of course, is only the beginning of the regulatory process. For a regulatory system to be effective, there must be a clear commitment to the enforcement of standards. Under OSHA, a worker can request workplace inspection if the request is in writing and signed. Anonymity is preserved on request. When an inspector visits a workplace, a representative of the workers can accompany the inspector on the "walk-around."

If specific requests for inspections are not made, OSHA makes random inspections of those workplaces with worse-than-average safety records. However, the inspection frequency is low. Furthermore, firms with significant exposures to chemicals may not be routinely inspected, simply because their record for *injuries* (which dominate the reported statistics) is good.

Inspections are usually conducted without advance notice, but an employer may insist that OSHA inspectors obtain a court order before entering the workplace. In 1987, federal OSHA had fewer than 1,100 inspectors (compared to 1,300 in 1980) and state agencies fewer than 2,000. Clearly not all 5 million workplaces covered by the act could be inspected.

OSHA can fine employers up to $1,000 for each violation of the act that is discovered during workplace inspection and up to $10,000 if the violation is willful or repeated. Management can appeal violations, amounts of fines, methods of correcting hazards, and deadlines for correcting hazards (abatement dates). Workers can appeal only deadlines. All appeals are processed through the Occupational Safety and Health Review Commission, which also was established by the OSHAct.

The act requires OSHA to encourage states to develop and operate their own job safety and health programs. State programs, when "at least as effective" as the federal program, can take over enforcement activities. Once a state plan is approved, OSHA funds half of its operating costs. About 20 state plans, which OSHA monitors, are in effect. State safety and health standards under such approved plans must keep pace with OSHA standards, and state plans must guarantee employer and employee rights as does OSHA.

During the 1980s OSHA inspection policy resulted in directives given to the field staff to deemphasize general duty violations. In addition, inspectors were actually evaluated by the managers of the establishments they inspected. Follow-up inspections after violations were often restricted to checks by telephone. Thus, incentives for aggressive inspection activity were not great under the Reagan and Bush administrations.

## The Right to Know

The transfer of information regarding workplace exposure to toxic substances has received considerable public attention. It is clear that workers need an accurate picture of the nature and extent of probable chemical exposures to decide whether to enter or remain in a particular workplace. Workers also need to have knowledge regarding past or current exposures to be alert to the onset of occupational disease. Regulatory agencies must have timely access to such information if they are to devise effective strategies to reduce disease and death from occupational exposures to toxic substances. Accordingly, laws designed to facilitate this flow of information have recently been promulgated at the federal, state, and local levels. Indeed, the Right to Know has become a political battleground in many states and communities and has been the subject of intensive organizing efforts by business, labor, and citizen-action groups.

In essence, the Right to Know embodies a democratization of the workplace. It is the mandatory sharing of information between management and labor. Through a variety of laws, manufacturers and employers are directed to disclose information regarding toxic substance exposure to workers, to unions in their capacity as worker representatives, and to governmental agencies charged with the protection of public health. The underlying rationale for these directives is the assumption that this transfer of information will prompt activity that will improve worker health.

Although the phrase *Right to Know* is a useful generic designation, it is an inadequate description of the legal rights and obligations that govern the transfer of workplace information on toxic substances. One cannot have a meaningful *right* to information unless someone else has a corresponding *duty* to provide that information. Thus, a worker's Right to Know will be secured by requiring a manufacturer or employer to disclose. The disclosure requirement can take a variety of forms, and the practical scope of that requirement may depend on the nature of the form chosen. In particular, a duty to disclose only such information as has been requested may provide a narrower flow of information than a duty to disclose all information, regardless of whether it has been requested. The various rights and obligations in the area of toxics information transfer may be grouped into three categories. Though they share a number of similarities, each category is conceptually distinct.

1. *The duty to generate or retain information* refers to the obligation to compile a record of certain workplace events or activities or to maintain such a record for a specified period of time

if it has been compiled. An employer may, for example, be required to monitor its workers regularly for evidence of toxic exposures (biologic monitoring) and to keep written records of the results of such monitoring.

2. *The right of access* (and the corresponding duty to disclose on request) refers to the right of a worker, a union, or an agency to request and secure access to information held by a manufacturer or employer. Such a right of access would provide workers with a means of obtaining copies of biologic monitoring records pertaining to their own exposure to toxic substances.

3. Finally, *the duty to inform* refers to an employer's or manufacturer's obligation to disclose, without request, information pertaining to toxic substance exposures in the workplace. An employer may, for example, have a duty—independent of any worker's exercise of a right to access—to inform workers whenever biologic monitoring reveals that their exposure to a toxic substance has produced bodily concentrations of that substance above a specified level.

In general, the broadest coverage is found in rights and duties emanating from the OSHAct. By its terms, that act is applicable to all *private* employers and thus covers the bulk of workplace exposures to toxic substances. Most private industrial workplaces are also subject to the National Labor Relations Act (NLRA). Farmworkers and workers subject to the Railway Labor Act, however, are exempt from NLRA coverage. TSCA provides a generally narrower scope. While many of the act's provisions apply broadly to both chemical manufacture and use, its information transfer requirements extend only to chemical manufacturers, processors, and importers. On the state level, the relevant coverage of the various rights and duties will depend on the specifics of the particular state and local law defining them. In general, common law rights and duties will evidence much less variation than will those created by state statute or local ordinance.

Under OSHA's Hazard Communication Standard, employers have a duty to inform workers of the identity of substances with which they work through labeling the product container and disclosing to the purchaser (the employer) using material safety data sheets (MSDSs).

Employers are under no obligation to amend inadequate, insufficient, or incorrect information provided by the manufacturer. Employers must, however, transmit certain information to their employees: (1) information on the standard and its requirements, (2) operations in their work areas where hazardous chemicals are present, and (3) the location and availability of the company's hazard communication program. The standard also requires that workers must be trained in (1) methods to detect the presence or release of the hazardous chemicals; (2) the physical and health hazards of the chemicals; (3) protective measures, such as appropriate work practices, emergency procedures, and personal protective equipment; and (4) the details of the hazard communication program developed by the employer, including an explanation of the labeling system and the MSDSs, and how employees can obtain and use hazard information.

Rights and duties governing toxic information transfer in the workplace can originate from a variety of sources. Some will be grounded in state common law, while others will arise out of specific state statutes or local ordinances. Although the states have been increasingly active in this field, the primary source of regulation is federal law. Most federal regulation in this area emanates from three statutes: the OSHAct, TSCA, and NLRA, administered by the National Labor Relations Board (NLRB).

The scope of a particular right or duty will depend on many factors. The first, and perhaps most important, is the nature of the information required to be transferred.

*Scientific* information refers to data concerning the nature and consequences of toxic substance exposures. These data, in turn, can be divided into three subcategories:

1. *Ingredients information* provides the worker with the identity of the substances to which he or she is exposed. Depending on the circumstances, this information may involve only the generic classifications of the various chemicals involved or may include the specific chemical identities of all chemical exposures and the specific contents of all chemical mixtures.
2. *Exposure information* encompasses all data regarding the amount, frequency, duration, and route of workplace exposures. This information may be of a general nature, such as the results of ambient air monitoring at a central workplace location, or may take individualized form, such as the results of personal environmental or biologic monitoring of a specific worker.
3. *Health effects information* indicates known or potential health effects of workplace exposures. This information may be general data regarding the effects of chemical exposure, usually found in an MSDS or a published or unpublished workplace epidemiologic study, or it may be individualized data, such as worker medical records compiled as a result of medical surveillance.

The federal standard preempts state Right-to-Know laws in the worker notification area in a minority of jurisdictions; it would appear to be coexistent with state requirements in most jurisdictions, although its stated intent is to preempt all state efforts.

Under OSHA's Medical Access Rule, an employer may not limit or deny an employee access to his or her own medical or exposure records. The current OSHA regulation, promulgated in 1980, grants employees a general right of access to medical and exposure records kept by their employer. Furthermore, it requires the employer to preserve and maintain these records for 30 years. There appears to be some overlap in the definitions of *medical* and *exposure* records, because both may include the results of biologic monitoring. Medical records, however, are generally defined as those pertaining to "the health status of an employee,"

while the exposure records are defined as those pertaining to "employee exposure to toxic substances or harmful physical agents."

The employer's duty to make these records available is a broad one. The regulations provide that upon any employee request for access to a medical or exposure record: "the employer *shall* assure that access is provided in a reasonable time, place, and manner, but in no event later than 15 days after the request for access is made."

An employee's right of access to medical records is limited to records pertaining specifically to that employee. The regulations allow physicians some discretion as well in limiting employee access. The physician is permitted to "recommend" to the employee requesting access that the employee (1) review and discuss the records with the physician; (2) accept a summary rather than the records themselves; or (3) allow the records to be released instead to another physician. Furthermore, where information in a record pertains to a "specific diagnosis of a terminal illness or a psychiatric condition," the physician is authorized to direct that such information be provided only to the employee's designated representative. Although these provisions were apparently intended to respect the physician-patient relationship and do not limit the employee's ultimate right of access, they could be abused. In situations in which the physician feels loyalty to the employer rather than the employee, the physician could use these provisions to discourage the employee from seeking access to his or her records.

Similar constraints do not apply to employee access to exposure records. Not only is the employee assured access to records of his or her own exposure to toxic substances, but the employee is also assured access to the exposure records of other employees "with past or present job duties or working conditions related to or similar to those of the employee." In addition, the employee has access to all general exposure information pertaining to the employee's workplace or working conditions and to any workplace or working condition to which he or she is to be transferred. All information in exposure records that cannot be correlated with a particular employee's exposure is accessible.

One criticism of the OSHA regulation is that it does not require the employer to compile medical or exposure information but merely requires employee access to such information if it is compiled. The scope of the regulation, however, should not be underestimated. The term *record* is meant to be "all-encompassing," and the access requirement appears to extend to all information gathered on employee health or exposure, no matter how it is measured or recorded. Thus, if an employer embarks on any program of human monitoring, no matter how conducted, he or she must provide the subjects access to the results. This access requirement may serve as a disincentive for employers to monitor employee exposure or health, if it is not clearly in the employer's interest to do so.

The regulations permit the employer to deny access to "trade secret data which discloses manufacturing processes . . . or . . . the percentage of a chemical substance in a mixture," provided that the employer: (1) notifies the party requesting access of the denial; (2) if relevant, provides alternative information sufficient to permit identification of when and where exposure occurred; and (3) provides access to all "chemical or physical agent identities including chemical names, levels of exposure, and employee health status data contained in the requested records."

The key feature of this provision is that it ensures employee access to the precise identities of chemicals and physical agents. This access is especially critical for chemical exposures. Within each "generic" class of chemicals, there are a variety of specific chemical compounds, each of which may have its own particular effect on human health. The health effects can vary widely within a particular family of chemicals. Accordingly, the medical and scientific literature on chemical properties and toxicity is indexed by specific chemical name, not by generic chemical class. To discern any meaningful correlation between a chemical exposure and a known or potential

health effect, an employee must know the precise chemical identity of that exposure. Furthermore, in the case of biologic monitoring, the identity of the toxic substance or its metabolite is itself the information monitored.

Particularly in light of the public health emphasis inherent in the OSHAct, disclosure of such information does not constitute an unreasonable infringement on the trade secret interests of the employer. In general, chemical health and safety data are the least valuable to an employer of all the "proprietary" information relevant to a particular manufacturing process.

TSCA imposes substantial requirements on chemical manufacturers and processors to develop health effects data. TSCA requires testing, premarket manufacturing notification, and reporting and retention of information. TSCA imposes no specific medical surveillance or biologic monitoring requirements. However, to the extent that human monitoring is used to meet more general requirements of assessing occupational health or exposure to toxic substances, the data resulting from such monitoring are subject to an employer's recording and retention obligations.

The EPA has promulgated regulations requiring general reporting on approximately 350 chemicals, including information related to occupational exposure. The EPA administrator may require the reporting and maintenance of those data "insofar as known" or "insofar as reasonably ascertainable." Thus, if monitoring is undertaken, it must be reported. The EPA appears to be authorized to require monitoring as a way of securing information that is "reasonably ascertainable."

In addition to the general reports required for specific chemicals listed in the regulations, the EPA has promulgated rules for the submission of health and safety studies required for more than 400 substances. A health and safety study includes "[a]ny data that bear on the effects of chemical substance on health." Examples are "[m]onitoring data, when they have been aggregated and analyzed to measure the exposure of humans . . . to a chemical substance or mixture." Only data that are "known" or "reasonably ascertainable" need be reported.

Records of "significant adverse reactions to [employee] health" must be retained for 30 years under Section 8(c). A recently promulgated rule implementing this section defines significant adverse reactions as those "that may indicate a substantial impairment of normal activities, or long-lasting or irreversible damage to health or the environment." Under the rule, human monitoring data, especially if derived from a succession of tests, would seem especially reportable. Genetic monitoring of employees, if some basis links the results with increased risk of cancer, also seems to fall within the rule.

Section 8(e) imposes a statutory duty to report "immediately . . . information which supports the conclusion that [a] substance or mixture presents a substantial risk of injury to health." In a policy statement issued in 1978, the EPA interpreted "immediately" in this context to require receipt by the agency within 15 working days after the reporter obtains the information. Substantial risk is defined exclusive of economic considerations. Evidence can be provided by either designed, controlled studies or undesigned, uncontrolled studies, including "medical and health surveys" or evidence of effects in workers. In the EPA's rule for Section 8(c), Section 8(e) is distinguished from Section 8(c) in that "[a] report of substantial risk of injury, unlike an allegation of a significant adverse reaction, is accompanied by information which reasonably supports the seriousness of the effect or the probability of its occurrence." Human monitoring results indicating a substantial risk of injury would thus seem reportable to the EPA. Either medical surveillance or biologic monitoring data would seem to qualify.

Section 14(b) of TSCA gives the EPA authority to disclose from health and safety studies the data pertaining to chemical identities, except for the proportion of chemicals in a mixture. In addition, the EPA may disclose information, otherwise classified as a trade secret, "if the Administration determines it necessary to protect . . . against an unreasonable risk of injury to health." Monitoring data thus seem subject to full disclosure.

In addition to the access provided by OSHA regulations, individual employees may have a limited right of access to medical and exposure records under federal labor law. Logically, the right to refuse hazardous work (see below), inherent in Section 7 of the NLRA and Section 502 of the Labor Management Relations Act, carries with it the right of access to the information necessary to determine whether or not a particular condition is hazardous. In the case of toxic substance exposure, this right of access may mean access to all information relevant to the health effects of the exposure and may include access to both medical and exposure records. These federal labor law provisions are clearly not adequate substitutes for OSHA access regulations, however, as there is presently no systematic mechanism for enforcing this right.

*Collective* employee access, however, is available to unionized employees through the collective bargaining process. In four recent cases, the NLRB has held that unions have a right of access to exposure and medical records so that they may bargain effectively with the employer regarding conditions of employment. Citing the general proposition that employers are required to bargain on health and safety conditions when requested to do so, the NLRB adopted a broad policy favoring union access: "Few matters can be of greater legitimate concern to individuals in the workplace, and thus to the bargaining agent representing them, than exposure to conditions potentially threatening their health, well-being, or their very lives."

The NLRB, however, did not grant an unlimited right of access. The union's right of access is constrained by the individual employee's right of personal privacy. Furthermore, the NLRB acknowledged an employer's interest in protecting trade secrets. While ordering the employer in each of the four cases to disclose the chemical identities of substances to which the employer did not assert a trade secret defense, the NLRB indicated that employers are entitled to take reasonable steps to safeguard "legitimate" trade secret information. The NLRB did not delineate a specific mechanism for achieving the balance between union access and trade secret disclosure. Instead, it ordered the parties to attempt to resolve the issue through collective bargaining. Given the complexity of this issue and the potential for abuse in the name of "trade secret protection," the NLRB may find it necessary to provide further specificity before a workable industrywide mechanism can be achieved.

The legal avenues for worker and agency access to information relevant to workplace exposures to toxic substances have been expanded substantially. Despite certain inadequacies in the current laws and despite current attempts by OSHA to narrow the scope of some of these even further, access to toxics data remains broader than it has ever been. By itself, however, this fact is of little significance. The mere existence of information-transfer laws will mean little unless those laws are employed aggressively to further the objective of the Right to Know: the protection of workers' health. Currently, the various rights and duties governing toxics information transfer in the workplace present workers, unions, and agencies with a magnificent opportunity. The extent to which they seize this opportunity over the next few years will be a true measure of their resolve to bring about meaningful improvement in the health of the American worker.

## The Right to Refuse Hazardous Work

The NLRA and the OSHAct provide many employees a limited right to refuse to perform hazardous work. When properly exercised, this right protects an employee from retaliatory discharge or other discriminatory action for refusing hazardous work and incorporates a remedy providing both reinstatement and back pay. The nature of this right under the NLRA depends on the relevant collective bargaining agreement, if there is one. Non-union employees and union employees whose collective bargaining agreements specifically exclude health and safety from a no-strike clause have the *collective* right to stage a safety walkout under Section 7 of the NLRA. If they choose to walk out based on a good-faith belief that working conditions are unsafe, they will be protected from any employer retaliation. Union employees who are subject to a comprehensive collective bargaining agreement may avail themselves of the provisions of Section 502 of the NLRA. Under this section, an employee who is faced with "abnormally dangerous conditions" has an *individual* right to leave the job site. The right may be exercised, however, only where the existence of abnormally dangerous conditions can be objectively verified. Both exposure and medical information are crucial here.

Under a 1973 OSHA regulation, the right to refuse hazardous work extends to all employees, *individually,* of private employers, regardless of the existence or nature of a collective bargaining agreement. Section 11(c) of the OSHAct protects an employee from discharge or other retaliatory action arising out of his or her "exercise" of "any right" afforded by the act. The Secretary of Labor has promulgated regulations under this section defining a right to refuse hazardous work in certain circumstances: where an employee reasonably believes there is a "real danger of death or serious injury," there is insufficient time to eliminate that danger through normal administrative channels, and the employer has failed to comply with an employee request to correct the situation.

Under the federal Mine Safety and Health Act, miners also have rights to transfer from unhealthy work areas if there is exposure to toxic substances or harmful physical agents or if there is medical evidence of pneumoconiosis.

## OCCUPATIONAL HEALTH AND SAFETY IN BRITISH COLUMBIA

The discussion in this chapter has focused on occupational health and safety in the United States. The system in British Columbia, Canada, is very different and provides another useful perspective.

### Profile of British Columbia

British Columbia is Canada's third largest province, with 1.4 million workers out of a total population of 3 million people. Thirty-seven percent of the workers are unionized, compared to about 15 percent in the United States. Ninety-five percent of the firms have 50 or fewer workers and 75 percent have five or fewer workers. In 1991 120 fatalities were reported from occupational accidents and 63 from occupational disease, and 200,000 claims were made for workplace injuries. Scaled up to U.S. size, this is equivalent to 8,400 accidental deaths, 4,500 deaths from occupational disease, and 14,000,000 claims for workplace injuries a year. This contrasts with the 2,800 deaths for accidents and illnesses and 6,000,000 injuries annually in the United States reported by the Bureau of Labor Statistics (BLS). Critical of the BLS, the National Safety Council reports 9,900 accidental deaths annually in the United States, and health and safety professionals argue that the BLS figures are gross underestimates of both occupational diseases and injuries.

### Administrative Structure

In British Columbia the occupational safety and health regulation and enforcement activities and the workers' compensation system are part of the same administrative public corporation, the Workers' Compensation Board (WCB), and both are funded by assessed premiums on employers (see box in Chap. 10). The WCB is administered by a 15-member Board of Governors representing employers, labor, and the public.

The Occupational Safety and Health (OSH) Division employs 374 persons, which would translate into 28,000 for the U.S. (compared to the actual number of 2,000). The annual OSH Division budget is $22 million (U.S.), which would translate into a $1.5 billion budget for OSHA, five times larger than the $290 million actually allocated in the U.S.

### Legal Structure/Basis

Two provincial pieces of legislation—the Workers' Compensation Act (see box in Chap. 10) and the Workplace Act—provide the basis for the WCB's standard-setting authority. The federal Workplace Hazardous Materials Information System (WHMIS) serves as the basis for provincial Right-to-Know activities. The Board of Governors, with the assistance of a tripartite Regulation Advisory Committee, is responsible for adopting regulations. Thereafter, there is no legal mechanism to challenge the regulations in the British Columbia system. Thus, the development of regulatory policy by the courts discussed for the U.S. system does not exist in British Columbia for all practical purposes.

### Enforcement

Historically, British Columbia standards have not been technology-forcing. For example, until 1993 the lead standard permitted exposures up to 150 $\mu g/m^3$, compared to the U.S. standard of 50 $\mu g/m^3$. First-instance citations (mandatory citations upon discovery of violations) exist only for a few, mostly safety, violations. There is pressure to include specific chemical exposures and failure of the employer to provide an adequate health and safety program/health and safety committee in the list of violations requiring first-instance citations. The OSH Division can and does impose penalty assessments; criminal penalties are rarely issued. Labor is generally dissatisfied with the extent of worker participation in the WCB's enforcement and appellate process (see below).

Inspection activity is targeted by a combination of industry hazard classification, payroll, and compensation claims. The construction and logging industries are targeted for special attention because of their high hazard nature and poor claims experience. In general, the OSH Division lacks sufficient data collection and analysis activities, criticisms often levied against OSHA and the U.S. Bureau of Labor Statistics. Accident reports often lack the information needed to focus prevention activities because they rarely describe the cause of the accident, but rather the cause of the injury.

### Consultation

Most inspection activity results in warnings and corrective orders, rather than monetary penalties on the employer. Some consultation and technical assistance is usually rendered by the inspector at the time of the inspection or closing conference. At times, inspectors are confused about the balance of their enforcement and consultant/facilitator roles. The OSHA Division provides engineering guidance and advice to employers in the form of technical bulletins and on-site consultation. The WCB also has an active first-aid certification program for workplace-based first-aid attendants, which is required by law. The WCB does not charge a fee for consulting advice or laboratory assistance/analysis.

### Worker Participation

Workplace safety and health programs are currently required to be provided by all employers with a workforce of 50 or more employees (i.e., 5 percent of the firms). For especially hazardous industries, the programs are required for employers with a workforce of 20 or more employees. Joint workplace safety and health committees are considered an essential part of these programs. There is pressure to expand the number of firms required to have such a program. Workers complain that they need more authority in the functions of the safety and health committees. They also complain of the inadequacy of the antidiscrimination provisions of the current law/structure, such as in relation to the right to refuse hazardous work.

### Comment

Features of the BC system suggest U.S. OSHA reforms, such as mandatory health and safety programs and committees, greater recognition of occupational disease, a streamlined standard-setting process, and a linkage of compensation and prevention activities. Support for OSHA reform is gaining momentum. The past 22 years have revealed both the strengths and weaknesses of the U.S. system, including the need to strengthen the connection between OSHA and EPA through the OSHAct and TSCA.

## OCCUPATIONAL HEALTH AND SAFETY IN THE EUROPEAN COMMUNITY

Occupational health and safety legislation in individual European countries is in a great deal of flux following the formation of the European Community (EC). The Single European Act establishing the EC was enacted in 1987. Article 118A of the Act addresses employment, working conditions, and occupational health and safety and provides a streamlined legislative process for the development of health and safety directives, and minimum health and safety standards, affecting about 150 million people. The EC directives have the force of law and set down general principles for the protection of workers. However, individual countries are obligated to adopt national legislation implementing these principles, with important technical details concerning enforcement and administration left to the EC Member States. Thus, programs may be expected to differ considerably among countries in the near future, although these differences may narrow as European integration becomes a reality. Therefore, it may be some time before innovations in health and safety regulatory approaches can be evaluated and serve as models for OSHA reform in the U.S. Nevertheless, the EC experience may be important for the United States because (1) with the formation of a North American Free Trade Zone the problems of harmonization of legislation may be similar, (2) the EC will be an important force in occupational safety and health, and (3) the EC will be a major trade competitor. The recent agreement between the EC and the European Free Trade Association (EFTA) countries to set up a free trade area means that the EC safety and health legislation is applicable in 19 countries in Europe.

### Legal Structure/Basis

Regulatory activity within the EC can include regulations, decisions, directives, resolutions, and recommendations, varying from commitments in principle to legally enforceable mandates on the Member States. The European Commission, aided by expert groups, makes formal proposals to the EC Council of Ministers. The Council, in consultation with the Economic and Social Committee and the European Parliament, adopts, rejects, or modifies the proposals and issues directives by a qualified majority vote of 54 of a total of 76. Individual Member States can maintain or introduce more stringent measures for the protection of working conditions than those contained in the directives.

Until 1988 EC directives, for example, those dealing with occupational exposure limits (OELs) for vinyl chloride, lead, asbestos, and benzene, were very detailed and prescriptive. Short-term exposure limits (STELs) were also specified. Af-

ter Article 118A was enacted, a more general Framework Directive 89/391/EEC "on the introduction of measures to encourage improvements in the safety and health of workers at work" was issued. This directive is the centerpiece of EC health and safety policy and establishes the guiding principles upon which more specific directives are issued. There are now seven so-called daughter directives to the Framework Directive. Directive 90/394/EEC addresses carcinogens at work. Directive 88/642/EEC addresses risks related to exposure to chemicals and physical and biologic agents at work and has led to some 27 indicative limit values (ILVs), which are advisory only. The enforcement of those limits is left to the individual regulatory systems and styles of the various Member States. Nevertheless, there is a preferred hierarchy of control for "dangerous substances and products." In order of preference, these are substitution of dangerous substances by safe or less dangerous ones, the use of closed systems or processes, local extractive ventilation, general workplace ventilation, and personal protective equipment.

Other EC directives address biologic agents, asbestos, video display terminals, work equipment, personal protective equipment, and handling of loads. In 1988 the European Parliament adopted a Resolution on Indoor Air Quality, which is receiving attention for development into a directive.

All Commission proposals are submitted to the Advisory Committee on Safety, Hygiene and Health Protection at Work, composed of representatives of employers, workers, and governments. Initially, an expert scientific group evaluates all scientific data relevant to protecting workers from a particular substance. The Commission makes a proposal and solicits Advisory Committee opinion. The Technical Progress Committee votes on the proposal. The limit values may be adopted as indicative values by Commission directive. If the exposure limits are mandatory, they are adopted by the Council of Ministers as directives pursuant to Article 118A. Compared with the United States, relatively few health standards have been established, reflecting the slowness of the tripartite process of participatory standard-setting envisioned by the EC.

The Framework Directive applies to all sectors of employment activity, both public and private. However, it excludes the self-employed and domestic workers. Employers have a general "duty to ensure the safety and health of workers in every aspect related to the work" (Article 5.1). Among the employer's specific duties are: (1) to evaluate risks in the choice of work equipment, chemicals, and design of the workplace; (2) to integrate prevention into the company's operations at all levels; (3) to inform workers and/or their representatives of risks and preventive measures taken; (4) to consult workers and/or their representatives on all health and safety matters; (5) to train workers on workplace hazards; (6) to provide appropriate health surveillance; (7) to protect especially sensitive risk groups; and (8) to keep records of accidents and injuries.

### Enforcement

Labor inspectorates in each Member State have the responsibility for ensuring employer compliance with health and safety requirements. However, beyond broad principles and duties, the EC Directives are often advisory and not many specific requirements are enforceable through EC channels. Attempts to place binding obligations on national governments to establish the necessary institutional elements to support proper implementation of safety and health regulations, such as health and safety technical centers, have been unsuccessful. The Commission established a Committee of Senior Labor Inspectors in 1982 to facilitate information exchange to encourage coordination of

policy. Recently, the Commission submitted a proposal for a regulation setting up a European Agency for Safety and Health at Work.

The Commission does have the authority to bring action against a Member State for failure to adhere to EC Directives, but the Commission does not yet have the institutional capacity to monitor compliance effectively. Action against a Member State has never been brought, however, even though some countries have not adopted national legislation to conform with specific mandatory exposure limits, for example, noise. No uniform policy on enforcement of standards, such as first-instance citations or penalty levels, exists at this time and it is likely that intercountry variations will be allowed.

### Worker Participation

The Framework Directive calls for "the informing, consultation, balanced participation . . . and training of workers and their representatives" to improve health and safety at the workplace (Article 1.2). The Directive gives workers the rights to consult in advance with their employers on health/safety matters, to be paid for safety activities, to communicate with labor inspectors, and to exercise the right to refuse dangerous work. Safety committees are not explicitly addressed by the Directive. Similarly, joint decision making is not mandated.

### Comment

The health and safety policy of the EC is evolving. While the general principles declared in EC legislation and specific directives are laudable, it remains to be seen what course implementation will take and how much variation will continue to exist among the different Member States. European regulatory systems tend to be more advisory. On the other hand, they are also more participatory, inviting decision making on a tripartite basis.

## CHILD LABOR: A CASE OF INADEQUATE REGULATION
Letitia Davis

A 16-year-old female cook, while moving a container of hot grease in a fast-food restaurant, was badly burned when she slipped, spilling the grease over her ankles, arms, chest, and face.

A 17-year-old boy working to compact boxes at a supermarket caught his head and shoulders in the trash compactor and was crushed to death.

An 11-year-old boy working on his family farm slipped into a grain wagon and was suffocated under 3 tons of corn.

A 15-year-old female migrant laborer was hospitalized with pesticide poisoning after being sent into a field that was still wet from crop spraying.

While occupational health and safety professionals have long been aware of the problems of child labor and its attendant workplace health risks, it was not until the economic recession of the late twentieth century that these professionals recognized that the problem was not limited to developing nations but was present throughout the world (Fig. 9-4). In response, the International Labor Organization (ILO), concerned about child labor since its inception, initiated a major new effort in 1993 called the International Program for the Elimination of Child Labor. The objective is that all countries abolish nonvoluntary child labor with the emergency priority to abolish child labor in dangerous types of employment, industries, and occupations and to protect all children who have to work.

As an example of the nature of the problem some of the developing information about child labor in the U.S. is instructive. Work is a pervasive feature of adolescent life in the U.S. According to federal statistics, nearly 4.5 million adolescents were employed sometime during 1988—on farms, in fast-food restaurants, in grocery stores, in nursing homes, and in factories. These official figures are believed to substantially underestimate the actual number of working children, particularly those who work under illegal conditions—in sweat shops, at home doing industrial work, in fields still wet with pesticides performing farm work.

To protect children from oppressive and dangerous working conditions, both state and federal laws regulate the hours of employment and occupations in which minors (persons less than 18 years old) can work. Nevertheless, working children routinely confront health and safety hazards on the job, and each year substantial numbers of children are killed and injured in the workplace. Unfortunately there is virtually nothing but anecdotal information to estimate the prevalence and incidence of either acute or chronic occupational disease among child laborers.

According to Occupational Safety and Health Administration (OSHA) records, at least 100 children suffer fatal occupational injuries in the U.S. each year; many of these deaths occur among those working in prohibited occupations. These figures do not include children working on farms. It is estimated that as many as 300 children are killed each year in the U.S. while doing farm work.

Nonfatal injuries far outnumber fatal injuries, and occupational injuries contribute significantly to the ongoing epidemic of injuries to adolescents. The U.S. Government Accounting Office identified almost 59,000 injuries among minors in the 2-year period 1987 to 1988, based on workers' compensation data from 26 states. New York State reported that more than 1,300 children under the age of 18 received workers' compensation for occupational injuries from 1980 to 1987. Over 40 percent of the reported injuries caused permanent disability.

Workers' compensation claims reveal only part of the problem. Not all industries, most notably agriculture, are covered by the workers' compensation system. In addition, although many injuries may result in a sufficient number of lost workdays to qualify for compensation, many children, especially those working illegally, may never enter the system. Based on a U.S. national sample of emergency department visits in 1992, more than 64,000 teenagers 14 to 17 years of age are treated for work-related injuries each year in hospital emergency departments. According to a Massachusetts study, between 7 and 13 percent of all medically treated injuries to teenagers 14 to 17 years of age occurred at work, and occupational injuries accounted for 26 percent of injuries with known location among 17-year-olds. A survey of teens in Saskatchewan identified work-related injuries as the leading cause of injuries to 16- and 17-year olds.

Work can be an important and positive experience for young people. However, it is crucial to assure that youth are working in situations where their health and well-being are protected. The prevention of illnesses and injuries among working children requires the combined efforts of government officials, business people, health workers, educators, and family members.

The existing laws restricting types of jobs and hours worked by minors should be improved and vigorously enforced. Better information is essential to guide prevention efforts. Surveillance systems should be established, and etiologic research to identify specific risk factors should be performed. Both school-based and workplace-based education regarding job health and safety is essential. In a recent study, fewer than half of interviewed teenagers with occupational injuries reported that they received any prior training on how to avoid injury at work. Engineering changes that reduce or eliminate hazards, generally considered the most effective means of prevention, may play an even more critical role for young people.

Clinicians treating children and adolescents, who in some states sign work permits for minors, have a potentially important role to play in providing guidance regarding safe, healthful, and appropriate work. This guidance should involve not only providing information about child labor laws, but also working with children and their parents to assess both the work environment and the fit between that environment and the child. The occupational health community, which, in recent years, has focused primarily on adult workers, faces the challenge of developing prevention strategies that take into account the development characteristics, both physical and psychosocial, of children and adolescents, as well as the environments in which they work.

### Bibliography

Am J Ind Med, vol. 24, no. 3, 1993. (*Entire volume is devoted to child labor and health issues.*)

Pollack SH, Landrigan PJ. Child labor in 1990: Prevalence and health hazards. Ann Rev Public Health 1990; 11:359–75.

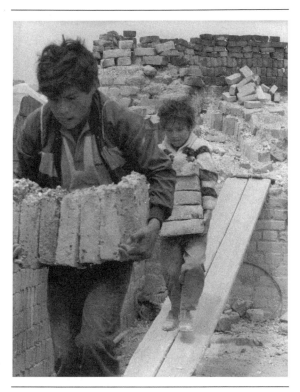

**Fig. 9-4.** Child labor is poorly regulated internationally. (Courtesy of International Labor Office.)

## Bibliography

Ashford A. Crisis in the workplace: Occupational disease and injury, a report to the Ford Foundation. Cambridge: MIT Press, 1976.
*A policy-focused overview of science, law, economics, and public policy dealing with occupational disease and injury.*

Ashford NA, Caldart CC. Technology, law and the working environment. New York: Van Nostrand Reinhold, 1991.
*A textbook of law and policy with court cases, law review articles, and policy analysis.*

Caldart C. Promises and pitfalls of workplace right-to-know. Semin Occup Med 1986; 1:81–90.
*Legal and ethical considerations concerning the transfer of toxic substances information in the workplace.*

Commission of the European Community. Social Europe: Health and safety at work in the European community. Brussels, February 1990.
*Text and explanation of EC Directives and legislation pertaining to occupational safety and health.*

Hecker S. Part 1: Early initiatives through the Single European Act. New Solutions 1993;3:59–69; Part 2: The Framework Directive: Whither harmonization? New Solutions 1993; 4:57–67.
*A critical look at EC health and safety policy.*

Hunter WJ. EEC legislation in safety and health at work. Ann Occup Hyg 1992; 36:337–47.
*Commentary by the Director of the EC Commission on Health and Safety.*

LaDou J. ed. Occupational health law. New York: Marcel Dekker, 1981.
*A collection of articles written by attorneys on various aspects of occupational health law.*

Rest KM, Ashford NA. Occupational safety and health in British Columbia: An administrative inventory. Cambridge: Ashford Associates, 1992.
*A review of Occupational Health and Safety Administration in British Columbia.*

U.S. Congress, Office of Technology Assessment. Preventing illness and injury in the workplace. Washington, D.C.: U.S. Government Printing Office, 1985.
*An update and comprehensive assessment of the political problems faced in preventing occupational disease and injury.*

U.S. Department of Labor. Protecting people at work, a reader in occupational safety and health. Washington, D.C.: U.S. Government Printing Office, 1980.
*A collection of short articles on various aspects of occupational health and safety written by authors in government, industry, labor, and academia.*

# 10
# Workers' Compensation

Leslie I. Boden

Workers' compensation is a legal system designed to shift some of the costs of occupational injuries and illness from workers to employers. Workers' compensation laws generally require employers or their insurance companies to reimburse part of injured workers' lost wages and all of their medical and rehabilitation expenses. This chapter describes workers' compensation systems in the United States, discusses the role of the physician, and analyzes the very difficult problems of compensating victims of chronic occupational disease.

## Historical Background

Prior to the passage of the first workers' compensation act in 1911, workers generally bore the costs of their work-related injuries. Injured workers and their families were forced to cope with lost wages and medical care and rehabilitation costs. Under the common law[1] workers had to prove in a court of law that their injuries were caused by employer negligence to recover these costs.

For several reasons it was extremely difficult for workers to win such negligence suits. The injured worker had the burden of proof and had to show that the employer was negligent, that there was a work-related injury, and that the negligence caused the injury. To sustain this burden of proof, the worker had to hire a lawyer (which was costly) and often had to rely on the testimony of fellow

workers (who, along with the suing worker, might be fired for their part in the suit). All of this was enough to deter most workers from bringing suit.

In addition, employers had three very strong defenses that usually protected them from losing negligence suits when they were brought:

*Doctrine of contributory negligence:* If employees were found by judges to have contributed in any way to their injuries, they were barred from winning.

*Fellow-servant rule:* If fellow employees' actions were found by judges to have caused the injuries, employers were not considered responsible.

*Assumption of risk:* If injuries were found to be caused by common hazards or unusual hazards of which workers were aware, they could not recover damages.

In the late nineteenth century, these defenses were widely used, and fewer than one-third of all employees who brought such negligence suits won any award. In one case a New York woman lost her arm when it was caught between the unguarded gears of the machine she had been cleaning. Unguarded gears were in violation of the laws of New York State at that time, and prior to the accident she had complained to her employer about this hazard. Still, her employer refused to guard the machine. After the accident the worker sued her employer, but the court held that she could not be compensated; she had obviously known about the hazard and of her own free will

---

[1]The common law is a body of legal principles developed by judicial decisions rather than by legislation. Legislation (statutory law) can override these judge-made laws.

had continued to work. This evidence showed that she had "assumed the risk" and that her employer was not responsible for the consequences.

The inability to hold employers responsible for their negligent actions persisted in the face of the high and increasing toll of occupational death and disability at the beginning of this century. After a disabling injury, workers and their families were left largely to their own resources and to assistance from relatives, friends, and charities.

By 1920 some efforts had been made to provide better means of compensation to injured workers and their families. Some of the larger corporations had established private compensation schemes, and several states and the federal government had enacted employers' liability acts. These laws retained the basic common law liability scheme but reduced the role of the three common law defenses.

Most injured workers, however, were not able to take advantage of these changes. They were not employed by companies with private programs and were still not able to win negligence suits. There was growing support for a major change in the law, not only from the social reformers of the Progressive Era but also from major corporations. It is not entirely clear why the major corporations were promoting legislative reform. Some observers believe that industrial leaders realized that the burden of workplace injuries could spur independent, radical political action by workers. Others believe that employer defenses were already being weakened by legislation and that corporate leaders feared a rapid rise in the costs of employer liability suits. Still others argue that the basic motives to support new laws were humanitarian in nature.

These pressures gave rise to the passage of the first workers' compensation law in New York State in 1911. Many other states rapidly followed suit, and by 1920 all but eight states had passed similar laws, although most did not cover occupational disease. Mississippi, in 1948, was the last state to establish a workers' compensation system.

## Description of Workers' Compensation

Workers' compensation provides income benefits, medical payments, and rehabilitation payments to workers injured on the job as well as benefits to survivors of fatally injured workers. There are 50 state and three federal workers' compensation jurisdictions, each with its own statute and regulations.

While state and federal systems are different in numerous ways, they have several characteristics in common. Benefit formulas are prescribed by law. Generally, medical care and rehabilitation expenses are fully covered, but lost wages are only partially reimbursed. Employers are legally responsible for paying benefits to injured workers. Some large employers pay these benefits themselves, but most pay yearly premiums to insurance companies, which process all claims and pay compensation to injured workers. Workers' compensation is a no-fault system. Injured workers do not need to prove that their injuries were caused by employer negligence. In fact, employers are generally required to pay benefits even if the injury is entirely the worker's fault.

The change to a no-fault system was established to minimize litigation. For a worker to qualify for workers' compensation benefits, only three conditions must be met: There must be an injury or illness, the injury or illness must "arise out of and in the course of employment," and there must be medical costs, rehabilitation costs, lost wages, or disfigurement. Clearly, these conditions are much easier for the injured worker to demonstrate than is employer negligence. For example, if a worker falls at work and breaks a leg, all three conditions are easily demonstrated. Unusual cases sometimes arise in which the question of the relationship of an injury to employment is difficult to resolve, and there may be questions about when a worker is ready to return to work. Such issues may result in litigation, but they are the exception, not the rule. In most cases a worker files a claim for compensation with the employer, and the claim is accepted and paid either directly by the employer or by the workers' compensation insurance carrier of the employer.

The following case is typical of the events that follow many minor claims for workers' compensation:

Mr. Fisher had a painful muscle strain while lifting a heavy object at work on Monday afternoon. He went to the plant nurse and described the injury. He was sent home and was unable to return to work until the following Friday morning. On Tuesday the nurse sent an industrial accident report to the workers' compensation carrier and a copy to the state workers' compensation agency. Two weeks after he returned to work Mr. Fisher received a check from the insurance company covering part of his lost wages—as mandated by state statute—and all of his out-of-pocket medical expenses related to the muscle strain.

Workers' compensation has wider coverage than did the common law system. Under workers' compensation workplace injuries and illnesses are compensable even if they are only in part work-related. Suppose, for example, a worker with preexisting chronic low back pain becomes permanently disabled as a result of lifting a heavy object at work. In this case the worker's preexisting condition might just as easily have been aggravated by carrying out the garbage at home, but the fact that the disabling event occurred at work is generally sufficient for compensation to be awarded.

Cases in which an occupational injury or illness becomes disabling as a result of non-work exposures are more complicated. A worker with non-disabling silicosis may leave a granite quarry job for warehouse work. Without further exposure the silicosis will probably never become disabling. However, the worker begins to smoke cigarettes and loses lung function until partial disability results. In most states this worker should receive compensation from the owner of the granite quarry if the work relationship can be demonstrated.

Generally, diseases are considered eligible for compensation if occupational exposure is the *sole cause* of the disease, is *one of several causes* of the disease, was *aggravated* by or aggravates a non-occupational exposure, or *hastens* the onset of disability (Table 10-1). Several states, including California and Florida, allow disability to be apportioned between occupational and nonoccupational causes. While at first this may seem like a sensible approach, apportionment creates some difficult decisions for workers' compensation administrators. Many disabilities are not additively caused by two separable exposures. With silica exposure or cigarette exposure alone, the worker in the above example would not have become disabled. Often, as in the case of lung cancer caused by asbestos exposure and smoking, the contribution to disability or death of two factors is many times greater than that of one alone. Such issues make the apportionment of disability very difficult if not impossible.

**Table 10-1.** Likelihood of compensation, by source of preexisting condition and source of ultimate disability

| Source of ultimate disability | Source of preexisting condition | |
| --- | --- | --- |
| | Work-related | Non-work-related |
| Work-related | Compensable | Generally compensable |
| Non-work-related | Generally compensable | Not compensable |

Source: Adapted from PS Barth, HA Hunt. Workers' compensation and work-related illnesses. Cambridge, MA: MIT Press, 1980.

When workers' compensation was introduced, workers gained a swifter, more certain, and less litigious system than existed before. In return, however, covered workers waived their right to sue employers through common law. They also accepted lower awards than those given by juries in negligence suits: Workers' compensation provides no payments for "pain and suffering" as there might be in a common law settlement. In addition, disability payments under workers' compensation are often much less than lost income, especially for more severe injuries.

The United States does not have a unified workers' compensation law. Each state has its own system with its own standards and idiosyncracies. In addition, federal systems cover federal employees, longshoremen and harbor workers, and workers employed in the District of Columbia. Almost all states require employers either to purchase insurance or to demonstrate that they are able to pay any claims that might be made by their employees. In most states private insurers underwrite workers' compensation insurance paid for by premiums from individual employers. In some states a non-profit state workers' compensation fund has been established; the state government therefore acts as an insurance carrier, collecting premiums and disbursing benefits. State funds seem to be very effective in delivering benefits: They disburse a higher percentage of premiums in the form of benefits than do private insurance carriers.

## Common Law Suits

While workers' compensation coverage bars workers from suing their employers at common law, it generally does not bar suits against a third party whose negligence caused a worker's injury or illness. If workers are injured by faulty machinery, workers' compensation coverage does not bar them from suing the manufacturer(s) of the equipment. Similarly, workers whose asbestosis is work-related may sue the asbestos manufacturer. In both circumstances, of course, negligence must be dem-

onstrated. In a case decided in the U.S. Eighth Circuit Court of Appeals it was ruled that the manufacturer of an "unreasonably dangerous" product, asbestos, was negligent because it did not warn exposed workers of the hazards of being exposed to this product.

## The Role of the Physician in Workers' Compensation

Workers' compensation is basically a legal system, not a medical system. The decision points for claims in this complex system are shown in Fig. 10-1. If a claim is rejected by the workers' compensation carrier or self-insured employer, it will generally be necessary for the injured worker to hire a lawyer. The worker's lawyer may then bargain with the lawyers for the insurance carrier in an attempt to settle the dispute informally. If this

**Fig. 10-1.** Decision points for workers' compensation claims.

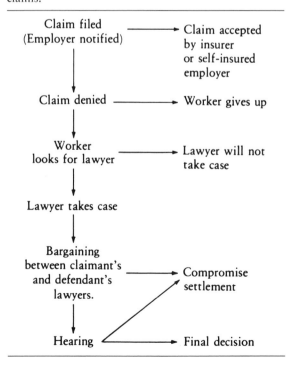

bargaining does not result in agreement, the claim must either be dropped or taken before an administrative board—a quasi-judicial body established by state statute—for a hearing. To the worker or to a physician who may be called to testify in such a hearing, such a proceeding may be indistinguishable from a formal trial: Witnesses are sworn, rules of evidence are followed, and testimony is recorded.

As a part of this legal proceeding medical questions are often raised. There may be disagreement about the degree of disability of a worker, when an injured worker is ready to return to work, or whether a particular injury or illness is work-related. To settle these disputes physicians may be called on to give their medical opinions about employees' disabilities. Many physicians do not like to testify in such hearings, and most are not prepared by their training or experience to assume this role. Their expertise may be challenged; moreover, they may be confused by the different meanings of legal and medical terminology.

In workers' compensation, decisions are based on legal definitions, and the legal distinction between disability and impairment is often unclear to physicians (see Chap. 11). A physician called in to testify about whether or not a worker is permanently and totally disabled may understand total disability as a state of physical helplessness and may therefore testify that the injured worker is not totally helpless. However, this standard is not what a workers' compensation board would apply; the term *disability* as used in workers' compensation proceedings means that wages have been lost, while *total disability* means that the injured worker loses wages as a result of not being able to perform gainful employment. This definition is in contrast to total *impairment,* which might imply that the injured worker could, in addition, not feed him- or herself or get out of bed. For example, a worker who has been exposed to silica at work may have substantially reduced pulmonary function and therefore impairment. However, if the worker continues to work at the same job, no wages have been lost and therefore no disability payment is made. Many states, however, offer specified payments for disfigurement or losses of sight, hearing, or limbs, with compensation based on impairment and not on disability (Table 10-2).

While physicians may feel that they have not been trained adequately for their role in workers' compensation, workers do need their support in this area. A lack of assistance may mean unnecessary financial hardship for the victim of an occupational injury or disease. The best way a physician can help identify a work-related disease or injury is by taking an occupational history (see Chap. 3). If the physician suspects a work-related disease or injury, the patient should be informed of the right to receive workers' compensation and the time limits on such claims. (The period for filing a claim generally begins when the patient is informed that the disease is work-related.) Physicians should also suggest the possibility of seeking legal counsel, and they can provide direct help by completing any required reports, including descriptions of the illness or injury and why it is believed to be work-related. The extent of probable disability should also be noted (see Chap. 11). None of these steps requires testimony before a workers' compensation board; most workers' compensation claims are either paid without contest or settled without a hearing.

The National Institute for Occupational Safety and Health has published *A Guide to the Work-Relatedness of Disease* (rev. ed., 1979; edited by S Kusnetz and MK Hutchison). It proposes that such a determination be made on the basis of evidence of disease, epidemiologic data, evidence of exposure, and validity of testimony. A primary care physician may be the only person willing and able to provide documentation for an employee wishing to file a workers' compensation claim. Support for valid compensation claims not only assists injured workers but also helps to ensure that employers and their insurance carriers will shoulder the costs that result from workplace hazards. If these costs are not paid under workers' compensation, they will be borne by workers and

Table 10-2. Income benefits for scheduled injuries in selected jurisdictions (as of January 1, 1993)*

| Jurisdiction | Location of injury | | | | |
| | Arm at shoulder | Hand | Thumb | First finger | Foot |
|---|---|---|---|---|---|
| Alabama | $ 48,840 | $ 37,400 | $13,640 | $ 9,460 | $ 30,580 |
| California | 62,345 | 46,028 | 7,595 | 3,360 | 35,668 |
| Connecticut | 239,928 | 193,788 | 73,055 | 41,526 | 144,572 |
| Delaware | 81,958 | 72,122 | 24,587 | 16,391 | 72,122 |
| Georgia | 56,250 | 40,000 | 15,000 | 10,000 | 43,250 |
| Illinois | 157,481 | 122,710 | 46,909 | 26,805 | 103,870 |
| Mississippi | 45,436 | 34,077 | 13,631 | 7,952 | 28,398 |
| New York | 124,800 | 97,600 | 30,000 | 18,400 | 82,000 |
| North Carolina | 105,080 | 88,400 | 33,150 | 19,890 | 63,648 |
| Washington | 54,000 | 48,600 | 19,440 | 12,150 | 37,800 |
| Wisconsin | 76,000 | 60,800 | 8,320 | 9,120 | 38,000 |
| Federal employees | 389,651 | 304,727 | 93,666 | 57,448 | 256,020 |
| U.S. longshoremen | 224,996 | 175,958 | 54,086 | 33,172 | 147,834 |

*Amounts in table reflect maximum potential entitlement.
Source: Reprinted with the permission of the Chamber of Commerce of the United States of America from Analysis of Workers' Compensation 1993. © 1993 Chamber of Commerce of the United States of America.

their families or by all of us through our share of the costs of third-party medical payments, welfare, Social Security, and other public support programs.

## The Adequacy of Workers' Compensation for Occupational Injuries

The fundamental problems of the common law scheme were that litigation was a necessary element of compensation and that it was very difficult for workers to win suits against their employers. Even when workers won negligence suits, payments were made long after they were injured, and a large amount of each settlement was diverted for legal fees. Today workers with minor injuries covered by workers' compensation generally can expect to receive payments promptly and without a contest. In fact, fewer than 10 percent

of all claims for occupational injuries—as opposed to occupational diseases—are contested.

Under workers' compensation, insurance carriers or self-insured employers have the right to contest a claim. A claim may be contested because the injury is not considered work-related, for example, or because the claim is for a larger settlement than the insurer is willing to pay. However, in most injury cases the employer or insurance carrier has little incentive to contest because proof of eligibility is easy, and the potential gain to the insurer of postponing or eliminating small payments is not enough to offset the legal costs of pursuing a claim. For expensive injury claims such as permanent total disability and death claims, insurance companies are much more likely to contest. Even if they do not win, a contest enables them to keep the settlement money temporarily, invest it, and receive investment income until the case is closed and the claimant paid. Since a contest delays the date of payment, this investment income is an incentive to contest even those cases that the insurer is very likely to lose. The higher the potential settlement, the stronger the incentive to contest. This analysis is supported by the fact that claims for permanent disability and death are contested five times more frequently than are claims for temporary disability.

Aside from the incentives to contest major claims, several other important problems can be cited in the more than 50 workers' compensation systems in the United States. In theory, workers' compensation should cover all employees; however, many states exempt agricultural employees, household workers, or state and municipal employees. Another problem is that, while compensation systems generally provide replacement for close to two-thirds of lost wages for temporary disability, benefits for victims of permanent disability are characterized by low maximum weekly ceilings and low statutory limits on total benefits, with the worker generally receiving the smaller of two-thirds of lost wages or the state maximum benefit. The maximum weekly benefit provided varies widely among the jurisdictions: The highest, on January 1, 1993, was for federal employees ($1,249) and the lowest was in Mississippi ($227) (Table 10-3). Many jurisdictions do not provide for cost-of-living adjustments, so that a person injured 30 years ago but still disabled may receive total disability payments of only $10 to $20 a week. They also do not account for the increased wages that would have been earned if the employee had continued to work.

Table 10-3. Maximum weekly benefits for total disability provided by workers' compensation statutes of selected states (as of January 1, 1993)

| Jurisdiction | Fraction of worker's wage | Maximum weekly benefit (to nearest dollar) |
|---|---|---|
| Alabama | $2/3$ | 400 (SAWW) |
| Alaska | $4/5$ of worker's spendable earnings | 700 |
| California | $2/3$ | 336 |
| District of Columbia | $2/3$ | 647 (SAWW) |
| Florida | $2/3$ | 425 (SAWW) |
| Iowa | $4/5$ of worker's spendable earnings | 755 (200% of SAWW) |
| Massachusetts | $2/3$ | 543 (SAWW) |
| Michigan | $4/5$ of worker's spendable earnings | 441 (90% of SAWW) |
| Mississippi | $2/3$ | 227 |
| New Hampshire | $2/3$ | 633 (150% of SAWW) |
| New York | $2/3$ | 350 ($2/3$ of SAWW) |
| North Carolina | $2/3$ | 442 (110% of SAWW) |
| Ohio | 72% first 12 weeks, then $2/3$ | 460 (SAWW) |
| Pennsylvania | $2/3$ | 475 (SAWW) |
| Texas | $7/10$ | 456 (SAWW) |
| West Virginia | $7/10$ | 405 (SAWW) |
| Federal employees | $2/3$ or $3/4$* | 1249 |
| U.S. longshoremen | $2/3$ | 721 (twice NAWW) |

Key: SAWW = state's average weekly wage; NAWW = national average weekly wage.
*Maximum is $3/4$ if one dependent or more.
Source: Reprinted with the permission of the Chamber of Commerce of the United States of America from Analysis of Workers' Compensation 1993, © 1993 Chamber of Commerce of the United States of America.

# Rising Workers' Compensation Medical Costs

In the period from 1975 to 1985 workers' compensation medical costs grew more than general medical care costs (Fig. 10-2). From 1980 to 1985 workers' compensation medical costs rose at an average annual rate of 14.7 percent, compared to an annual increase of 9.8 percent in other systems. If this trend has continued, the disparity in cost growth probably has widened since 1985.

A recent study provides additional evidence that workers' compensation medical costs are even more of a problem than non–workers' compensation costs. The Minnesota Department of Labor and Industry analyzed medical cost data from a matched sample of claims from Minnesota's largest workers' compensation insurer, the Liberty Mutual Insurance Company, and the major non–workers' compensation insurer, Blue Cross/Blue Shield [1]. The results are fascinating—and consistent with the data on rapidly rising workers' compensation costs.

The Minnesota study found that workers' compensation medical charges were generally higher than Blue Cross charges for the same types of in-juries. Disparities were greatest where medical care providers had the most discretion, for back injuries. They were smallest where treatment options were limited, for lacerations and fractures.

Table 10-4, Part A, shows the ratio of average workers' compensation charges to non–workers' compensation charges for all injuries and for four common types of workplace injuries. For all injuries in the Minnesota sample, workers' compensation charges were 75 percent higher on average than non–workers' compensation charges. Workers' compensation paid about one-third more to treat fractures but 2½ times as much to treat back injuries.

The averages displayed in Part A do not account for factors that may affect treatment costs but are not part of the two-payment systems. These factors include such claimant characteristics as age, gender, and urban/rural residence. Part B displays the ratios in Part A after adjusting for these claimant characteristics; it shows that, with patient characteristics accounted for, medical care for workers' compensation injuries costs more than for non–workers' compensation injuries. Averaged over all injuries, workers' compensation treatment is more than twice as expensive. As in

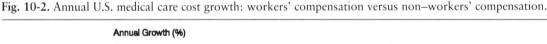

Fig. 10-2. Annual U.S. medical care cost growth: workers' compensation versus non–workers' compensation.

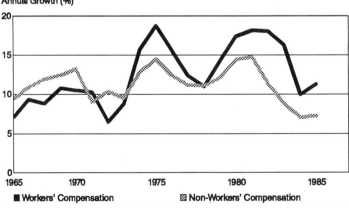

**Table 10-4.** Ratio of workers' compensation medical charges to non–workers' compensation charges

| Injury type | Ratio |
| --- | --- |
| **Part A** **Average charges** | |
| All injuries | 1.75 |
| Back injuries | 2.49 |
| Sprains and strains | 2.23 |
| Lacerations | 1.55 |
| Fractures | 1.34 |
| **Part B** **Charges controlled for patient characteristics** | |
| All injuries | 2.40 |
| Back injuries | 2.43 |
| Sprains and strains | 2.37 |
| Lacerations | 1.39 |
| Fractures | 1.18 |
| **Part C** **Charges controlled for patient characteristics and utilization** | |
| All injuries | 2.04 |
| Back injuries | 2.30 |
| Sprains and strains | 1.95 |
| Lacerations | 1.55 |
| Fractures | 1.00 |

Source: Minnesota Department of Labor and Industry (1990); and L Thornquist. Health care costs and cost containment in Minnesota workers' compensation program. John Burton's Workers' Compensation Monitor 1990; 3:3–26.

Part A, fractures cost only a little more, but back injuries continue to cost almost 2½ times as much in workers' compensation.

Differences in the two systems may cause differential medical care utilization; that is, medical care providers may use more diagnostic tests on workers' compensation claimants and may hospitalize them more frequently. On the other hand, the type and intensity of medical care services used may reflect differences in injury severity. We do not know if this is attributable to inherent differences between workers' compensation and non–workers'

compensation medical care. Controlling for differential utilization may in part control for the systemic differences in the two systems. To measure these differences conservatively, data in Part C of Table 10-4 display workers' compensation medical costs relative to non–workers' compensation costs, controlling for both claimant characteristics and medical care utilization.[2] The patterns displayed in Table 10-4, Parts A and B, persist, even when controlling for provider and service use.

The disparities between workers' compensation and non–workers' compensation medical costs appear to reflect a substantial difference between payments for the same injuries in the two systems. Alternatively, they might reflect unusually high workers' compensation medical costs in Minnesota relative to other states' systems. The Minnesota study suggests that this is not true [1]. The authors compared Minnesota's workers' compensation medical costs with those of six other states (Iowa, Missouri, Illinois, Pennsylvania, Oregon, and Wisconsin) and found them similar. Also, Minnesota's average 1984 workers' compensation medical costs ranked eleventh of 42 states; its 1980 to 1985 medical cost growth rate ranked as twenty-first of 43 states [2]. Minnesota's disparities between workers' compensation and non–workers' compensation medical costs thus provide additional grounds for concern that workers' compensation systems are facing medical cost problems even greater than those faced in the wider medical care system.

## Causes of Higher Workers' Compensation Medical Costs

Factors specific to workers' compensation may have caused its medical costs to accelerate. Certain cost control techniques are absent in workers'

[2]Measures of utilization include the types of providers (physicians, chiropractors, physical therapists, and so on) and the quantity of medical services rendered (number of x-rays, blood tests, physical examinations, physical therapy visits, inpatient hospital days, surgery, and so on).

compensation, and others are more difficult to carry out. For example, copayments and deductibles are used regularly outside workers' compensation to reduce the demand for medical care and thus its cost. Yet workers' compensation systems traditionally have paid all medical costs resulting from covered injuries and illnesses.

Workers' compensation insurers or self-insured companies may find discounts for medical care difficult to negotiate for two reasons. First, workers' compensation has only a small share of the medical care market (about 2 percent), and therefore has less bargaining power. Second, workers have the legal right to choose a treating physician in about half the states, making it more difficult for employers to direct them to lower-cost providers. Evidence about the impact on costs of who chooses the treating physician is equivocal, with some studies suggesting that employer choice reduces costs [3] and others showing no impact [2].

Litigation also increases the medical costs of workers' compensation beyond those that might be incurred in other settings. Litigation can complicate care and delay recovery, prolonging the duration of medical treatment paid for by workers' compensation. In addition, most states allocate the expense of medical evaluations used to resolve legal disputes, which are often substantial, as medical costs.

Another factor that could influence the comparison is the relationship between economic conditions and reported workplace injuries. Unemployment was much higher between 1980 and 1985 than it was between 1965 and 1970. Reported injury rates rise as unemployment falls and fall as unemployment rises [4]. If average injury severity also has a cyclical component, the more rapid increase in workers' compensation medical costs may reflect greater injury severity, not just changes in the underlying structure of medical costs. Contrary to injury rates, the duration of workers' compensation claims and the consequent utilization of medical services may rise with unemployment, increasing average medical costs per claim.

## Workers' Compensation Medical Cost Control

Rapidly increasing medical costs have driven many states to implement controls on medical costs. The most common of these are:

- Fee schedules that list maximum reimbursement levels for health care services or products
- Limited employee initial choice of medical care provider, or limitations on changing medical care providers
- Mandatory bill review for proper charges, generally tied to a fee schedule
- Mandatory utilization review of the necessity and appropriateness of admissions and procedures, length of hospitalization, and consultations by specialists before, during, or following an inpatient admission
- Managed care programs that seek to ensure the appropriateness of treatment, the delivery of care in a cost-effective manner, and the prevention of health problems that can be caused by the uncoordinated utilization of medical services (for example, health maintenance or preferred provider organizations)

Over the past several years, many states have adopted one or more of these methods of containing medical costs. Between mid-1990 and mid-1991, 15 states added one or more new cost-containment initiatives or were developing them [5].

## Medicolegal Roadblocks to Compensation for Occupational Diseases

The burden of proving that occupational injuries arose "out of and in the course of employment" is usually straightforward. However, workers with occupational illnesses face a different situation (Table 10-5). The workers' compensation system expects a physician to say whether or not a worker's illness was caused by or aggravated by work.

**Table 10-5.** Roadblocks to compensation for occupational disease

| Limitations of medical science | Statutory limitations | Other limitations |
| --- | --- | --- |
| Difficulty of differential diagnosis | Time limits | Lack of exposure records (duration and intensity) |
| Lack of epidemiologic and toxicologic studies | Burden of proof | |
| Multiple causal pathways | Restrictive definitions of disease | |
| Limitations of physician training | | |

Physicians are asked, "Was this illness caused by workplace conditions?" This is a question for which medical science often does not have a simple answer.

Many aspects of occupational diseases make the disabled worker's burden of proof difficult to sustain. Physicians may not realize that their patients may have become ill as a result of workplace exposures. Many physicians are not able to identify occupational diseases because their medical training in this has been inadequate; many have not even been trained in taking occupational histories. Furthermore, the signs and symptoms of most occupational diseases are not uniquely related to an occupational exposure. Medical and epidemiologic knowledge may be insufficient to distinguish clearly a disease of occupational origin from one of nonoccupational origin. For example, shortness of breath, an important symptom of occupational lung disease, is also associated with other chronic lung diseases (Fig. 10-3).

Another complicating factor is that a disease may have multiple causes, only one of which is occupational exposure. A worker who smokes and is exposed to ionizing radiation at work may develop lung cancer. Since both cigarette smoke and ionizing radiation are well-established risk factors for lung cancer, it may be impossible to say which of these two factors "caused" the disease. In many cases occupational disease may develop many years after exposure began, and perhaps many years after exposure ceased. Consequently, memories of

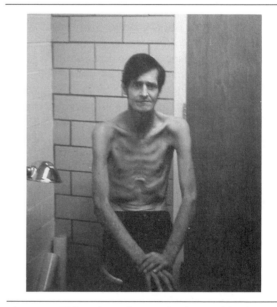

**Fig. 10-3.** Although workers with silicosis, like this rock driller, generally qualify for workers' compensation, most workers with chronic occupational *diseases* often find their claims denied. (Reprinted from DE Banks, et al. Silicosis in surface coal mine drillers. *Thorax* 1983; 30:275.)

events and exposures may be unclear, and records of employment may not be available.

Some occupational injuries occur as a result of extended exposure to a hazard. These are "cumulative trauma" injuries, such as carpal tunnel syndrome, noise-induced hearing loss, and chronic low back pain. As with chronic occupational diseases, it may be difficult to prove the work-relatedness of these injuries. Moreover, records of exposure to occupational hazards are not often kept, so that even when a worker knows the type, level, and duration of exposure, no written evidence of this can be presented.

These aspects of occupational disease mean that many victims do not even suspect that their disease is job-related. For those who do and wish to make a claim, the causal relationship between disease and workplace exposures may be very difficult to establish. These are major reasons why so few claims for compensation for occupational disease are filed. A study of occupational disease in Washington and California revealed that, of the 51 probable cases of occupational respiratory conditions, only one was reported as a workers' compensation claim.

When claims for chronic occupational disease are filed, many are contested by the insurance carrier or self-insured employer (Table 10-6). Therefore, payments to disabled workers are delayed and uncertain (Table 10-7). Workers with chronic occupational diseases wait an average of more than a year to receive compensation payments. In

Table 10-6. Percent of alleged occupational disease cases controverted (contested) by category of disease

| Category | Percent |
| --- | --- |
| Dust disease | 88 |
| Disorders due to repeated trauma | 86 |
| Respiratory conditions due to toxic agents | 79 |
| Cancers and tumors | 46 |
| Poisoning | 37 |
| Skin diseases | 14 |
| Disorders due to physical agents | 10 |
| Other | 54 |
| All diseases | 63* |

*In contrast, the percentage for all injuries is 10 percent.
Source: Adapted from PS Barth, HA Hunt. Workers' compensation and work-related illnesses. Cambridge, MA: MIT Press, 1980.

Table 10-7. Delays in compensation for occupational disease by category of disease

| Category | Mean number of days from notice to insurer to first payment |
| --- | --- |
| Skin diseases | 59 |
| Dust diseases | 390 |
| Respiratory conditions due to toxic agents | 389 |
| Poisoning | 111 |
| Disorders due to physical agents | 79 |
| Disorders due to repeated trauma | 362 |
| Cancers and tumors | 260 |
| Other illnesses | 180* |

*In contrast, the mean delay for all injuries is 43 days.
Source: Adapted from PS Barth, HA Hunt. Workers' compensation and work-related illnesses. Cambridge, MA: MIT Press, 1980.

addition, administrative and legal costs absorb many of the resources devoted to compensating occupational diseases.

## Establishing Work-relatedness for Compensation

The burden of proving that disease is occupational in origin lies with workers. They must find physicians who are convinced that their illnesses are occupational in origin or that their illnesses were aggravated or hastened by occupational exposures. Physicians must then be able to convince referees who hear the cases that the diseases are indeed work-related.

The burden of proof might at first seem to be impossible for those diseases that are not uniquely occupational in origin. For example, lung cancer may be caused by smoking, air pollution (although not definitely established), occupational or non-occupational radiation exposure, or all of these factors.

Suppose that a worker with lung cancer has smoked cigarettes, has had diagnostic x-rays, and has also been occupationally exposed to ionizing radiation in a uranium mine. Since occupational lung cancer does not have distinctive clinical features, an expert medical witness, using clinical judgment, cannot say that the disease is without question occupational in origin. The expert witness cannot even say with certainty that occupational exposure to ionizing radiation was one of several causes or if it hastened the onset of the cancer. At best all that can be determined is that the worker has an increased risk of lung cancer as a result of the job. In this case the legal standard is that there must be a "preponderence of evidence"

that the disease is occupational in origin, or the case is unlikely to be settled in favor of the disabled worker. A "preponderence of evidence" means that it is more likely than not (probability greater than 50 percent) that the illness in question was caused by, aggravated by, or hastened by workplace exposure.

In some cases workers' compensation laws have been written so that payment of a claim may be denied even though convincing evidence is presented that the illness was caused by or aggravated by the worker's employment. Some states require that a disease not be "an ordinary disease of life." In other words, diseases such as emphysema and hearing loss may not be compensable because they

**Table 10-8.** Time limits on filing occupational disease claims in selected jurisdictions (as of January 1, 1993)

| Jurisdiction | Time limit on claim filing |
|---|---|
| Alabama | Disability: within 2 years after last exposure or last payment; death: within 2 years of death or last payment; radiation: within 2 years after disability or death and when claimant knows or should know relation to employment. |
| California | Disability: within 1 year from injury or last payment; death: within 1 year after death and in no case more than 240 weeks after injury, except for asbestos-related disease claims. Date of injury is defined as when claimant is disabled and knows or should know of relation to employment. |
| Colorado | Within 2 years after commencement of disability or death; within 5 years in case of ionizing radiation, asbestosis, silicosis, or anthracosis. |
| Massachusetts | Within 1 year after injury or death; delay excusable. |
| Michigan | Within 2 years after claimant knows or should know of relation to employment. |
| New York | Within 2 years after disability or death, or 2 years after the claimant knows or should know of relation to employment. |
| North Carolina | Within 2 years after final determination of disability. Within 6 years after death from an occupational disease. |
| Oregon | Within 1 year of worker's discovery of the disease, after disablement, or physician informs worker of disease. |
| Utah | Within 6 years after cause of action arose, but no later than 1 year after death. |
| Virginia | Within 2 years after diagnosis is first communicated to worker or within 5 years after exposure, whichever is first; within 3 years after death, occurring within limit for disability. |
| Federal employees | Within 3 years after injury, death, or disability and claimant knows or should know relation to employment; delay excusable. |
| U.S. longshoremen | Within 2 years of knowledge of relation to employment or 1 year after last payment. |

Source: Reprinted with the permission of the Chamber of Commerce of the United States of America from Analysis of Workers' Compensation 1993. © 1993 Chamber of Commerce of the United States of America.

often occur among people with no occupational exposure. More than 20 states have a related requirement that diseases are only compensable if they are "peculiar to" or "characteristic of" a worker's occupation.

All jurisdictions have a statute of limitations (often one or two years) on claims for workers' compensation. A two-year statute of limitation means that the claim must be filed by the worker within two years of a given event. A time limit of two years after the worker has learned that a disease is work-related imposes no particular hardship on occupational disease victims. In some states, however, the time period begins when the disease becomes symptomatic, even if this takes place before the disease is diagnosed or determined to be work-related. The latter policy for starting the statute of limitation may be a special problem if the worker's physician is not familiar with the occupational disease. The most burdensome statutes require that a claim be filed one or two years after exposure. Since chronic occupational diseases commonly do not manifest themselves until 5, 10, 20, or more years after exposure, such rules effectively eliminate the possibility of compensation for workers with these illnesses. In a recent study, occupational disease compensation among a group of asbestos insulators was only half as great in states with these restrictive statutes of limitation as in other states. Time limits for filing workers' compensation claims are described in Table 10-8.

## The Problem of Compromise Settlements

A workers' compensation claim that is denied by the employer or insurer does not automatically go to a hearing. The injured worker must first find a lawyer who will take the case. The lawyer's fee is often based on the portion of the award attributed to lost wages, which means that the lawyer's fee will be small in a small award and that the lawyer will receive nothing if the claim is denied. Thus, it is hard for injured or ill workers to find lawyers to represent them when claims are small or success is unlikely.

Lawyers generally prefer to bargain informally with the defendant's lawyers rather than go to trial. If a compromise settlement can be reached prior to trial, no preparation for a hearing is necessary, and the lawyer will therefore have more time to work on other cases and earn additional income. A settlement reached outside the courtroom is called a compromise settlement because the amount paid to the claimant generally is a compromise between the maximum amount that the claimant could receive in a court decision and the amount (if any) of the settlement if the claimant lost.

In the face of protracted litigation with uncertain results, a compromise settlement may seem very attractive to an injured worker who may have no wage income for a considerable period and may be facing large medical bills. The injured worker may therefore prefer a small settlement paid immediately to a much larger but uncertain settlement that would not be available for one or two years. Especially where the worker does not foresee a quick return to work, a settlement may be accepted that might seem quite small to an outside observer. Insurers may use their knowledge of the financial pressures on the claimant to obtain a small settlement; they will thus contest, delaying the time when the case is closed in the hope of obtaining a small compromise settlement.

The compromise settlement will usually be paid in a lump sum to the injured worker and the attorney. This lump sum settlement will take the place of future payments for lost earnings and medical and rehabilitation costs. Many compromise settlements also release the insurer from future liability: If the claimant's condition should change at a later date or if future medical needs were inadequately estimated, the insurer would not incur the costs of any increased disability or medical or rehabilitation expenses. The injured worker who has accepted a "compromise and release" settlement may later need additional medical care but not have the resources to pay for that care.

For example, a worker with a back injury was denied compensation by his employer, who claimed that the injury was not work-related. He then took action that led to his being offered a lump sum settlement:

I went to my union representative and filled out the forms for the industrial accident board, and about three weeks later they sent me an award which was about $600 . . . and I wouldn't take it.

But then I applied for an attorney and talked to my attorney, and then filed suit. They turned around and told my attorney that they would consider [the injury] an industrial accident. So, I never did go to court. All they did was talk to my lawyer. They settled out of court. My lawyer told me while I was in the hospital that they wanted to settle it for $7,500. The fee for him [would be] $2,500.[3]

If the settlement of $7,500 was the result of a compromise and release agreement, the insurer or employer will not be liable for any future disability or medical costs resulting from this injury.

## Recommendations of the National Commission

As part of the Occupational Safety and Health Act of 1970 Congress established the National Commission on State Workmen's Compensation Laws to "undertake a comprehensive study and evaluation of State workmen's compensation laws in order to determine if such laws provide an adequate, prompt, and equitable system of compensation." In 1972 the Commission released its report, which described many problems of workers' compensa-

[3]Adapted from Subcommittee on Labor, Committee on Labor, and Public Welfare, U.S. Senate. Hearings on the National Workers' Compensation Standards Act, 1974. Statement of Lawrence Barefield.

tion and made recommendations for improving state workers' compensation systems. This report, still relevant today, included these seven "essential" recommendations:

1. Compulsory coverage. Employees could not lose coverage by agreeing to waive their rights to benefits.
2. No occupational or numerical exemptions to coverage. All workers, including agricultural and domestic workers, should be covered. All employers, even if they have only one employee, should be covered.
3. Full coverage of work-related diseases—the elimination of arbitrary barriers to coverage such as highly restrictive time limits, occupational disease schedules, and exclusion of "ordinary diseases of life."
4. Full medical and physical rehabilitation services without arbitrary limits.
5. Employees' choice of jurisdiction for filing interstate claims.
6. Adequate weekly cash benefits for temporary total disability, permanent total disability, and fatal cases.
7. No arbitrary limits on duration or sum of benefits.

Since this report was issued, many states have changed their statutes to follow the recommendations of the National Commission. By increasing coverage and raising benefits, they have substantially improved the value of workers' compensation to injured employees. However, general changes in coverage have done little to discourage the litigation of occupational disease claims and costly occupational injury claims.

## The Future of Workers' Compensation

The common law system in effect during the nineteenth century was time-consuming, inefficient (because of litigation costs), and uncertain. Workers' compensation was designed to minimize litigation, but in spite of the change to a no-fault system more than 80 percent of all compensation claims for chronic occupational diseases are contested (see Table 10-6), and almost half of all injury claims for permanent total disability or death are also contested. This process of contests leads to delays of a year or more in settling workers' compensation claims (see Table 10-7). The settlements may be compromised and may thereby leave claimants seriously undercompensated. Also, legal fees, commonly 15 to 20 percent of the compensation award for lost wages, must be paid by the claimant. For cases of permanent total disability from occupational disease, for which the average award for lost wages was about $9,700 in 1975, the average worker received only about $8,000 after legal costs were paid.

Two essential elements of workers' compensation that lead to so many contested cases are (1) the necessity of proving that a disease is work-related, and (2) the fact that large medical and wage replacement payments to compensated workers come directly from their employers or employers' insurance carriers. The first element leaves room for much legal argument; the second gives considerable incentive for employers or their insurance carriers to pursue such arguments. If contesting claims were less rewarding, more difficult, and less likely to be successful, employers might instead find it cheaper to pay them, thereby reducing the amount of litigation in the system.

In one proposed reform aimed at eliminating incentives for litigation, benefits would be paid from industry-wide funds rather than by individual employers or their insurance carriers. This plan would mean that individual employers or carriers would not gain financially by contesting an award and would thereby have little incentive to do so. A concern about such an arrangement, however, is that if workers submit claims for nonoccupational injuries and illnesses, insurers would have little incentive to screen out such claims.

A second proposed reform would establish expert medical boards to make decisions about the compensability of each contested case of alleged occupational disease as soon as a claim was denied by the employer's insurance carrier. If the medical board ruled that a disease was occupational in origin, the burden of proof would be lifted from the worker. The employer or insurer would be able to contest the decision of the medical board, but there would remain a strong presumption that the claim was valid.

Another way of reducing the burden of proof of causation would be to establish presumptive standards. A presumptive standard defines a level of evidence sufficient to demonstrate legally a causal relationship between occupation and disease. For example, a history of 10 years of work in a coal mine, combined with specific medical test results consistent with coal workers' pneumoconiosis ("black lung"), could be defined as legally sufficient evidence to presume that a specific disease is work-related. An employer or insurance company would then have the burden of proving that the disease was not work-related to avoid paying the claim.

The compensation of victims of occupational disease may also be improved through publicly funded programs such as Social Security Disability Insurance (SSDI). Currently, SSDI offers disability payments to people suffering from total disability, whether or not that disability is work-related. If SSDI were broadened to cover partial disability, those unable to receive workers' compensation disability payments would still receive income support. Similarly, a mandatory medical insurance program would assure medical benefits for treatment of injuries and illnesses regardless of cause.

Other countries have workers' compensation systems with considerably less controversy surrounding compensation for occupational diseases (see box). Part of the reason for this is these countries have social programs that provide medical benefits and disability benefits that are substantially greater than those provided to many Ameri-

## ANOTHER NORTH AMERICAN SYSTEM: WORKERS' COMPENSATION IN BRITISH COLUMBIA*

Canadian workers' compensation systems are administered at the provincial level, just as most workers' compensation systems in the United States are state systems (see box in Chap. 9). The workers' compensation system in British Columbia is similar to U.S. systems in states with exclusive state funds. The Workers' Compensation Board (WCB) of British Columbia is the only organization allowed to offer workers' compensation insurance to employers in that province.

The British Columbia workers' compensation system offers the same types of benefits to injured employees as systems in the U.S.: temporary and permanent disability benefits, fatality benefits for survivors, medical benefits, and vocational rehabilitation benefits. Benefits to replace lost wages are high compared with most U.S. jurisdictions. This is, in part, because maximum benefits are high. Also, British Columbia has no waiting period for wage replacement benefits; in contrast, U.S. jurisdictions have waiting periods ranging from 3 to 7 days. Therefore, more workers are paid wage replacement benefits in British Columbia than in the United States.

British Columbia provides payments through its Medical Services Plan to cover health care for all its citizens. Yet the workers' compensation system pays the medical expenses of injured workers. Providers are paid fees that are 10 percent higher than those in the private sector, to cover the additional paperwork required by the workers' compensation system.

*Unless otherwise noted, the source of the information presented here is HA Hunt, PS Barth, MJ Leahy. Workers' compensation in British Columbia: An administrative inventory at a time of transition. Kalamazoo: W.E. Upjohn Institute for Employment Research, 1991.

Four separate organizations within the Ministry of Labour and Consumer Services administer the workers' compensation act. The WCB provides insurance and administers the payment of claims. The Workers' Compensation Review Board (WCRB) adjudicates disputed claims, as do workers' compensation commissions and industrial accident boards in the U.S. Two other agencies provide services that generally have no parallel in U.S. systems. The Workers' Adviser Service (WAS) helps workers to bring claims and may represent them before the WCB or WCRB. The WAS also trains union personnel to represent their members in disputed claims. The Employers' Adviser Service (EAS) provides similar services to employers. Outside the Ministry of Labour and Consumer Services, the Ombudsman of British Columbia responds to complaints and provides oversight of the other agencies.

The last three agencies have no counterpart in U.S. workers' compensation jurisdictions, although some workers' compensation agencies in the U.S. do provide information about the law to workers and employers. These agencies reflect a less litigious approach to workers' compensation, an approach that is reflected in statistics. Compared with U.S. jurisdictions, British Columbia has many fewer appealed claims. In 1990 workers or employers appealed only 3.1 percent of new claims filed, or 7.7 percent of claims with lost wages in British Columbia. In Wisconsin, a low-litigation state, 10 percent of claims with lost wages involve a request for hearing. This rate is 10 percent in North Carolina, 19 percent in Pennsylvania, 25 percent in Georgia, and 43 percent in Missouri.

In 1989 only 12 percent of workers in appealed claims were represented by attorneys. Of these workers, 30 percent were unrepresented, 5 percent were represented by the WAS, and 26 percent had union representation. Virtually all U.S. workers with appealed claims hire attorneys. This difference between the British Columbia system and the U.S. systems is probably produced in part by the availability of assistance from the WAS and the EAS. A study of the British Columbia system[†] suggests that another reason is "the strong posture in the Act and by the WCB that it should administer the law in an inquiry, rather than an adversarial, manner."

Another interesting feature of the British Columbia workers' compensation system is the Medical Review Panel (MRP). When a medical issue is in dispute, a worker or employer can appeal that issue to an MRP. The provincial government (with advice from the British Columbia College of Physicians and Surgeons) appoints and keeps a list of 14 private physicians who can chair panels. Chairs are chosen sequentially from this list. When a physician's name comes up, that physician is chosen to head a panel. The chair then sends the worker and employer a list of specialists in relevant disciplines from which they can each choose one. This panel of three physicians sees the worker, reads relevant records, and can order additional medical testing. The decision of the panel on medical issues is binding; it cannot be appealed. This feature probably would not survive a legal challenge in the U.S. A Massachusetts law that established medical referees that could issue binding opinions was overturned in the Massachusetts state court because it limited the parties' access to appeals and therefore to due process [Meunier's Case, 319 Mass. 421, 66 N.E.2d 198 (1946)].

Medical payments are much lower in the British Columbia workers' compensation system than in U.S. systems. In 1989 medical payments were 40.5 percent of all workers' compensation benefits in the U.S. [7]; in that year they were 19.0 percent of all benefits paid in British Columbia. The reason for this is not clear. It may reflect generally lower Canadian medical costs. Perhaps higher litigation rates in the U.S. lead to more medical care or reduce the effectiveness of medical care, thus leading to greater utilization. Also, this ratio may be lower in British Columbia because wage-replacement benefits are high.

In British Columbia, unlike U.S. jurisdictions, the workers' compensation agency has authority to develop and enforce workplace safety and health regulations. WCB inspectors can require correction of hazards, recommend penalties, or issue 24-hour closure orders where imminent dangers exist. For firms above a certain size and hazard level, the law in British Columbia requires occupational health and safety programs, including labor-management health and safety committees. WCB inspectors review these programs, decide whether they are adequate, and provide advice on improving them.[†]

[†]KM Rest, NA Ashford, Occupational safety and health in British Columbia: An administrative inventory. Cambridge, MA: Ashford Associates, 1992.

can workers; thus, a worker who does not receive workers' compensation still can pay for needed medical care and continue to help support the family through disability payments. Countries with national health systems such as Great Britain and Sweden provide free medical care whether or not illnesses are occupational; Belgium and Denmark have excellent social insurance and disability programs, which provide a significant amount of wage replacement for disabled workers whether or not their disability is work-related.

Alternate sources of free medical care in these countries reduce litigation and provide a medical "safety net" for victims of occupational disease. Yet, workers' compensation still may not provide benefits, and for the same reasons as in the U.S.

Physicians do not identify occupational diseases, workers are unaware of their exposures to workplace hazards, and, when they are, they find that exposures are difficult to document. Also, legislation and regulations may be restrictive in covering occupational diseases [6].

# References

1. Thornquist L. Health care costs and cost containment in Minnesota's workers' compensation program. John Burton's Workers' Compensation Monitor 1990; 3:3–26.
   *A comparison of medical costs in Minnesota between workers' compensation and Blue Cross/Blue Shield.*
2. Boden LI, Fleischman CA. Medical costs in workers' compensation: Trends and interstate comparisons. Cambridge, MA: Workers' Compensation Research Institute, 1989.
   *This book describes growth in workers' compensation and non–workers' compensation medical costs. It also compares costs among states.*
3. National Council on Compensation Insurance. Cost containment. NCCI Digest. 1989; 4:25–49.
   *A study of system features affecting workers' compensation medical costs.*
4. Robinson J. The rising long-term trend in occupational injury rates. Am J Public Health 1988; 78: 276–80.
5. Boden LI, Johnson SM, Smith JCH. Medical cost containment in workers' compensation: A national inventory 1992. Cambridge, MA: Workers' Compensation Research Institute, 1993.
   *This book describes workers' compensation medical cost-containment programs in place in the 50 states and the District of Columbia in 1992.*
6. Mony AT. Compensation of occupational illnesses in France. New Solutions, 1993; 4:57–61.
7. Nelson W Jr. Workers' compensation coverage, benefits, and costs, 1989. Social Security Bulletin 1992; 55(1).
   *This is the latest in an annual summary of workers' compensation benefits and costs in the United States.*

# Bibliography

Ashford NA. Economic issues. II. Workmen's compensation. In crisis in the workplace. Cambridge, MA: MIT Press, 1976.
   *Provides a good summary of the goals of workers' compensation, the problems in meeting these goals, and how well they are actually met. The shortest overview among the references cited here.*
Barth PS, Hunt HA. Workers' compensation and work-related illnesses. Cambridge, MA: MIT Press, 1980.
   *The most complete description available of how workers' compensation programs handle occupational diseases. Describes how different states compensate occupational diseases and gives an overview of litigation and settlement of workers' compensation disease claims in the United States. Also reviews workers' compensation in other countries.*
Chamber of Commerce of the United States. Analysis of workers' compensation laws. Washington, D.C. 1993.
   *An annual review of workers' compensation laws in the United States and Canada. Compensation statutes are continually changing, and reading this review is one way of keeping up-to-date on the coverage, payment levels, and administrative arrangements of different laws.*
Kusnetz S, Hutchison MK. eds. A guide to the work-relatedness of disease. revised ed. Washington, D.C.: NIOSH, 1979.
   *Designed primarily as an aid to state agencies and others concerned with occupational disease compensation, this presents one method for assembling and evaluating evidence that may be relevant in determining the work-relatedness of a disease in an individual. Information on 14 disease-producing agents is presented to illustrate the decision-making process.*
National Commission on State Workmen's Compensation Laws. Report and compendium on workmen's compensation. Washington, D.C.: U.S. Government Printing Office, 1972 and 1973.
   *The National Commission was created by the Occupational Safety and Health Act of 1970 to evaluate the status of workers' compensation. It undertook a 2-year study. The Compendium is a descriptive report on workers' compensation in 1973, while the Report makes recommendations to upgrade workers' compensation programs.*
Selikoff IJ. ed. Disability compensation for asbestos-associated disease in the United States. New York: Mt. Sinai School of Medicine, 1983.
   *Reviews the asbestos occupational health problem in detail and discusses the workers' compensation and tort litigation experience of asbestos-exposed workers.*
Somers HM, Somers AR. Workmen's compensation. New York: Wiley, 1954.

*A general description of workers' compensation, written from a policy perspective, which was so well done that it is still worth reading decades later.*

U.S. Department of Labor, Assistant Secretary for Policy, Evaluation and Research. An interim report to Congress on occupational diseases. Washington, D.C., 1980.

*Report of a task force in the U.S. Department of Labor that conducted a study of the compensation of occupational respiratory diseases. Discusses the problems of compensating occupational diseases and suggests ways of improving that compensation.*

# 11
# Ability to Work and Disability Evaluation

Jay S. Himmelstein and Glenn S. Pransky

Over the years, industrialized societies have taken two basic approaches to dealing with the problems of poverty and social isolation that frequently befall people with disabilities who have been unable to achieve gainful employment. One approach, disability compensation, provides income support for those who are unable to work because of a disability: This approach is typified by the Social Security Disability Income system in the United States, described later in this chapter, and by various "workers' compensation" systems (see Chap. 10) designed to compensate those whose disability resulted from workplace injury or disease.

An increasingly popular approach seeks to promote the independence of people with disabilities through equal opportunity for employment. In general, these laws entitle people with disabilities to obtain rehabilitation services intended to facilitate or maintain employment (for example, the United States Rehabilitation Act of 1973) and remove barriers to employment by regulating employment practices and workplace conditions that have tended to exclude people with disabilities (for example, the Americans with Disabilities Act, or ADA [see Chapter Appendix]).

In both of these approaches, physicians and other health care providers play a key role in the generation and evaluation of medical information that is used to determine eligibility for income replacement under the first approach, or entitlement to services and legal protection under the second. This chapter offers clinicians a review of the theoretical basis and practical aspects of their role in

evaluating work ability and disability. The health care provider willing to become more informed about the rationale and process of these evaluations can provide an important service to patients.

Clinicians' effectiveness in dealing with work ability and disability evaluations will be enhanced by a clear understanding of (1) key definitions related to the evaluation process, (2) common features of insurance plans and antidiscrimination legislation affecting disabled workers, (3) the clinician's role in the evaluation of work ability, and (4) unresolved controversies and potential role conflicts for the clinician.

In reviewing the variety of compensation plans and the associated roles for the health care provider, it is important to recognize a few key concepts. Most important is the distinction between *impairment* and *disability.*

*Impairment* is commonly defined as the loss of function of an organ or part of the body compared to what previously existed. Ideally, impairment can be defined and described in purely medical terms and quantified in such a way that a reproducible measurement is developed (for example, severe restrictive lung disease with a total lung capacity of 1.6 liters).

*Disability,* on the other hand, is usually defined in terms of the impact of an impairment on societal or work functions. A disability evaluation would therefore take into account the loss of function (impairment) *and* the patient's work requirements and home situation. Certain agencies use a more restrictive definition of disability; for example, the Social Security Administration defines disability as "inability to perform any substantial gainful work." Often, private disability insurance defines disability as an "inability to perform the essential tasks of the usual employment." However, the determination of disability is always predicated on an assessment of impairment, followed by a determination of the loss in occupational or societal functioning that results from the impairment. In general, the determination of impairment is performed by a health care professional (usually a physician); most often, nonphysician administrators use this information to determine the presence and extent of disability.

Disability compensation systems frequently request a determination of the *extent* and *permanence* of a disability condition. An injured worker who cannot do *any* work because of a medical condition is considered to be *totally disabled*. If this person can work but has some limitations and cannot do his or her customary work, a *partial disability* exists. Either type of disability is considered to be *temporary* as long as a resolution of the disability is expected. When no significant functional improvement is expected, or a condition has not changed over a one-year period, it is inferred that a medical end-result (sometimes called maximal medical improvement) has been achieved. A *temporary* (partial or total) *disability* would then be regarded by most systems as a *permanent disability*.

Workers' compensation insurance systems usually require determination of the work-relatedness of a disability. A *work-related* injury or disease refers to conditions that are thought to result from some exposure (physical, chemical, biologic, or psychological) in the workplace. In acute traumatic injuries, the relationship of the injury to the workplace is usually clear (Fig. 11-1). In chronic conditions, however, it may be difficult to be certain of the relationship between work and disease. It is recommended that the physician's determination of work-relatedness should be based on the evidence of disease, the exposure history, and the

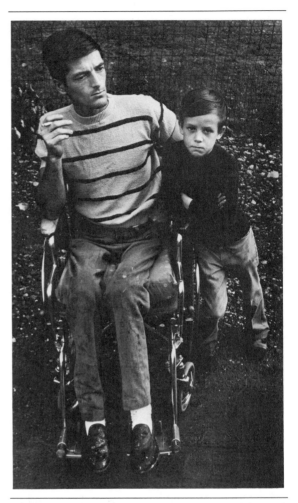

**Fig. 11-1.** Coal miner disabled from mine roof fall and his son. (Photograph by Earl Dotter.)

epidemiologic evidence linking exposure and disease [1].

Health professionals must be aware, however, that the legal definition of cause may be less exacting than the medical definition, and that most disability systems are based on the legal standard. One legal definition of a work-related condition is one ". . . arising out of or in the course of employment" or "caused or exacerbated by . . . employment" [2]. Thus, a preexisting condition, unrelated to work, that becomes substantially worse because of work may legally be work-related. A typical legal standard of proof is that a condition is work-related if it is "more likely than not" that the condition would not have been present or would have been substantially better had the work exposure not occurred. (See Chaps. 3 and 10 for more discussion of work-relatedness.)

## Disability Compensation Systems

Some of the confusion regarding disability assessment stems from the multitude of disability compensation systems and plans, since each may have its own definition of disability and criteria for assessing impairment. Different countries have designed verifying approaches to providing income security to those who find their wage-earning capacity compromised by injury or disease [3]. In the United States, most compensation systems fall into one of thee major categories (Table 11-1).

Occupational physicians are most familiar with workers' compensation insurance, which provides coverage of most federal, state, and private employees. These plans compensate for medical expenses and lost wages due to work-related conditions.

The federal government sponsors the major compensation programs for the severely disabled, through Social Security Disability Insurance. These programs pay a limited amount of compensation to those who are unable to achieve any gainful employment, regardless of the cause of disability.

Private disability insurance is often purchased by individuals or provided as an employer or union benefit and is designed to provide compensation for those who are unable to work at their regular jobs regardless of the cause of disability, or to supplement Social Security benefits.

Thus, a patient who can no longer work because of injury or illness might receive support from his or her employer's insurer, a federal or state agency, and/or an insurance policy that has been purchased privately.

Although each plan has different eligibility criteria and levels of payment, all share a few common features:

1. Every plan incorporates *shared risk*. Many people or employers at risk of financial losses contribute to a pool, from which a few individuals are reimbursed. The cost of entering the pool is partially determined by the actuarial risk of future events for that person or insured group. Thus, private disability insurance is much more expensive per year for a 55-year-old than for a 20-year-old, since the older worker has a higher risk of disabling medical illness. Workers' compensation insurance is more expensive per employee for a construction company (higher risk of injury to employees) than for a stock brokerage firm.

2. Because payments into the pool are predictable, *finite resources* are available to all potential recipients of each plan. Therefore, eligibility criteria are structured so that the limited resources go to those in greatest need. Workers' compensation plans often do not replace lost wages for fewer than 6 days of absence from work, since doing so might greatly increase the cost of the program. Many private disability insurance plans do not begin coverage until 30 days to 6 months of illness absence has occurred. The SSDI plan usually does not begin payments until a year of sickness absence has occurred.

3. Before medical evaluation of impairment, a potential recipient of benefits must first demonstrate *legal eligibility*. The basis for eligibility is different in each plan. For example, to be eligible for SSDI, one must have worked and contributed to Social Security for 5 of the past 10 years. Workers' compensation covers only regular employees, not consultants or subcontractors. Private disability insurance often does not cover illness that occurs during the first 60 to 90 days of enrollment.

Table 11-1. Compensation systems

| Program | Eligibility | Source of benefits | Basis for claim | Clinician's role |
|---|---|---|---|---|
| 1. WORKERS' COMPENSATION (WC) SYSTEMS—"CAUSE" OF DISABILITY IS DETERMINANT. | | | | |
| State<br>Federal<br>Railroad workers | Private employees<br>Federal employees<br>Railroad employees | Employer insurance<br>Taxes<br>Employer | Work-related illness or injury | Evaluate work-relatedness, impairment, and disability |
| Black lung benefits | Coal miners | Tax on coal | Lung disease | Report chest x-ray, pulmonary and function tests, and examination results only |
| 2. PROGRAMS FOR SEVERELY DISABLED—INABILITY TO PERFORM GAINFUL ACTIVITIES IS DETERMINANT. | | | | |
| Social Security Disability Insurance (SSDI) | Contributing workers | Workers' contributions | Severe disability | Evaluate and report impairment |
| Supplemental Security Income (SSI) | The aged, blind, and severely disabled | Taxes | | |
| 3. PRIVATE DISABILITY PLANS—REGARDLESS OF CAUSE, PROTECT INCOME IF UNABLE TO PERFORM REGULAR JOB. | | | | |
| Short-Term Disability (STD)<br>Long-Term Disability (LTD) | Enrolled workers | Payments by employee, employer, or union | Any illness preventing usual employment | Evaluate impairment and disability |

4. *Medical information* on impairment is requested once a legal basis for a claim has been established. In every system, a medical diagnosis is necessary; in the worker's compensation system, physicians are often asked their opinions on the *work-relatedness* of employees' conditions, the prognosis for eventual return to work, and the restrictions or job accommodations that might be necessary to return the worker to employment.

5. The information from the physician, however, does not determine whether benefits are awarded or how much is paid; all of these systems are under *administrative control*. In the Social Security system, an administrator-physician team reviews medical information from the evaluating physician and compares it with specific criteria for eligibility. In the worker's compensation systems, if there is a significant discrepancy between the employer's report of an injury and the physician's report, benefits may be withheld pending an investigation by the insurance company.

6. *Benefits are limited* and are intended to provide only a proportion of lost wages, medical expenses related to the specific impairment, and vocational rehabilitation. Only in rare circumstances are worker's compensation benefits intended to punish gross negligence by an employer in causing the injury; in all other instances, *fault has no bearing on benefit levels*.

7. Applicants generally have a *right of appeal* of an administrative or medical decision, with review by a third party. In the Social Security system, applicants who are initially denied benefits can appeal to a second administrator-physician team, then to a Social Security benefits coordinator, then to an administrative law judge, and finally to the federal courts, if desired. In most worker's compensation plans, the claimant can request an administrative hearing and be represented by an attorney. The agencies that provide benefits also conduct periodic reviews of cases to verify that continued eligibility (disability) exists.

8. Recently, there has been an increased emphasis on developing resources for *retraining and rehabilitation,* closely allied with each system. Beneficiaries are often required to participate in programs to maximize their potential for return to alternative, gainful employment.

*Worker's compensation insurance* is reviewed in Chap. 10. The United States does not have a federal workers' compensation law, and each state has developed its own system. In addition, there are a number of workers' compensation programs that are occupation-specific; these programs often have developed their own definitions of disability and related eligibility criteria. The Black Lung Program, for example, provides payments to coal miners with a documented work history and respiratory insufficiency who meet certain criteria. All disabling respiratory insufficiency is assumed to be related to mining if the miner meets a standard of number of years worked in the mines. Other examples of occupation-specific workers' compensation programs include those of railroad workers, longshoremen, military veterans, and municipal workers such as police and firefighters.

The purpose of each plan is to reimburse workers for medical expenses, rehabilitation expenses, and lost wages that result from a work-related injury or illness. Plans are generally designed to be nonadversarial so that, in most cases, limited benefits are paid to injured workers without the necessity of a formal hearing. In most cases of acute traumatic injuries (for example, fractures or lacerations occurring at work), the relationship to work is unquestionable and the system works reasonably well at compensating the injured worker. In many cases, however, the relationship to work is less clear, and the demand on the clinician more complicated, as the following case illustrates.

A 50-year-old truck driver followed by his physician for 6 years because of chronic low back pain came to the physician stating "I cannot take it anymore." Although he could not recall a specific injury, he found that the requirements of driving a long-haul tractor trailer caused him severe discomfort that was no longer relieved by rest or analgesics. His back discomfort generally improved while he was on vacation but was clearly aggravated after more than 2 hours of driving or after any heavy lifting (at home or at work). He had been out of work for one week because of his discomfort and required a note from the physician before returning to work. Physical examination revealed a mild decrease in forward flexion. X-rays were consistent with osteoarthritis of the spine. The patient wanted to know the physician's opinion on whether his back problems were due to his work as a truck driver, whether he should change his vocation because of his discomfort, and whether he should file a workers' compensation claim for work-related injuries.

This case illustrates some of the difficulties in evaluating and treating the patient with work incapacity. The patient went to the physician because his back discomfort was interfering with his ability to do his job. Like most patients with chronic low back pain, his symptoms and examination findings were nonspecific. The standard recommendations of rest and avoidance of exacerbating activities met with transient success, but his symptoms reappeared with his return to work. It is logical at this point to explore with the patient any opportunity for job accommodations at work, and, if no alternatives are available, for him to seek employment that would not exacerbate the symptoms. The patient, for a variety of reasons, however, may be reluctant to consider changing to another line of work, despite the discomfort associated with the current job.

With regard to causality, the high prevalence of nonspecific low back pain in the general population and the multifactorial etiology of this common condition make it impossible to say with medical certainty that this patient's back discomfort was caused in its entirety by his work. Several epidemiologic studies, however, have linked truck driving with a higher incidence of chronic disabling low back pain and have attributed this increase to excessive vibration, sitting, and heavy lifting. Despite medical uncertainty, it is likely that most compensation systems would recognize this patient's low back pain as a condition that is aggravated by work and that the patient's medical bills and lost wages related to his back pain would be covered by workers' compensation insurance.

The Social Security Administration, in the U.S. Department of Health and Human Services, administers two plans that provide benefits to those unable to work regardless of the cause of disability.

*Social Security Disability Insurance (SSDI)* is a true insurance plan in that all nongovernmental employees in the United States contribute to the plan through mandatory deductions from wages. Eligibility requires 5 years of contributions to the plan over the previous 10 years, and is determined by the federal Social Security Administration. State rehabilitation commissions are given the responsibility of determining whether the applicant's impairment qualifies for benefits. To qualify, an impairment must be the result of a documented medical illness and must be expected to result in at least one year of inability to work, or death, but does not have to be a consequence of work. Once a claim is accepted, there is a 6-month waiting period until benefits begin. Claims are reevaluated periodically to determine whether a severe impairment continues to exist, and updated medical information is requested. The condition must be as severe as the standard description listed in the Social Security Administration's publication *Disability Evaluation Under Social Security*. If a condition is not listed in the regulations, it must be medically equivalent to one that is listed. A sufficient impairment must result in inability to perform any gainful employment, not only the person's usual job. In cases in which the impairment does not meet the established criteria, the examiner will take into account age, education, and prior work history in determining the likelihood that an applicant would be able to find any future employment. The following case illustrates the basic medical considerations involved in the Social Security disability determination process.

A 60-year-old man was referred for Social Security disability for evaluation related to chronic lung disease. The patient had been a maintenance worker since age 25 and had moderate exposure to asbestos when he worked as a "fireman" on a Navy ship during World War II. He smoked one to two packs of cigarettes a day for the past 42 years until quitting 6 months before this evaluation. He had been short of breath for 7 years. He became exhausted by merely dressing himself in the morning. Physical examination revealed him to be thin, with a respiratory rate of 18 at rest. His breath sounds were distant posteriorly and there was no clubbing or cyanosis of the nail beds. Chest x-ray showed flattened diaphragms, emphysematous changes, and bilateral pleural plaques. His pulmonary function tests showed severe obstructive lung disease with an $FEV_1$ of 1.1 liters (35 percent of predicted), and FVC of 3.1 liters (68 percent of predicted), a TLV of 5.4 liters (80 percent of predicted), and an $FEV_1/FVC$ ratio of 35 percent.

In this case, a patient with severe chronic lung disease was being evaluated for disability under Social Security. His exposure history was significant for occupational exposure to asbestos and nonoccupational exposure to cigarette smoke. His physical examination, chest x-ray, and pulmonary function tests were consistent with diagnoses of (1) severe obstructive lung disease and possible restrictive lung disease, and (2) asbestos-related pleural plaques.

A number of systems have been developed for evaluation of severe pulmonary impairment. These systems are not identical in the level of impairment that is considered severe. For 40- and 60-year-old men who are each 70 inches tall, the $FEV_1$ values for "severe impairment" are different for each system (Table 11-2). Comparison of this patient's pulmonary function tests with the guidelines for SSDI demonstrates that people of this height who have an $FEV_1$ of less than 1.4 liters are considered disabled under Social Security.

The patient's occupational exposure to asbestos might have played a small etiologic role in the development of pulmonary insufficiency. It is worth noting, however, that this would have no effect on the patient's application for SSDI.

**Table 11-2.** Comparison of levels of $FEV_1$ required for severe impairment for 40- and 60- year-old white men, 70 in. (178cm) tall, using different criteria

| Criteria | Actual $FEV_1$ and percent of predicted value* | |
|---|---|---|
| | Age = 40 | Age = 60 |
| Social Security Administration (1986) | 1.5 (36%) | 1.5 (40%) |
| American Medical Association (1993) | 1.68 (40%) | 1.49 (40%) |
| Gaensler et al. (1966) | 1.59 (38%) | 1.37 (37%) |
| Department of Labor Black Lung Benefits (1978) | 2.38 (56%) | 2.06 (56%) |

*Percent predicted is based on RO Crapo, AH Morris, RM Gardner. Reference spirometric values using techniques and equipment that meet ATS recommendations. Am Rev Respir Dis 1981; 123:659–66.

The other Social Security Administration plan, *Supplemental Security Income* (SSI), is a program, funded through federal taxes (not by employee contributions), for blind, disabled, or elderly people who do not qualify for SSDI. Although criteria for disability are identical to those for SSDI, benefits are generally lower and do not begin until the claimant's assets and benefits from all other sources are exhausted.

*Private disability insurance* is available from many insurers in the United States and may be purchased individually or through an employer or union. These programs provide benefits to supplement SSDI and have much less stringent criteria for acceptance of claims. Usually, the claimant need only have his or her physician state that an impairment exists that prevents working at the usual job. Most plans provide a percentage of regular income for the first 2 years of disability if one is unable to work at his or her usual job because of a medical condition. Afterward, full benefits are paid only if the claimant is totally disabled from any type of work; if the claimant can do work with lower wages than previously, the difference between current potential wages and prior wages may be used to determine the reimbursement level. Programs usually provide for maintenance of health insurance and certain other employee benefits, and benefits usually end at retirement age. Many variations and supplements exist that can be purchased by an employee. The next case illustrates a typical situation that would be covered through private disability insurance.

A 60-year-old male maintenance worker, who formerly smoked cigarettes, was referred by his employer for a return-to-work evaluation. The patient had been out of work for 3 months following hospitalization for myocardial infarction (MI). Despite an adequate medical regimen, the patient continued to have fatigue after minimal exertion, but had no chest pain. His home activities were limited to 20 minutes of walking twice a day. On physical examination he was in no acute distress, with a resting heart rate of 80 beats per minute. His lungs were clear to auscultation, and his heart sounds showed a normal rate and rhythm without murmur or gallop. The electrocardiogram showed evidence of his previous MI. A recent exercise test had been discontinued after 4 minutes because of the patient's fatigue, but he had no signs of active ischemia or arrhythmia. His job as a maintenance worker involved walking long distances in the plant, pushing a 45-kg (100-lb) maintenance cart, and performing scheduled and unscheduled machinery repair.

In summary, this patient showed evidence of cardiopulmonary deconditioning after a myocardial infarction. He demonstrated decreased exercise capability by his symptoms and exercise tolerance test performance. This deconditioning would probably prevent him from performing his normal job tasks. Most likely he had not achieved a medical end-result by the time of his evaluation. It would, therefore be appropriate to refer this patient to a cardiac rehabilitation program in an attempt to increase his exercise tolerance before making any judgment about permanent impairment. He would be supervised in a progressive exercise program,

which might restore much of his exercise capacity. Until fit enough to return to work, this patient would be eligible for continued short-term disability compensation from his company-sponsored plan. He would *not* be eligible under Social Security because the disability was not expected to last more than one year and did not meet the relevant guidelines. Since outcome of rehabilitation efforts may be difficult to predict at the outset, the treating physician would want to monitor the patient's progress and reevaluate his disability once a plateau in reconditioning has been reached.

## Steps in the Disability Evaluation Process

The following questions are involved in disability evaluation:

1. What is the patient's medical diagnosis?
2. Does the individual have any impairment related to this diagnosis? If an impairment is present, is it temporary or permanent?
3. What is the extent of any impairment? (See box.)
4. Is the patient's impairment or disease caused or aggravated by work?
5. What is the impact of this impairment on the individual's ability to obtain employment in specific occupations and to perform specific jobs? Alternatively, in the context of the ADA, what are this person's current capabilities? Might accommodations allow for employment?
6. What other sources of information on work capabilities or possible accommodations should be considered?
7. In consideration of the answers to the previous questions, to what, if any, economic benefit is the individual entitled?

Physicians generally play a major role in answering the first four questions. The ADA encourages their participation in the fifth and sixth ques-

## STANDARDIZED MEASURES OF IMPAIRMENT

Most sytems that provide disability benefits require objective evidence of functional loss. However, clinicians' assessments tend to integrate subjective impressions with objective data in their evaluations, since this integrative model has proved useful in treating patients. Therefore, impairment measurements may differ considerably among evaluators. A number of systems to standardize impairment measurement have been developed, such as the American Medical Association (AMA) *Guidelines to the Evaluation of Permanent Impairment,* to limit these differences. Any system that attempts to evaluate work disability in the absence of detailed information on job requirements, however, will be seriously flawed.

Why bother to develop standardized measures of impairment? First, since most reimbursement systems rely on objective medical data (physical examination findings and laboratory test results) to verify impairment, standardization might allow for a common method of reporting this information. Second, consistent examination methods and reliance on objective findings rather than on subjective descriptions would eliminate much of the conflict over degree of functional loss and resulting compensation benefits. Third, quantifiable measurements of residual function in various organ systems should be linked with data on functional ability required by various jobs; this linkage might be helpful in designing individualized rehabilitation programs. Finally, objective measurements of function have been shown to aid in measuring progress in a rehabilitation program, or lack of progress when a medical end-result has been reached.

For over 30 years, the AMA and the Social Security Administration (SSA) have worked to develop guides for objective impairment quantification. Both organizations' guides divide evaluations by organ systems, specifying the medical information required for the evaluation. The SSA guide provides threshold criteria for impairments sufficient for eligibility; the AMA guides express impairment as a percentage of total body function that has been lost. For example, the AMA guides provide reproducible information for impairment from hand injuries, allowing documentation of functional changes over time. The validity of these so-called standardized measures of impairment in predicting actual functional losses in other organ systems has not been established.

A number of problems frustrate attempts to develop measures of impairment that are reproducible, valid, and standardized. The absence of a "pre-injury" baseline evaluation usually forces the examiner to use population-derived norms to predict degrees of functional loss. For example, the results of simple lung function tests are often compared to the distribution of test results in a population, standardized by age, sex, height, and race, to determine what percentage of a predicted value is present in an individual. An individual who originally had large lung volumes and lost a significant percentage of function because of disease might have a substantial respiratory impairment but may still have "normal" lung volumes by testing. Conversely, another person may have always had lung volumes below the population-derived norm, and a slight decrease on lung function tests may result in a misleading label of "abnormal lung function." Exercise testing with oxygen uptake monitoring provides a much better measure of how well the lungs perform in their essential function of oxygen transport; these tests can reveal critical limitations of gas exchange that are not shown by simple spirometric testing [6]. Therefore, a static test of lung volume might be quick and inexpensive but would not reveal information about actual ability that a test of function, such as exercise testing, shows. Inaccuracies caused by poor cardiovascular conditioning, lack of understanding, fear of test procedures, or poor motivation can confound even the best test in providing estimates of actual functional ability. A determination of medical end-result may be frustrated by an illness with a variable course of presentation, where signs and symptoms wax and wane.

Several devices have been developed to quantify musculoskeletal function. These devices measure ability to exert a rotational or linear force against a mobile or stationary object. Output of the device, which is usually reproducible, generally indicates the degree or distance of motion and the maximum force applied. Many programs have used these devices in assessment and rehabilitation of extremity injuries. To date, these devices have not been shown to accurately predict ability to perform occupational tasks, since the actions required to operate them are usually unrelated to job tasks. When considering purchase and use of these devices, the clinician should carefully review the scientific data supporting any advantages over existing forms of assessment and rehabilitation.

The following case is an example of an impairment and disability evaluation, where standardized measurement of impairment had been attempted:

A physician had been treating a 58-year-old clerk for apparently non–work-related carpal tunnel syndrome of both hands, mainly the right (dominant) hand. Her job required filing, answering phones, and occasional typing. Six months after successful right carpal tunnel surgery, her pain and numbness largely resolved, although she still complained of considerable weakness of the right hand. Physical examination showed a well-healed scar and considerable loss of sensation in a median nerve distribution on the right, normal sensation on the left. Pinch strength by dynamometer was 5.4 kg (12 lb) with the left hand, and 2.7 kg (6 lb) with the right. She had been out of work for 6 months, and the physician believed that her condition had stabilized. She was concerned that "no one will hire me because I have hand problems" and wanted the physician to examine her for Social Security Disability Insurance (SSDI) eligibility.

1. What was the patient's medical diagnosis?

Carpal tunnel syndrome: status—post–right carpal tunnel release, with residual median nerve damage.

2. Was impairment present?

Yes. There was loss of normal function of the right hand, and the information suggested that no further return of function was likely to occur.

3. What was the level of impairment?

One could first quantify the impairment using the AMA guides. History and examination revealed that the left hand was normal; however, there was evidence of considerable sensory loss of the right hand. She stated that she could do most of the activities of self-care but had difficulty with digital dexterity; physical examination revealed considerable loss of two-point discrimination, pain sensation, and sensation to fine touch over the affected area, as well as decreased oppositional strength between the thumb and other fingers. According to the charts in the AMA guides, she had a 2 percent loss of motor function in the upper extremity caused by median nerve motor injury (20 percent loss of median nerve motor function in the hand, multiplied by 10 percent maximal loss of upper-extremity strength due to median neuropathy). Similar calculations revealed a 23 percent loss of function in the upper extremity from sensory deficit. These values are combined to yield a 27 percent impairment of the upper extremity, or a 16 percent impairment of the whole person. This calculation has limited medical significance, although the structured examination could be repeated in the future to aid in determining whether any medical progress has been made.

For the SSDI application, the physician must provide a description of the patient's functional status by history and examination; it would be helpful to describe her attempts to move objects in the office. The evaluation report should also include a copy of the nerve conduction studies and the statement that a medical end-result had been reached.

4. Was the patient's impairment caused or aggravated by work?

No report of forceful or repetitive movements required at work was indicated. A careful review of the job tasks with the patient might have uncovered a history of unusual activities that might have exacerbated or even caused the carpal tunnel syndrome, such as folding large quantities of paper, typing on a manual typewriter, or using scissors extensively. Work-relatedness, however, is not an issue in SSDI.

5. What was the impact of the impairment on the individual's ability to obtain employment or perform specific jobs?

The amount of impairment here may have interfered with typing and filing but may not have interfered with other duties. If these activities were required in the job, then the physician might have had to ask the patient to demonstrate her ability to perform these skills; the exercise in the AMA guides would not have been helpful in determining disability. The actual abilities of the patient over an 8-hour workday are difficult to determine by a cursory office examination and are best decided by a vocational evaluation specialist with a thorough understanding of a patient's functional ability and job demands. The history of current household activities may also aid in assessment of functional ability.

6. To what, if any, economic benefits was this patient entitled?

It is unlikely that she would have initially received SSDI, since the threshold in *Disability Evaluation Under Social Security* requires a process that "results in sustained disturbance of gross and dexterous movements in *two* extremities." If on case review she demonstrated limited education and work experience, and impairment preventing performance of practically any job, her claim might have been accepted. The physician's input in this regard is not considered; Social Security disability determination services often employ vocational assessors to perform this function. However, if the patient were applying for private disability insurance, the physician might have to determine whether the essential job tasks could be performed by the patient.

tions, along with other professionals. The answer to the fifth question often depends on the specialized skills of a vocational evaluation unit and input from the employer, and may be based on legal-administrative criteria. The last question is usually resolved by administrators using legal guidelines.

Physical examination findings that support the degree of impairment and the stated diagnosis are important. For example, SSDI claims without positive objective physical findings (symptoms without physical or laboratory findings) are rejected. Evaluations often include measurement of strength and endurance, length of scar, degree of visual impairment, and other relevant items. Serial measurement of these findings over time provides an objective basis for deciding whether a medical end-result has been achieved. Since the physician's office usually has meager resources to fully evaluate functional capacity, referral to an occupational therapist or vocational evaluation specialist for work capacity evaluation may be appropriate. A

series of standardized tasks can be performed to document functional impairment.

The physician is often asked to determine whether the impairment is permanent or whether a medical end-result has been achieved. For example, in the first case, it is likely that the patient would feel better once he had been away from work for a few weeks. However, his physician's experience showed that this patient consistently developed back pain soon after returning to this type of work. Although some improvement of the symptoms is likely, the patient probably would not improve enough medically to allow him to continue working as a truck driver. Therefore, in terms of functional ability, a medical end-result has been achieved; although his discomfort is not likely to be permanent, the medical limitations to his working as a truck driver probably will not change.

At times, insurance companies or lawyers ask for a determination of permanency that seems to require a crystal ball. In many cases, the prognosis for functional improvement is uncertain. Pressures from a lawyer or insurer may be present to declare a medical end-result so that a case can be settled. However, it is important to communicate uncertainty, both to the patient and to others involved with the case; patients do not benefit from a premature medical determination of permanent disability.

In workers' compensation and in private insurance disability cases, the physician is often asked whether the impairment is disabling and to describe how the impairment impedes the performance of usual job tasks. A clear job description is the basis for evaluating whether the employee can perform the essential functions of the job. Often, this cannot be determined without knowing what accommodations at work might be available. Thus, in the second case, it cannot be determined whether the patient is totally disabled until it is known whether any alternate work or accommodations are available. The same considerations apply to determining disability for private insurance. A visit to the workplace usually will resolve the lack of clarity that frequently is present in standard job descriptions and may have an important role in encouraging an employer to provide accommodations for the disabled employee.

Most insurance systems reimburse individuals for loss of earning capacity caused by objective impairment. It is often difficult to determine whether sufficient impairment exists for one to qualify for benefits under a given plan. Physicians usually lack the experience, technical facilities, and ability to accurately estimate vocational potential; in these situations, early involvement with a qualified vocational rehabilitation specialist is worthwhile. Specialized skills and a broad database are required to predict residual earning capacity when an employee is no longer able to return to previous work. For example, factors related to worker autonomy, such as the availability of self-paced work, educational and experience levels, and self-employment, have been shown to be more important in determining disability status in patients with rheumatoid arthritis than the extent of med-

ical findings [4]. In workers' compensation plans and in most private disability plans, the treating or reviewing physician is required only to determine that the impairment is sufficient to prevent work. However, in the Social Security, Veteran's Administration, and Black Lung programs, there are often specific criteria for impairment that determine whether one is eligible for benefits, which vary from plan to plan. For example, the Black Lung and Social Security programs have threshold pulmonary function values; if an applicant's lung function is better than the threshold, then he or she does not qualify for disability. In the Veteran's Administration system, the degree of lost function is expressed as a percentage of total lung function. Benefits are assigned based on the percentage of function lost; in contrast, the Social Security and Black Lung programs usually provide a fixed amount of benefits only if a worker is totally disabled according to the threshold criteria. Physicians are often frustrated with the arbitrary nature of the determination process. Under these criteria, some individuals with truly disabling impairments will be refused compensation, while others capable of gainful employment will receive benefits.

## The Clinician's Role

Within the disability evaluation process, three different and potentially conflicting roles for the clinician become clear: patient advocate, provider of information, and medical adjudicator. It is important to understand the requirements of each of these roles so that the patient can best be served.

Clinicians must not neglect their role as patient advocate in treating patients with work incapacity and, when appropriate, assisting them in obtaining accommodations at work, or benefits to the extent entitled by a particular disability system. The clinician should not let personal feelings about a specific disability or impairment rating system interfere with judgment in assisting patients.

As patient advocates, clinicians need to be aware of their role in preventing complications in patients with work disability (see box). Patients frequently are limited financially and socially by their work incapacity, and social isolation frequently accompanies isolation from the workplace. Patients may be upset at how they have been handled by the "system," especially if benefits have been delayed or denied. They may be angry at the apparent insensitivity of their employer, insurer, or physician and this anger often complicates their evaluation and treatment. Patients are often afraid of returning to the workplace where a serious in-jury occurred, or they may be afraid of being dismissed once they have successfully returned to work. Being aware of the complicated social, legal, and psychological state of disabled workers is an essential aspect of assisting their recovery. Appropriate referral for psychological diagnosis and treatment should be considered in every case of prolonged work incapacity. Mindful of the adverse psychological, physical, and economic consequences of disability, the clinician should be careful to avoid removing patients from gainful employment whenever possible.

Patients may also have significant concerns

---

## REHABILITATION MANAGEMENT FOR WORK-RELATED INJURIES
—Charles D. DelTatto and
  Edward C. Swanson

The physical restoration and ultimate reorientation of injured workers has become a multifocal process involving a multidisciplinary team of professionals (Fig. 11-2). Members of this team include physicians, physical therapists, occupational therapists, occupational health nurses, and safety personnel. In large corporations, all team members may be within the same health unit. For small employers, the team members may be consultants to the workplace or be professionals practicing in the community. Regardless of the setting, it is essential that the team be clearly identified and utilized.

Historically, occupational injuries have been grouped together with other injury cases and have been expected to respond to similar interventions. However, analysis of case outcomes reveals the need to rethink current management models and to give occupational injuries a more specialized approach.

On the surface, this approach may appear no different from any other acute medical model. However, here the processes of triage, diagnosis, and treatment are predicated on unique information: (1) a clear understanding of the worker's job, especially those physical demands contributing to the injury; and (2) environmental and other physical demands the worker will encounter.

Each member of the team must consider this information when designing an effective rehabilitation program that will result in return to work and avoidance of reinjury. This goal is achieved by early integration of physical restoration and injury prevention measures.

To facilitate this approach an early referral to physical or occupational therapy is desirable. In so doing, critical information required by the team will be gathered in a systematic way.

First, the job description at the time of injury should be requested from the occupational nurse or other appropriate person at the workplace. This description will form the baseline measurement for the physical restoration program and provide the framework for any specific medical release. Initial investigation of the factors that contributed to the injury should also begin. This information can be collected by the workplace safety officer or industrial nurse. A plan to eliminate or minimize factors that contributed to the injury should be implemented prior to the worker's return and should be coordinated with the physical restoration process. The therapist may also be able to assist in task redesign and worker instruction in proper material handling techniques, if deemed appropriate [1, 2].

Because the therapist, in most cases, will spend the greatest amount of time with the injured worker, he or she must act as investigator, mediator, and sounding board for the rest of the team.

Program design must be specific to the nature of the injury and expected physical demands. Simulated work tasks should also be incorporated into any restoration plan [3]. These tasks will serve as an objective measure of the workers' progress and form the basis of specific return-to-work recommendations.

Modification of treatment approach may be necessary and will largely depend on the team's ability to identify both the physical and emotional signs of any delayed recovery [4].

Frequent communication of critical information must be made among team members, allowing for a clear mutual understanding of where the injured worker is in the recovery process and when return-to-work planning should begin.

Any breakdown in communication among team members leads to misunderstanding and often unnecessarily protracts the restoration process. Nowhere is this breakdown more evident than at the time of medical release. Often the employer receives little information at this point, usually in the form of a physician's vague order to "return to light duty" or "do not lift over 15 lb." It is very difficult for the employer to translate this into functional terms, and consequently the employee is often not allowed back to the workplace without a medical release stating that he or she is 100 percent fit for duty.

What makes return to work optimal is a medical release that addresses specific alternative jobs or tasks that the worker can safely perform and includes a timetable for progressive reemployment, if the worker is unable initially to sustain a full workday. This kind of specific medical release is only possible if the restoration program is designed to yield this type of information from its start.

The successful rehabilitation of injured workers depends on a team approach. Program design must address expected physical demands while the contributing factors of the original injury are identified and controlled, if not totally eliminated, prior to return to work. Communication among all involved parties is most critical and will ultimately determine the success of the entire process.

## References

1. Ayoub MA. Control of manual lifting hazards: Training in safe handling. J Occup Med 1982; 24:573–7.
2. Ayoub MA. Control of manual lifting hazards: Training in safe handling. J Occup Med 1982; 24:668–76.
3. Matheson L. Work capacity evaluation, 1986, VI: pp. 2–26; VII: pp. 2–23. Anaheim, CA: Employment Rehabilitation Institute of California.
4. Tullis W, Devebery VJ. Delayed recovery in the patient with a work compensable injury. J Occup Med 1983; 25:829–35.

## Bibliography

Cyriax J. Diagnosis of soft tissue lesions. In Textbook of orthopedic medicine. Vol. 1, 8th ed. London: Balliere-Tindall, 1979.
*Manual of techniques for the systematic approach to evaluation and treatment of soft tissue lesions.*
Saunders H. Orthopedic physical therapy evaluation and treatment of musculoskeletal disorders. 1982.
*Saunders' evaluation and treatment planning of musculoskeletal conditions including indication for, contraindication to, and effects of physical exercise and physical agents.*
Alexander D, Palat BM. Industrial ergonomics, a practitioner's guide. Norcross, GA: Industrial Engineering & Management Press, 1985.
*This text explains through example and illustration the use of ergonomics in the industrial setting. All articles are original works or adaptations written especially for this book.*
Mayer et al. Objective assessment of spine function following industrial injury. JAMA 1987; 258: 1763–7.
*This article details comprehensive assessment and treatment of patients with low back pain: compared with a control group of chronic patients who did not participate in a treatment program.*

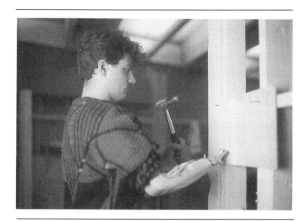

Fig. 11-2. Highly trained professionals take advantage of advanced technology in prosthetics and retaining equipment in worker rehabilitation to achieve the best possible function for an injured individual, such as this man who is relearning his trade as a carpenter using a prosthetic arm. The immensity of the effort and its inherent limitations emphasize the importance of all possible efforts to prevent the initial injury. (Courtesy of Liberty Mutual Medical Services)

about the disability evaluation itself. Since they are aware that the outcome of the evaluation may determine their access to or continuation of benefits, they may feel the need to emphasize the extent of the disability to "prove" their case. They may have residual anger from previous examinations in which clinicians seemed unsympathetic or doubted their "true" disability.

As a patient gradually loses function because of a progressive disease process, the physician should anticipate the possibility that earning capacity may be lost and discuss this potential with the patient. Patients should be made aware of the potential loss of self-esteem and income and the uncertainty of receiving benefits while out of work. Actively assisting patients in vocational rehabilitation and early selection of jobs that will not conflict with physical limitations can avoid unnecessary time out of work. Physicians should learn of possible accommodations in the workplace by contacting the personnel manager or the patient's

supervisor, and seek input from specialists in job accommodation. With this information, the physician can often help the employee return to work earlier, thus preserving earning capacity and often providing an additional stimulus to recovery.

In the routine care of patients, clinicians will frequently be asked to provide information relating to their patient's medical condition for the purposes of determining impairment or disability. Such requests may originate from employers, insurance companies, state agencies, or patients. When such requests are accompanied by the patient's signed requests for release of information, it is appropriate to supply information that is relevant to the request. (However, it would not be appropriate, for example, to comment on or release records about a patient's diabetes or epilepsy when the request was for information about impairment from an injury to the lower back.) Since records relating to workplace injuries must be routinely supplied in workers' compensation cases, it may be worthwhile to make and provide office notes that are separate from the notes relating to other, non–work-related problems. Since a worker's reimbursement is frequently tied to the receipt of records from the attending clinician, it is important that clinicians be prompt in responding to such requests to minimize financial difficulties for their patients.

Several sources of information can aid in the provision of relevant information. For example, most private disability plans have a short guide on eligibility requirements for clinicians, state workers' compensation boards often publish free guidebooks, and the Social Security Administration office will provide a free copy of the *Disability Determination Guide*.

The greatest potential conflict arises between the primary clinician's traditional role as patient advocate and his or her gatekeeper or adjudicator role, brought about by a request from an employer or insurance company for professional evaluation of impairment. This situation can lead to hostility between patient and clinician because of unrealistic expectations and inexperience with disability systems. Frequently, patients are not aware of the requirements of different systems and will blame their clinicians if benefits are denied. Clinicians will frequently share their patients' frustration with the arbitrary nature of a particular disability system. Clinicians occasionally resent their patients for "trying to take advantage" of an insurance system, and patients may rightly resent the need to "prove" their illness. All of these feelings may interfere with a satisfactory clinician-patient relationship.

When a clinician is acting as an adjudicator, therefore, it is important to clarify the purpose of the evaluation and the limitations of the clinician's situation. It may be appropriate for the clinician to refer the patient to a social worker, lawyer, or union representative for clarification of the social, legal, and financial issues surrounding application for disability. It is often appropriate for a clinician to seek an independent opinion about impairment and disability when there is a potential for conflict with a patient or significant uncertainty about the cause or extent of disability [5].

## References

1. Kusnetz S, Hutchinson MK. eds. A guide to the work-relatedness of disease. Revised ed. (NIOSH publication no. 79-116). Washington, D.C.: U.S. Government Printing Office, 1979.
2. Barth PS, Hunt HA. Workers' compensation and work-related illnesses. Cambridge, MA: MIT Press, 1980.
3. Hadler NM. Disability backache in France, Switzerland, and the Netherlands: Contrasting sociopolitical constraints on clinical judgment. JOM, 1989; 31: 823–30.
4. Yelin E, et al. Work disability in rheumatoid arthritis: Effects of disease, social and work factors. Ann Intern Med 1980; 95:551–6.
5. Sullivan MD, Loeser JD. The diagnosis of disability: Treating and rating disability in a pain clinic. Arch Intern Med 1992; 152:1829–35.
6. Becklake MR. Organic and functional impairment:
Overall perspective. Am Rev Respir Dis 1984; 129: (Suppl.) S96–S100.

## Bibliography

Committee on Mental and Physical Impairment, American Medical Association. Guidelines to the evaluation of permanent impairment. 4th ed. Chicago: American Medical Association, 1993.
*These guidelines offer a quantitative approach to the measurement of permanent impairment. They are easy to use and well illustrated. There is no documentation concerning the validity of the impairment ratings. However, the guidelines are a useful starting point in impairment evaluations.*
Becklake MR. Organic and functional impairment: Overall perspectives. Am Rev Respir Dis 1984; 129:(Suppl.) S96–S100.
*Thorough, yet concise, discussion of the problems inherent in development and use of "normal" values for interpretation of lung function tests and methods of cardiopulmonary disability determination.*
Care TS, Hadler NM. The role of the primary physician in disability determination for Social Security and workers' compensation. Ann Intern Med 1986; 104:706–10.
*A good overview of the physician's role in these systems.*
Social Security Administration. Disability evaluation under Social Security, Social Security Administration publication no. 05-10089. Washington, D.C.: U.S. Department of Health and Human Services, 1986.
*A guide to SSA medical criteria for disability.*

---

APPENDIX

# A Human Rights Approach to People with Disabilities: The Americans with Disabilities Act

Jay S. Himmelstein, Glenn S. Pransky, and David Fram

---

The employment provisions of the Americans with Disabilities Act (1990) seek to promote the inde-

David Fram is an ADA Policy Attorney in the Office of Legal Counsel, U.S. Equal Employment Opportunity Commission. This article was cowritten by Fram in his private capacity. No official support or endorsement by the Commission or any other agency of the U.S. Government is intended or should be inferred.

pendence of people with disabilities through equal opportunity for employment. As such, this act promotes a "human rights" approach—as opposed to a "compensation" approach—to the problems confronted by people with disabilities. The Appendix reviews the major employment provisions of the Americans with Disabilities Act (ADA) and discusses opportunities for health professionals to support appropriate employment opportunities for people with disabilities and to thereby help *prevent* the tertiary consequences of disability such as poverty and social isolation.

## Employment Provisions of the ADA

Title I of the ADA prohibits employment discrimination against "a qualified individual with a disability" on account of his or her disability. An individual with a disability is defined in the ADA as someone who (1) has a physical or mental impairment that substantially limits one or more major life activities, (2) has a record of such impairment, or (3) is regarded as having such an impairment. An individual is "qualified" if she or he meets the basic job prerequisites and can perform the "essential functions" of the job with or without "reasonable accommodation." This prohibition reaches to all aspects of the employment relationship, including application procedures, hiring, promotion, compensation, training, and discipline. The ADA also requires employers to make reasonable accommodations for qualified individuals with disabilities.

Under the ADA, employers may not conduct medical examinations or make inquiries regarding the existence, nature, or severity of an applicant's disability before she/he is extended a conditional offer of employment. After an individual is offered a job, but before he/she starts work, an employer may require such examinations and may make such inquiries, if this applies equally to all applicants in the job category. Although an employer may obtain medical/disability-related information at the postoffer stage, the ADA restricts employ-

ers' subsequent actions based on this information. An employer may withdraw a conditional job offer because of an individual's disability *only* if the employer can show one of the following:

1. The individual cannot perform the essential functions of the job despite reasonable accommodations.
2. The individual poses a "direct threat" to self or others in the position, which cannot be reasonably accommodated.
3. Other federal laws or regulations (for example, those administered by the Federal Aviation Administration [FAA] and the Department of Transportation [DOT]) require the employer to withdraw the job offer because of the individual's medical condition.

Therefore, to avoid liability under the ADA, an employer must analyze the following key issues, frequently with input from medical personnel:

1. *Does the individual have a disability protected by the ADA?* This requires the employer to examine whether the individual has a "physical or mental impairment," and whether the impairment "substantially limits" a "major life activity." It also requires the employer to analyze whether the individual has a "record of" or is "regarded as" having such an impairment.
2. *Is the individual qualified to perform the job?* This requires the employer to examine whether the individual can perform the "essential functions" of the job, with "reasonable accommodation," if needed.
3. *Does the individual pose a "direct threat" and,* if so, can the risk of harm be reduced below the direct threat level through a reasonable accommodation? This requires the employer to examine whether the individual poses a "significant risk of substantial harm" to himself or others, and whether that risk can be reduced through a reasonable accommodation.

# The Role of the Health Professional Under the ADA

The ADA places requirements on employers aimed at providing equal employment opportunities for people with disabilities. The role of medical professionals in this process is primarily to provide guidance on issues of whether an individual has a covered disability, to determine whether the individual poses a direct threat, and to make recommendations regarding workplace accommodations.

## Does the Individual Have a Covered Disability?

The health professional can assist the employer in determining whether an individual has a physical or mental impairment and whether the impairment substantially limits a major life activity, without revealing information unrelated to the diagnosis of disability. In the simplest case, this role can be fulfilled merely by providing information regarding an impairment that limits one or more major life activities. For example, a patient who has multiple sclerosis that substantially interferes with walking would have an impairment that "substantially limits one or more major life activities" and therefore would have a covered disability. Likewise, a potential employee who has fully recovered from back surgery but is limited by his inability to lift objects weighing more than five pounds from floor level may be considered to have a covered disability. A physician's determination that someone has no actual disability does not completely resolve the matter; an individual may have a covered disability if an employer simply "regards" him or her as having a disability.

## Does the Individual Pose a Direct Threat?

An employer may require that an individual not pose a "direct threat" to the health or safety of self or others in performance of the job. However, the requirements to meet the "direct threat" threshold as specified under the ADA are quite stringent. The risk and adverse outcome of concern must be specific, significant (severe), and highly probable; the risk factors must be based on objective medical data, not speculation or generalization from studies of large groups or similar persons; the risk must be constant, not temporary; and finally, the risk must be one that cannot be eliminated through reasonable accommodations. Each one of these areas should be addressed by an evaluating health professional in advising the employer whether the "direct threat" standard has been met. The consideration of whether an individual constitutes a direct threat to self or others is probably the most complicated aspect of the ADA that is likely to be confronted by clinicians. We strongly recommend that clinicians familiarize themselves with the examples offered by the technical assistance manual published by the United States Equal Employment Opportunity Commission on this subject [1].

## What Accommodations Are Appropriate?

An important and positive role for medical personnel is the recommendation of reasonable accommodations that would allow a person to perform the essential functions of the job. This, of course, requires that the evaluating health provider has detailed information about the job requirements or has personal knowledge of the job through visiting the workplace. In the example of the patient with multiple sclerosis described previously, it may be that the only accommodation needed is wheelchair access to his desk so that he can perform his job as a data entry clerk. In the case of the patient after back surgery, the recommendations for accommodation may be more complex. For example, assuming that "lifting" is not an essential function of the job, reassigning the lifting duties to another employee would likely be an appropriate accommodation. If "lifting" is an essential function, then the clinician might suggest that certain equipment be obtained so that the employee can perform this function, despite his physical limitations. Regardless of the clinician's suggestion, it is ultimately up to the employer to provide the reasonable accommodation.

It should be obvious from the above description that active participation in enhancing employment of people with disabilities requires an expanded base of information for practicing clinicians. Several caveats are worth emphasizing:

1. *The evaluation of workers must be individualized to a specific person and a specific set of job tasks.* Except for certain situations, there are overriding health and safety requirements established under federal laws; physicians and employers will be prohibited from relying on nonspecific "physical standards" unless it has been demonstrated that those who fail to meet the standards because of a disability constitute a "direct threat" to themselves or others or cannot perform essential job tasks with reasonable accommodations.

2. *A person's ability to do a job is often best determined by job simulation or job trial.* Many of the best methods for determining fitness, therefore, will be nonmedical in nature, and the role of the medical examination may be minimal in determining employability. Moreover, determining a person's future risk of injury or disease progression is especially complicated and filled with potential liability for the evaluating clinician and the employer. In relating to employers and employees, therefore, the physician should be careful to ensure that employers are aware of the very limited benefit of preplacement worker fitness and risk evaluations.

3. *Clinicians are health care providers, not lawyers or personnel managers.* Although health professionals need to become conversant with their role under the law, it is not their duty to act as legal counsels to employers or employees. Although providers should communicate with employers, they must remember that it is not their responsibility to make employment decisions. The physician's responsibility is to provide *medical opinions* and guidance regarding disability status, functional capability, and direct threat, and, where appropriate, to recommend modifications and accommodations to mitigate risk or enhance capabilities. The responsibility for making employment decisions or deciding whether or not it is possible to make a reasonable accommodation for a person with a disability lies with the employer, who is expected to incorporate insight from a variety of sources (including other health professionals and disability experts) in making employment decisions.

The ultimate impact of the ADA on the make-up of the American workplace will not be known for many years. However, it seems likely that if the ADA is successful in removing barriers to people with disabilities, occupational health practitioners, with their unique training and experience, and their familiarity with medicine and demands of work, will play a distinct and vital role in enhancing their opportunities and safety at work. To accomplish this, clinicians must shift from their traditional focus on diagnosing disability to recognizing and enhancing capability, consistent with the vision of occupational health as a true subspecialty of preventive medicine.

## Reference

1. A technical assistance manual on the employment provisions (Title I) of the Americans with Disabilities Act, Equal Employment Opportunity Commission. Washington, D.C.: US Government Printing Office, January 1992.

# 12
# Ethics in Occupational and Environmental Health

Kathleen M. Rest

*Case 1:* A company is seeking a permit to build an incinerator in a poor community with a large minority population. The company's risk assessment shows that the incinerator will pose no health risk to the community. A local environmental group presents a risk assessment that suggests otherwise.

*Case 2:* A government agency is considering whether to lower the permissible workplace exposure limit of a chemical because a recently completed epidemiologic study demonstrated adverse reproductive health effects at the current exposure level. The epidemiologists who conducted the study are reluctant to get involved in the policy debate, but other experts from industry, labor, and academia are asked to comment about the need for such action. They present conflicting interpretations of the new study, different views about the findings from prior studies, and widely divergent opinions on the need for more stringent regulation.

*Case 3:* A company decides to move its pesticide manufacturing operations to another country because labor costs are cheaper and because the other country's environmental and occupational regulations are much less stringent and virtually unenforced. The other country's ministry of commerce and development welcomes the company.

*Case 4:* A team of university scientists (epidemiologists, physicians, industrial hygienists, toxicologists, and statisticians) is funded to conduct a large industry-sponsored epidemiologic study. The team wants to establish an independent advisory board to oversee study design, conduct, analysis,

interpretation, and dissemination. The industry is reluctant to agree.

*Case 5:* A hospital-based occupational health program has a contract to provide clinical and consultation services to a local furniture manufacturer. The company has many ergonomic problems, and many workers have suffered musculoskeletal and repetitive strain injuries. Although the company physician, nurse, and safety engineer have recommended ergonomic changes in the work environment many times, the company has taken no action. Instead, the company has asked the nurse to institute a weight reduction program and a class on safe lifting techniques for the workers.

*Case 6:* A company has asked a local family physician to conduct its preplacement physicals, periodic screening examinations, and return-to-work evaluations and to provide all medical information to the company. The company has its own ideas about what the examinations should include. The physician has never visited the plant and has little information about workplace conditions and job demands.

*Case 7:* An occupational medicine resident conducts an "independent medical evaluation" on an individual who has been out of work for six months with a work-related injury. She tells her preceptor that she cannot understand why the patient seems hostile to her medical evaluation.

These cases illustrate the range of issues and types of ethical and moral questions that occupational and environmental health professionals, researchers, regulators, and others can expect to encounter on a regular basis. Because the environment in which these health and safety professionals function is one characterized by competing goals and interests and differential power structures, thorny ethical issues are common.

As a field of study, ethics comprises a complex discipline that attempts to analyze, define, and defend the moral basis of human action. For our purposes, we can use the term *ethics* to refer to the rightness and wrongness of human behavior. Ethics entails a sense of "ought"; that is, ethics helps us decide how we ought to act or what ought to be done. Ethics is not law, social custom, personal preference, or consensus of opinion, although any of these may derive from ethical considerations. Rather, ethics and ethical analyses help provide guides for action that are consistent; justifiable by appeal to commonly held values, principles, or rules; and able to withstand close moral scrutiny [1].

In occupational and environmental health, conflict and disagreement are common at many levels and sectors of activity and decision making—public, private, community, and individual. Difficult questions abound: What is the level of risk? What level should trigger action? What are the costs and benefits of regulating or not regulating, screening or not screening? How safe is safe enough? How much information are people entitled to? How should tradeoffs between health, environmental protection, and economic development be made? Not all aspects of these conflicts and decisions are ethical in nature; some may reflect simple disagreements about facts, methods, processes, or desired outcomes. Much of the disagreement, however, will have some underlying moral dimension, even when the arguments are framed in technical or economic terms.

This chapter provides a brief and basic discussion of the ethical dimensions of and the moral principles relevant to common occupational and environmental health issues in both policy and practice. Ethical analyses can make unique contributions to decision making and action. Readers may find such analyses helpful when they encounter situations similar to those raised in this chapter.

## Ethical Issues in Science and Policy

Science, technology, public and private business policy, and professional practice are common breeding grounds for heated debate and disagreement about occupational and environmental health issues.

In occupational and environmental health, most debates in science and public policy focus on the regulation and control of health and safety hazards. Beneath the thin veneer of technical and economic arguments over the basis, process, and content of regulation lie clear differences in values and in the deference given to widely held moral principles.

Although science, in its pursuit of truth, is often held to be "objective," it is now rather widely accepted that individual, social, and cultural values influence scientists in many aspects of their work [2]. These values may influence what scientists decide to study, how they frame research questions and design studies, what data they collect, how they analyze and interpret data, how they report study results, and how they participate in policy debates that involve the use of their findings. When scientists are honest with themselves and with the public about the influence of their own values or those of relevant interest groups on their activities and pronouncements, this is actually a good thing; it adds an important dimension to public and private decision making. However, there have been cases in which science and scientists have been bought (directly or indirectly) to serve political or ideological interests under the guise of "objectivity" [3].

Several cases mentioned at the beginning of this chapter illustrate common ethical issues in science and policy (public and private). In these cases, we find scientists and experts with different opinions about what a study means or which risk assessment reveals "the truth." Their differing views may involve honest disagreements about methodology, but may also reflect different understandings of the duties imposed by several widely held moral principles and concepts, such as beneficence, nonmaleficence, autonomy, justice, and responsibility [1, 4].

In deciding whether to approve the siting of an incinerator (in Case 1, the site is a poor community) or to lower the permissible exposure limit of a potential workplace reproductive toxin (as in Case 2) or to move a hazardous operation to a country with less stringent environmental controls (as in Case 3), scientists, regulators, government officials, and employers are dealing with concepts of *nonmaleficence* (the duty to do no harm), *beneficence* (the duty to do or promote good), *autonomy* (the duty to respect people's rights to self-determination), *justice* (the duty to be fair), and moral *responsibility* (the duty to secure a good outcome in matters for which one is responsible). The latter is said to arise either from interpersonal relationships, such as the responsibility a parent has for a child, or from the special knowledge that one person has relevant to the welfare of another [5]. Consideration of and deference to these moral concepts are particularly important in decisions involving health and safety regulations, which, to a large extent, transfer choice about "acceptable" risk from individuals to other entities, such as governments or corporations.

While there is a debate about the extent to which individuals are morally obligated to take positive action to contribute to the welfare of others, there is little disagreement that individuals should refrain from doing harm and, in some cases, take positive action to prevent harm from occurring. If the incinerator is sited, the health and well-being of community members may be harmed. If a chemical is not regulated more stringently, the reproductive health of workers in Case 2 may be endangered. If the hazardous facility is moved abroad, residents and workers in the new host country may be harmed.

On the other hand, one could argue that the incinerator will create new jobs for the poor community and that public welfare demands that it be sited somewhere, that more stringent regulation of a chemical will adversely affect the financial resources of some manufacturers and may even cause some workers to lose their jobs, and that the economy of the other country will be improved by the migration of the potentially hazardous industry.

Many disagreements are likely to revolve around issues relating to uncertainty, an inherent element in many areas of occupational and environmental health research, policy, and practice. Risk assessments will vary by orders of magnitude, depending on the models and assumptions made by the investigators [6]. Most epidemiologic studies show associations, not causation, and reported mortality risks are bounded by confidence intervals of varying widths. Of course, the models chosen, the assumptions made, and the designs employed may reflect the investigator's values or the values and interests of the study sponsors.

The comments of scientists and the decisions of policy-makers often reflect their value-laden approach to issues of uncertainty. What level of proof is needed to trigger action, and who bears the burden of proof? Should we wait for certain evidence of harm before we take action, or is a reasonable suspicion enough? Should consumers or workers be responsible for showing that a product is dangerous, or should the manufacturer or employer show that the product is safe before it is allowed into the market or workplace?

While science may contribute information and even define the parameters of the debate, the answers to these questions reflect policy judgments that invariably are influenced by values. Some scientists, regulators, and members of the public will prefer to wait for additional evidence and to take the risk of future harm rather than expend potentially unnecessary resources to impose costly regulation now. These individuals will likely frame their arguments in economic terms and focus their critiques on the design flaws and technical limitations of individual studies bearing on the question. A recent, novel, but ultimately confusing, approach employed a so-called risk-risk analysis, which suggested that stricter regulation designed to save lives will actually lead to increased mortality by lowering workers' incomes [7].

Other scientists, regulators, and members of the public will prefer to err on the side of caution in protecting worker and public health and will seek to impose regulation or deny siting permits, even at the risk of being found wrong at some future date. Their arguments will focus on human health or environmental impacts and are more likely to synthesize the available data, overlook the design flaws of individual studies, and give weight to the aggregate suggestive evidence. How much of these determinations is "scientific" and how much is driven by different views of one's duty to prevent harm or do good?

Cases 1 and 3 also illustrate issues of *justice*. Many policy decisions reflect a utilitarian approach to policy-making; that is, decisions are made to maximize benefit or confer the greatest good on the greatest number. This approach, deeply rooted in ethical theory, often has salutary effects and can justify actions that harm a few while helping many. However, this approach often fails to consider issues of distribution. *Distributive justice* relates to fairness in the distribution of risks, costs, and benefits. Who benefits? Who bears the risks or costs? Who gets to make the decision? What is the relationship between those who bear the costs, those who reap the benefits, and those who make the decisions?

The growing environmental justice movement has documented case after case of environmental inequity where hazardous waste landfills are located in and around predominantly poor and minority communities and where poor and minority populations suffer excess burdens of environmentally related health problems, such as lead and pesticide poisoning [8–10]. In these cases, it seems that the most vulnerable members of society are asked to bear a disproportionate share of environmental pollution and associated health risk. The principle of justice requires us to ask if this is fair.

The principle of *autonomy* can also provide guidance in occupational and environmental health science and policy. Autonomy concerns respect for persons and the individual's right to self-determination. In biomedical ethics, discussions about autonomy usually center on the concept of informed consent. In research, the concept of informed consent is well established. Research subjects should be informed of the risks and benefits of their *voluntary* participation in any study. In occupational and environmental health research, there may be additional requirements. For example, subjects should be informed about reasons for the study, the sponsors of the study, the timetable for the completion of the study, and how the results will be disseminated and used [11]. Study subjects should also be informed about possible economic risks of participation, for both themselves and their employers.

The autonomy of the researcher is also a significant factor in occupational and environmental health. Because research findings can have serious consequences for many of the interest groups involved, any of them may seek to influence the researcher and his or her work. In the past, industry sponsors have tried to influence the design, conduct, and interpretation of research as well as the dissemination and publication of results [3]. For this reason, it would behoove independent researchers to institute structural safeguards before conducting a study sponsored by an industry or other interest group. Case 5 illustrates how one research team sought to protect the integrity and independence of their industry-sponsored research project. The sponsor's reluctance should signal the need to examine the potential for interference or influence very carefully.

The principle of autonomy also has important implications for policy decisions about regulation and control of occupational and environmental hazards. Respect for persons requires their informed and meaningful participation in decisions that will affect them. In the past, public agencies and private corporations have employed a "decide, announce, defend" strategy when making decisions affecting public health and safety. By ignoring the rights of individuals and communities to be informed about and participate in decisions that would affect them, public agencies and employers have found themselves increasingly distrusted by and at odds with local citizens [12].

The principle of autonomy is the ethical underpinning of regulations regarding worker and community Right-to-Know laws, discussed later in this chapter. While public agencies may sometimes need to make unpopular decisions, real community involvement in the debate at least provides an element of fairness to the process.

*Applications in Public Policy*

The application of ethical principles to occupational and environmental health policy is more than just the fodder for interesting debate. We can actually see their reflection in many of the regulatory decisions taken by governmental agencies.

For example, the Occupational Safety and Health Administration (OSHA) lead standard addresses issues of autonomy, justice, nonmaleficence, and beneficence. The regulatory debate on lead included scientific questions about safe airborne levels and the merits of using blood levels as the primary measure of compliance with the standard. An interesting part of the debate centered on the establishment of medical removal protection with (hourly) rate retention for workers found to have elevated blood-lead levels. There was little argument about the wisdom of removing workers with high blood-lead levels from exposure. Rather, the conflict arose over a proposal that obligated employers to maintain the workers' hourly rates and seniority rights during the period of removal. The Lead Industries Association argued against such medical removal protection on legal grounds, stating that Congress did not intend OSHA to have the power to require such policies and that it violated provisions of the Occupational Safety and

Health Act. Workers' representatives focused on issues of autonomy and fairness, noting that workers would choose not to participate in a blood-lead screening program that might threaten their livelihoods. Although medical removal was in the best interest of the workers' health, their representatives argued that it was unfair to penalize them by putting their wages and seniority benefits at risk in an exposure situation over which they have little, if any, control. The courts ruled in favor of the medical removal with rate retention policy, but the ethical issues surrounding the regulation of lead did not abate.

Recognizing the reproductive effects of lead, some employers began to institute "fetal protection" policies. Such policies ostensibly seek to protect actual and potential fetuses of women who are pregnant or of reproductive capacity. These policies involve the principles of beneficence and nonmaleficence, which may clash with the principles of autonomy and justice. In weighing options, employers who adopted such policies placed a higher value on protecting the fetus from harm (and also protecting themselves from future liability) than providing autonomous choices to female workers, who could take steps to control their fertility. In addition, lead is known to have toxic effects on both men and women. Thus, one could question the fairness of differentially protecting female and male employees.

The U.S. Supreme Court recently ruled against the use of "fetal protection" policies on the basis of sex discrimination (fairness), upholding the autonomy of women workers [United Automobile Workers (UAW) v. Johnson Controls, U.S., 111 S. Ct. 1196 (1991)]. The Court stated that such policies force female workers "to choose between having a child and having a job" and that "it is no more appropriate for the courts than it is for individual employers to decide whether a woman's reproductive role is more important to herself and her family than her economic role." Rather, the Court found that "Congress has left this choice to the woman as hers to make." Thus, the Court gave overriding weight to the woman's autonomy.

Freedom and noninterference are tightly guarded and highly cherished rights in the United States. In occupational and environmental health, the principle of autonomy is reflected in Right-to-Know laws and regulations. In this context, the principle of autonomy suggests that individuals have a right to know about their workplace or environmental exposures in order to make decisions and take individual or political action. Such decision making requires information—in this case, information about the exposures, their potential health effects, methods of protection, and, ideally, possible substitutes or alternatives.

In the United States, the concept of Right-to-Know has been embodied in both occupational and environmental legislation. The OSHA Medical Access Rule provides workers with access to their own medical records and to records pertaining to their exposure to toxic substances to the extent that the employer compiles such records. Under this rule, information is provided upon request. The OSHA Hazard Communication Standard obliges employers to educate and train workers about the hazardous chemicals in the workplace. Employers must provide this information as a matter of course, even without a request. Congress extended the right to know about toxic hazards to communities in 1986 with the enactment of the Emergency Planning and Community Right-to-Know Act. Its many provisions provide local citizens with access to information about the location, use, and release of toxic chemicals in their communities.

In promulgating these Right-to-Know laws and regulations, the government recognized workers' and citizens' needs for information about toxic substances in their workplaces and communities, granted them a right to such information, and conferred on manufacturers and employers the duty to provide it. However, provisions were also enacted to balance these needs with the needs of employers and manufacturers to protect their trade secrets.

Concern about the adequacy of Right-to-Know legislation surfaced soon after its passage. One author suggested that "to contribute to worker autonomy in any real sense, Right-to-Know must facilitate enough of a change in the employer-employee relationship to enable the worker to effect changes in workplace technology (or changes in the way in which workplace technology is employed in the workplace) . . . If all Right-to-Know does is provide a mechanism whereby workers are able to summon the courage to risk occupational disease . . . , it will be an empty exercise" [13]. More recently, there have been calls to empower workers and communities with the "right-to-know more" [14] and the "right-to-act" [15, 16]. The former would provide communities with additional information on plants' production processes; the latter would, among other things, give inspection authority to one or more worker(s) in every plant and expand workers' influence over health and safety programs through meaningful participation on joint committees with management.

### Applications in Private Policy

Public policy and regulation can go only so far in protecting workers and communities from occupational and environmental hazards. Corporate and business policies and decisions have the most immediate impact on health, safety, and the environment—they can promote good (beneficence) or result in significant harm. Although many corporations and individual employers have excellent health, safety, and environmental programs and function as responsible corporate citizens, there have been too many cases of business policies and practices that demonstrate wanton disregard for worker and community health and the principle of nonmaleficence. While historical examples abound—from the Triangle Shirtwaist Company and Gaulley Bridge to the Johns-Manville asbestos debacle [17]—there is no paucity of more recent events. Coal mine operators tamper with dust samples [18], 25 workers lose their lives in a fire at a poultry processing plant because managers bolted emergency exits to prevent theft of chicken parts [19], and corporations' irresponsible waste disposal practices continue to present risks to the health and environments of communities across the country [20].

The public is well aware of and disillusioned by these corporate failures. Surveys indicate that the public considers industry the least trusted (but most knowledgeable) source of information about chemical risk [21]. Recognizing the impact of this public perception, private industry has developed a variety of initiatives and policies to upgrade its practices and reassure a skeptical public. For example, the Chemical Manufacturers Association instituted a voluntary program (Responsible Care) for its member companies, which provides codes for management practices and guidelines for community and employee outreach activities. Individual employers also may have refined their policies and practices to improve their health, safety, and environmental programs; facilitate Right-to-Know and worker training; and eliminate discriminatory practices against its female workers. Business schools have instituted courses in "Business Ethics."

Obviously, the employer community plays a significant role in creating ethical problems relating to occupational and environmental health. What is needed are opportunities and incentives for employers to enhance their abilities to recognize, understand, and respond to their ethical obligations and responsibilities.

Workers and their representatives, including organized labor, also have ethical duties and responsibilities to prevent harm, do good, be fair, and tell the truth. However, most workers in the United States and other countries are not in the position to enact and enforce policies and programs in the workplace. Like everyone else, their individual conduct, on and off the job, should be guided by the same moral considerations discussed above. While individual workers (and labor organizations) can and sometimes do create ethical dilemmas for occupational health professionals, they are not, in most cases, a powerful and organized group, and thus are not treated as such in this chapter.

## Occupational Health Practice

Most occupational and environmental health professionals encounter difficult ethical issues in the routine activities of their work—issues that test their allegiance and independence as professionals. These professionals include those directly involved in providing occupational and environmental health services, such as occupational physicians, nurses, industrial hygienists, safety professionals, and occupational ergonomists. In addition, professionals from a variety of other disciplines have roles and responsibilities that, directly or indirectly, affect workplace and environmental health. These include engineers, architects, lawyers, manufacturers, advertisers, reporters, managers, organizational consultants, and others. Although not trained as health and safety specialists, these professionals are not relieved of their ethical obligations to prevent harm; and neither are workers, supervisors, and employers. Indeed, the actions and decisions of many of these individuals will have tremendous impact on occupational and environmental health and safety. However, the following discussion focuses on those occupational and environmental health specialists who provide direct health and safety services. These individuals have clear professional and moral responsibilities that derive from their special knowledge of occupational and environmental health and safety and from the special relationships they develop with workers and employers. The section examines the ethical dimensions of several situations commonly encountered by these professionals.

In exploring these issues, it is important to appreciate the very real and personal consequences that these individuals may experience as a result of their work. Their actions can enhance their own reputation, status, and esteem or incur the wrath and distrust of their employers, patients, and colleagues. Their decisions can affect their income, employability, standing in their professional community, and respectability in the eyes of individuals for and to whom they are responsible. The difficulty of "doing the right thing" in these situations should not be underestimated.

### Working for Companies

Health and safety professionals who work for companies—full-time, part-time, or on a contractual basis—frequently face a host of ethical issues that call their loyalty and allegiance into question. The goals and interests of their professional practice may differ significantly from those of their employers and workers/patients. The company's primary purpose and interest is to profitably manufacture a product or provide a service and to stay in business. The workers are primarily interested in earning a living, providing for their families, and finding personal gratification in their work. When the health care provider and the patient share the same employer and the interests of the employer and patient diverge, what is the role of the provider? Any semblance of the traditional provider-patient relationship is surely strained.

Within this complicated structure, the practice of occupational medicine, nursing, safety, or industrial hygiene is inherently difficult and challenging. Employers may expect physicians and nurses to function as agents of social control, making determinations about when, where, and if an individual can work. They may limit the ability of their industrial hygienists and safety officers to take action on workplace hazards. Workers, on the other hand, may expect occupational health professionals to protect their interests and function as their advocates when problems arise. The worker and health professional may not always agree on issues relating to return-to-work or job restrictions. When the employer/client's interests differ from those of the worker/patient, it is not surprising that skepticism, distrust, and hostility arise on all fronts. The occupational medicine resident in Case 7 has probably failed to appreciate the complex social and power structures that often come into play when a worker is injured on the job and compensation or return-to-work issues are raised.

The issue of confidentiality also arises when a health care professional provides a service at the request of a company. How much of the personal and medical information obtained by the health care provider is the company entitled to? Should employers be informed that a job applicant has diabetes or a history of back pain? Should the employer be told that the executive being considered for promotion has cardiac disease or is seeing a psychiatrist? As in Case 6, physicians and nurses may encounter direct or indirect pressure to release this type of information to help the company protect its legitimate business interests. However, such disclosure invades the workers' privacy and may threaten their job status. How should the provider reconcile these competing interests? To begin to answer this question, the provider might try to clarify any legal requirements and restrictions (especially in light of the Americans With Disabilities Act; see Chap. 11) and then assess what the employer really needs to know. In most cases, the employer does not need diagnostic or medical data, but information about the employee's ability to work and the need for job modifications or work restrictions.

A larger and even more difficult problem relates to the extent to which these professionals are obligated to take action on suspected or known health and safety problems. The physician, nurse, and safety engineer in Case 5 have expressed their concern about the company's ergonomic problems and have made numerous recommendations for correcting them. The company has taken no action. Having expressed their concern (perhaps even in writing), do these professionals have any further obligation to follow up on these problems? Do the principles of nonmaleficence and beneficence impose an ethical duty on these professionals to do more than make recommendations? Workers have already been injured, and there is every reason to believe that the injuries will continue. Should the physician, nurse, or safety officer notify OSHA? Try to organize the workers to take action? Quit? How far should the company-employed health and safety professional go to protect the workers? Similarly, if the company's environmental engineer is aware that the company is violating federal or state regulations on waste disposal, should he or she notify the appropriate authorities if the company continues to break the law?

### Participating in Screening Programs

In almost any practice setting, physicians and nurses may be asked to conduct or participate in some sort of worker screening program—from preplacement and return-to-work physicals to OSHA-mandated, exposure-specific examinations and the more controversial testing for drug use, human immunodeficiency virus (HIV), and genetic imperfections. Screening activities give rise to a host of ethical issues [22, 23] (see Chap. 3).

Worker screening is usually done for one of two reasons: (1) to assess an individual's ability to perform a job, including making recommendations on worker fitness and work restrictions, and (2) to predict an individual's risk of future health problems that would inhibit job performance or result in large economic expenditures for the company [24]. Such predictions are usually based on certain genetic, behavioral, physiologic, or biochemical factors. A variety of descriptive terms are commonly used and frequently confused in discussions of worker screening. These include medical monitoring, surveillance, genetic testing, and biologic monitoring. Each has a precise definition. For our purposes, they will not be differentiated, but rather considered under the broad rubric of worker screening.

Issues of privacy, confidentiality, fairness, informed consent, and informed refusal pervade almost every form of worker screening. They may relate to the purpose and content of the screening program itself or to the use of the results generated by the screening program.

As in Case 6, many employers require individuals to undergo medical screening before and during the course of employment. It is helpful

to ascertain why the employer wants the workers screened. To help assure that the worker can do the job without injury to himself or herself or to others? To comply with government regulations? To help evaluate the effectiveness of workplace controls? (For example, is the ventilation adequately protecting workers from lead exposure?) To weed out applicants who may pose a future liability risk to the employer? To find medical reasons to justify the removal of a troublemaker or a frequently absent employee?

Decisions about what the screening program or examination should include can also be problematic. Sometimes these examinations and their content are mandated by OSHA regulations; sometimes the company has its own ideas about what the examination should include, such as back x-rays and blood tests; and sometimes the physician makes the decision without any input whatsoever. Many worker screening programs are ill-conceived from both a scientific and ethical point of view [25]. Problems with test validity (sensitivity and specificity) and predictive value may weaken any appeal to beneficence. For example, some employers may insist on using lumbosacral x-rays to screen out individuals with back problems, despite the low predictive value of these x-rays to forecast future back injury. The use of this test provides no real benefit to the company and exposes the worker to unnecessary radiation as well as to the risk of job loss. The use of cardiovascular stress testing in healthy young adults applying for jobs in the hazardous waste industry is another questionable practice.

In all cases, the physician or nurse should be aware that a worker's participation in a screening program or consent to a medical examination does not necessarily reflect an entirely autonomous decision. Individuals may consent to these examinations simply because they need a job. During the examination, they may knowingly or unknowingly (through testing) divulge highly personal and sensitive information to the health care provider. They may not know how or even if the information will be passed on to others and used for their benefit or to their detriment.

In Case 6, the employer wants to dictate the contents of the preplacement, return-to-work, and other periodic screening evaluations to a community physician, who has agreed to provide these services although he or she has never visited the plant. Can physicians exercise their professional and ethical responsibility to practice competently when, in making judgments about a worker's ability to perform a job, they have neither seen the job nor are well acquainted with the real job demands? Even if the physician understands the nature of the job, how will he or she balance fairness to the employer with the protection of the prospective or current employee? Will the workers be informed that the results of the medical evaluation may adversely affect their employability, remuneration, or advancement in the company? Will they be informed of their test results and counseled about their meaning? Will results of medical evaluations be used to help improve workplace conditions or simply to weed out "unfit" employees? If the screening program is the employer's sole approach to controlling workplace illness and injury, health care providers should weigh their involvement very carefully.

These factors place stringent ethical obligations on physicians and nurses who participate in worker screening programs. They must decide if the purpose and content of the proposed screening program is medically reasonable and ethically justifiable. They must decide how much information employers need and are entitled to. The concepts of nonmaleficence, beneficence, and responsibility must also be considered in decisions about the use of screening information and the need for follow-up action. Any action or inaction may adversely affect the employer, the worker, and, possibly, the provider's own standing with the company.

In considering these and other issues relating to worker screening, one group of authors suggests that such testing be used only if: (1) it is an appro-priate preventive tool that addresses a specific workplace problem; (2) it is used in conjunction with environmental monitoring; (3) it is not used to divert attention and resources from reducing worker exposure to toxic substances and improving workplace conditions; (4) the tests are accurate, reliable, and have a high predictive value in the population screened; and (5) medical removal protection for earnings and job security is provided [26]. Others have noted the importance of voluntary, informed consent and of providing workers with information about the purpose of the testing, who has access to the results, how the results may be used, what actions may be taken in response to the results, and how employee confidentiality will be maintained [26]. Because workers involved in medical screening have few legal protections, occupational health professionals must take care in designing and participating in worker screening programs.

### Workplace Health Promotion

In addition to the types of screening activities mentioned above, employers may ask health professionals to develop and deliver a variety of wellness or health promotion programs in the workplace, or health care professionals who work for a company may be approached by outside groups that sell these types of programs. Employers are increasingly attracted to wellness programs because of rising health care costs, concerns about declining productivity, and the recognition that behavioral risk factors have a significant impact on worker health and medical care costs.

In many ways, the workplace is an ideal site for such intervention programs. It is a place where large numbers of relatively healthy people spend a significant amount of time. The workplace is a locus for exercising a variety of social controls that may influence personal behavior, such as no-smoking and vending machine policies, contests and financial incentives, peer pressure, and accessible information and services [27]. By helping workers change their unhealthful habits, these health promotion programs are buttressed by the principle of beneficence. Yet because they have the potential for misuse, they can present ethical challenges to the unwary provider [28].

For example, there is concern that a focus on the lifestyle risks of the individual worker will divert attention from the workplace risks that are under the direct control of the employer. This appears to be happening in Case 5. The employer has ignored recommendations for ergonomic changes in the workplace and has decided to institute weight reduction and safe lifting classes for the workers instead. Is this the best way of preventing musculoskeletal injury in this workplace? Is it fair to place the sole burden on the workers? Should the nurse agree to conduct these health promotion programs in the absence of workplace ergonomic changes? Should the nurse encourage workers to participate in these wellness programs without also informing them of their substantial job-related risks and the actions the employer could take to reduce or eliminate them?

The debate has been framed as one between health promotion and health protection—or between the behavioralist and the environmentalist approach to public health [28, 29]. The priority and emphasis given these approaches by occupational health professionals may reveal something of their primary allegiance. One commentator has noted that occupational physicians are a "scarce resource" whose central role relates to the recognition, treatment, and prevention of *job-related* disease. As such, their attention to behavioral risk factors should be a "second-order" concern [29].

This brief discussion is not meant to disparage workplace wellness programs. They can help address important public health problems, and can be beneficial to and well received by both workers and employers. However, in the absence of effective health and safety programs targeted on workplace hazards, they should be subject to close ethical scrutiny.

## Codes of Ethics and Decision Making

Professional organizations of occupational and environmental health specialists have acknowledged and tried to provide guidance to these difficult ethical problems through the development of ethical codes. The American College of Occupational and Environmental Medicine (formerly the American Occupational Medical Association), the American Association of Occupational Health Nurses, the American Academy of Industrial Hygiene, and the National Society of Professional Engineers have adopted codes of ethics for their respective fields (see boxes). The International Commission on Occupational Health has adopted an international and interdisciplinary code of ethics for occupational health professionals.

These codes have many features in common and clearly reflect attention to the principles of nonmaleficence and autonomy. For example, the code for occupational physicians exhorts them to give the health and safety of the worker the highest priority and to treat as confidential whatever is learned about the individual unless the law or an overriding public health concern dictates otherwise. The hygiene code advises hygienists to hold their responsibilities to the employer subservient to their ultimate responsibility of protecting employee health. The nursing code clearly makes the worker the primary focus. The engineering code is quite detailed and provides guidance on many issues, including what to do when a client or employer insists on unprofessional conduct or on designs that threaten public safety, health, or welfare. The engineering code is also guided by the principle of beneficence; it advises engineers to seek opportunities to act in the public interest. The international code is also detailed, providing guidance on issues relating to competence, remedial action and follow-up, information transfer, biologic monitoring, health surveillance, and confidentiality.

Although often vague, these codes can be helpful. Indeed, they could be appended to any contract or agreement that occupational and environmental health professionals enter into with companies or other organizations. Ethical codes, however, cannot solve the very real moral dilemmas that arise in the day-to-day practice of occupational and environmental health. Further, they do not provide the protection that health professionals may need when they take action that is contrary to the wishes of their employers. In the final analysis, these professionals will have to make their own decisions.

In addition to clarifying legal responsibilities, conflict resolution can be informed by a close examination of all the options in light of the ethical principles discussed in this chapter. Who will benefit or be harmed by each alternative? Who is the least advantaged individual or group in this situation? Are their needs and preferences known, and have they been given the appropriate weight? What are the long-term consequences of each action? What will happen if a particular action is *not* taken? Why does the health professional feel reluctant to do one thing or another? What does the professional stand to lose or gain from each possible alternative? Can the professional exercise independent judgment or is pressure being exerted? Would the professional make a different decision or determination if he or she were practicing in another setting? Although these questions may not provide definitive answers, especially in situations where alternative actions have merit and ethical justification, they can help clarify the values involved in the process.

---

## AMERICAN COLLEGE OF OCCUPATIONAL AND ENVIRONMENTAL MEDICINE CODE OF ETHICAL CONDUCT

This code establishes standards of professional ethical conduct with which each member of the American College of Occupational and Environmental Medicine (ACOEM) is expected to comply. These standards are intended to guide occupational and environmental medicine physicians in their relationships with the individuals they serve; employers and workers' representatives; colleagues in the health professions; and the public and all levels of government, including the judiciary.

Physicians should:

1. accord the highest priority to the health and safety of individuals in both the workplace and the environment;
2. practice on a scientific basis with integrity and strive to acquire and maintain adequate knowledge and expertise upon which to render professional service;
3. relate honestly and ethically in all professional relationships;
4. strive to expand and disseminate medical knowledge and participate in ethical research efforts as appropriate;
5. keep confidential all individual medical information, releasing such information only when required by law or overriding public health considerations, or to other physicians according to accepted medical practice, or to others at the request of the individual;
6. recognize that employers may be entitled to counsel about an individual's medical work fitness, but not to diagnoses or specific details, except in compliance with laws and regulations;
7. communicate to individuals and/or groups any significant observations and recommendations concerning their health or safety; and
8. recognize those medical impairments in oneself and others, including chemical dependency and abusive personal practices, which interfere with one's ability to follow the above principles, and take appropriate measures.

Source: Adopted October 25, 1993, by the Board of Directors of the American College of Occupational and Environmental Medicine.

AMERICAN ACADEMY OF INDUSTRIAL
HYGIENE CODE OF ETHICS
FOR THE PROFESSIONAL PRACTICE
OF INDUSTRIAL HYGIENE

*Purpose*

This code provides standards of ethical conduct
to be followed by industrial hygienists as they
strive for the goals of protecting employees'
health, improving the work environment, and
advancing the quality of the profession. Industrial hygienists have the responsibility to practice their profession in an objective manner following recognized principles of industrial
hygiene, realizing that the lives, health, and welfare of individuals may be dependent upon their
professional judgment.

*Professional Responsibility*

1. Maintain the highest level of integrity and
   professional competence.
2. Be objective in the application of recognized
   scientific methods and in the interpretation
   of findings.
3. Promote industrial hygiene as a professional
   discipline.
4. Disseminate scientific knowledge for the benefit of employees, society, and the profession.
5. Protect confidential information.
6. Avoid circumstances where compromise of
   professional judgment or conflict of interest
   may arise.

*Responsibility to Employees*

1. Recognize that the primary responsibility of
   the industrial hygienist is to protect the
   health of employees.

2. Maintain an objective attitude toward the
   recognition, evaluation, and control of
   health hazards regardless of external influences, realizing that the health and welfare of
   workers and others may depend upon the industrial hygienist's professional judgment.
3. Counsel employees regarding health hazards
   and the necessary precautions to avoid adverse health effects.

*Responsibility to Employers and Clients*

1. Act responsibly in the application of industrial hygiene principles toward the attain-
   ment of healthful working environments.
2. Respect confidences, advise honestly, and report findings and recommendations accurately.
3. Manage and administer professional services
   to ensure maintenance of accurate records to
   provide documentation and accountability in
   support of findings and conclusions.
4. Hold responsibilities to the employer or
   client subservient to the ultimate responsibility to protect the health of employees.

*Responsibility to the Public*

1. Report factually on industrial hygiene matters of public concern.
2. State professional opinions founded on adequate knowledge and clearly identified as
   such.

Source: Am Ind Hyg Assoc J (40), June 1979.

EXCERPTS FROM THE AMERICAN ASSOCIATION OF OCCUPATIONAL HEALTH NURSES (AAOHN) CODE OF ETHICS AND INTERPRETIVE STATEMENTS

*Preamble*

The AAOHN Code of Ethics has been developed in response to the nursing profession's acceptance of its goals and values, and the trust conferred upon it by society to guide the conduct and practices of the profession. As a professional, the occupational health nurse accepts the responsibility and inherent obligation to uphold these values.

1. The occupational health nurse provides health care in the work environment with regard for human dignity and client rights, unrestricted by considerations of social or economic status, national origin, race, religion, age, sex, or the nature of the health status.
2. The occupational health nurse promotes collaboration with other health professionals and community health agencies in order to meet the health needs of the workforce.
3. The occupational health nurse strives to safeguard the employee's right to privacy by protecting confidential information and releasing information only upon written consent of the employee or as required or permitted by law.
4. The occupational health nurse strives to provide quality care and to safeguard clients from unethical and illegal actions.
5. The occupational health nurse, licensed to provide health care services, accepts obligations to society as a professional and responsible member of the community.
6. The occupational health nurse maintains individual competence in occupational health nursing practice, recognizing and accepting responsibility for individual judgments and actions, while complying with appropriate laws and regulations (local, state, and federal) that impact the delivery of occupational health services.
7. The occupational health nurse participates, as appropriate, in activities such as research that contribute to the ongoing development of the profession's body of knowledge while protecting the rights of subjects.

Source: Am Assoc Occup Health Nurses J, August 1991.

In conclusion, the fields of occupational and environmental health are charged with ethical problems and dilemmas that are not easy to solve. Consideration of the principles of autonomy, nonmaleficence, beneficence, justice, and responsibility can help guide decision making but may not make hard choices any easier in the practical sense. Advances in medicine, science, and technology presage a growing number of complex ethical problems. The need for structural safeguards for occupational and environmental health professionals is clear. Unless these professionals can somehow be insulated from personal and economic reprisals, it will remain difficult for them to make the bold decisions that are needed to ensure worker and community environmental health. The development of these structural safeguards will require creativity and, most likely, legislative action. Constructive solutions will also demand honest dialogue and a clear understanding by all parties of how their actions and expectations can contribute to both the creation and the resolution of ethical issues in occupational and environmental health.

EXCERPTS FROM THE CODE OF ETHICS
FOR ENGINEERS, NATIONAL SOCIETY
OF PROFESSIONAL ENGINEERS

*Preamble*

Engineering is an important and learned profession. The members of the profession recognize that their work has a direct and vital impact on the quality of life for all people. Accordingly, the services provided by engineers require honesty, impartiality, fairness, and equity, and must be dedicated to the protection of the public health, safety and welfare. In the practice of their profession, engineers must perform under a standard of professional behavior which requires adherence to the highest principles of ethical conduct on behalf of the public, clients, employers, and the profession.

I. *Fundamental canons*

Engineers, in the fulfillment of their professional duties shall

1. Hold paramount the safety, health and welfare of the public in the performance of their professional duties.
2. Perform services only in areas of their competence.
3. Issue public statements only in an objective and truthful manner.
4. Act in professional matters for each employer or client as faithful agents or trustees.
5. Avoid deceptive acts in the solicitation of professional employment.

II. *Rules of practice*

1. Engineers shall hold paramount the safety, health and welfare of the public in the performance of their professional duties.
   a. Engineers shall at all times recognize that their primary obligation is to protect the safety, health, property and welfare of the public. If their professional judgment is overruled under circumstances where the safety, health, property or welfare of the public is endangered, they shall notify their employer or client and such other authority as may be appropriate.

   e. Engineers having knowledge of any alleged violation of this Code shall cooperate with the proper authorities in furnishing such information or assistance as may be required.
3. Engineers shall issue public statements only in an objective and truthful manner.

III. *Professional obligations*

1. Engineers shall be guided in all their professional relations by the highest standards of integrity.
   a. Engineers shall admit and accept their own errors when proven wrong and refrain from distorting or altering the facts in an attempt to justify their decisions.
2. Engineers shall at all times strive to serve the public interest.
   a. Engineers shall seek opportunities to be of constructive service in civic affairs and work for the advancement of the safety, health and well-being of their community.
   b. Engineers shall not complete, sign, or seal plans and/or specifications that are not of a design safe to the public health and welfare and in conformity with accepted engineering standards. If the client or employer insists on such unprofessional conduct, they shall notify the proper authorities and withdraw from further service on the project.
3. Engineers shall avoid all conduct or practice that is likely to discredit the profession or deceive the public.
5. Engineers shall not be influenced in their professional duties by conflicting interests.
7. Engineers shall not attempt to obtain employment or advancement or professional engagements by untruthfully criticizing other engineers, or by other improper or questionable methods.

Source: NSPE publication No. 1102 as revised January 1987.

## EXCERPTS FROM THE INTERNATIONAL CODE OF ETHICS FOR OCCUPATIONAL HEALTH PROFESSIONALS

### Basic Principles

The three following paragraphs summarize the principles of ethics on which is based the International Code of Ethics for Occupational Health Professionals, prepared by the International Commission on Occupational Health (ICOH).

*Occupational health practice* must be performed according to the highest standards and ethical principles. Occupational health professionals must service the health and social well-being of the workers, individually and collectively. They also contribute to environmental and community health.

*The obligations of occupational health professionals* include protecting the life and the health of the worker, respecting human dignity and promoting the highest ethical principles in occupational health policies and programs. Integrity in professional conduct, impartiality, and the protection of the confidentiality of health data and of the privacy of workers are part of these obligations.

*Occupational health professionals are experts* who must enjoy full professional independence in the execution of their functions. They must acquire and maintain the competence necessary for their duties and require conditions which allow them to carry out their tasks according to good practice and professional ethics.

### Duties and Obligations of Occupational Health Professionals

1. The primary aim of occupational health practice is to safeguard the health of workers and to promote a safe and healthy working environment. In pursuing this aim, occupational health professionals must use validated methods of risk evaluations, pro-

pose efficient preventive measures, and follow up their implementation. . . .

2. Occupational health professionals must continuously strive to be familiar with the work and the working environment as well as to improve their competence and to remain well informed in scientific and technical knowledge, occupational hazards and the most efficient means to eliminate or reduce the relevant risks. . . .

4. Special consideration should be given to rapid application of simple preventive measures which are cost-effective, technically sound and easily implemented. . . . When doubt exists about the severity of an occupational hazard, prudent precautionary action should be taken immediately.

5. In the case of refusal or of unwillingness to take adequate steps to remove an undue risk or to remedy a situation which presents evidence of danger to health or safety, the occupational health professionals must make, as rapidly as possible, their concern clear, in writing, to the appropriate senior management executive, stressing the need for taking into account scientific knowledge and for applying relevant health protection standards, including exposure limits, and recalling the obligation of the employer to apply laws and regulations and to protect the health of workers in their employment. Whenever necessary, the workers concerned and their representatives in the enterprise should be informed and the competent authority should be contacted.

6. Occupational health professionals must contribute to the information of workers on occupational hazards to which they may be exposed in an objective and prudent manner which does not conceal any fact and emphasizes the preventive measures. . . .

8. The objectives and the details of the health surveillance must be clearly defined and the

workers must be informed about them. The validity of such surveillance must be assessed and it must be carried out with the informed consent of the workers. . . . The potentially positive and negative consequences of participation in screening and health surveillance programs should be discussed with the workers concerned.

9. The results of examinations . . . must be explained to the worker concerned. The determination of fitness for a given job should be based on the assessment of the health of the worker and on a good knowledge of the job demands and the worksite. . . .

10. The results of the examinations prescribed by national laws or regulations must only be conveyed to management in terms of fitness for the envisaged work or of limitations necessary from a medical point of view in the assignment of tasks or in the exposure to occupational hazards. . . .

14. Occupational professionals must be aware of their role in relation to the protection of the community and of the environment. . . .

### Conditions of Execution of the Functions of Occupational Health Professionals

16. Occupational health professionals must always act, as a matter of priority, in the interest of the health and safety of the workers. . . .

17. Occupational health professionals must maintain full professional independence and observe the rules of confidentiality in the execution of their functions.

18. All workers should be treated in an equitable manner without any form of discrimination. . . . A clear channel of communication must be established and maintained between occupational health professionals and the senior management executive responsible for decisions at the highest level about the conditions and the organization of work and the working environment in the undertaking, or with the board of directors.

19. Whenever appropriate, occupational health professionals must request that a clause on ethics be incorporated into their contract of employment. . . .

21. Occupational health professionals must not seek personal information which is not relevant to the protection of workers' health in relation to work. . . .

Source: International Commission on Occupational Health, 1992.

# References

1. Beauchamp TL, Childress JF. Principles of biomedical ethics. New York: Oxford University Press, 1983.
2. Ashford NA. Science and values in the regulatory process. Statis Science 1988; 3:377–83; and Shrader-Frechette K. Values, scientific objectivity, and risk analysis—five dilemmas. In J Humber and RF Almeder. eds. Biomedical ethics reviews, quantitative risk assessment, vol. 4. Clifton, NJ: Humana Press, 1986.
3. Soskolne CL. Epidemiology: Questions of science, ethics, morality, and law. Am J Epidemiol 1989; 129:1–18.
4. Ladd J. The task of ethics. In WT Reich. ed. Encyclopedia of bioethics. New York: The Free Press, 1978.
5. Center for Technology, Policy and Industrial Development, Massachusetts Institute of Technology. Monitoring the community for exposure and disease: Scientific, legal, and ethical considerations. Report prepared for and available from the Agency for Toxic Substances and Disease Registry,

U.S. Department of Health and Human Services, 1991.

6. For excellent critiques of quantitative risk assessment, see Ginsberg R. Quantitative risk assessment and the illusion of safety. New Solutions 1993; 3:8–15; Wartenberg D and Chess C. The risk wars: Assessing risk assessment. New Solutions 1993; 3:16–25; and Shrader-Frechette K, as in [2].

7. Kenney RL. Mortality risks induced by economic expenditures. Risk Analysis 1990; 10:147–59.

8. General Accounting Office. Siting of hazardous waste landfills and the correlation with racial and economic status of surrounding communities. Washington, D.C.: General Accounting Office, 1983.

9. Office of Emergency and Remedial Response. Hazardous waste sites on Indian lands. Washington, D.C.: Environmental Protection Agency, 1987.

10. Environmental Protection Agency, Environmental Equity Task Force. Environmental equity: Reducing risk for all communities (2 volumes). Washington, D.C.: Environmental Protection Agency, 1992.

11. Thar WE. The epidemiologist's responsibilities to research subjects in the occupational setting. J Clin Epidemiol 1991; 44 (Suppl. 1):91S–94S.

12. Ozonoff D, Boden LI. Truth and consequences: Health agency responses to environmental health problems. Sci Technol Hum Values 1987; 12:70–7.

13. Caldart CC. Promise and pitfalls of workplace right-to-know. *Semin Occup Med* 1986; 1:81–90.

14. Working Group on Community Right-to-Know. Tracking toxics for pollution prevention. Working notes on community right-to-know. Washington, D.C.: Working Group on Community Right-to-Know, November-December 1991.

15. Roundtable on OSHA at 20: What now? New Solutions 1991; Spring:60–65.

16. Robinson JC. Toil and toxics—workplace struggles and political strategies for occupational health. Berkeley: University of California Press, 1991.

17. Berman DM. Death on the job: Occupational health and safety struggles in the United States. New York: Monthly Review Press, 1978.

18. Weeks JL. Tampering with dust samples in coal mines (again). Am J Indus Med 1991; 20:141–4.

19. McAteer JD, Whiteman L. Learning from Hamlet: The case for a national safety and health board. New Solutions 1993; 3:54–9.

20. Brown P, Mikkelsen EJ. No safe place: Toxic waste, leukemia, and community action. Berkeley: University of California Press, 1990.

21. McCallum DB, Covello VT. What the public thinks about environmental data. EPA J 1990; 113:467–73.

22. Lappe M. Ethical concerns in occupational screening programs. J Occup Med 1986; 28:930–4.

23. Derr P. Ethical considerations in fitness and risk evaluations. Occup Med: State of the Art Rev 1988; 3:193–208.

24. Rothstein MA. Medical screening: A tool with broadening use. *Bus Health* 1986; 3:7–9.

25. Ashford NA, Spadafor CJ, Hattis DB, Caldart CC. Monitoring the worker for exposure and disease: Scientific, legal, and ethical considerations in the use of biomarkers. Baltimore: Johns Hopkins Press, 1990.

26. Matte TD, Fine L, Meinhardt TJ, Baker EL. Guidelines for medical screening in the workplace. Occup Med: State of the Art Rev 1990; 5:439–56.

27. Walsh DC, Jennings SE, Mangione T, Merrigan DM. Health promotion versus health protection: Employees' perceptions and concerns. J Public Health Pol 1991; 12:148–64.

28. Allegrante JR, Sloan RP. Ethical dilemmas in workplace health promotion. Prev Med 1986; 15:313–20.

29. Walsh DC. The vanguard and the rearguard: Occupational medicine revisits its future. J Occup Med 1988; 30:124–34.

# III
# Hazardous Workplace Exposures

# 13
# Toxins and Their Effects

Howard Frumkin

With cases by James Melius

A toxin is generally understood to be a substance that is harmful to biologic systems, but within this simple concept lies a great deal of variability. A substance that is harmful at a high dose may be innocuous or even essential at a lower dose. A toxin may damage a specific body system, or it may exert a general effect on an organism. A substance that is toxic to one species may not be toxic to another because of different metabolic pathways or protective mechanisms. And the biologic damage may be temporary, permanent over the organism's lifetime, or expressed over subsequent generations.

Toxicology is the study of the harmful effects of chemicals on biologic systems. It is a hybrid science built on advances in biochemistry, physiology, pathology, physical chemistry, pharmacology, and public health. Toxicologists describe and quantify the biologic uptake, distribution, effects, metabolism, and excretion of toxic chemicals. A subfield, environmental toxicology, focuses on exposures to toxic substances in the atmosphere, in food and water, and in occupational settings. These exposures have important effects both on humans and on the ecosystem in which we live.

The course of most toxicologic interactions takes the form of uptake → distribution → metabolism → excretion. Storage and biologic effects are other important events that may, but need not, occur. A knowledge of each of these steps is essential for a complete understanding of the effects of a chemical.

## Classes of Toxic Substances

Toxic or harmful substances encountered in the workplace may be classified in various ways. A simple and useful classification is given below, along with definitions adopted by the American National Standards Institute (ANSI).

*Dusts* Solid particles generated by handling, crushing, grinding, rapid impact, and detonation of organic or inorganic materials such as rocks, ore, metal, coal, wood, and grain. Dusts do not tend to flocculate except under electrostatic forces; they do not diffuse in air but settle under the influence of gravity.

*Fumes* Solid particles generated by condensation from the gaseous state, generally after volatilization from molten metals, and often accompanied by a chemical reaction such as oxidation. Fumes flocculate and sometimes coalesce.

*Mists* Suspended liquid droplets generated by condensation from the gaseous to the liquid state or by breaking up a liquid into a dispersed state, such as by splashing, foaming, or atomizing.

*Vapors* The gaseous form of substances that are normally in the solid or liquid state and can be changed to these states by either increasing the pressure or decreasing the temperature. Vapors diffuse.

*Gases* Normally formless fluids that occupy the space of enclosure and can be changed to the

## ASPHYXIANTS: CARBON MONOXIDE POISONING AMONG WORKERS AT AN ONION FARM

In December, a 50-year-old woman was brought to the emergency room of a small rural hospital after having collapsed at work. She reported no previous problems with syncopal episodes or chest pain and had no significant past medical history other than treatment for mild hypertension. She was doing her ordinary work at the farm's warehouse, packing onions for shipment, when she suddenly became dizzy and passed out. Her electrocardiogram (ECG) showed mild ischemic changes, and she was admitted to the intensive care unit for observation.

The next afternoon, two other workers from the same farm were brought to the emergency room complaining of headaches, dizziness, and nausea. Blood samples were drawn for determination of carboxyhemoglobin levels, and both had slightly elevated levels (around 10 percent). Interpretation of these levels was complicated by the length of time for the two patients to reach the hospital from the farm (over 30 minutes). The emergency room physician called the farm, and the owner reported that he had called the gas company to send people to check the propane heaters used in the barn. They had tested the barn with a "gas meter" and found no problem with carbon monoxide or other gases.

The two workers went back to work the next morning and again became ill. They returned to the emergency room. This time, their carboxyhemoglobin levels were more elevated (14 to 16 percent). A nurse from a local occupational health program was notified and visited the farm that afternoon. In discussing the situation with the farmer and other workers, she found a number of potential problems. Temperatures in the barn were kept very cold, and there was little ventilation. Several small propane heaters provided some heat. More importantly, a propane-powered fork lift was used intermittently in the barn. Because of weather conditions, the doors to the barn had been kept closed at all times for the last several days.

The nurse requested that an industrial hygienist visit the facility to conduct further air sampling. He came the next day. Although long-term personal samples taken that day only showed acceptable car- bon monoxide levels (up to 24 ppm, with the OSHA standard at 50 ppm), short-term samples taken in different places in the facility showed higher levels (up to 100 ppm), especially around the fork lift. Doors in the facility were kept open the day that the sampling took place. Based on these findings, the farmer obtained a battery-powered fork lift and took other steps to improve ventilation in the facility.

Possible carbon monoxide (CO) exposure should be considered in patients who collapse at work or report sudden headaches or light-headedness. In this case, the emergency room physician was alerted by occurrence of the same symptoms in two individuals from the same facility and by the person admitted the previous day. Interpretation of carboxyhemoglobin levels can be difficult if some time has passed since the original exposure, if oxygen has been given to the patient recently, or if the patient smokes cigarettes. Normal levels in a nonsmoker usually range up to 4 percent while smokers may have levels ranging up to 8 percent.

Headaches, lightheadedness, and nausea are typical symptoms of mildly elevated carboxyhemoglobin levels. More serious problems usually do not occur unless levels reach 20 percent or above. However, ischemic ECG changes have been found to occur in patients with preexisting heart disease during exercise after carbon monoxide exposures equivalent to carboxyhemoglobin levels of approximately 4 percent.

Intermittent or episodic exposures to elevated levels of carbon monoxide can be difficult to detect. In this case, the original testing by the "gas meter" might have occurred after the barn had been better ventilated or the instruments might not have been capable of detecting slightly elevated levels. Sampling with better instrumentation revealed the source of elevated levels. A worker's exposure from this source (the fork lift) could vary with time and location in the facility.

This case is only one of the many cases of carbon monoxide poisoning that occur every year and serves to illustrate several important principles. First, not every toxic exposure is exotic or mysterious. Second, workers, when exposed to an asphyxiant or intoxicant, become less alert and less able to react briskly to hazards. In a manner analogous to chemical synergy, their risk of accidents is enhanced markedly. Third, in an environment with very high gas concentrations every breath boosts the blood level of the gas, and toxicity can develop remarkably rapidly. Such acute exposures are common in enclosed spaces such as reaction tanks; other workers who rush to the victim's aid can be quickly overcome as well. Finally, when a worker is found unconscious or dead following an unknown exposure, a blood sample should always be taken. Carboxyhemoglobin concentration can be determined, as can evidence of numerous other toxicities.

Asphyxiants are usually grouped into two major categories. Simple or inert asphyxiants, such as propane or hydrogen, act by displacing oxygen in the atmosphere at the workplace. The most common scenario for this type of asphyxiation is someone working in a confined space, such as a manhole, where an inert asphyxiant has replaced the oxygen in the atmosphere of that confined space. The Occupational Safety and Health Administration (OSHA) recently promulgated a new standard for confined space work that should help to reduce the incidence of this common cause of workplace fatalities.

Chemical or toxic asphyxiants include a number of chemicals that interfere with the transport, delivery, or utilization of oxygen in the body. Common examples include carbon monoxide, hydrogen cyanide, and hydrogen sulfide. While these materials are sometimes used in a workplace, more commonly they are produced as a result of some other process, such as combustion, or chemical mixing, and the asphyxiation occurs "accidentally" as a result of that process.

Carbon monoxide is the most common chemical asphyxiant. Most acute incidents related to carbon monoxide occur secondarily from a source of combustion, such as heating device or fork lift. Carbon monoxide has a very strong affinity for hemoglobin, forming carboxyhemoglobin, which interferes with oxygen transport and delivery to tissues. In acute exposure incidents, the first symptoms are usually headache progressing to nausea, weakness, and decreased alertness. As carboxyhemoglobin levels climb above 35 percent, coma occurs. For young, healthy individuals, death occurs at levels above 50 percent, but in older persons with heart disease or other significant health problems, death may occur at lower concentrations.

Measurement of carboxyhemoglobin levels provides a good method of assessing the severity of the acute exposure. However, at lower exposure levels, cigarette smoking by the individual or delay between the time of exposure and the time of testing may interfere with interpretation of the results. Hyperbaric oxygen is indicated for severe carbon monoxide poisoning. Even with such treatment, permanent neurologic damage may occur from severe poisonings. Chronic exposures to lower levels of carbon monoxide increase the risk of cardiovascular disease among groups such as highway tunnel toll collectors.

Hydrogen cyanide (HCN) exposure may occur in several industries including electroplating and manufacture of certain specialty chemicals. Hydrogen cyanide is most commonly produced as a result of acids coming into contact with cyanide compounds. The burning of acrylonitrile plastics can also produce significant levels of hydrogen cyanide. The substance acts by inhibiting the enzyme cytochrome oxidase, which is necessary for tissue respiration. Exposure to levels around 100 ppm for 30 to 60 minutes can be fatal. Initial symptoms include headache and palpitations, progressing to dyspnea and then convulsions. Treatment with sodium nitrite, sodium thiosulfate, and amyl nitrite can be effective but must be started almost immediately. Blood cyanide levels can be utilized to monitor the effectiveness of treatment.

Acute hydrogen sulfide ($H_2S$) poisoning may occur in a number of workplace settings, including leather tanneries, sewage treatment plants, and oil-drilling sites, usually as a by-product of another process or as a contaminant. The latter is a common cause of work-related fatalities in the oil fields in the southwestern U.S., where natural gas has high levels of hydrogen sulfide contamination.

Hydrogen sulfide acts by interfering with oxidative enzymes, resulting in tissue hypoxia. Although at lower levels hydrogen sulfide has a characteristic "rotten egg" odor, at levels above 100 to 150 ppm, the exposed person's olfactory sense is diminished, which can provide a false sense of security. Initial symptoms of acute exposure include eye and respiratory irritation progressing to dyspnea and convulsions (from anoxia). Similar to hydrogen cyanide, rapid treatment with nitrites is effective. Delayed pulmonary edema has also been reported in some people after acute exposures.

Diagnosis of exposure to asphyxiants is dependent on rapid recognition of the potential source of exposure combined with the clinical presentation. Diagnosis of health problems from chronic or intermittent exposures to carbon monoxide can be difficult, but recognition of this substance as a possible source of symptoms such as headaches is important.

Prevention is usually dependent on procedures to limit production of these compounds from accidental mixing of chemicals or from combustion sources. For the latter, proper ventilation of combustion sources is important. Another important preventive measure is the testing of confined spaces before entry and the use of safety equipment and procedures, such as rescue lines.

liquid or solid state only by the combined effect of increased pressure and decreased temperature. Gases diffuse.

This classification does not include the obvious categories of solids and liquids that may be harmful, nor does it encompass physical agents that cannot be considered "substances." Living agents such as bacteria and fungi constitute another group of "substances" that would appear in a comprehensive classification of occupational health hazards.

## Absorption

In the workplace chemicals are taken up by three main routes: the respiratory system, the skin, and the gastrointestinal tract. Other routes of absorption, generally of less importance, include mucous membranes and open lesions. If these routes of exposure are remembered by a health professional while taking an occupational history, the importance of each can be evaluated with appropriate questions (see Chap. 3).

### Respiratory Tract

Inhalation is the major route of entry of the gases, vapors, mists, and airborne particulate matter encountered in the workplace. To analyze this process we need to consider gases, vapors, and mists separately from particles.

*Gases, Vapors, and Mists.* Gases, vapors, and mists can damage the respiratory tract; they can pass from the lungs to the bloodstream for distribution to other parts of the body; or both may occur.

Irritant gases are an important example of respiratory tract toxins (see Chap. 22). Their effects may be immediate or delayed. Gases that are very water soluble like hydrogen fluoride, ammonia, and sulfuric acid tend to dissolve in the moist lining of the upper respiratory tract, often producing immediate irritation, which forces an exposed worker to flee the area. Less soluble irritant gases, such as nitrogen dioxide, ozone, and phosgene, reach the bronchioles and alveoli where they dissolve slowly and may cause acute pneumonitis and pulmonary edema hours later. Long-term exposure at low concentrations may lead to chronic changes such as emphysema and fibrosis. Whether acute or chronic, the effects of irritant gases are seen mainly in the respiratory tract.

Asphyxiants are inhaled substances that exert toxicity by interrupting the supply or use of oxygen. *Simple asphyxiants* such as methane or nitrogen have relatively little direct physiologic effect, but by displacing oxygen in ambient air, they can cause severe hypoxia. This is a common problem in enclosed spaces such as silos and storage tanks. *Chemical asphyxiants* block the delivery or use of oxygen at the cellular level through one of several mechanisms. One example is carbon monoxide, a product of incomplete combustion found in foundries, coke ovens, furnaces, and similar facilities. It binds tightly to hemoglobin, forming a carboxyhemoglobin complex (COHb) that is ineffective at oxygen transport. Another example is cyanide, which is used in plastic production, metallurgy, electroplating, and other processes. Cyanide inhibits the cytochrome oxidase enzymes, compromising oxidative metabolism and phosphorylation. A third example, hydrogen sulfide, a gas found in mines, petrochemical plants, and sewers, also inhibits cytochrome oxidase. Unfortunately, occupational fatalities from all these exposures remain common.

Gases, vapors, and mists that are fat soluble can cross from the alveoli to the bloodstream and migrate from there to binding or storage sites for which they have a special affinity. Substances that are readily absorbed following inhalation and exert their effects elsewhere include carbon disulfide, volatile aliphatic and aromatic hydrocarbons, volatile halogenated hydrocarbons, and aliphatic saturated ketones such as methyl ethyl ketone. Because of the impressive variety of substances involved and the wide spectrum of acute and chronic effects that may result, this is an important pathway of absorption in workplace settings.

The toxic action of some inhaled gases, vapors, and mists may be considerably enhanced when they are adsorbed to respirable particles. Presumably, the particles transport these toxins to deep parts of the respiratory tree, which would otherwise be inaccessible. An example is radon gas: This substance increases lung cancer incidence among uranium miners, but, if it is experimentally inhaled in dust-free air, then almost none is retained by the lung and little or no carcinogenic effect is seen.

Several other variables influence the delivery of gases, vapors, and mists to the lower respiratory tract. With rapid, deep breathing, as occurs during strenuous exertion, the delivered dose increases. When a respirator is incorrectly chosen, poorly fit, or inadequately maintained, significant amounts of airborne toxins can reach workers' lungs (see Chap. 6).

*Particles.* Inhaled particles, unlike most gases and vapors, are of interest primarily for their pathologic effects on the lungs. Their deposition, retention, and clearance are influenced by several well-defined factors.

One factor is inertia, which tends to maintain moving particles on a straight course. A second is gravity, which tends to move particles earthward, promoting the early settling out of larger and denser particles. A third is Brownian diffusion, the random motion that results from molecular kinetic energy. When these forces cause a particle to strike the airway wall or alveolar surface, deposition occurs.

Three factors influence the location and extent of deposition: anatomy of the respiratory tract, particle size, and breathing pattern. Branching, angling, and narrowing at each point in the airways define the local velocity and flow characteristics of the inspired air, which in turn influence particle deposition. For example, the nasopharynx features sharp bends, nasal hairs, and narrow cross-sections with resulting high linear velocities, which together promote the impaction of inhaled particles.

This principle has some well-known applications. Nasal cancers are rare in the general population, but they occur with an increased incidence in certain occupational groups, probably due to nasal deposition of inhaled dusts that contain carcinogens. Examples include workers in furniture manufacturing who are exposed to wood dust, and workers in leather shoe and boot manufacturing who are exposed to leather, fiberboard, rubber, and cork dusts. A similar phenomenon is thought to occur farther along the airways. Most bronchogenic carcinomas arise at airway branch points, where particle deposition is promoted by locally turbulent air flow.

The effective anatomy of the respiratory tract changes significantly with a simple shift from nose-breathing to mouth-breathing, as occurs normally during physical exertion. This bypasses the more efficient filtration of larger particles by the nasopharynx and results in greater deposition in the tracheobronchial tree. Through such a transition workers performing physical labor may lose the benefit of a major natural defense mechanism.

Since particle density and shape also influence deposition, these parameters are subsumed in a conceptual measure of size, the *effective aerodynamic diameter*. Comparisons among unlike particles, as if they were spherical and of unit density, are thus possible. As Fig. 13-1 shows, deposition is very efficient for particles with an effective aerodynamic diameter above several microns ($\mu$), reaches its minimal level at about 1.0 $\mu$, and increases again below 0.5 $\mu$. Particles with an effective aerodynamic diameter of between 0.5 and 5.0 $\mu$ (the respirable fraction) can persist in the alveoli and respiratory bronchioles after deposition there, the first step in the development of pneumoconiosis. Smaller particles are cleared by macrophages, lymphatics, and the bloodstream, while larger particles are filtered out in the upper airways. The size of a particle is not always constant; hygroscopic particles such as some salts can expand significantly when hydrated in the upper airways. The result is a higher proportion of upper airway deposition.

As minute volume increases, the deposition of particles in the airways increases, especially of larger particles. In contrast, a change to rapid, shallow breathing diminishes the residence time of airborne particles in the lungs and hence the probability of deposition. Deep breathing, as during strenuous exertion, delivers a larger proportion of inhaled air to the distal airways and promotes alveolar deposition. Thus, with some basic knowledge of the particles in question and the nature of the inhalation exposure, one can evaluate, in general terms, the seriousness of a workplace exposure.

Filtration of particles in the upper airways and clearance of particles that do arrive distally are accomplished mainly by the mucociliary escalator. Particles that impact on ciliated regions of the airways are carried toward the pharynx within hours and thus have little chance to dissolve or undergo leaching. However, particles deposited in nonciliated regions may be more persistent. If they are removed from surface sites by alveolar macrophages, they reach the mucociliary escalator and are cleared within 24 hours. (Materials that are carried to the pharynx by the mucociliary escalator are then swallowed, resulting in gastrointestinal exposure and possibly explaining the elevated incidence of gastrointestinal cancer among asbestos workers.)

Alternatively, particles that reach nonciliated regions may penetrate into fixed tissue, such as connective tissue or lymph nodes, where they may reside for years, sometimes eliciting pathologic reactions. This penetration is especially likely when the performance of the mucociliary escalator is somehow compromised, as it is in smokers or in some chronically exposed workers. In general, the mucociliary escalator is an effective defense against the retention of most inhaled particles. When it is overrun, however, particles are retained and the stage is set for subsequent pathology.

### Skin

Human skin consists of three layers (the epidermis, dermis, and subcutaneous fat) and three kinds of glandular structures (sebaceous glands, apocrine sweat glands—both part of the "pilosebaceous unit"—and eccrine sweat glands) (see Fig. 24-1).

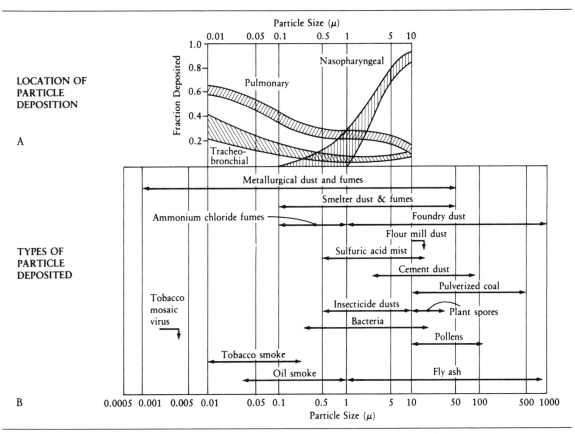

**Fig. 13-1.** A. Fractional deposition plotted against particle size (effective aerodynamic diameter) for three functional parts of the respiratory tree, based on the model of the International Committee on Radiation Protection. The broad bands reflect large standard deviations. B. Examples of inhaled particles, classified by size. By comparing (A) and (B), one can generate approximate predictions of the deposition pattern of each particle. (Adapted from JD Brain, PA Valberg. Aerosol deposition in the respiratory tract. Am Rev Respir Dis 1979; 120:1325–73.)

The outermost layer of the epidermis, the stratum corneum or horny layer, provides some of the skin's structural stability and much of its chemical resistance. This layer consists mainly of thickened cell envelopes and a combination of sulfur-rich amorphous proteins and sulfur-poor fibrous proteins known as keratin.

There are two forms of percutaneous absorption: *transepidermal* (through the epidermal cells) and *appendageal* (through the hair follicles and sebaceous glands). The appendageal route offers greater permeability and plays an important role early in exposure and in the diffusion of ions and polar nonelectrolytes. However, the transepidermal route is generally more prominent because of its far greater absorbing surface.

Transepidermal transport occurs by passive diffusion, and several mechanisms have been hypothesized. According to one theory, the intracellular keratin matrix of the stratum corneum provides the main resistance to penetration by toxins, with polar and nonpolar molecules appearing to permeate through distinct channels. Alternatively, a two-phase series model postulates a protein-rich "cytoplasm" and a lipoidal "cell wall" to describe the passage of alcohols and steroids through the stratum corneum. A third possibility is that the stratum corneum limits the passage of polar molecules, while aqueous "boundary layers" prevent the diffusion of more lipophilic substances. Even very soluble substances encounter a relative barrier at the skin; in one experiment mustard gas was found fixed in the epidermis and dermis of human skin 24 hours after application. (An interesting possibility is that the skin acts as a reservoir due to in situ fixation. After exposure ceases, toxins could continue to enter the bloodstream from skin stores. This process has been documented with some steroids.)

A tremendous variety of aliphatic and aromatic hydrocarbons, metals, and pesticides can undergo at least some percutaneous absorption. Generally, fat-soluble substances show a greater flux than water-soluble ones, and substances that are soluble in both fat and water show the greatest flux. For any substance the relative importance of percutaneous absorption must be evaluated in light of other significant routes of entry: Although volatile solvents such as trichloroethylene and toluene are absorbed through the skin, inhalation would be far more significant in most occupational settings; on the other hand, for a substance such as benzidine, which is readily absorbed by the skin but has low volatility, percutaneous absorption may be the major route of entry.

A variety of factors can influence the extent of percutaneous absorption. Some are properties of the skin such as wetness, location on the body, and vascularization. Prior damage, such as abrasion or dermatitis, can dramatically increase absorption. Certain organic solvents, such a dimethyl sulfoxide (DMSO), and mixtures, such as ethanol/ether or chloroform/methanol, are efficient delipidizing agents, which compromise the barrier function of the stratum corneum. Occlusion is often used to promote the absorption of medications, but in the workplace occlusion can have untoward results. For example, if a worker wears rubber gloves that contain a solvent, absorption may be enhanced.

Other factors that influence percutaneous absorption reside in the substance being absorbed and included concentration, phase (aqueous or dry), pH, molecular weight, and vehicle. In fact, the best single determinant of the flux of a substance across the skin is its *partition coefficient* between stratum corneum and vehicle, which varies with the vehicle.

Skin absorption, of course, is necessary but not sufficient for the development of percutaneous toxicity. Cutaneous exposure may be followed by local effects (as discussed in Chap. 24), by systemic effects (as discussed later in this chapter), or by no effects at all.

### Gastrointestinal Tract

Ingestion of hazardous substances is generally not a major route of workplace exposure, although there are important exceptions. Workers who mouth-breathe or who chew gum or tobacco can absorb appreciable amounts of gaseous materials during a workday. Inhaled particulates swept upward by ciliary action from the airways can be swallowed. And materials on the hands may be brought to the mouth during on-the-job eating, drinking, and smoking.

Several features of the gastrointestinal (GI) tract help to minimize toxicity by this route. Gastric and pancreatic juices can detoxify some substances by hydrolysis and reduction. Absorption into the bloodstream may be inefficient and selective. Food and liquid present in the GI tract can dilute toxins and can form less soluble complexes with them. Finally, the portal circulation carries absorbed materials to the liver, where metabolism can begin promptly. As a result, the most serious GI exposures to consider are those with slowly cumulative action such as mercury, lead, and cadmium.

## Distribution

Some toxins exert their effects at the site of initial contact. For example, the skin can be "burned" by strongly acidic or basic solutions or delipidized by some solvents, inhalation of phosgene can lead to delayed pulmonary edema, and inhalation of cadmium fume can lead to pneumonitis. However, many toxins are taken up by the bloodstream and transported to other parts of the body, where they may exert biologic effects or be stored. The destination of a chemical is largely determined by its ability to cross various membrane barriers and by its affinity for particular body compartments.

Membranes are the main obstacle to the free movement of chemicals among the various compartments of the body. The mammalian cell membrane consists of a lipid layer sandwiched between two protein layers, with a combined thickness of about 100 Å. Large protein molecules, freely mobile in the plane of the membrane, can penetrate one or both faces, and small pores 2 to 4 Å in diameter traverse the membrane. There are thus three mechanisms by which a chemical can cross a membrane: simple diffusion of lipid-soluble substances through the membrane; filtration through the pores by small molecules that accompany the bulk flow of water; and binding by specialized carrier molecules, which transport polar molecules actively or passively through the lipid layer.

In a steady-state situation, the solute concentrations on the two sides of a membrane reach an equilibrium. This equilibrium is described by Fick's first law of diffusion, which states that the amount of solute (ds) that diffuses across an area (A) in time (t) is proportional to the local concentration gradient (dc/dx):

$$\frac{ds}{dt} = - DA \frac{dc}{dx}$$

The proportionality constant (D) is the diffusion coefficient. This constant is inversely proportional to the cube root of the molecular weight for a spherical molecule. Accordingly, many small molecules that ordinarily cross membranes without difficulty are unable to cross the same membranes once bound to large serum molecules. The diffusion coefficient also reflects the lipid/water partition coefficient. The result is an important gener-

alization: Molecules that are fat-soluble cross membranes far more readily and far more rapidly than compounds that are water-soluble.

This generalization not only describes the distribution of toxins in the body; it has clinical applications as well. Manipulating the pH on one side of a membrane can alter the extent of ionization of a solute, which, in turn, modifies its membrane solubility. This practice can be used to "trap" solute in a desired body compartment—in effect changing the flux by changing the diffusion coefficient. For example, patients who ingest large amounts of salicylates are treated with bicarbonate, in part because the resulting alkaline urine ionizes the filtered salicylate and prevents reabsorption by renal tubular cells.

Movement from one body compartment to another may not entail traversing membrane bilayers. Each of three morphologic forms of capillaries—continuous, fenestrated, and discontinuous—provides an alternative way for solutes to leave the bloodstream. Thus, various mechanisms exist by which membrane-insoluble substances and fluids can cross capillary walls, leave the vascular compartment, and reach target cells. The importance of these mechanisms is unclear, as most chemicals are thought to pass directly through capillary cells. However, in the face of local conditions such as acidosis, or in organs like the liver with discontinuous capillaries, these mechanisms may contribute significantly to the extravasation of toxins.

Two barriers to distribution deserve special attention. First, the *blood-brain barrier* hinders the passage of many toxins from central nervous system (CNS) capillaries into the brain. Its anatomic identity is not precisely known, but it probably involves the glial connective tissue cells (astrocytes), very tight junctions between endothelial cells, or an unusually low capacity for pinocytosis by endothelial cells. The blood-brain barrier is not uniform throughout the brain; for example, the cortex, lateral hypothalamic nuclei, area postrema, pineal body, and neurohypophysis are relatively less protected, perhaps due to a richer blood supply, a more permeable barrier, or both. Radiation, inorganic and alkyl mercury, and several other toxins and diseases can damage the blood-brain barrier and impair its performance.

Chemical passage across the blood-brain barrier is governed by the same rules that describe membrane crossing elsewhere in the body. Only molecules that are not bound to plasma proteins can cross into the brain. Greater fat solubility helps a molecule permeate the barrier; thus, nonionized molecules enter the brain at a rate proportional to their lipid/water partition coefficient, while ionized molecules are essentially unable to leave the CNS capillaries. The blood-brain barrier, then, is distinctive mainly in its quantitatively greater protective effect compared to the body's other capillary beds.

The second barrier of particular interest is the *placenta*. In the placentas of humans and other primates, three layers of fetal tissue (trophoblast, connective tissue, and endothelium) separate the fetal and maternal blood. Some species such as the pig have six cell layers in the placental barrier, while others—the rat, rabbit, and guinea pig— have only one. These structural differences may correspond to differences in permeability, and therefore animal data on transplacental transport must be interpreted with caution.

The placenta has active transport systems for vital materials like vitamins, amino acids, and sugars. However, most toxins appear to cross the placenta by simple diffusion. In addition, a variety of nonchemical agents can cross the placenta, including viruses (such as rubella), cellular pathogens (such as the syphilis spirochete), antibody globulins (IgG, but not IgM), fibers (including asbestos!), and even erythrocytes. There is evidence suggesting that the placenta actively blocks transport of some substances into the fetus, perhaps through chemical biotransformation mechanisms. Substances that do diffuse into the fetal circulation observe the laws discussed above, and in a steady state their maternal and fetal plasma concentrations are equal. Of course, since maternal and fetal tissues may have different affinities for some substances, the concentrations in specific kinds of tissues may differ. For example, the fetal blood-brain barrier is incompletely formed, and lead can accumulate in the fetal CNS far faster than in the maternal CNS; workplace exposure to lead thus poses a special problem for pregnant women.

## Storage

Most foreign substances that reach the plasma water are excreted fairly promptly, either intact or following chemical modifications. However, some substances, while being distributed as described above, reach sites for which they have a high affinity, where they accumulate and persist. The result is storage depots.

These depots may occur at the sites of toxic action. For example, carbon monoxide has a very high affinity for its target molecule, hemoglobin, and the herbicide paraquat, which causes pulmonary fibrosis, accumulates in the lungs. More commonly, however, the storage depot is different from the site of toxic action. For example, lead is stored in bone but exerts its toxic effects on various soft tissues. There is an equilibrium between plasma and depot concentrations of any stored substance, and therefore a depot can slowly release its content into the bloodstream long after exposure has ended.

One important storage depot is adipose tissue. Most chlorinated solvents like carbon tetrachloride and chlorinated pesticides like DDT and dieldrin migrate from the blood to the fat due to their high lipid solubility. Storage of such substances appears to involve simple physical dissolution in neutral fats, which constitute about 20 percent of a lean individual's weight and up to 50 percent of an obese individual's weight. The fat reservoir can therefore protect an obese person by sequestering a toxin from circulation; conversely, a rapid loss of weight through illness or dieting might release toxic amounts of a stored substance back into the bloodstream.

A variety of proteins can bind exogenous molecules and thereby function as a storage depot.

STORAGE OF DDT.

TERATOGENS: BIRTH DEFECTS IN
CHILDREN OF MOTHERS EXPOSED TO
CHEMICALS AT WORK

*Case A:* A 19-year-old woman, who worked in the
reinforced plastics industry and whose husband was
a 26-year-old carpenter in the same factory, gave
birth to her first child, a 3,900-gm, 54-cm boy, 18
days before her predicted delivery date. The child
was found to have congenital hydrocephalus, anomaly of the right ear, and bilateral malformations of
the thoracic vertebral column and ribs. Antibody
tests for rubella, *Toxoplasma,* and *Listeria* in mother
and child, and mumps and herpes simplex in the
mother, were negative.

In the third month of pregnancy the mother had
had bronchitis, and she was given 3 days sick leave
and treated with penicillin. Otherwise her pregnancy
was normal, and she had taken no drugs except for
iron and vitamin preparations. The mother worked
regularly during pregnancy; she ground, polished,
and mended reinforced plastic products and was exposed to styrene, polyester resin, organic peroxides,
acetone, and polishes. In her second trimester she
was heavily exposed to styrene for about 3 days
when she cleaned a mold without a face mask.

*Case B:* A 24-year-old woman, who worked in the
reinforced plastics industry and whose husband was
a 22-year-old welder-plater in the metal industry,
gave birth to her first child, a 2,200-gm, 47-cm girl,
6 weeks before her predicted delivery date. The baby
died during delivery; anencephaly was diagnosed. Serologic tests of the mother for *Toxoplasma* and *Listeria,* and placental culture for *Listeria,* were all negative.

The pregnancy had been normal except for contractions during the second month. At that time 10
mg of isoxsuprine was prescribed three times a day
for 7 days. Slight edema occurred in the seventh
month of pregnancy, and 500 mg of chlorthiazide a
day was prescribed for 7 days. The mother worked
during most of her pregnancy. In the third month of
pregnancy she did manual laminating for about 3
weeks with no face mask and was then exposed to
styrene, polyester resin, organic peroxides, and acetone. After this period she did needlework in the
same workshop for about 1 month and then lami-
nated again at varying intervals [1].

These cases were identified during an investigation of congenital malformations in Finland. They were reported when the investigators found an overrepresentation of workers in
the reinforced plastics industry among the parents of affected infants.

Teratogenesis due to industrial chemicals
may well have occurred in these cases. Styrene
(vinyl benzene) is metabolized to styrene oxide,
a known bacterial mutagen. Styrene is also a
structural analogue of vinyl chloride, which is
associated with lymphocyte chromosomal aberrations and hepatic angiosarcomas among exposed workers (see Chap. 14). These molecules
are sufficiently fat-soluble to cross membranes
and could have passed from the maternal to the
fetal circulation. Of course, the women had
multiple chemical exposures, and the possibility
of combined effects cannot be excluded.

However, as is typical when a chemical exposure is clinically associated with teratogenic
or carcinogenic effects, no causal relation can
be proven in these cases. In fact, for any particular substance it may be impossible ever to assemble a large enough group of exposed subjects to conduct an epidemiologic study that
would yield statistically significant results (see
Chap. 5). Health professionals must therefore
use available toxicologic knowledge to evaluate
case reports such as this one, identify potential
hazards, and advise their patients on appropriate precautionary measures.

Probably the best known example is serum albumin, which binds and transports many pharmacologic agents. Recent evidence suggests that environmental agents such as DDE (the principal
metabolite of DDT) and some dyes may compete
for the albumin-binding sites. Molecules that are
bound to albumin or to other plasma proteins like
ceruloplasmin and transferrin are unavailable for
toxic action elsewhere as long as they remain
bound. A more deleterious form of protein binding

occurs with mercury and cadmium: Both metals complex with renal tubular proteins, and mercury complexes with CNS proteins as well, causing dysfunction at these sites. Finally, carcinogenic hydrocarbons appear to complex with proteins on contact with the skin and lung wall, and they initiate transformation by their continued presence (see Chap. 14).

Several important toxins are stored as insoluble salts. Lead, strontium, and radium form phosphates, which are deposited in bone. Lead has a toxic effect on marrow (see Chap. 29), and it can be mobilized during acidosis to cause acute lead poisoning. Strontium, if deposited as a radioactive isotope (especially strontium 90), releases ionizing radiation, and radium is an alpha-emitter; both are associated with osteosarcomas and hematologic neoplasms (see Chap. 15). Finally, fluoride is stored in the bones and teeth as an insoluble calcium salt; high levels can lead to bone and joint distortion, joint dysfunction, and mottling of dental enamel in children.

An unusual example of storage is the lymphatic accumulation of crystalline silica in the lung. Macrophages that engulf the silica migrate to lymph nodes, where they are destroyed. Continued irritation by the silica then induces inflammation and fibrosis (see Chap. 22).

## Biotransformations

Between initial absorption and final excretion many substances are chemically converted by the body. Although many different metabolic conversions have been described, they can be characterized by a few simple generalizations and divided into a small number of categories.

Metabolic transformations are mediated by enzymes. The liver is rich in metabolic enzymes, and most biotransformation occurs there. All cells in the body, however, have some capacity for metabolizing xenobiotics (chemicals foreign to the body).

In general, metabolic transformations lead to products that are more polar and less fat-soluble,

consistent with the eventual goal of excretion. This process usually entails a change from more toxic to less toxic forms: For example, benzene is oxidized to phenol, and glutathione combines with halogenated aromatics to form nontoxic mercapturic acid metabolites.

However, metabolic transformations sometimes yield increasingly toxic products. One example is the oxidation of methanol to formaldehyde. Another example is the solvent methyl n-butyl ketone (MBK), which produces peripheral neuropathy ("cabinet finisher's neuropathy") in exposed workers (see Chap. 26). Animal toxicology studies have revealed that a γ-diketone metabolite of MBK, 2,5-hexanedione, is probably the actual neurotoxin. N-hexane is also oxidized to 2,5-hexanedione, which helps explain the neurotoxicity of that solvent (Fig. 13-2). In contrast, other hexacarbons such as methyl isobutyl ketone (MIBK) and methyl ethyl ketone (MEK) cannot give rise to

**Fig. 13-2.** The metabolic transformation of *n*-hexane. (From PS Spencer et al. On the specific molecular configuration of neurotoxic aliphatic hexacarbon compounds causing central-peripheral distal axonopathy. Toxicol Appl Pharmacol 1978; 44:17. Modified from GD Divincenzo, et al. Characterization of the metabolites of methyl-*n*-butyl ketone, methyl isobutyl ketone, and methyl ethyl ketone in guinea pig serum and their clearance. Toxicol Appl Pharmacol 1976; 36:511.)

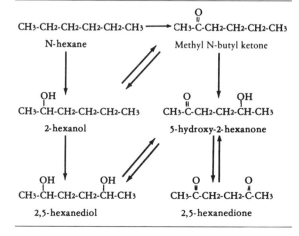

## ORGANIC SOLVENTS: CASE OF A CAR PAINTER WITH NONSPECIFIC CNS SYMPTOMS

During a routine medical examination, a 24-year-old man reported problems with concentration: He frequently lost his train of thought, forgot what he was saying in midsentence, and had been told by friends that he seemed forgetful. He also felt excessively tired after waking in the morning and at the end of his workday. He had occasional listlessness and frequent headaches. At work he often felt drunk or dizzy, and several times he misunderstood simple instructions from his supervisor. These problems had all developed insidiously during the previous 2 years. The patient thought that other employees in his area of the plant had complained of similar symptoms. He had noted some relief during a recent weeklong fishing vacation. He denied appetite or bowel changes, sweating, weight loss, fever, chills, palpitations, syncope, seizures, trembling hands, peripheral tingling, and changes in strength or sensation. He was a social drinker and denied drug use and cigarette smoking.

The patient had worked for 3½ years as a car painter in a railroad car repair garage. He had compiled a list of substances to which he had been exposed.

| PAINT SOLVENTS | PAINT BINDERS | OTHER SUBSTANCES |
|---|---|---|
| Toluene | Acrylic resin | Organic dyes |
| Xylene | Urethane resin | Inorganic dyes |
| Ethanol | Bindex 284 | Zinc |
| Isopropanol | Solution Z-92 | Chromates |
| Butanol | | Titanium dioxide |
| Ethyl acetate | | Catalysts |
| Ethyl glycol | | |
| Acetone | | |
| Methyl ethyl ketone | | |

His plant had been inspected by OSHA 1 year previously, and the only citations issued were for minor safety violations.

Physical examination, including a careful neurologic examination, was completely normal. The erythrocyte sedimentation rate was 3 mm/hr. Routine hematologic and biochemical tests, thyroid function studies, and heterophile antibody assay were all negative, except for slight elevations of serum gamma glutamyl transpeptidase (SGGT) and alkaline phosphatase [2].

This case illustrates some of the many problems that confront a health care provider in applying occupational toxicology. The patient reported vague, nonspecific symptoms, which a busy clinician might easily dismiss. Unfortunately, many toxins have just such generalized effects. Furthermore, the patient had multiple chemical exposures, and no one toxin could be readily identified as the agent causing his symptoms. This patient was unusual in that he was able to provide a list of his exposures, but even this list had its limitations. Note the presence of two (fictional) trade names on the list; their identities are unknown and may be off limits even to an inquiring physician (see Appendix A, How to Research the Toxic Effects of Chemical Substances). The absence of OSHA citations a year earlier may mean that all exposures were currently at permissible levels, but one cannot be certain of this fact. The inspection might have been directed only at safety hazards, the plant may have been temporarily cleaned up for the inspector's benefit, conditions could have deteriorated in the subsequent year, and new production processes could have been initiated or new materials introduced. In any event, all the symptoms reported by this patient have been associated with "safe" levels of solvent exposure, so even a well-maintained plan might offer cause for concern (see also Chap. 26).

Organic solvents are commonly used industrial chemicals. Exposures occur in a variety of workplace settings, including oil refining and petrochemical facilities, plastics manufacturing, painting, and building maintenance. Often several different solvents may be used in a given product, and multiple products containing solvents may be used in a facility. The formulation of products containing solvents has changed over time because of economic factors and concern about the toxicity of specific solvents. These factors may make the identification of the specific exposure of an individual worker difficult to ascertain. This is particularly a problem for solvent use in the construction industry, where multiple employers and products may be involved.

As illustrated in the case outlined above, the neurologic system is affected by many different organic solvents, causing both acute effects (narcosis) and chronic neurobehavioral effects in some individuals. In addition, several specific solvents, including carbon disulfide, *n*-hexane, and methyl *n*-butyl ketone (MEK), cause a peripheral neuropathy characterized by loss of distal sensation, progressing to include motor weakness and even paralysis. The disease may progress for several months after exposure has ceased, and permanent damage may occur.

Long-term exposures to a number of solvents, including toluene, xylene, and trichloroethane, may cause chronic neurobehavioral changes, ranging from mild changes in affect and ability to concentrate to severe loss of intellectual function. Some individuals appear to develop more severe disease than others, and the exact relationship to exposure history or to specific solvent exposure has been difficult to determine. As most workers exposed to solvents are exposed to a mixture of solvents, the effects of individual solvents are difficult to separate.

Several organic solvents cause other toxic effects. Benzene was a commonly used industrial and commercial solvent. High exposures suppress bone marrow production, sometimes leading to anemia or pancytopenia. Benzene is also a potent carcinogen, leading to leukemia and other hematopoietic malignancies. Due to this toxicity, benzene is used much less commonly today, although exposures continue to

occur in the petrochemical and some other industries. Several other hydrocarbons, including ethylene oxide, the chloromethyl ethers, and epichlorohydrin, are also carcinogenic. Many other solvents are suspected of being carcinogenic, including several halogenated compounds.

Several organic solvents are hepatotoxic. Carbon tetrachloride, chloroform, and tetrachloroethane may cause hepatic necrosis. Long-term exposure to carbon tetrachloride has been associated with the development of cirrhosis. Dimethyl formamide and 2-nitropropane have been responsible for outbreaks of chemically induced liver disease in exposed workers.

Several organic solvents, including the glycol ethers and ethylene oxide, have been shown to affect the reproductive system.

Skin irritation also commonly results from solvent exposures. These chemicals dry the skin by removing natural skin oils. Many organic solvents are also acute respiratory irritants.

The diagnosis of health problems related to solvent exposure is very dependent on a good exposure history. Due to the variety of health effects from different individual organic solvents, identification of the person's exposure is critical. Biologic monitoring may be helpful for some solvents, but only if the person is currently being exposed to the substance.

Control of solvent exposure often depends on a careful evaluation of how the exposure occurs. Work procedures and practices are often important determinants of solvent exposure for many groups that work with organic solvents such as painters. Personal protective equipment and changes in work practices may be needed to limit exposures. In some settings, traditional engineering methods, such as ventilation, may also be useful.

2,5-hexanedione and would thus be preferable to MBK as solvents.

The concept of toxic metabolites is especially salient with regard to carcinogens (see Chap. 14). Vinyl chloride, a causative agent of liver, lung, lymphatic, and central nervous system tumors, is

oxidized to a reactive epoxide intermediate, which is actually the proximate carcinogen. The same is probably true for trichloroethylene, vinylidene chloride, vinyl benzene, and chlorobutadiene. In fact, a major mechanism of carcinogenicity of aromatic compounds is conversion to reactive epoxides, which in turn combine with cellular nucleophiles like DNA and RNA.

Classically, metabolic transformations are divided into four categories: oxidation, reduction, hydrolysis, and conjugation. The first three reaction types, which are known as phase I reactions, increase the polarity of substrates and can either increase or decrease toxicity. In conjugation, the only phase II reaction, polar groups are added to the products of phase I reactions. Most chemicals are handled sequentially by the two phases, although some are directly conjugated. The spectrum of reactions of each type can be found in any toxicology text, and only a few examples of occupational health interest are presented here.

*Oxidation* is the most common biotransformation reaction. There are two general kinds of oxidation reactions: direct addition of oxygen to the carbon, nitrogen, sulfur, or other bond; and dehydrogenation. Most of these reactions are mediated by microsomal enzymes, although there are mitochondrial and cytoplasmic oxidases as well. Examples of oxidation include:

Hydroxylation:

Benzene   to   Phenol

N-Hydroxylation:

Aniline   to   Phenylhydroxylamine

Desulfuration:

$(C_2H_5O)_2$ –P–O– –$NO_2$   $(C_2H_5O)_2$ –P–O– –$NO_2$

Parathion   to   Paraoxon

The thiophosphate insecticides, such as parathion, are relatively nontoxic until the S is replaced by O through this reaction.

Deamination:   $CH_3-(CH_2)_3-NH_2$     $CH_3-(CH_2)_2-C\overset{H}{\underset{O}{}} + NH_3$

N-Butylamine   to   Butaldehyde and Ammonia

*Reduction* is a much less common biotransformation than oxidation, but it does occur with substances whose redox potentials exceed that of the body. Examples include:

Azo reduction:

()-aminoazotoluene   to   Aniline derivatives

The azo dyes have been known since the 1930s to include many mutagens and carcinogens. Reduction of the azo bond yields aromatic amines, such as aniline and benzidine, which are probably the active carcinogens. In mammalian test species, the principal target sites are the bladder and liver. Not all azo dyes are carcinogenic; extensive investigation of these compounds has yielded a rich body of information about structure-activity relationships.

Aromatic nitro reduction:

Nitrobenzene   to   Aniline

*Conjugation* involves combining a toxin with a normal body constituent. The result is generally a less toxic and more polar molecule, which can be more readily excreted. However, conjugation can be harmful if it occurs in excess and depletes the body of an essential constituent. Examples of conjugation reactions include:

Sulfation:

Phenol   to   Its sulfate conjugate

Sulfation is the major means of preparing phenol for excretion. It is also used for alcohols, amines, and other groups.

Acetylation:

Aniline    to    Its acetyl conjugate

The above two reactions exemplify the sequential processing of substances by phase I and phase II reactions. Phenol and aniline can themselves be metabolites of other toxins, as previously illustrated; they are then conjugated and excreted.

Mercapturic acid addition:

COOH
S—CH₂—CH
HN—COCH₃

Naphthalene    to    Its mercapturic acid conjugate

The addition of mercapturic acid (*N*-acetylcysteine) is a multi-step process, which proceeds through the addition of glutathione and subsequent cleavage to cysteine derivatives. This reaction is extremely important in handling reactive electrophilic compounds, the products of exogenous exposure or of endogenous metabolic processes. Polyaromatic hydrocarbons (PAHs) and polyhalogenated hydrocarbons are predominantly excreted in this way.

*Hydrolysis* is a common reaction in a variety of biochemical pathways. Esters are hydrolyzed to acids and alcohols, and amides are hydrolyzed to acids and amines.

As mentioned above, various combinations of these reactions may be assembled in response to the same toxin. Metabolic strategies for a particular toxin may vary widely among species, and therefore an animal study, to be applicable to humans, must use a species with pathways similar to those of humans.

The most prominent enzyme system for performing phase I reactions is the cytochrome 450 system, also known as the mixed-function oxygenase system. These enzymes are found in the endo-plasmic reticulum of hepatocytes and other cells. In recent years, advances in molecular biology have greatly expanded our understanding of cytochrome P-450. Over 70 distinct P-450 genes have been identified, and many have been sequenced. They have been grouped into eight distinct families, and for many, specific functions have been identified. For example, the enzyme CYP1A1 metabolically activates polycyclic aromatic hydrocarbons; the enzyme CYP2D6 is responsible for metabolizing such medications as beta-blockers, tricyclic antidepressants, and debrisoquin; and the enzyme CYP2E1 bioactivates vinyl chloride, methylene chloride, and urethane.

These insights, in turn, have helped explain why people may vary widely in their metabolic activity following similar exposures. Polymorphism in the genes that code for various P-450 proteins has been shown to result in different metabolic phenotypes. For example, people whose CYP2D6 phenotype makes them poor metabolizers of debrisoquin are at risk of various adverse drug reactions, while extensive metabolizers are at increased risk of lung cancer, probably because of carcinogenic metabolites they produce.

Any enzyme system has a finite capacity. When a preferred pathway is saturated, the remaining substrate may be handled by alternative pathways. (Most substrates can be metabolized by more than one enzyme system.) However, in some instances when a preferred metabolic pathway is saturated, the substrate may persist in the body and exert toxic effects. An example is dioxane metabolism. Dioxane (cyclic-$OCH_2CH_2OCH_2CH_2$) is a solvent with a variety of industrial applications, including painting, printing, and textile manufacturing. High-dose exposure in rats causes hepatocellular and renal tubular cell damage as well as hepatic and nasal carcinoma. Based on rat studies, the principal human metabolite of dioxane has been identified as β-hydroxyethoxyacetic acid (HEAA). HEAA is found in the urine of exposed workers at over 100 times the concentration of dioxane, suggesting that at low exposures the dioxane is rapidly converted to HEAA. However, the metabolic pathway from dioxane to HEAA can be saturated by high-dose exposure, and in rats this event has been correlated with toxicity. Thus, the effects of dioxane appear to be most pronounced when the ordinary metabolic pathway is saturated, allowing high levels of the solvent to accumulate. (All of this, however, does not prove that low-dose workplace exposure to dioxane is harmless, since dioxane is a carcinogen for which no safe threshold can be demonstrated.)

A particular form of enzyme saturation is *competitive inhibition,* which may be a mechanism of toxicity, as when organophosphate pesticides compete with acetylcholine for the binding sites on cholinesterase molecules, or when metals such as beryllium compete with magnesium and manganese for enzyme ligand binding. However, competitive inhibition is important as well in the metabolic processing of toxins. For example, methyl alcohol is oxidized by the enzyme alcohol dehydrogenase to the optic nerve toxin formaldehyde. This process can be blocked by large doses of ethanol, which competes for the binding sites of the enzyme and slows the formation of the toxic metabolite.

A less salutary example of competitive inhibition is the synergy demonstrated by two organophosphate pesticides, malathion and EPN (ethyl *p*-nitrophenyl phenylphosphonothionate). Although they are structurally similar, EPN is far more toxic than malathion. When the two pesticides are present together, the EPN competes for the enzyme that would ordinarily hydrolyze and thus detoxify the malathion. As a result malathion persists at unusually high concentrations, and the combined toxicity is far greater than would be expected. Other pairs of organophosphates that interact similarly are malathion and trichlorfon (Dipterex), and azinphos-methyl (Gusathion) and trichlorfon. Since most workplace exposures involve multiple substances, such synergistic effects are common but probably go unrecognized most of the time. This synergism is important to remember when evaluating reports on the toxicity of individual substances.

The enzyme systems that metabolize xenobiotics are not static. When the demand is high, their synthesis can be enhanced in a process called *enzyme induction.* The resulting increase in enzyme activity helps the organism respond to subsequent exposures not only to the original xenobiotic but to similar substances as well. DDT and methyl cholanthrene are examples of substances known to induce metabolic enzymes.

People vary in their capacity for biotransformation in several ways. Two have already been mentioned: genetic differences and enzyme induction. Other factors also account for interindividual differences in metabolism; among them are general health, nutritional status, and concurrent medications.

## Principles of Biologic Effects

The aspect of toxic substances of greatest medical concern is their biologic effects. Several concepts have been developed to help classify and account for these effects.

Exposure to a toxic agent, and likewise the biologic response, may be *acute* or *chronic.* An acute exposure often evokes an acute response, and a chronic exposure a chronic response, but neither sequence is invariable. For example, a short-term exposure to asbestos may cause mesothelioma, a fatal neoplasm, to develop many years later.

A biologic effect may be *reversible* or *irreversible,* independent of its time course. Chronic lead poisoning can cause hematologic, renal, neurologic, gastrointestinal, and reproductive effects, and all but the late renal and neurologic effects are reversible. On the other hand, acute mercury poisoning can produce irritability, tremors, delirium, or outright psychosis, which may all be irreversible. Reversibility is a function of the nature of the damage done and the regenerative capacity of the damaged tissue.

## HEAVY METALS: RECURRENT STOMACH PAINS IN A WORKER INVOLVED IN DELEADING

A 29-year-old handyman who is intermittently employed in commercial deleading operations was seen by his family physician with complaints of intermittent stomach pains over the last few weeks. The episodes of pain were not associated with meals. Onset had been gradual, and he had no associated systemic or gastrointestinal symptoms. He had not experienced any unusual stress at home or work. He reported drinking one or two cans of beer per day. His physician treated him with antacids.

Approximately 9 months later, he saw his physician again with the same complaints. His earlier pains had resolved approximately 1 month after being treated, and he had been feeling fine until a few weeks earlier when his stomach pains started to recur. This time, the pains were more severe and were associated with loss of appetite and generalized fatigue. There was no consistent association with mealtimes or with other activities. He had no other significant symptoms and reported no recent changes in his personal life or habits. His physical examination was normal. His doctor sent him for an upper GI series that was scheduled approximately 1 week later. He was again treated with antacids and dietary restrictions.

His doctor saw him again approximately 1 week after the x-ray. The x-ray had been normal, and his symptoms had improved slightly over the past week. He was seen again 4 weeks later, with continued improvement. However, he still reported intermittent epigastric pains. At this time, his physician became concerned about possible exposures to lead from his occupation. Although the patient knew that lead had been an ingredient in house paints, he thought this was no longer a problem and was poorly informed about the risks of lead paint removal (deleading). He reported no other hobbies that might expose him to lead. The physician obtained a complete blood count and a blood-lead level. The blood count was normal, and the blood-lead level was 15 μg/dL (also reported as normal). The physician continued antacid and dietary treatment.

Approximately 2 months later, the patient returned complaining of more severe epigastric pains, this time associated with abdominal cramping, headaches, and fatigue. He had been getting better but then started work at a new site, where he was scraping and torching paint from the exterior and the interior woodwork of an older house. In reviewing the history of these episodes of pain, the patient reported that all three had occurred a few weeks after he started a similar type of job. After consultation with an occupational physician, the family physician obtained another blood-lead level, which was 53 μg/dL. The patient stopped doing paint removal work, and his symptoms gradually improved. Within 2 weeks, his blood-lead level was reduced to 43 μg/dL. The handyman bought a respirator for use on paint removal work, and quarterly monitoring of his blood-lead level showed a gradual decline.

Although the use of lead pigment was discontinued in most paints by the 1970s, older lead-containing paints still cover many interior and exterior surfaces in older buildings and continues to be used on steel structures such as bridges. Not only does this exposure account for many cases of childhood lead poisoning, but also painters and other workers conducting renovation work on these buildings may have significant exposure to lead. Burning or torching the surface to remove the paint produces a lead fume that increases lead exposure through the respiratory tract.

The time course of lead exposure is important. In this case, the handyman's exposure was intermittent. By the time the first blood-lead level was obtained, the exposure had ceased for a few weeks, and the blood-lead level had returned to a lower level. If the level had been taken at the time of the first visit, it would have been higher and the suspected occupational etiology confirmed. This illustrates the importance of a good occupational history, inquiring not only about usual activities but also changes in workplace activities or possible exposures.

Most occupational lead exposure occurs by inhalation, although ingestion may also contribute, especially through contamination of food or cigarettes at work. Lead is initially absorbed into the blood and then gradually stored in the bones. Blood-lead levels reflect a complex equilibrium between very recent exposure, tissue levels, and bone stores. Blood-lead levels are a good indicator of recent exposure but may not reflect past exposures. Newer x-ray fluorescence (XRF) techniques provide a better assessment of lead storage in bones.

Most metals, including lead, exert their biologic effects through enzyme ligand binding, and for many metals excretion can be hastened by chelation therapy with agents such as dimercaprol (British antilewisite, or BAL) and ethylenediaminetetraacetic acid (EDTA). Beyond these generalizations, however, metal toxicology is as varied as the metals themselves.

Lead affects a number of organ systems, including the hematopoietic, renal, and nervous systems. Typical early signs of exposure in adults include abdominal colic, headache, and fatigue, as evidenced by the handyman in this example. At even higher levels of exposure, lead may cause a peripheral motor neuropathy with wrist or foot drop. Higher levels of exposure may also lead to an anemia related to the inhibition of several enzymes involved in the production of hemoglobin. Chronic exposure to lead may lead to interstitial fibrosis and eventually renal failure. Lead exposure is also associated with adverse reproductive effects in both men and women.

The current OSHA lead standard is 50 $\mu g/m^3$ over an 8-hour day. Routine exposure at this level leads to a blood-lead level of approximately 40 $\mu g/dL$. The standard requires routine blood-lead monitoring and removal of a worker from exposure if his or her blood-lead level is elevated. OSHA recently applied this standard to the construction industry in the U.S., where many lead poisoning cases are being reported, especially in workers who remove lead paint from highway bridges and similar structures.

Mercury is another important metal used in the manufacture of monitoring instruments and in certain industrial processes. It is important to distinguish the form of mercury (organic or metallic) in evaluating toxic effects. Metallic mercury exposure affects mainly the central nervous system, leading to tremor, irritability, and personality changes. The kidney is also affected by mercury, usually manifested as renal tubular dysfunction. Gingivitis is another classic sign of severe mercury poisoning. Exposure to metallic mercury is usually monitored through urine mercury levels although blood levels may also be useful.

Organic mercury compounds (usually methyl mercury) are sometimes encountered in workplace settings, but are better known from outbreaks related to environmental contamination (usually human exposure to contaminated fish). These exposures have been associated with severe neurologic disease (both central and peripheral) and birth defects among children of pregnant women exposed to high levels of methyl mercury.

Arsenic is utilized in some industrial and chemical processes. Exposure also occurs in the smelting of some metal ores. Exposure to arsenic may cause a symmetrical distal polyneuropathy. High exposures to arsenic cause liver damage and skin lesions. Arsenic is also carcinogenic, causing lung, liver, and skin cancer. Exposure to arsenic is usually monitored through urinary arsenic levels.

Cadmium exposure occurs in many different industrial processes. Its main effect is on renal function leading to renal tubular dysfunction as cadmium accumulates in the kidney. Cadmium also causes lung cancer. Cadmium exposure can be monitored with either urine or blood concentrations.

Beryllium is a metal used in electronics and some other industrial applications. Exposure leads to a fibrotic lung disease similar to—and often mistaken for—sarcoidosis. Lymphocyte transformation testing of blood or bronchoalveolar lavage can assist with the early diagnosis of this illness.

Other important toxic metals include nickel, which is carcinogenic and is a very common cause of contact dermatitis; chromium, which similarly causes contact dermatitis and is believed to be carcinogenic, but only in the hexavalent form; and manganese, which causes a neurologic condition similar to Parkinson's disease.

Prompt medical diagnosis is very important for our current control of metal poisonings. Many current exposures are in small businesses or involve exposures secondary to other work such as lead exposure from removing lead paint. Biologic monitoring tests and a careful exposure history are critical for proper diagnosis and follow-up of people working in these industries. In larger industries, routine industrial hygiene control techniques are applied, including better ventilation and use of personal protective equipment.

Generally, higher levels of toxic exposure will lead to greater responses. They may occur within an individual—as when higher concentrations of inhaled carbon monoxide lead to higher concentrations of carboxyhemoglobin—or within a population—as when higher levels of benzidine dye exposure cause an elevation in the incidence of bladder cancer. Either relationship may be depicted with the familiar *dose-response curve* (Fig. 13-3).

The dose-response curve quantifies the dependence of biologic effects on dose levels. Note that the curve in Fig. 13-3 has a sigmoidal shape. This shape is common. At the lower end the beginning of a linear increase reflects the existence of a *threshold dose* below which variations in exposure presumably have no effect. At the upper end the flattening of the curve reflects a *ceiling* level of maximal response that cannot be increased by greater doses. This level might correspond to death in an individual or to 100 percent cumulative incidence of disease in a population.

Several additional toxicologic concepts emerge from the dose-response curve. The $LD_{50}$ is the dose that is lethal to 50 percent of a population; it is a measure of the *potency* of a compound, or the dose required to produce a certain effect. Potency should be distinguished from another pharmacologic measure, *efficacy,* which reflects the maximal effect a drug can produce (the ceiling on a dose-response curve). There are other standards that might be used. For example, cell killing by radiation is sometimes quantified by the "$D_o$" which corresponds to an $LD_{63}$ on the exponential cell-kill curve.

Individual departures from the expected dose-response pattern can take several forms. *Hypersusceptibility* indicates an unusually high response to some dose of a substance. This term requires very careful interpretation, however, since it is used in several different ways. It may refer to a genetic predisposition to a toxic effect, as discussed above; it may indicate a statistically defined deviation from the mean; it may reflect an observer's subjective impression; or it may be used, incorrectly, as a synonym for hypersensitivity. *Hypersensitivity* is one form of hypersusceptibility, characterized by an acquired, immunologically mediated sensitization to a substance. In workplace settings this sensitization is most commonly manifested in pulmonary or dermatologic responses with features of all four Gell and Coombs immunologic reaction types [3,4]. For example, toluene diisocyanate (TDI), a major ingredient in polyurethane manufacture, will evoke asthmatic reactions in a small percentage of exposed workers even at permissible exposure levels (see Chap. 22), and workers exposed to nickel can develop a skin reaction that resembles chronic eczema (see Chap. 24). It is important to remember that such so-called hypersensitivities need not be aberrant or even unusual. Among epoxy workers, for instance, the incidence of skin sensitization to resins is approximately 50 percent, and at least 75 percent of long-term employees relate a history of dermatitis.

*Hyposusceptibility,* conversely, indicates an unusually low response to some dose of a substance, and it also is defined in a variety of ways. One form of hyposusceptibility is *tolerance,* a diminished response to a given dose of a chemical following repeated exposures. Tolerance classically involves an attenuation of the immune response to

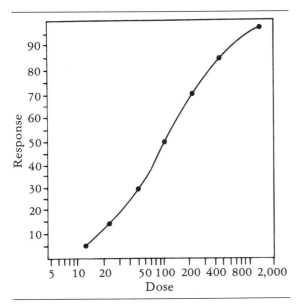

Fig. 13-3. The dose-response curve. (From M Amdur, J Doull, C Klaassen. eds. Casarett and Doull's toxicology. 4th ed. New York: Pergamon, 1991.)

a specific antigen and appears graphically as a shift to the right of the dose-response curve. In experimental animals tolerance can be induced by administering antigen in certain forms or doses and this process may well occur in workplace settings following chronic low-dose exposures. However, several equally conceivable events could yield an empirically similar result; these include the impairment of absorption, the induction of metabolizing enzymes, and the enhancement of excretion. Typically, such acquired resistance to a chemically induced response can be overcome with sufficiently large doses. *Tachyphylaxis,* in contrast, is a rapidly acquired resistance that persists even with a large subsequent dose. In view of the variety of mechanisms of hyper- and hyposusceptibility, an individual worker may readily show a dose-responsiveness that differs significantly from the mean of the larger population.

Many factors, some already mentioned, determine the *localization of effect* of a chemical exposure. These include translocation barriers such as membranes, which limit migration of the chemical; chemical affinities that concentrate the chemical on certain molecules; and regional differences in metabolic activity, in susceptibility to a given toxic effect, or in capacity for repair.

A useful classification of chemical-induced toxic effects, based in part on the work of Loomis [5], is as follows:

Normal (or expected) effects, depending on:
   Physical actions
   Nonspecific caustic or corrosive actions
   Specific toxicologic actions
   Production of pathologic sequelae
Abnormal (or unexpected) effects:
   Immune mechanisms
   Genetic susceptibility

Normal effects can be repeatedly induced, do not require preconditioning, and occur with an incidence that is primarily dose-dependent. These range from simple physical phenomena, such as the displacement of oxygen by asphyxiants, to more elaborate pathophysiologic events. Immune mechanisms, in contrast, require preconditioning (sensitization) and may not be inducible in the majority of members of a population simply by increasing the exposure. Finally, genetic susceptibility is in most cases not based on sensitization and may be nothing more than a quantitatively greater propensity for developing some "normal" response. An example is the elevated risk of hemolysis among people with glucose 6-phosphate dehydrogenase (G6PD) deficiency following exposure to oxidants such as naphthalene. Immune and genetic effects may coincide as inheritable immunodeficiency diseases.

## Excretion

Since biotransformation tends to make compounds more polar and less fat-soluble, the happy outcome

## PESTICIDES: ACUTE POISONING IN GREENHOUSE WORKERS

A 38-year-old woman was seen in the emergency room at a rural hospital on Saturday evening. She complained of a severe rash. The rash initially appeared on her forearms several weeks earlier, but in the last 2 weeks, it had become more severe, spreading to her face and neck. She indicated that the itching from the rash had become so severe that she had had great difficulty in sleeping for the last three nights. She came to the emergency room on a Saturday night because that was the only time she had off from work. She had never previously had this type of rash and thought that it might be due to the chemicals at work. She worked in a greenhouse growing flowers and was exposed to many different chemicals there. Her medical examination showed a severe maculopapular rash on her hands, forearms, face, and neck. The emergency room physician treated her with topical steroids and an antihistamine for the itching and referred her to a local community clinic for follow-up.

Two weeks later, she was seen at the community clinic. The rash was still quite severe. She had used the medication provided by the emergency room but was unable to fill the prescriptions due to lack of funds. The physician asked her about the chemicals used at work, but she knew only that they were pesticides used in the growing of the flowers. She did not use them herself but was exposed to them when the greenhouses were sprayed before she arrived at work and from handling the flowers. She knew none of the names of the pesticides. The physician provided her with medication for her dermatitis and asked her to return in 2 weeks and to try to get the names of the pesticides that were used at work.

The patient did not return to the clinic until 4 weeks later. By this time, her dermatitis was much more severe. She reported that the medications had initially helped but that in the past week they had used many more pesticides at work and that she and several other workers had become ill with headaches and nausea a few days ago. The greenhouse that they were working in that day had been sprayed the night before, and they could smell a strong odor when they went to work. About 1 hour after entering the greenhouse, she and her two fellow workers became very ill with nausea and headaches. They left the greenhouse. After resting outside for an hour, they felt better and returned to work. By that time, the patient's dermatitis was so bad that she decided to quit the job. She had requested information on the pesticides from the owner, but he told her that the information was too complicated for her to understand.

The physician from the community clinic treated the patient for the dermatitis, which slowly cleared up. After two more workers from the greenhouse came to the clinic reporting an episode of acute illness (headaches and nausea), the physician reported the problem to the state pesticide enforcement agency, which then inspected the facility. Although it found problems with the labeling of the pesticides used at the facility and with disposal practices, no serious violations of current regulations were found. The owner did change some application practices, and the patient was later able to return to work in another area of the facility without problems.

The diagnosis of pesticide-related illnesses can be very difficult. Some pesticides have systemic effects such as interfering with cholinergic nerve conduction (cholinesterase inhibitors). Exposure to these pesticides could have been responsible for the acute symptoms experienced by the workers. These effects can be measured through cholinesterase levels, but interpretation of results of these tests is difficult due to the wide range of normal levels. Levels may return to normal quite quickly after exposure ceases. This test may be more useful for periodic monitoring of exposed employees using a pre-exposure baseline for comparison.

Skin absorption is an important route of exposure for many pesticides. The exposure experienced by the workers in this example probably included both inhalation (from the pesticide fogging) and dermal exposure from contact with pesticide-contaminated plants and surfaces.

Skin problems are also common from exposure to pesticides or the materials used to dilute them for application. Some pesticides cause contact dermatitis. In this case, the patient had probably developed skin sensitization to fungicides used in the cultivation of the flowers.

Pesticides include a wide range of chemicals used for the control of insects and other pests. While most pesticide use takes place in agricultural settings, many people may also be occupationally exposed from the use of these chemicals for structural pest control. While pesticides, as a class of chemicals, affect nearly every organ system, individual pesticides usually have a more limited and more specific toxicity.

Organophosphate pesticides are among the most widely used in agricultural and structural applications. These compounds act by inhibiting the enzyme acetylcholinesterase at the nerve-to-nerve synapse or nerve–to–muscle motor end-plate, leading to increased levels of the neurotransmitter acetylcholine at many different sites in the body.

The worker in this case was most likely acutely exposed to one of the organophosphates. Any of these pesticides can be absorbed by the respiratory, percutaneous, and gastrointestinal routes, the first two of which were likely of importance here. Once absorbed, the organophosphate is then metabolized by hepatic microsomal enzymes. For one of the most studied of these pesticides, parathion, the first major conversion it undergoes is replacement of its sulfur by oxygen to form paraoxon, the actual anticholinesterase. Subsequent oxidation and hydrolysis result in detoxification.

Paraoxon binds with acetylcholinesterase molecules at cholinergic nerve endings, both centrally and peripherally. The organophosphates and the carbamates both act through this mechanism; a major difference is that the carbamate complexes dissociate spontaneously, while the organophosphate complex formation is virtually irreversible. Thus organophosphate poisoning causes a predictable constellation of muscarinic, nicotinic, and central nervous system symptoms. Severe cases can progress to coma and death.

Typical symptoms include miosis, salivation, sweating, and muscle fasciculation; at higher exposures, diarrhea, incontinence, wheezing, bradycardia, and even convulsions may occur. Depressed plasma or red blood cell cholinesterase levels may be used to confirm the poisoning, but these tests are less useful for assessing chronic or less overtly toxic levels of exposure. Acute poisoning can be treated with atropine or pralidoximine.

A delayed neurotoxicity syndrome, with weakness, paresthesias, and paralysis of the distal lower extremities, has been found in people exposed to organophosphate pesticides, and other chronic neurotoxicity syndromes also have been reported. These syndromes usually occur in people with chronic exposure or after a very high acute exposure.

Another frequently used category of pesticide is the carbamates. Carbamates also inhibit the enzyme acetylcholinesterase, but this inhibition is more readily reversed than for organophosphate pesticides. Hence, effects tend to be less severe. Because of the rapid reversal, serum and red blood cell cholinesterase levels tend to be less useful in the diagnosis of exposure to this type of pesticide.

Organochlorine pesticides, such as DDT, were more widely used in the past, but their use has been limited due to their persistence in the environment. However, some are still commonly used (such as lindane). Organochlorine pesticides are metabolized very slowly and accumulate in fat and other tissues. Their major toxicity is on the nervous system, leading to anorexia, malaise, tremor, hyperreflexia, and convulsions. Biologic monitoring with blood or fat levels is useful for assessing exposure to these compounds.

Many other individual pesticides have significant toxicity. For example, paraquat (a herbicide) may cause a severe pulmonary fibrosis. Dibromochloropropane (DBCP), used in the past to control nematodes, caused sterility among male workers exposed to high levels of this chemical. Many pesticides are carcinogenic: A series of studies have found a high incidence of non-Hodgkin's lymphoma among midwestern U.S. farmers who use large amounts of herbicides. Dermatitis is also common among people working with pesticides, although some of this incidence is due to exposure to other materials mixed with the pesticides.

Diagnosis of pesticide toxicity is dependent on a very careful medical and exposure history.

Laboratory testing is helpful for some pesticides, but a good understanding of the time frame of exposure is necessary in interpreting these tests. Prevention strategies for control of pesticide-related health risks are covered in Chap. 35.

of this process is that toxins can be more readily excreted from the body. The major route of excretion of toxins and their metabolites is through the kidneys (see Chap. 31). The kidneys handle toxins in the same way that they handle any serum solutes: passive glomerular filtration, passive tubular diffusion, and active tubular secretion. The daily volume of filtrate produced is about 200 liters—five times the total body water—in a remarkably efficient and thorough filtration process.

Smaller molecules can reach the tubules through passive glomerular filtration, since the glomerular capillary pores are large enough (40 Å) to admit molecules of up to about 70,000 daltons. However, this excludes substances bound to large serum proteins; these substances must undergo active tubular secretion to be excreted. The tubular secretory apparatus apparently has separate processes for organic anions and organic cations, and, like any active transport system, these can be saturated and competitively blocked. Finally, passive tubular diffusion out of the serum probably occurs to some extent, especially for certain organic bases.

Passive diffusion also occurs in the opposite direction, from the tubules to the serum. Like any of the membrane crossings discussed previously, lipid-soluble molecules are reabsorbed from the tubular lumen much more readily than polar molecules and ions, which explains the practice, already mentioned, of alkalinizing the urine to hasten the excretion of acids.

A second major organ of excretion is the liver (see Chap. 30). The liver occupies a strategic position, since the portal circulation promptly delivers compounds to it following gastrointestinal absorption. Furthermore, the generous perfusion of the liver and the discontinuous capillary structure within it facilitate its filtration of the blood. Thus, excretion into the bile is potentially a rapid and efficient process.

Biliary excretion is somewhat analogous to renal tubular secretion. These are specific transport systems for organic acids, organic bases, neutral compounds, and possibly metals. These are active transport systems with the ability to handle protein-bound molecules. Finally, reuptake of lipid-soluble substances can occur after secretion, in this case through the intestinal walls.

Marked variation in biliary secretion can exist. Liver disease can compromise the process, while some chemicals such as phenobarbital and some steroids, in addition to inducing hepatic metabolic enzymes, can actually increase bile flow and hence biliary excretion. The effects of different chemicals may have practical applications; certain steroids have been demonstrated to decrease mercury toxicity in animals, which is attributed, at least in part, to their effect on biliary excretion.

Toxins that are secreted with the bile enter the gastrointestinal tract and, unless reabsorbed, are secreted with the feces. Materials ingested orally and not absorbed and materials carried up the respiratory tree and swallowed are also passed with the feces. All of this process may be supplemented by some passive diffusion through the walls of the gastrointestinal tract, although it is not a major mechanism of excretion.

Volatile gases and vapors are excreted primarily by the lungs. The process is one of passive diffusion, governed by the difference between plasma and alveolar vapor pressure. Volatiles that are highly fat-soluble tend to persist in body reservoirs and take some time to migrate from adipose tissue to plasma to alveolar air. Less fat-soluble volatiles, on the other hand, are exhaled fairly promptly, until the plasma level has decreased to that of ambient air. Interestingly, the lungs can sustain alveolar and bronchial irritation when a vapor such as gasoline is exhaled, even if the initial exposure occurred percutaneously or through ingestion.

Other routes of excretion, although of minor significance quantitatively, are important for a variety of reasons. Excretion into mother's milk obviously introduces a risk to the infant, and since milk is more acidic (pH of 6.5) than serum, basic compounds are concentrated in milk. Moreover, owing to the high fat content of breast milk (3–5 percent), fat-soluble substances such as DDT can also be passed to the infant (see Chap. 32). Some toxins, especially metals, are excreted in sweat or laid down in growing hair, and these may be of use in diagnosis. Finally, some materials are secreted in the saliva and may then pose a subsequent gastrointestinal exposure hazard.

This chapter has presented basic principles of toxicology that are fundamental to the understanding of the effects of toxic substances and the treatment and prevention of these effects. In the chapters that follow (particularly Chaps. 14, and 22 through 31), the types of biologic effects caused by workplace toxins are explored in detail. Readers interested in particular toxins should refer to Appendix A, How to Research the Toxic Effects of Chemical Substances, and the Index, both at the back of the book.

# References

1. Holmberg PC. Central nervous defects in two children of mothers exposed to chemicals in the reinforced plastics industry. Scand J Work Environ Health 1977; 3:212.
2. Husman K. Symptoms of car-painters with long-term exposure to a mixture of organic solvents. Scand J Work Environ Health 1980; 6:19.
3. Newman L, Storey E, Kreiss K. Immunologic evaluation of occupational lung disease. Occup Med: State of the Art Rev 1987; 2:345.
4. Coombs RAA, Gell PGH. Classification of allergic reactions responsible for clinical hypersensitivity and disease. In PGH Gell, RAA Coombs, PJ Lachmann. eds. Clinical aspects in immunology. Oxford: Blackwell, 1963, p. 363.
5. Loomis T. Essentials of toxicology. Philadelphia: Lea & Febiger, 1974.

# Bibliography

Amdur MO, Doull J, Klaassen CD. eds. Casarett and Doull's toxicology: The basic science of poisons. 4th ed. New York: Pergamon, 1991.
*The standard toxicology text with chapters on general principles, individual body systems, and specific families of toxins.*
Brain JD, Valberg PA. Aerosol deposition in the respiratory tract. Am Rev Respir Dis 1979; 120:1325–73.
*The "classic" review article on airways deposition, with a discussion of major classes of inhaled particles and their effects on health.*
Clayton GD, et al., eds. Patty's industrial hygiene and toxicology. 3rd ed. vol. 3, 4th ed. vols. 1 and 2. New York: Wiley, 1991 (vol. 1), 1993 (vol. 2), 1994 (vol. 3).
*An encyclopedic reference text of toxicology.*
Gonzolez FJ, Crespi CL, Gelbrin HV. DNA-expressed human cytochrome P450: A new age of molecular toxicology and human risk assessment. Mutat Res 1991; 247:113–27.
*A useful review linking classical toxicology with advances in molecular biology.*
Hayes AW. ed. Principles and methods of toxicology. 2nd ed. New York: Raven Press, 1989.
*An alternative basic text with strong emphasis on toxicology testing methods.*
Lauwerys RR, Hoet P. Industrial chemical exposure: Guidelines for biological monitoring. 2nd ed. Boca Ratan, FL: Lewis, 1993.
*A review of the metabolism and excretion of various substances geared toward rational use of biologic monitoring tests.*
Loomis T. Essentials of toxicology. 3rd ed. Philadelphia: Lea & Febiger, 1978.
*Dated, but still the best short introductory toxicology text. Clear writing and lucid organization of basic principles.*

# 14
# Carcinogens

Howard Frumkin

In early 1972, 43-year-old Bob Pontious, newly diagnosed with lung cancer, was referred to a young pulmonary physician in Philadelphia, Dr. William Figueroa. Mr. Pontious worked at a Philadelphia chemical company, and according to the referring physician, some of his coworkers had succumbed to lung cancer. Figueroa later described his first encounter with the patient: "He came in, told me that he believed he had lung cancer, the same thing that had killed 13 other men he'd worked with. What excited me was that he had oat cell carcinoma, which is very rare among nonsmokers, and he'd never smoked. Oat cell is the wild, undifferentiated kind. It spreads fast. It's usually found among smokers. But [the patient] swore he'd never smoked and neither had three of the other men who'd died. Most of the others were very light smokers, he said. They were young. Cancer is an old man's disease, usually among men in their fifties and sixties who've smoked at least a pack a day for 20 to 30 years" [1].

Figueroa recognized that an occupational carcinogen might be involved, and he decided to investigate further. Many of the workers, it turned out, were exposed to chloromethyl methyl ether (CMME), an intermediate in the manufacture of ion-exchange resins. CMME is invariably contaminated with bis(chloromethyl) ether (BCME); animal data suggesting that BCME was a carcinogen had appeared in 1967, and well-designed experiments verified this by 1971. Figueroa appealed to company management for the exposure records of a cohort of workers in order to determine if BCME was associated with human lung cancer. Unfortunately, the records were not made available to him.

Faced with a similar situation several years earlier, another Philadelphia physician had not pursued the matter. "I had a feeling that four cases in 125 was excessive . . ." he explained. "I didn't go any further because I didn't know if it was significant. [The company] said there were no exposure data and I didn't know what to do" [1]. Figueroa, however, turned to another source of data—his patient.

"I decided to trust the memory of this guy, of one honest American worker," recalled Figueroa. "We stood next to [his] bed as he lay there, dying of cancer, in an oxygen mask. I read him all the names and he told me which had been exposed and who had died." Through this investigation Figueroa was able to suggest that BCME exposure was associated with a marked elevation in lung cancer mortality. His results were soon published [2], and together with subsequent corroborating data, produced both local and national effects. In 1974 the widows of BCME victims were informed that they could file for workers' compensation benefits based on the work-relatedness of their husbands' deaths. That same year, the Occupational Safety and Health Administration (OSHA) promulgated a series of regulations designed to control exposure to 14 carcinogens, one of which was BCME.

The BCME story illustrates six important principles:

1. Alert clinicians have a valuable role to play in occupational health through both clinical observation and appropriate follow-up.
2. Accurate information about occupational etiologies can benefit not only populations affected by preventive measures but also individual patients and their families.
3. Accurate exposure histories are often difficult to obtain, especially in cancer cases—when exposure predates disease by many years—and in situations involving proprietary interests.
4. One of the best sources of information on occupational hazards is one of the most frequently overlooked—exposed workers.
5. Animal data on carcinogenicity correlate well with the human experience and are usually available before epidemiologic data can be developed.
6. Confounding variables, such as smoking, can obscure carcinogenic associations. If all of the BCME victims had been smokers, their oat cell carcinomas might have been attributed to smoking, and the carcinogenicity of BCME could have remained unnoticed.

In terms of morbidity and mortality, work-related malignancies are an important category of occupational disease. Certainly, few diseases have raised as much public concern as cancer. With few exceptions, progress in treating cancer has been disappointing, and therefore public health interventions such as prevention and education are critical.

Health care providers confront occupational cancer in many ways. They have a vital role in recognition, as the BCME example illustrates. As clinicians, they care for patients with cancers. Patients may ask their providers to evaluate whether their cancers resulted from workplace exposures. When an occupational cancer is discovered, the clinician can be a valuable source of information, not only to the patient seeking compensation but also to coworkers, managers, and representatives of government agencies. Similarly, clinicians can educate and advise their patients on avoiding ex-

posure to proven or suspected occupational carcinogens, and can actively contribute to efforts to prevent further exposure to carcinogens. Finally, the study and understanding of carcinogens in the workplace have important implications for the control of similar (although lower-dose) exposures in the general environment and consumer products.

## Introduction

Cancer is the name given to dozens of diseases that arise in various organs and tissues throughout the body. Cancer cells have several features in common: They grow and divide in a rapid, uncontrolled manner, they lose their differentiation, and they survive for abnormally long periods of time.

Cancer is a major cause of morbidity and mortality worldwide. Among developing nations that have completed the "epidemiologic transition," cancer accounts for one in five deaths, most commonly affecting the lungs, the gastrointestinal tract, the breasts, and the prostate. In the United States, with an annual age-adjusted cancer mortality of 171 per 100,000, just over half a million people die of cancer every year. Among developing nations, where infectious diseases continue to play a major role, other cancers, such as those of the liver, cervix, and stomach, have greater relative importance, but mortality from "developed nation" sites such as lung and breast is rising.

Mortality is only one measure of cancer burden; others include incidence (the rate at which newly diagnosed cases arise in a population), years of potential life lost, disability-adjusted life years lost, and cost. If a region or country has a cancer registry it can tabulate the population's cancer incidence, usually stratified by age, race, gender, and cancer site. In the U.S., the National Cancer Institute's Surveillance, Epidemiology and End Results (SEER) program includes about 10 percent of the population, and many more people are included in state cancer registries. In other countries, various kinds of registries exist; the results are compiled by the International Agency for Research on Cancer in its series, *Cancer Incidence in Five Continents.*

## Cancer as an Environmental Disease

Most cancers are now believed to have an important environmental component, a view that evolved from centuries of clinical, epidemiologic, and laboratory observation. The first modern clinical report of environmental carcinogenesis was probably that of a London physician, Dr. John Hill, who in 1761 described the elevated prevalence of cancer of the nasal passages among tobacco snuff abusers. In 1775 a perceptive surgeon of the same city, Dr. Percival Pott, reported the first occupational cancer, an increased prevalence of scrotal skin cancer among chimney sweeps, who were heavily exposed to soot in their work. In the 1800s skin cancer was linked with occupational exposure to inorganic arsenic, to tar, and to paraffin oils (now known to contain polycyclic aromatic hydrocarbons [PAHs]), and bladder cancer was linked with occupational exposure to certain dyes. In 1935 the first case report of bronchogenic carcinoma in a patient with asbestosis was published.

Observational epidemiology has contributed much evidence. One example is *geographic comparisons,* which reveal vast differences in cancer mortality among nations. For example, age-adjusted stomach cancer mortality among men in 1986 to 1988 was 54.6 per 100,000 in Korea, 37.9 in Japan, 25.6 in Poland, 14.1 in the Netherlands, 5.3 in the United States, and 1.1 in Thailand. This variability likely reflects differences among populations in exposure to environmental factors (including diet), although differences in genetic susceptibility, diagnosis, treatment, and reporting also play a role. Cancer mortality is found to vary markedly among regions of the United States (Fig. 14-1). *Gender comparisons* may reveal quite disparate cancer rates between men and women in the same region. These differences may relate, in

part, to different environmental exposures of men and women, including occupational exposures. *Migration studies* have strongly implicated environmental factors, including diet, in cancer incidence. For example, native Japanese who migrate to the United States (Issei) experience a threefold increase in intestinal cancer mortality and a 35 percent decrease in gastric cancer mortality, compared to those Japanese who remain in Japan, bringing their rates much closer to those of the general U.S. population. The U.S.-born children of Japanese immigrants (Nissei) have rates that approximate U.S. rates even more closely. *Temporal trends* are also revealing. The lung cancer mortality among men in the U.S. increased tenfold from the 1930s to the 1980s, a trend that can only be explained by a change in environmental factors, especially smoking. Although claims of a cancer "epidemic" are probably overstated, recent investigations have suggested that among older people, cancer incidence and mortality at multiple sites are continuing to rise, suggesting an ongoing role for environmental exposures [3].

Studies in analytical epidemiology, designed to test specific hypotheses that link environmental exposures with cancer, have contributed important insights. Now that powerful computer software is widely available, further progress may be predicted. Such studies have provided convincing evidence of numerous associations: cigarette smoke and lung cancer, hepatitis B virus and liver cancer, ultraviolet radiation and skin cancer, hormone therapy and uterine cancer, diet and colon cancer, ionizing radiation and leukemia.

Finally, laboratory evidence has confirmed that environmental agents may cause cancer. A good example is mouse skin carcinogenesis, one of the oldest experimental systems. In 1918 two Japanese scientists, Yamagiwa and Ichikawa, reported causing skin cancer by applying coal tar to mouse skin. Numerous experimental systems have been developed since then, both in animals and in cell systems. In fact, many of these are now used to test chemicals for their carcinogenic effects, as described below.

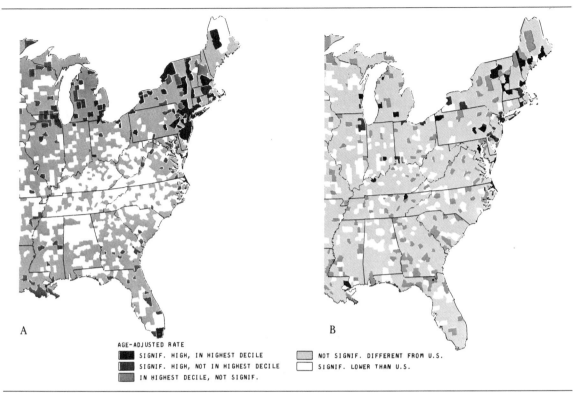

AGE-ADJUSTED RATE

■ SIGNIF. HIGH, IN HIGHEST DECILE

■ SIGNIF. HIGH, NOT IN HIGHEST DECILE

■ IN HIGHEST DECILE, NOT SIGNIF.

□ NOT SIGNIF. DIFFERENT FROM U.S.

□ SIGNIF. LOWER THAN U.S.

**Fig. 14-1.** Analyses of cancer mortality by geographic area may yield hypotheses that lead to specific research studies on cancers of occupational and/or environmental origin. These maps show U.S. bladder cancer mortality by county from 1950–1969. There is a concentration in petrochemical industry centers for men (A) but not for women (B), consistent with an occupational etiology. (Abridged from TJ Mason et al. Atlas for cancer mortality for U.S. counties, 1950–69. Bethesda, MD: National Cancer Institute, 1975.)

## Cancer as an Occupational Disease

Observations such as the above have confirmed the role of environmental carcinogens. What about occupational carcinogens? Some of the highest environmental exposures occur in workplaces. As a result, not only have environmental cancers been observed in workplace settings, but workers are often the "canaries in the coal mine" who first demonstrate that a chemical is carcinogenic. The same methods noted above—clinical observation, epidemiologic study, and laboratory testing—have helped identify a number of occupational carcinogens that cause a variety of tumors (Table 14-1).

Examples include vinyl chloride (which caused a cluster of hepatic hemangiosarcomas in a chemical plant), benzene (which was linked with high leukemia rates in the Turkish shoe industry), and coke oven emissions (which were found to cause lung cancer elevations among coke oven workers). Epidemiologic studies have also identified industries in which cancer risks are present but no specific carcinogen has yet been identified (Table 14-2).

How big a problem is occupational cancer? This has been a matter of considerable debate. Doll and Peto, in their 1981 *The Causes of Cancer* (see Bibliography), estimated that between 2 and 8 percent

Table 14-1. Some occupational carcinogens

| Carcinogen | Industry setting | Human cancer site |
|---|---|---|
| Acrylonitrile | Acrylic fiber, chemical, and pesticide production | ?Lung, ?colon, ?brain, ?stomach, ?prostate |
| 4-aminobiphenyl | Formerly used as rubber antioxidant and dye intermediate | Bladder |
| Arsenic and arsenic compounds | Smelting, metallurgy, pigment and glass production, and pesticide | Lung, skin |
| Asbestos | Insulation: for example, ships, buildings, pipes, brake shoes | Lung, pleura, peritoneum, larynx, gastrointestinal tract |
| Benzene | Multiple uses in chemical products: for example, adhesives, rubber, petrochemicals | Leukemia |
| Benzidine and salts | Plastic, rubber, dye, chemical industries | Bladder |
| Beryllium and certain beryllium compounds | Mining, electronics, chemical, electric, ceramics industries | Lung |
| Bis(chloromethyl) ether (BCME) | Contaminant of CMME | Lung |
| Chloromethyl methyl ether (CMME) | Ion exchange resin, organic chemical manufacturing | Lung, nasal cavity |
| Chromium | Welding, etching, plating; steel and metal industries | Lung, skin, ?kidney, ?prostate |
| Coal tars and coal tar pitches; soot | Petrochemical and steel industries; fossil fuel combustion by-product | Lung, bladder, skin |
| Coke oven emissions | Steel industry | |
| 1,2-dibromo-3-chloropropane (DBCP) | Former nematocide | A |
| 1,2-dibromoethane, ethylene dibromide (EDB) | Gasoline additive, solvent, pesticide | A |
| 3,3'-dichlorobenzidine and salts | Polyurethane and pigment workers | A |
| 1,4-dioxane | Solvent, degreaser | A |
| Epichlorohydrin | Chemical production | A |
| Ethylene oxide | Sterilizing agent | A |
| Formaldehyde | Manufacture of woods, resins, leather, rubber, metals | A |
| 4,4'-methylene-bis-2-chloroaniline (MBOCA) | Polyurethane, epoxy resin, elastomer manufacturing | A |
| Mineral oils (certain ones) | Lubricant in metal-working; solvents in printing | Skin, scrotum |
| Alpha-naphthylamine | Chemical, textile, dye, rubber industries | Bladder |
| Beta-naphthylamine | No longer in commercial use | Bladder |
| Nickel compounds | Nickel refining and smelting | Lung, nasal cavity |
| Polychlorinated and polybrominated biphenyls (PCBs and PBBs) | Flame retardants (PBBs); transformer and capacitor fluids, solvents (PCBs) | A |
| Beta-propiolactone | Production and use of plastics, resins, and viricides | A |
| Vinyl chloride | Polyvinyl plastic production | Liver |

Key: A = only animal evidence of carcinogenicity is currently satisfactory.

**Table 14-2.** Industries with cancer risk*

Aluminum production
Auramine manufacture
Boot and shoe manufacture and repair (certain
  exposures)
Coal gasification (older processes)
Coke production (certain exposures)
Furniture manufacture (wood dusts)
Iron and steel founding
Isopropyl alcohol manufacture (strong acid processes)
Magenta manufacturing
Painting
Rubber industry
Underground hematite mining (with radon exposure)

*According to the International Agency for Research on
Cancer.

of cancers can be attributed to workplace exposures. In the United States, this would represent between 23,000 and 92,000 new cases of cancer each year. Other estimates have been higher. All of these estimates pertain to the entire population; within high-risk groups, such as chemical workers, the proportion of cancers related to work is substantially higher. The cancers most closely associated with workplace exposures include common types, such as lung cancer and skin cancer, and less common types, such as bladder cancer, leukemia, and brain cancer. In developing nations, where agriculture is a major part of the economy and where aflatoxin contamination of many food products is common, one of the most common cancers, liver cancer, may be considered an occupational disease of people who live and work on farms.

## The Process of Carcinogenesis

A *carcinogen* is a substance that causes cancer. Carcinogens may be chemicals, physical agents such as ionizing radiation, or biologic agents such as viruses or aflatoxin. In some cases, such as in parts of the rubber industry, elevated rates of cancer have been detected, but a specific carcinogen has not been identified.

Current knowledge of the mechanisms of carcinogenesis remains incomplete. Based on experimental work with mouse skin in the 1940s, two stages in carcinogenesis were identified: initiation and promotion. *Initiation* was defined as the first event, when an irreversible change occurred to the cell's genetic material. *Promotion* consisted of one or more subsequent steps, when intra- and extracellular factors allowed the transformed cell to develop into a focal proliferation such as a nodule, then to a malignant tumor, and finally to metastases. Advances in molecular biology have revealed that carcinogenesis is a *multistep* process, and that specific genes play an important role.

The initiation of a cancer involves damage to cellular DNA, giving rise to an irreversible, heritable genetic lesion termed a *mutation*. Mutations can be induced by direct-acting carcinogens or by indirect-acting agents. Direct-acting carcinogens require no metabolic or chemical changes to produce lesions in DNA. Bis(chloromethyl) ether, for example, directly binds to DNA, creating DNA *adducts* that are known to be processed into mutations at a high frequency. Another example of a direct-acting agent is ionizing radiation, which acts by causing DNA strand breakage. Other chemicals, such as the polycyclic aromatic hydrocarbons (PAHs) generated by coke ovens or foundry operations and beta-naphthylamine used to make dyes, need to be converted to electrophilic metabolites before they bind DNA and potentially induce mutagenic changes.

The genes of critical importance in causing cancers generally fall into two classes: oncogenes and tumor suppressor genes. *Oncogenes* were originally recognized during studies of RNA viruses. Some of these viruses were noted to code for genetic sequences that, when inserted into host genomes, could cause malignant transformation. Those sequences were called oncogenes. It soon became clear that nascent forms of oncogenes, called *proto-oncogenes*, are common in many human and animal cells, encoding proteins that regulate normal cell growth and differentiation. However, if transformed into oncogenes, their products code for *oncoproteins* that act as growth factors, membrane receptors, protein kinases, or in other ways, resulting in rapid cell growth and de-differentiation. One of the best-studied examples is the *ras* oncogene, which was first identified in rat sarcomas. The *ras* oncogene can be activated by polycyclic aromatic hydrocarbons, N-nitroso compounds, and ionizing radiation, and has been found in a wide variety of human cancers, including bladder cancer, lung cancer, and others of occupational and environmental importance.

A second kind of gene important in carcinogenesis is the *tumor suppressor gene*, or anti-oncogene. Tumor suppressor genes function normally to regulate cell growth and stimulate terminal differentiation. When inactivated, they fail to perform those functions, and increase the probability of neoplastic transformation. The most commonly identified example is the p53 gene, located on chromosome 17. p53 mutations have been identified in various cancers, including those of the colon, lung, liver, esophagus, breast, and reticuloendothelial and hematopoietic tissues, and in the Li-Fraumeni syndrome of familial multiple cancer susceptibility. Of special interest, carcinogenic exposures such as aflatoxin and hepatitis B virus have been associated with specific mutations on the p53 gene, suggesting that each carcinogen may leave a unique genomic "signature." This may have clinical applications, as discussed below.

The initiation, promotion, and progression of cancers are now understood to consist of multiple genetic events that "activate" proto-oncogenes (to active oncogenes) and "inactivate" the tumor suppressor genes. The initial mutation in a proto-oncogene or in a tumor suppressor gene is thought to confer a growth advantage to the cell, leading to its proliferative *clonal expansion*. The population of clonally expanded mutant cells is then at increased risk for subsequent mutations in other critical target genes. These further mutations, in turn, lead to further growth of the cells, and eventually to the transformed cell that appears clinically as cancer. Any of these subsequent genetic lesions becomes more likely with exposure to carcinogens or other factors that enhance the growth advantage of the cells with the initiating mutations.

An important issue in carcinogenesis is *latency*. Latency refers to the period of time between the onset of exposure to a carcinogen and the clinical detection of resulting cancers. This period presumably corresponds to the stages of initiation, promotion, and progression between the first DNA mutation and the ultimate appearance of a malignant tumor. Because of latency considerations, screening of workers at risk of cancer should focus on the time after the initiating lesion and before clinical presentation. If surveillance is conducted too soon after the onset of exposure, when no increase in risk is expected, the yield will be low, the expense is avoidable, and there is a danger that negative results will be falsely reassuring. The correct timing of screening varies with the natural history of each cancer. The latency period for hematologic malignancies is in the range of 4 or 5 years, whereas the latency period for solid tumors is at least 10 to 20 years, possibly as long as 50 years.

Whether *threshold* levels of exposure to carcinogens exist has been a controversial topic. A threshold is a safe level of exposure to a carcinogen below which carcinogenesis does not occur. Since a single mutation in a single cell can theoretically initiate a malignancy, it has been argued that no safe level of exposure exists. Definitive evidence on this point is elusive, since both epidemiologic and experimental data are inherently uninformative at very low exposure levels. However, several arguments in support of thresholds have been advanced. First, there are known repair mechanisms that correct DNA damage, at least at low levels of exposure. Second, certain carcinogens, such as trace elements and hormones, are ubiquitous and even essential at low doses; it is argued that these substances are carcinogenic only at higher doses. Third, factors that act epigenetically rather than directly affecting DNA, such as promoters that stimulate cell division, typically have reversible effects, implying a threshold phenomenon. This question is important for regulators. If there are no safe thresholds of exposure, then no level of exposure can be regarded as absolutely safe. On the other hand, if thresholds do exist, then exposures below that level could readily be permitted. On the theory that no safe thresholds can be demonstrated, regulators have often made conservative assumptions, and have banned carcinogen exposures altogether. More recently, the trend has been to attempt to define some "acceptable" level of risk, and permit low-level exposures.

*Interaction* is another important concept in occupational carcinogenesis. This phenomenon occurs when the joint effect of two or more carcinogens is different than what would have been predicted based on the individual effects. *Synergy*, in which joint effects exceed the combined individual effects, and *antagonism*, in which joint effects are less than combined individual effects, are two examples of interaction. A classic example is the relationship between asbestos exposure and cigarette smoking revealed in early studies by Selikoff and colleagues: The relative risk of dying from lung cancer was elevated about 5-fold following asbestos exposure alone, about 10-fold following smoking alone, and about 80-fold following both exposures [4].

Interaction is a complicated concept, in part because statisticians, biologists, and lay people use different language to describe it. For the statistician, interaction is defined by mathematical models. If a combined effect departs from that predicted by a model, then synergy is said to exist. Since logistic regression is commonly used in modern epidemiologic analyses, synergy is signaled by the presence of a statistically significant interaction term. Epidemiologists call this "effect modification," and because of the assumptions of logistic regression, it implies multiplicative relations between different causes of cancer. On the other hand, additive relationships between different causes of cancer may be more important in the public health context. If the combined effect of two agents is greater than the sum of their effects, then eliminating either exposure would be quite effective in preventing disease.

In some cases, interaction may be nothing more than the combined effects of an initiator and a promoter. Individually, these substances may be predicted to have a certain magnitude of effect, but following sequential exposure, a much more potent carcinogenic effect may result.

## Clinical Applications of Molecular Biology

Insights gained from molecular biology have several applications to health care decisions for individual workers. One such application is in detecting markers of risk, and another is in detecting markers of exposure and early effect.

*Markers of risk* have been recognized for many years; disease states such as xeroderma pigmentosum carry an unusually high risk of cancer, because of defects in the ability to repair DNA damage. Increasingly, we are recognizing another dimension of increased risk, based on individual differences in metabolic enzymes. As noted above, many of the carcinogenic compounds found in the workplace are metabolized to active forms, usually electrophiles, that then bind covalently with DNA. The enzymes primarily responsible for this activation are those of the cytochrome P450 system. Others include *N*-acetyltransferase, epoxide hydrolase, and glutathione S-transferase. These enzyme systems evolved primarily to render xenobiotics more polar and therefore more readily excretable. However, their products are often reactive electrophiles that can bond with DNA to form adducts and cause mutations.

Considerable variation in these metabolic functions has been noted among species, and among different people. For example, people vary several thousandfold in their levels of aryl hydrocarbon hydroxylase (AHH), an enzyme of the cytochrome P450 system that helps metabolize PAHs. High levels of AHH have been associated with increased risk of lung cancer. Variations in AHH levels reflect genetic factors, but can also result from environmental exposures such as cigarette smoking and diet that induce enzyme activity. Another highly variable factor is the cytochrome P450 enzyme responsible for hydroxylating the antihypertensive drug debrisoquin. People who are "extensive hydroxylators" have several thousand times more enzyme activity than "poor hydroxylators." The extensive hydroxylator phenotype has been associated with a markedly increased risk of lung cancer. A third example, this one involving a repair enzyme, is $O^6$-methyltransferase deficiency. People with this deficiency are at increased risk of liver and intestinal cancers.

What is the significance of differential susceptibility? Some have suggested that more susceptible workers should be kept from jobs that have carcinogenic exposures, while less susceptible workers should preferentially work in such jobs. While this approach has a certain logic, there are compelling counterarguments. First, the more definitive and therefore preferred approach is to modify the workplace instead of the workforce (see Chap. 4). Second, the sensitivity and specificity of various enzyme phenotypes are not nearly high enough to support confident predictions of cancer risk. Third, barring people of certain phenotypes from employment is discriminatory and probably illegal under the Americans with Disabilities Act (see Chap. 11). Despite these arguments, identifying high- and low-risk individuals may find a future clinical role in worker placement, in counseling prospective workers about job choices, in tailoring medical surveillance programs according to individual risk levels, and in other ways.

*Markers of exposure,* often called biomarkers, will also grow in importance in occupational health, both in clinical practice and in epidemiologic study. For many years carcinogens or their metabolites have been directly measured in biologic media such as blood and urine. For example, benzene exposure can be monitored directly in expired air and blood and through urinary phenol levels, and exposure to the aromatic amine 4,4'-methylenebis(2-chloroaniline) (MBOCA) can be monitored through urinary MBOCA levels. More recently assays have measured the level of mutagenicity in urine; the basis for this approach is that carcinogens, when metabolized to active forms and excreted, should be detectable in urine, and should reflect the individual exposure. Perhaps the most promising way to measure carcinogen exposure is to assess the dose at the ultimate target, DNA, by measuring DNA adducts.

DNA *adducts* may be long-lived or short-lived and may vary greatly in form. They can be measured using a variety of techniques. One is immunoassay, which utilizes specific antibodies against DNA adducts. Another is DNA digestion, in which individual bases of digested DNA are separated with two-dimensional chromatography after radiolabeling with $^{32}P$, and adducts are visualized with autoradiography. The study of DNA adducts has several limitations, including the absence of DNA in the most readily available tissue, red blood cells (RNA adducts and protein adducts may also be studied), the instability and unknown clearance rates of DNA adducts, and the lack of good dose-response data. Most importantly, the significance of the various kinds of adducts and their associated conformational changes in DNA are still not well understood. However, data from ethylene oxide workers, welders, hazardous waste workers, and others suggest that DNA adducts may reflect biologically effective dose in exposed workers.

Another approach to biomarkers is to measure the level of chromosome aberrations or disturbances in the cells of exposed workers. Strictly speaking, this is a measurement of *early effect* rather than exposure. Cultured lymphocytes are the usual cells of choice, and the observations of interest may be sister chromatid exchanges (SCEs), micronuclei, or mutations at so-called reporter genes. SCEs are four-stranded exchanges of genetic material that are efficiently induced by DNA adducts. Micronuclei are induced by gross chromosomal damage that is not integrated into the nucleus at mitoses. Mutations induced in vivo, most commonly assessed at the *hprt* gene locus, reflect DNA-based lesions and can also be quantified. The *hprt* gene encodes a purine salvage pathway, which is the primary source of purines for DNA synthesis, and therefore the *hprt* gene can be used as a marker of induced mutations.

The precise relationship of these phenomena to the exposure-induced genetic changes of interest, mutations in proto-oncogenes and tumor suppressor genes, remains unclear. As the genes directly involved in the carcinogenic process become better understood, the biomarkers available for use in occupational studies of cancer risk will become more varied and more directly associated with specific disease risk.

It is important to note that biomarkers of exposure, whether simple blood levels of a chemical or sophisticated genetic measures, should never replace environmental monitoring as a check on workplace exposure levels. However, they have an important role as a "backup" means of monitoring exposure levels and identifying excessive exposures that require abatement.

## Testing and Evaluation of Carcinogens

Several methods have emerged by which carcinogens are identified (Table 14-3). These methods include epidemiologic studies, animal studies, in vitro test systems, and analysis of structure-activity relationships.

*Epidemiologic studies* are potentially the most definitive source of information on human carcinogenicity since they are based on human exposures in "real-life" situations. However, occupational cancer epidemiology is limited in important ways. One challenge is cohort definition and follow-up; if a group of workers was exposed to a suspected carcinogen years ago, it can be difficult to enumerate them and trace their health outcomes. Another limitation pertains to exposure assessment. Job designations and even direct measurements may not accurately reflect worker ex-

posures, making it difficult to test whether differing levels of exposure are associated with differing levels of cancer risk. Another limitation pertains to outcome information. Death certificates, a major source of diagnostic information in occupational cancer epidemiology, may be inaccurate. They are also limited because they provide information only on mortality, and not on incidence. Still another problem is confounding. For many cancers of interest, both occupational and nonoccupational exposures play a role, but information on the relevant nonoccupational exposures is often unavailable. Most of these limitations bias results toward the null hypothesis, or a finding of no effect. For this reason, great caution is necessary in interpreting epidemiologic results.

Moreover, epidemiologic studies are expensive and time-consuming, and they yield evidence of carcinogenicity only after the fact, when workers have already been affected. In fact, given the long latency period of most cancer, by the time epidemiologic studies conclusively identify a carcinogen, many thousands of workers may have been exposed. For these reasons, animal and in vitro studies have gained wide importance.

Animal studies for carcinogenicity use species that range from *Drosophila* to higher mammals. In accordance with National Cancer Institute guidelines, a substance is usually tested at two doses in both sexes of two strains of rodents, with at least 50 animals in each test group (2 doses × 2 sexes × 2 strains = 8 test groups). Therefore, at least 400 animals are usually studied, in addition to the 100 or more control animals that receive a placebo. The testing usually takes about 2 years, but 4 years can elapse from the initial planning of such a study until the final report has been completed, at a cost of several hundred thousand to more than one million dollars.

With test groups limited by cost to usually 50 animals each, small elevations in cancer incidence tend to be statistically insignificant. However, even a small elevation in incidence rate, when multiplied by a large exposed human population, could imply a substantial number of preventable

**Table 14-3.** Relative advantages of the major methods of carcinogenicity testing[a]

| Advantage | In vitro bioassay | Animal bioassay | Epidemiologic study |
|---|---|---|---|
| Low cost | + + + | + + | + |
| Rapidity | + + + | + + | + |
| Ease of performance | + + + | + + | + |
| Ability to control for multiple chemical exposures | + + + | + + + | + |
| Ability to demonstrate threshold level of carcinogen exposure | 0 | 0 | 0 |
| Validity of results as predictor of human carcinogenesis | + | + + | + + + |
| Validity of results in identifying locus of human carcinogenesis (i.e., organ specificity) | NA | + | + + + |
| Provides absolute proof of human carcinogenicity | 0 | 0 | 0[b] |

[a]The grading scale used in this table is qualitative only. Specific methodologic features and appropriate applications of each method are discussed in the text.
[b]Although by formal standards there may be no "absolute proof" of carcinogenicity, evidence from multiple well-designed epidemiologic studies is generally accepted to be a functional equivalent of proof.

cancers. Consequently, to ensure that positive results will not escape notice, every effort is made to detect the carcinogenic effect of a test substance. One way this is done is by using as one of the test doses the *maximum tolerated dose* (MTD), the highest dose that will not kill or acutely poison test animals. (Often the other test dose is one-fourth of the MTD.) Critics have noted that the MTD introduces an element of unreality to bioassays: Such a large dose far exceeds human exposure levels, may create an unrepresentative biochemical milieu in test animals, and may overwhelm natural protective mechanisms such as detoxification and repair systems. Further, the MTD clearly causes cell death with subsequent mitogenic stimulation (stimulation of cells to divide) of surrounding, surviving cells. This mitogenesis, rather than the direct carcinogen interaction with DNA, could be critical to the carcinogenic process; cells with a limited amount of genetic damage may be intensely promoted by the repopulation that follows MTD-induced cell death, causing additional genetic changes critical to tumor formation. However, even with the use of MTDs, most chemicals tested show no carcinogenic activity. This finding suggests that the use of high doses is reasonable and refutes the belief that "everything causes cancer."

Another controversial issue raised by animal testing is the existence of *threshold* levels of exposure. Since animal tests necessarily use high-dose exposures, our conclusions about the effects of low-dose exposures must come from downward extrapolation of observed dose-response patterns. Uncertainty about the mechanisms of carcinogenesis makes this extrapolation speculative (Fig. 14-2). It is largely for this reason and for analogous considerations in epidemiology that no safe threshold for carcinogen exposure can be demonstrated with certainty.

A related issue concerns the *potency* of a carcinogen. In animal testing, different chemicals vary quantitatively in their ability to induce tumors. Such results can help identify the most worrisome human exposures. However, there is less basis to believe that they quantitatively predict human cancer incidence, as assumed in risk assessment calculations. Similarly, the target organ in a test species may differ from that in humans, due mostly to differing metabolic pathways. Benzidine, for example, causes bladder cancer in humans, hepatomas in mice, and intestinal tumors in rats.

The major questions about animal bioassays, of course, concern their accuracy at predicting human carcinogenesis. Some argue that animal studies

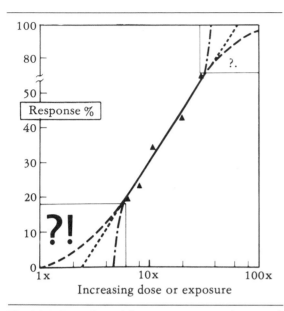

**Fig. 14-2.** Hypothetical dose-response curve for animal carcinogenicity study. These results are usually obtained at relatively high levels of exposure, as indicated by the triangles. The problem in estimating human risks is trying to determine what happens at lower exposures. As indicated on the diagram, there are several possible ways to extrapolate. In most cases, extrapolation of the observed results with a straight line will yield a result suggesting no response at low doses—that is, a threshold. Most scientists, however, now think that the actual response is indicated by the smooth curve passing through zero dose and zero response. (From PJ Gehring, Dow Chemical Co. Published in TS Maugh II. Chemical carcinogens: How dangerous are low doses? Science 1978; 202:37.)

are of limited value because animals and humans often have different sensitivities to carcinogens, and because the ability to activate and detoxify carcinogens may vary markedly among species. Of the several hundred chemicals that have been formally bioassayed, about half have given positive results. Not all of these animal carcinogens have been shown to cause cancer in humans, but most have not been studied epidemiologically. On the other hand, every human carcinogen, with the possible exception of benzene, is an animal carcino-

gen. In general, therefore, properly conducted and replicated animal bioassays are reasonable predictors of human cancer risk.

*In vitro* testing involves the use of bacterial or human tissue cultures. Suspected carcinogens are added to these systems, and endpoints that reflect DNA damage, such as DNA alteration, increased repair, or altered gene expression, are monitored. The prototype *in vitro* assay is the Ames test, first described in 1966. This test uses special strains of *Salmonella typhimurium* that cannot synthesize the amino acid tryptophan. Mutant strains synthesize tryptophan and show growth on a tryptophan-free medium, an endpoint easily detectable by examining the medium for bacterial growth.

*In vitro* assays such as the Ames test determine mutagenicity, not carcinogenicity. However, both theoretical and empirical evidence suggests that mutagenicity and carcinogenicity are closely linked. The theoretical link lies in the molecular event that is common to both: alteration of DNA. The empirical link is that nearly all known carcinogens are mutagenic. However, recent reports have emphasized that many naturally occurring substances not regarded as carcinogenic, including common plant products, food constituents, and hormones, are also mutagenic in the Ames test. Some observers have therefore questioned the assumption that in vitro mutagenicity predicts human carcinogenicity.

Numerous modifications of the Ames test have been made, including the addition of liver microsomes to test systems in order to metabolize substances that may not be mutagenic in their original form. Other short-term in vitro assays include such tests as the induction of chromosomal aberrations, SCEs, and micronuclei, as well as the malignant transformation of cultured cells that produce tumors when inoculated into an appropriate host. Short-term assays, in addition to suggesting potential human carcinogenicity tests in animals, are used to help identify both mutagens in complex mixtures and active metabolites of mutagens in human body fluids, and to study mechanisms of chemical carcinogenesis.

Finally, in analyzing structure-activity relationships (SARs), investigators review chemical configurations for their similarity to those of known carcinogens. Such analysis can direct suspicion to chemicals that may have carcinogenic potential; further testing will generally be necessary.

Based on these four types of data, regulatory and research agencies have developed standardized ways to classify chemical carcinogenicity. The most widely used scheme is that of the International Agency for Research on Cancer (IARC), which designates three categories [5]. Group 1 includes chemicals and processes established as human carcinogens based on "sufficient evidence," usually epidemiologic data. Group 2 includes chemicals and processes that are "probably" (group 2A) or "possibly" (group 2B) carcinogenic to humans. Group 2A reflects limited evidence of carcinogenicity in humans and sufficient evidence of carcinogenicity in experimental animals, while group 2B reflects limited evidence in humans without sufficient evidence in animals, or sufficient evidence in animals without any human data. IARC policy has been to recommend treating group 2 chemicals as if they presented a carcinogenic risk to humans. Group 3 includes agents that are not classified, and group 4 includes agents that are probably not carcinogenic to humans. Using this classification, IARC has evaluated approximately 750 chemicals, industrial processes, and personal habits. More than 50 have been placed in group 1, and almost 250 have been placed in group 2. The American Conference of Governmental Industrial Hygienists (ACGIH), the National Toxicology Program (NTP), and the National Institute for Occupational Safety and Health (NIOSH) have all adopted analogous schemes.

## Risk Assessment and Regulation of Workplace Carcinogens

OSHA's approach to carcinogen regulation was set forth in 1980 in its generic carcinogen standard, "Identification, Classification, and Regulation of Potential Occupational Carcinogens" [29 CFR 1990]. This standard defines a protocol for interpreting test data on carcinogenicity and classifying chemicals accordingly. Which chemicals are then regulated is decided based on several criteria:

1. The estimated number of workers exposed
2. The estimated levels of human exposure
3. The exposure levels reported to be carcinogenic
4. The extent to which regulation might also reduce occupational risks other than cancer
5. Whether the molecular structure of a chemical resembles that of a known carcinogen
6. Whether substitutes are available, or other evidence suggests that the costs of regulation would be small
7. The actions of other agencies in regulating the chemical

Despite this well-defined scheme, the carcinogen standard has not been utilized by OSHA since its promulgation in 1980. Consequently, most known carcinogens that are regulated by OSHA are regulated through earlier consensus standards and not in accordance with the generic carcinogen standard.

## Risk Assessment

An important component of regulation is risk assessment. Risk assessment has been defined as a four-part process: hazard identification, exposure assessment, dose-response assessment, and risk characterization. Hazard identification asks whether a chemical is carcinogenic to humans, based on data from epidemiologic studies, animal studies, short-term bioassays, and SARs. Exposure assessment asks how many people are exposed, for how long, and through what routes. Dose-response assessment combines data from the first two steps to estimate quantitatively the magnitude of human cancers at specific dose levels, generally below the observable range. This involves extrapolation across species and down the dose-response curve, and often relies on complex mathematical models. Finally, risk characterization provides the "bottom line": a quantitative estimate of human cancer risk at known exposure levels.

Risk assessment has been widely debated. It represents a methodical approach to quantifying risks, and it is especially useful in comparing risks between or among different exposures. However, many argue that available data are rarely adequate to support quantitative estimates of human risk. Extrapolation from high exposures to low exposures is based on a number of assumptions, most of which are unverifiable. The same is true of extrapolation from animal tests to human experience. Moreover, risk is generally calculated based on a single chemical exposure, while exposures are more often to mixtures of chemicals. However, at present risk assessment is a key component of carcinogen regulation in the U.S., both by OSHA and by other agencies.

## Clinical Encounters with Carcinogens

A health care provider may face questions about occupational cancer risk in several ways, both in treating individuals and in considering populations. The remainder of this chapter poses situations and discusses responses to them.

*"Is this chemical carcinogenic?"* This question is best answered according to defined criteria, such as those discussed above. The primary animal and epidemiologic data on a chemical may be accessed through standard reference sources. Formal evaluations of carcinogenicity may be found in the IARC monographs on the Evaluation of the Carcinogenic Risk of Chemicals to Humans, in annual reports of the NTP, and in other publications and databases.

*"I am exposed to a carcinogen. What should I do?"* This query has two components: One pertains to the carcinogenic exposure and one to the patient.

Ideally, there should be no workplace exposure to a carcinogen. As previously discussed, safe threshold exposure levels cannot currently be demonstrated. A clinician who becomes aware of an ongoing carcinogenic workplace exposure should take appropriate steps to end that exposure, which will often involve contacting responsible individuals at the workplace and government agencies. Exposure may be ended through substitution of the carcinogen, enclosure of the process or other engineering techniques, or, when necessary, personal protective equipment.

The worker who reports being exposed to a carcinogen should be advised to terminate the exposure, to avoid concomitant carcinogenic exposures such as smoking, and to seek appropriate medical monitoring.

*"Did my exposure cause my cancer?"* Patients with cancer who have been exposed to carcinogens often inquire about the possibility that the exposures were causal. The question sometimes arises in the context of litigation or may simply reflect a patient's psychological need to explain a catastrophic life event. The issue of cancer causation in an individual patient is difficult to address because it entails the application of epidemiologic and statistical data (which derive from groups) to individuals. This process is as much philosophical as scientific.

Certain requirements must be met before it may be said that an exposure has "causally contributed" to a cancer. There must be evidence that the exposure has indeed occurred. The tumor type in question must be associated with the exposure, based on prior studies. Finally, the appropriate temporal relationship must hold; in particular, a sufficiently long latency period must have elapsed between the onset of exposure and the diagnosis of cancer.

When these requirements have been met, additional issues should be considered. Suppose that the baseline incidence of lung cancer in unexposed adult men is 80 cases per 100,000 per year. Suppose further that a particular occupational exposure has been associated with a relative risk of lung cancer of 1.8. Therefore, the incidence among exposed men would be 144 cases per 100,000 per year. If an exposed man develops lung cancer and wonders whether his exposure caused his cancer, what should he be told?

The simplest analysis is qualitative. Any exposure that markedly increases risk may be considered to contribute to the development of cancer in an exposed individual. A "marked" increase has no firm definition; relative risks as low as 1.3 have been considered in this category. By this analysis, the patient could be told that his exposure contributed to his cancer.

A second qualitative approach is to ask whether the patient's cancer would have occurred "but for" the exposure. In the above example, over half the cases of lung cancer in the exposed population would occur even without the exposure. It might then be concluded that any individual case is "more likely than not" to have occurred irrespective of exposure. Similarly, a relative risk of 2.2 would lead to the conclusion that any individual case of cancer would not have occurred "but for" exposure.

This approach is obviously unsatisfactory. It accounts for no cancer causation when the relative risk is below 2.0, and it accounts for all cancer causation when the relative risk exceeds 2.0. This violates common-sense notions of causation, and it places far too much weight on the precision of the relative risk estimate.

Finally, in the quantitative approach, causation is allocated to various causes, including occupational exposures. In the above example, the patient might be told that the occupational exposure was "responsible" for 44 percent (0.8/1.8) of his lung cancer. On the other hand, if he were a smoker, with a consequent tenfold increase in lung cancer risk, he might be told that smoking accounted for 83 percent (9/10.8) of his cancer, that the job exposure accounted for 7 percent (0.8/10.8), and that baseline population risk factors accounted for 9 percent (1/10.8).

This approach has intuitive appeal, since it confronts the multiplicity of exposures and attempts to quantify the relative importance of each. However, the data needed for this approach are rarely available. Interaction of multiple exposures, such as synergy, often occurs but is rarely quantitated. Consequently, even if a population relative risk can be estimated for an occupational exposure, the relative causal contribution of several factors in an individual is usually impossible to quantitate.

The latter two approaches outlined above are often demanded in legal settings, but as noted, they generally have inadequate scientific basis. Until further data or analytical methods are available, the first approach is recommended. It accords with common sense, stays within the confines of available data, and is understandable to patients and their families.

*"How should a screening program for cancer be designed?"* The theory and practice of screening have advanced in recent years. With regard to cancer, three goals are sought by screening programs: (1) identifying susceptible individuals, presumably before exposure; (2) identifying markers of exposure (biologic monitoring); and (3) identifying early signs of disease (medical surveillance). Some screening tests fall between the second and third category, since they identify physiologic changes related to exposure but of uncertain pathologic significance. The first two kinds of screening were discussed above, and this section focuses only on the third (see Chap. 3).

Cancer surveillance in occupational settings has been best explored with regard to bladder cancer and lung cancer. Among workers exposed to beta-naphthylamine, benzidine, or benzidine congeners such as o-toluidine, two methods have been primarily used: urinalysis for microscopic hematuria and urine cytology. Hematuria is relatively sensitive in detecting both superficial and invasive bladder cancer, but its low specificity results in a high false-positive rate, requiring a large number of invasive studies on healthy individuals. Urine cytology has good sensitivity and specificity for invasive bladder cancer, but no firm evidence demonstrates a survival advantage for patients whose disease is detected through such screening. More advanced techniques such as flow cytometry and quantitative fluorescence image analysis remain unvalidated, but appear to have suboptimal sensitivity and/or specificity. The International Conference on Bladder Cancer Screening in High-Risk Groups, sponsored by NIOSH in 1989, concluded that urinalysis and cytology might be appropriate, especially following high exposure to known or suspected bladder carcinogens, but that further data were necessary [6]. Ongoing studies of high-risk groups such as the Drake Health Registry [7] should support further recommendations in the near future.

Lung cancer surveillance consists of interval chest radiography or sputum cytology, or both. These approaches were evaluated in a series of trials at the Mayo Clinic, Johns Hopkins University, and the Memorial Sloan-Kettering Cancer Center in the 1970s. The combination of chest x-rays and sputum cytology tests three times a year yielded a significant increase in lung cancer detection and resectability compared to control subjects (who were merely advised to be tested once a year). However, no significant decrease was found in lung cancer mortality. These results, in combination with other data, have supported the recommendation that no routine surveillance for lung cancer be offered, even to high-risk populations [8, 9].

Evidence does not support other specific approaches to medical surveillance for occupational cancer. Most tests carry a high risk of false-positives, a low positive predictive value, high cost, worker unacceptability, and/or morbidity. The major exceptions are tests that are generally recommended for the larger population, and that might be easily provided in the workplace setting; these include Papanicolaou (Pap) smears for cervical cancer, stool guaiac testing and sigmoidoscopy for colorectal cancer, physical examination and mammography for breast cancer, and possibly digital examination and prostate-specific antigen for prostate cancer.

*"We have a cluster of cancer in our plant. How should we respond?"* Suspected excesses of cancer, clustered in time or space, may be noted by workers or by the workplace medical department. These situations arouse a great deal of concern, and it is essential that they be handled openly, methodically, and expeditiously. A multidisciplinary approach is necessary, drawing on the experience and knowledge of workers, physicians, epidemiologists, industrial hygienists, and managers. The following sequence is suggested:

First, the presence of a cluster should be confirmed or refuted. Each case of cancer should be confirmed, and tissue type, date of diagnosis, demographic data, and exposure data should be obtained. The worker population should be enumerated and subdivided into age, sex, and other pertinent categories. (If information on retirees is available, it should be included.) Age- and sex-specific cancer incidence rates for the state should be obtained from the state cancer registry, if one exists. With this information, an age-standardized cancer rate can be computed for the workplace and compared with the expected rate, based on state data. Confidence intervals can be calculated for the workplace cancer rate; these will usually be broad because of small numbers. However, even a statistically insignificant elevation in the cancer rate in the workplace should prompt further evaluation.

Next, the tissue types of the cancer cases should be reviewed. An excess of unusual tumors, or tumors known to be environmentally induced, should prompt further concern.

Then the latency periods of each cancer case should be reviewed. If many of the workers began their plant employment only shortly before diagnosis, an exposure-related cluster is less plausible.

Next, confounders should be reviewed. Other factors that may contribute to an elevation of cancer should be noted. However, care should be taken not to let the presence of confounders obscure one's view of an occupational carcinogen.

Next, the occupational histories of the cases should be reviewed. Detailed personnel histories of each affected worker may reveal that a particular job title is associated with cancer. It is important that jobs in the distant past, not just recent ones, are examined.

An occupational hygiene review should be made to determine whether any particular exposures are common among the affected workers. A variety of job titles may share a common chemical contact, which may help explain the cluster. Early exposures may need to be reconstructed, which may involve interviewing older workers or reviewing production records.

Next, the same analysis should be made with regard to worksites. If many of the cases arise from a single building or location, an environmental cause is suggested. Any worksites in question should be subjected to a thorough occupational hygiene evaluation, which should include both the production process and "incidental" exposure such as the heating, ventilation, and air-conditioning system (HVAC) and the drinking water.

Based on the above analysis, an initially suspected cancer cluster may be found to be (1) not actually present, (2) present but not consistent with occupational causation, (3) possibly related to occupational exposures, or (4) definitely related to occupational exposures. The results should be carefully and thoroughly communicated to all those concerned. If an occupational cause is implicated, aggressive corrective action is in order. Whatever the conclusion, careful ongoing surveillance of both the workplace and the workforce should continue.

A health care provider who analyzes an apparent cancer cluster may require further assistance. The most appropriate sources are NIOSH, a state health department, or a qualified consultant group, such as a university-based occupational health program.

## Conclusion

Occupational cancer is a feared consequence of certain workplace exposures. It differs from other occupational diseases in several ways: No safe level of exposure to carcinogens is recognized, many different forms of cancer exist, cancer develops many years after exposure, occupational cancer generally resembles cancer of nonoccupational origin, and competing carcinogenic exposures are present in many cases. On the other hand, occupational cancer shares at least important features with other occupational diseases: there are large data gaps in relating exposure to disease, and most cases are preventable.

The health care provider's role in confronting occupational cancer is varied. He or she should maintain a high index of suspicion of workplace causes when treating cancer, especially lung, bladder, and brain cancer and leukemia. The clinician should work to identify past exposures, utilizing the patient's knowledge, toxicologic resources, and consultants. In case of ongoing exposures, he or she should assume a public health role, working to end these exposures. Finally, it is important to educate patients, employee and employer groups, and communities about the hazards of carcinogenic exposures and ways to prevent them.

## References

1. Randall WJ, Solomon S. Building six: The tragedy at Bridesburg. Boston: Little, Brown, 1976.
2. Figueroa WG, Raszkowski R, Weiss W. Lung cancer in chloromethyl methyl ether workers. N Engl J Med 1973; 288:1096–7.
3. Hoel DG, et al. Trends in cancer mortality in 15 industrialized countries, 1969–1986. J Natl Cancer Inst 1992; 84:313–20.
4. Selikoff IJ. Asbestos exposure, smoking, and neoplasia. JAMA 1968; 204:104.
5. Vainio H, Wilbourn J. Identification of carcinogens within the IARC monograph program. Scand J Work Eviron Health 1992; 18(Suppl.):64.
6. Halperin W, et al. Final discussion: Where do we go from here? J Occup Med 1990; 32:936.
7. Marsh GM, et al. A protocol for bladder cancer screening and medical surveillance among high-risk groups: The Drake Health Registry experience. J Occup Med 1990; 32:881.

8. Eddy DM. Screening for lung cancer. Ann Intern Med 1989; 111:232.
9. Strauss GM, Gleason RE, Sugarbaker DJ. Screening for lung cancer re-examined. A reinterpretation of the Mayo Lung Project randomized trial on lung cancer screening. Chest 1993; 103 (Suppl. 4):337S.

# Bibliography

Alderson M. Occupational cancer. London: Butterworths, 1986.
*An excellent review of chemicals and industrial processes, with evidence for carcinogenicity. Current through 1985.*

Bailar JS, Smith EM. Progress against cancer? N Engl J Med 1986; 314:1226–32.
*A sobering argument that cancer treatment and prevention have not been very successful.*

Bishop JM. Molecular themes in oncogenesis. Cell 1991; 64:235–48.
*An excellent review of the molecular biology of cancer.*

Brandt-Rauf PW. New markers for monitoring occupational cancer: the example of oncogene proteins. J Occup Med 1988; 30:399–404.
*Reviews the role of oncogenes in occupational medicine.*

Davis DL, Hoel D. eds. Trends in cancer mortality in industrial countries. Ann NY Acad Sci, Vol. 69, 1990.
*A collection of papers that discuss and analyze cancer rates in North America, Europe, and Japan.*

Doll R, Peto R. The causes of cancer. New York: Oxford University Press, 1981.
*A brief monograph reviewing and synthesizing epidemiologic and laboratory data.*

Harris CC. Chemical and physical carcinogenesis: Advances and perspectives for 1990. Cancer Res 1991; 51:(Suppl)5023s–44s.
*An excellent review of mechanisms of carcinogenesis.*

Hart RW, Hoerger FD. Carcinogen risk assessment: New directions in the qualitative and quantitative aspects. Banbury Report 31. Cold Spring Harbor: Cold Spring Harbor Laboratory, 1988.
*Proceedings of a conference on risk assessment, with papers that discuss methodologic difficulties and other problems.*

Hemminki K. Occupational cancer and carcinogenesis. Scand J Work Environ Health 1992; 18 (Suppl. 1):1–117.
*A monograph with up-to-date papers on all aspects of occupational cancer.*

Higginson J, Muir CS, Muñoz N. Human cancer: Epidemiology and environmental causes. Cambridge: Cambridge University Press, 1992.
*A brief but comprehensive general text on cancer and its causes.*

International Agency for Research on Cancer. IARC monographs on the evaluation of carcinogenic risks to humans, suppl. 7. Overall evaluations of carcinogenicity: An updating of IARC monographs vols. 1–42. Lyon, France: IARC, 1987.
*The latest in-depth summary of IARC monographs. This is updated briefly in [5].*

National Academy of Sciences. Managing the process: Risk assessment in the federal government. Washington, D.C.: National Academy Press, 1983.
*Explains the components of risk assessment as used by federal agencies.*

Office of Science and Technology Policy. Chemical carcinogens: A review of the science and its associated principles. Fed Register 1985; 50:10372–442. Reprinted in Environ Health Perspect 1986; 67:201–82.
*This source and the next one explain the basis for federal regulatory approaches.*

Office of Technology Assessment. Identifying and regulating carcinogens, OTA-BP-H-42. Washington, D.C.: U.S. Government Printing Office, 1987.

Schottenfeld D, Fraumeni JF. eds. Cancer epidemiology and prevention. 2nd ed. Philadelphia: Saunders, 1993.
*The best reference on cancer epidemiology, reviewing causal factors and clinical aspects.*

Siemiatycki J. Risk factors for cancer in the workplace. Boca Raton, FL: CRC Press, 1991.
*Both a basic text and a report of a massive series of studies in Montreal.*

Wogan GN. Markers of exposure to carcinogens. Environ Health Perspect 1989; 81:9–17.
*A thorough review of biomarkers of carcinogen exposure.*

# 15
# Ionizing Radiation

Arthur C. Upton

Chernobyl, USSR, April 27, 1986. An explosion and fire occurred in a large, uranium-fueled, graphite power reactor during a test in which the emergency cooling, regulating, and shutdown systems had been deliberately turned off. The resulting damage to the reactor caused the release of large quantities of radioactive fuel and fission products, which contaminated the plant site and areas downwind from it for hundreds of miles. Two plant workers died immediately after the accident from burns and traumatic injuries, and hundreds were hospitalized later for radiation sickness, 29 of whom died within subsequent weeks.

Although no other radiation accident thus far has been as serious as the one at Chernobyl, scores of other accidents have occurred, some of which also have caused fatalities [1]. Even in the absence of accidents, moreover, mortality from cancer and other diseases has been increased in radiation workers in the past. Today, even the smallest doses of radiation are considered to pose some risk of injury. Therefore, in view of the large number of workers at risk (Tables 15-1 and 15-2), the recognition, treatment, and prevention of radiation injury command an important place in occupational health.

Preparation of this report was supported in part by Grants ES 00260 and CA 13343 from the U.S. Public Health Service and Grant SIG 09 from the American Cancer Society.

## Nature and Measurement of Ionizing Radiation

Ionizing radiations are of two main types: electromagnetic and particulate. The former include x-rays and gamma rays; the latter include electrons, protons, neutrons, alpha particles, and other corpuscular radiations of varying mass and charge (Table 15-3). Ionizing radiations are produced in the release of energy that occurs when atoms disintegrate. This process takes place in the disintegration of naturally unstable elements, such as uranium, thorium, and radium, and in the disintegration of elements that are disrupted by bombardment in an "atom smasher," atomic reactor, or other such device. After their release, x-rays and gamma rays travel with the speed of light, whereas particulate radiations vary in initial velocity, depending on their energy and mass.

As ionizing radiation penetrates matter, it collides with atoms and molecules in its path, disrupting them in the process, and thereby giving rise to ions and free radicals—hence, its designation *ionizing* radiation. The collisions tend to be clustered densely along the track of an alpha particle, causing the radiation to give up all of its energy in traversing only a few cells. With an x-ray, on the other hand, the collisions tend to be distributed so sparsely along its track that the radiation may traverse the entire body. The average amount of energy deposited per unit length of track (expressed in KeV/$\mu$) is called the linear energy transfer (LET) of the radiation.

**Table 15-1.** Estimated numbers of U.S. workers occupationally exposed to ionizing radiation

| Types of work | Number of workers exposed annually | Average dose per year (mSv) |
|---|---|---|
| Nuclear energy (fuel cycle) | 62,000 | 8.4 |
| Naval reactor | 36,000 | 2.2 |
| Healing arts | 500,000 | 1.2 |
| Research | 100,000 | 1.2 |
| Manufacturing and industrial | 7,000,000 | 0.07 |

Source: Department of Health, Education, and Welfare. Interagency task force on the health effects of ionizing radiation. Report of the work group on science. Washington, D.C.: Department of Health, Education, and Welfare, 1979.

**Table 15-2.** Types of workers who may be occupationally exposed to ionizing radiation

| | |
|---|---|
| Airline crews | Nuclear submarine workers |
| Atomic energy plant workers | Oil well loggers |
| Cathode ray tube makers | Ore assayers |
| Dental assistants | Petroleum refinery workers |
| Dentists | Physicians |
| Electron microscope makers | Pipeline oil flow testers |
| Electron microscopists | Pipeline weld radiographers |
| Electrostatic eliminator operators | Plasma torch operators |
| Fire alarm makers | Radar tube makers |
| Gas mantle makers | Radiologists |
| High-voltage television repairmen | Radium laboratory workers |
| High-voltage vacuum tube makers | Television tube makers |
| High-voltage vacuum tube users | Thickness gauge operators |
| Industrial fluoroscope operators | Thorium-aluminum alloy workers |
| Industrial radiographers | Thorium-magnesium alloy workers |
| Inspectors using, and workers located near, sealed gamma ray sources (cesium-137, cobalt-60, and iridium-192) | Thorium ore producers |
| | Uranium mill workers |
| Klystron tube operators | Uranium miners |
| Liquid level gauge operators | X-ray aides |
| Luminous dial painters | X-ray diffraction apparatus operators |
| | X-ray technicians |
| | X-ray tube makers |

Source: Based on data from MM Key et al. eds. Occupational diseases: a guide to their recognition. Washington, D.C.: NIOSH, 1977, 471–472.

Radiations of high LET, such as alpha particles, tend to cause greater injury for a given total amount of energy deposited in a cell than do radiations of low LET, such as x-rays [2]. The high relative biologic effectiveness (RBE) of high-LET radiation results from the capacity of each densely ionizing particle to deposit enough energy in a critical site within the cell (for example, a DNA molecule or a chromosome) to cause biologically significant molecular damage. Hence, although alpha particles generally travel only a short distance (Table 15-3) and thus pose little risk if emitted outside the body, they may be highly injurious to those cells that they penetrate.

**Table 15-3.** Principal types and properties of ionizing radiation

| Type of radiation | Relative mass | Charge | Range in soft tissue* |
|---|---|---|---|
| Gamma ray | 0 | 0 | Centimeters |
| X-ray | 0 | 0 | Centimeters |
| Beta ray (electron) | 1/1,840 | −1 | Millimeters |
| Neutron | 1 | 0 | Centimeters |
| Proton | 1 | +1 | Microns |
| Alpha particle | 4 | +2 | Microns |

*Range depends on the energy of the radiation; values shown are typical for radiations commonly encountered in the workplace.

When a radionuclide is taken into the body, its tissue distribution and retention depend on its physical and chemical properties. Radioactive iodine, for example, is normally concentrated in the thyroid gland, whereas strontium-90 is deposited primarily in bone. After deposition of a given amount of radioactivity, the quantity remaining in situ decreases with time through both physical decay and biologic removal. The time taken for a radionuclide to lose one-half of its radioactivity by physical decay varies from a fraction of a second in the case of some radionuclides to millions of years in the case of others. With iodine-131, for example, the physical half-life is seven days, whereas with plutonium-239 it is over 24,000 years. Biologic half-lives also vary, tending to be longer for bone-seeking radionuclides (for example, radium, strontium, and plutonium) than for

QUANTITIES AND UNITS

The *amount of radioactivity* that is present at any one time in a given sample of matter is expressed in *becquerels*. One becquerel (Bq) correponds to that quantity of radioactivity in which there is one atomic disintegration per second. Another unit that has been used for the same purpose is the *curie* (Ci). One Ci represents that quantity of radioactivity in which there are $3.7 \times 10^{10}$ atomic disintegrations per second ($1 \text{ Bq} = 2.7 \times 10^{-11}$ Ci).

The unit that is generally used for expressing the *dose of radiation* that is absorbed in tissue is the *gray* (Gy). Another unit used for the same purpose is the *rad* (1 Gy = 1 joule per kg of tissue = 100 rad).

The *sievert* (Sv) is the unit that expresses the so-called *dose equivalent*. This unit is used in radiologic protection to enable doses of different types of radiation to be normalized in terms of biologic effectiveness, since particulate radiations generally cause greater injury than x-rays or gamma rays for a given dose in Gy. Another unit that has been used for the same purpose is

the *rem* (1 Sv = 100 rem). The dose equivalent of any radiation in sieverts is the dose in Gy multiplied by an appropriate RBE-dependent quality factor Q. In principle, therefore, one sievert of any radiation represents that dose which is equivalent in biologic effectiveness to one gray of gamma rays.

For expressing the *collective dose* to a population, the *person-Sv* (or *person-rem*) is used. This unit represents the product of the average dose per person times the number of people exposed. For example, 1 sievert to each of 100 people equals 100 person-sievert (= 10,000 person-rem).

For measuring *exposure* to x-rays, the classic unit is the *roentgen*. One roentgen (R), defined loosely, is the amount of x-radiation that produces one electrostatic unit of charge in one cubic centimeter of air under standard conditions of temperature and pressure. Exposure of the surface of the skin to 1 R of x-rays deposits a dose of slightly less than 10 mGy (1 rad) in the underlying epidermis.

radionuclides that are deposited predominantly in soft tissue (for example, iodine, cesium, and tritium).

## Sources and Levels of Radiation in the Environment

All living organisms have evolved in the presence of natural background radiation. This radiation consists of (1) cosmic rays, which come from outer space; (2) terrestrial radiation, which emanates from the radium, thorium, uranium, and other radioactive elements in the earth's crust; and (3) internal radiations, which are emitted by the potassium-40, carbon-14, and other radionuclides contained within living cells themselves (Table 15-4). The average total dose received annually from all three sources by a person residing at sea level in the United States is slightly less than 1 mSv (100 mrem); however, a dose up to 30 percent larger may be received by a person residing at a higher elevation, where cosmic rays are more intense, or by a person residing in an area where the radium content of the soil is comparatively high. Also substantially higher is the average dose to the bronchial epithelium from inhaled radon and its daughters (Table 15-4).

A nuclear power plant worker who measured his radioactivity immediately on entering the plant found it to be unexpectedly high. On investigation, the source of his radioactivity was found to be the radon in his home, which was present at concentrations thousands of times higher than average. The discovery that his house contained such high levels of radon prompted the worker to take steps to reduce the levels, by improving the ventilation of the house and blocking the entry of radon from the underlying soil. His discovery also prompted a survey of radon levels in other houses throughout the U.S., preliminary results of which indicate radon levels to be well in excess of the recommended limits (4–8 pCi/liter) in a significant percentage of houses.

People are exposed to radiation from artificial as well as natural sources. The major source of ex-

**Table 15-4.** Estimated average soft tissue dose of radiation received annually by members of the U.S. population[a]

| Source of radiation | Dose/year (mSv) |
| --- | --- |
| Natural | |
|   Radon | 24[a] |
|   Cosmic | 0.27 |
|   Terrestrial | 0.28 |
|   Internal | 0.39 |
|   Total natural | 0.94[b] |
| Artificial | |
|   Medical | |
|     X-ray diagnosis | 0.39 |
|     Nuclear medicine | 0.14 |
|     Consumer products | 0.10 |
|   Other | |
|     Occupational | 0.009 |
|     Nuclear fuel cycle | <0.01 |
|     Fallout | <0.01 |
|     Miscellaneous[c] | <0.01 |
|   Total artificial | <0.66 |
|   Total natural and artificial | <1.60[b] |

[a]Dose equivalent to bronchi from radon daughter products.
[b]Excluding dose to bronchial tract
[c]Department of Energy facilities, smelters, transportation, etc.
Source: National Council on Radiation Protection and Measurements (NCRP). Ionizing radiation exposures of the population of the United States. Report no. 93. Washington, D.C.: National Council on Radiation Protection and Measurements, 1987.

posure to artificial radiation is the use of x-rays in medical diagnosis (Table 15-4). The average annual dose to the population from medical and dental examinations in developed countries now is a substantial fraction of that from natural background irradiation (Table 15-4). Smaller doses of artificial radiation are received from radioactive minerals in building materials, phosphate fertilizers, and crushed rock; radiation-emitting components of TV sets, smoke detectors, and other consumer products; radioactive fallout from atomic weapons; and nuclear power.

To protect radiation workers against excessive occupational irradiation, their working conditions are generally designed in such a way as to minimize their exposure; nevertheless, the dose they receive occupationally varies, depending on their particular work assignment and operating conditions (see Table 15-1). The average dose of whole-body radiation received occupationally by workers in the U.S. is less than 5 mSv (0.5 rem) per year, and fewer than 1 percent of workers exposed to ionizing radiation approach or exceed the maximum permissible limit (50 mSv) in any given year [3].

## Types of Radiation Injury

Irradiation can cause many types of effects on the human body, depending on the dose and the conditions of exposure. For purposes of radiologic protection, two types of radiation effects are distinguished: (1) *stochastic* effects, which vary in frequency but not severity with dose; and (2) *nonstochastic, or deterministic*, effects, which vary both in frequency and severity with dose [4]. Since the production of nonstochastic effects requires doses large enough to kill many cells, there are thresholds for such effects. The production of stochastic effects, on the other hand, can conceivably result from random injury to a single cell, with the result that no threshold for such effects is presumed to exist [4].

Stochastic effects include mutagenic effects, carcinogenic effects, and teratogenic effects. Nonstochastic effects include erythema of the skin, cataract of the lens, impairment of fertility, depression of hemopoiesis, and various other types of radiation-induced tissue injury. Both types of effects are end-results of radiation-induced changes at the cellular level, which are discussed briefly in the following section.

## Effects of Radiation on Cells

At the cellular level, radiation injury may include inhibition of cell division, damage to chromosomes, damage to genes (mutations), neoplastic transformation, and various other changes, all of which result from macromolecular lesions initiated by radiation-induced ions and free radicals. Any molecule in the cell can be altered by irradiation, but DNA is the most critical target since damage to a single gene can profoundly alter or kill the cell.

A dose of x-radiation that is sufficient to kill the average dividing cell (for example, 1–2 Sv) produces dozens of strand breaks and other changes in the cell's DNA molecules. Most of the changes in DNA are reparable, but those that are caused by high-LET radiation are likely to be less reparable than those caused by low-LET radiation. The ultimate fate of the DNA, in any case, is likely to depend on the effectiveness of the cell's repair processes as well as on the nature of the initial lesions themselves.

The susceptibility of cells to radiation-induced killing increases with their rate of proliferation. Dividing cells are thus radiosensitive as a class. The percentage of cells surviving, as measured by their ability to proliferate, tends to decrease exponentially with increasing dose. A rapidly delivered dose of 1 to 2 Sv generally reduces the surviving fraction to 1/e, or 37 percent; however, if the same dose of low-LET radiation is divided into two or more exposures separated by several hours, fewer cells are killed because some of the sublethal damage is repaired between exposures [2].

## Damage to Chromosomes

Radiation-induced changes in chromosome number and structure are among the most thoroughly studied effects of radiation. These changes result from the breakage and rearrangement of chromosomes, as well as from interference with the normal segregation of chromosomes to daughter cells at the time of cell division. The majority of such aberrations interfere with mitosis, causing the affected cell to die when it attempts to divide.

The frequency of chromosomal aberrations increases in proportion to the radiation dose in the low-to-intermediate dose range, the increase being steeper with high-LET radiation than with low-LET radiation. Also increased in frequency by irradiation are sister chromatid exchanges. In human blood lymphocytes irradiated in culture, the frequency of chromosomal aberrations approximates 0.1 per cell per Sv. The frequency of acentric and dicentric aberrations in such cells is also increased in radiation workers and other irradiated populations, in whom they can serve as a crude biologic dosimeter [5]. Only a small percentage of all chromosome aberrations in members of the general population is attributable to natural background radiation; the majority result from other causes, including certain viruses, chemicals, and drugs.

## Damage to Genes

Mutagenic effects of radiation have been investigated extensively in many types of cells, including human somatic cells, but heritable effects of radiation are yet to be documented in human germ cells. The increased frequency of mutations per locus amounts to about $10^{-6}$ per Sv in human lymphocytes and by about $10^{-5}$ Sv in mouse spermatogonia and oocytes, depending on the conditions of irradiation [6]. In view of the small magnitude of the increase per unit dose, it is not astonishing that no heritable abnormalities have been detectable in the children of atomic bomb survivors, given the limited number of such children (78,000) who have been available for examination and the relatively small average gonadal dose (0.5 Sv) that was received by their parents [6].

On the basis of the available data, the dose required to double the frequency of mutations in the human species has been estimated to lie between 0.2 and 2.5 Sv. Hence, it is inferred that only a small percentage (0.1–2.0 percent) of all genetically related diseases in the human population is attributable to natural background irradiation [6].

## Effects on Tissues

Effects of radiation on tissues include a wide variety of reactions, some of which are delayed. Mitotic inhibition and cytologic abnormalities, for example, may be detectable immediately in irradiated tissues, whereas fibrosis and other degenerative changes may not appear until months or years after exposure. Tissues in which cells proliferate rapidly are generally the first to exhibit injury [7].

In tissues capable of rapid cell turnover, the killing of dividing cells by irradiation tends to elicit the compensatory proliferation of surviving cells. As a result, a given dose causes less depletion of cells when spread out in time than when received in a single brief exposure. By the same token, the effects of a given dose are generally less severe if only a fraction of the cells in the tissue are irradiated than if the entire tissue is exposed [7].

Depending on the specific tissue or organ irradiated and the conditions of exposure, the effects of irradiation may vary greatly. Since it is beyond the scope of this chapter to review such effects comprehensively, only those reactions that are particularly relevant to occupational irradiation are discussed briefly in the following section.

### Skin

Because of the superficial location of the skin, its response to radiation has been investigated more thoroughly than that of any other organ. Erythema is the earliest outward reaction of the skin, and it may occur within minutes or hours after exposure, depending on the dose. After rapid exposure to a dose of 6 Sv or more, the reaction typically lasts only a few hours, to be followed 2 to 4 weeks later by one or more waves of deeper and more prolonged erythema. After a dose of 10 Sv or more, dry desquamation, moist desquamation, necrosis of the skin, and epilation may ensue, followed eventually by pigmentation. Sequelae, which may develop months or years later, include atrophy of the epidermis and its adnexae, telangiectasia, and dermal fibrosis [7].

### Bone Marrow and Lymphoid Tissue

Hemopoietic cells are highly radiosensitive and show degenerative changes within minutes after a dose in excess of 1 Sv. If a dose as high as 2 to 3 Sv is received rapidly by the whole body, a sufficient percentage of such cells is killed so that the normal replacement of aging leukocytes, platelets, and erythrocytes is impaired. As a result, the blood count declines gradually, leading to maximal depression of the leukocyte and platelet counts in 3 to 5 weeks (Fig. 15-1). After rapid exposure to a dose above 5 Sv, leukopenia and thrombocytopenia are likely to be severe enough to cause fatal infection, hemorrhage, or both [8]. Doses larger than 5 Sv can be tolerated only if they are accumulated gradually, over a period of months, or delivered to only a small portion of the total marrow.

Lymphocytes also are highly radiosensitive, degenerating rapidly after intensive irradiation. A

**Fig. 15-1.** Hematologic values, symptoms, and clinical signs in five men exposed to whole-body irradiation in a criticality accident. (The blood counts are average values for the five men; the figures in parentheses denote the number showing the symptoms and signs indicated). (From GA Andrews, EW Sitterson, AL Kretchmar, M Brucer. Criticality accidents at the Y-12 plant. In Diagnosis and treatment of acute radiation injury. Geneva: World Health Organization, 1961, pp. 27–48.)

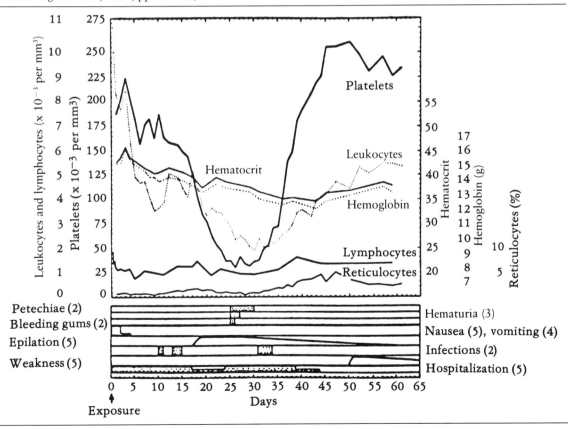

dose of whole-body irradiation in excess of 2 to 3 Sv thus causes severe aplasia of lymphoid tissues, with profound depression of the immune response.

### Gastrointestinal Tract

In many respects, the reaction of the gastrointestinal tract to irradiation resembles that of the skin. Dividing cells in the mucosal epithelium of the small intestine are highly radiosensitive and are killed in sufficient numbers by a dose of 10 Sv to interfere with normal renewal of the epithelium. The resulting depletion of epithelial cells, if sufficiently severe, may lead within a few days to ulceration and, ultimately, denudation of the mucosa. Hence rapid delivery of a dose in excess of 10 Sv to a large part of the small intestine, as may happen in the event of a radiation accident, can cause a fatal dysentery-like syndrome [8].

### Gonads

Because of the high radiosensitivity of spermatogonia, the seminiferous tubules are among the most radiosensitive organs of the body. Acute exposure of the testes to a dose as low as 0.15 Sv suffices to depress the sperm count for months, and a dose of more than 2 Sv may cause permanent sterility [7].

Oocytes also are highly radiosensitive. Acute exposure of both ovaries to a dose of 1.5 to 2.0 Sv can cause temporary sterility, and a dose of 2.0 to 3.0 Sv can result in permanent sterility, depending on the age of the woman at the time of exposure.

### Lens of the Eye

Irradiation of the lens can cause the formation of lens opacities, or cataracts, which may not become evident until months or years later. The frequency, severity, and timing of the opacities depend on the dose and its distribution in time and space. The threshold for a vision-impairing opacity is estimated to vary from 2 to 3 Sv received in a single brief exposure, to 5.5 to 14.0 Sv received in repeated exposures over a period of months [7].

In the 1940s, a number of pioneer cyclotron physicists developed radiation cataracts as a result of their occupational exposure to neutrons. The occurrence of cataracts in these workers provided the first indication of the high relative biologic effectiveness of neutrons for injury to the lens [7].

## Radiation Sickness

Intensive irradiation of a major part of the hemopoietic system or the gastrointestinal tract can kill sufficient numbers of cells in these tissues to cause radiation sickness ("acute radiation syndrome"), as mentioned previously. The associated prodromal symptoms characteristically include anorexia, nausea, and vomiting during the first few hours after irradiation, followed by a symptom-free interval until the main phase of the illness [7, 8] (Table 15-5).

In the intestinal form of the syndrome, the main phase of the illness typically begins 2 to 3 days after irradiation, with abdominal pain, fever, and increasingly severe diarrhea, dehydration, disturbance of salt and fluid balance, prostration, toxemia, and shock, leading to death within 7 to 14 days [7, 8].

In the hemopoietic form of the syndrome, the main phase typically begins in the second or third week after irradiation, with granulocytopenia, thrombocytopenia, and other complications of radiation-induced aplasia of the bone marrow. If damage to the marrow is sufficiently severe, death may ensue between the fourth and the sixth week after irradiation, from septicemia, exsanguination, or other complications [7, 8]. At midlethal dose levels, the probability of survival varies among individuals, depending on differences in hemopoietic reserve, resistance to infection, and other variables [8].

Within hours after performing maintenance work in a large industrial radiography facility that was subsequently found to have a defective safety interlock system, a pipefitter experienced transitory nausea and vomiting. One to two weeks later, generalized erythema developed, followed within several days by loss of hair, sore throat, bleeding from the gums, diarrhea, and

**Table 15-5.** Symptoms of acute radiation sickness

| Time after exposure | Lethal dose (6–10 Gy) | Median lethal dose (3–5 Gy) | Moderate dose (1–2 Gy) |
|---|---|---|---|
| First hours | Nausea and vomiting within several hours | | |
| First week | Diarrhea, vomiting, inflammation of throat | No definite symptoms | |
| Second week | Fever, rapid emaciation, leading to death in all exposed | | |
| Third week | | Loss of hair begins, loss of appetite, general malaise, fever, hemorrhages, pallor | |
| Fourth week | | Leading to rapid emaciation and death for 50 percent of the exposed population | Loss of appetite, sore throat, pallor and diarrhea. Recovery begins (no deaths in absence of complications) |

weakness. On examination, 3 weeks after his initial onset of symptoms, his lymphocyte count was 1,100 per mm$^3$, leukocyte count 2,200 per mm$^3$, platelet count 27,000 per mm$^3$, hematocrit 40 percent, and reticulocyte count 1 percent. On cytogenetic analysis, his blood lymphocytes revealed an increased frequency of chromosomal aberrations, consistent with whole-body ionizing irradiation. Following treatment with platelet transfusions and antibiotics, his symptoms subsided in 2 to 3 weeks.

A third form of the acute radiation syndrome, the cerebral form, can result from acute exposure of the brain to a dose in excess of 50 Sv. In this syndrome, the same prodromal symptoms—anorexia, nausea, and vomiting—occur almost immediately after irradiation, but are followed within minutes or hours by increasing drowsiness, ataxia, confusion, convulsions, loss of consciousness, and death [7, 8].

## Effects on Growth and Development of the Embryo

Embryonal and fetal tissues are extremely radiosensitive, in keeping with their highly proliferative character. Rapid exposure to 0.25 Sv during a critical stage in organogenesis has been observed to cause malformations of many types in experimental animals [6]. Comparable effects have been observed after larger doses in prenatally irradiated children. Mental retardation, for example, was greatly increased in frequency in children who were exposed to atomic bomb radiation at Hiroshima and Nagasaki between the eighth and fifteenth weeks of prenatal development [6].

## Effects on Cancer Incidence

Observations on atomic bomb survivors, patients exposed to radiation for medical purposes, and early radiation workers (such as radiologists, radium dial painters, and pitchblende miners) indicate that many types of cancer can be increased in frequency by irradiation, depending on the conditions of exposure [6, 8]. The cancers resulting from irradiation, however, do not appear until years or decades later and have no distinguishing features by which they can be recognized as radiation-induced. Hence, the occurrence of a given cancer in an irradiated individual cannot be attributed with certainty to his or her previous irradiation.

The epidemiologic data came predominantly from observations at relatively high doses (0.5–2.0 Sv) and do not define the shape of the dose-incidence curve in the low-dose domain. Thus, the carcinogenic risks of low-level irradiation can be estimated only by interpolation or extrapolation, based on assumptions about the relationship between incidence and dose.

The most extensive dose-incidence data pertain to leukemia and cancer of the female breast. For leukemias other than the chronic lymphocytic type, the overall incidence increases with dose during the first 5 to 25 years after irradiation, by approximately three cases per year per 10,000 persons at risk per Sv to the bone marrow [6, 8]. The relationship between the total cumulative incidence and the dose can be represented by various mathematical functions, including a linear-nonthreshold function, but interpretation of the dose-incidence data is complicated by unexplained variations among different types of leukemia in the magnitude of the increase for a given dose, age at irradiation, and time after exposure (Fig. 15-2). It is noteworthy that the incidence of chronic lymphocytic leukemia is apparently unaffected by irradiation [6, 8].

For cancer of the female breast, the incidence appears to increase in proportion to the dose (Fig. 15-3), and the magnitude of the increase for a given dose seems to be essentially the same whether the radiation is received instantaneously (as in the atomic bomb survivors), over 1 to 4 days

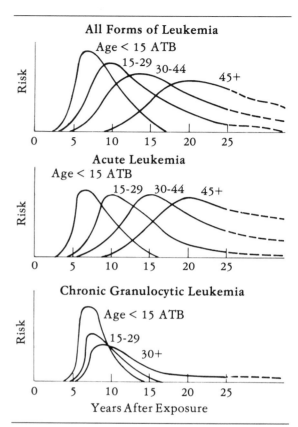

Fig. 15-2. Schematic representation of the time distribution of the increase in absolute risk of leukemia in atomic bomb survivors in relation to age at time of irradiation. (ATB = at time of bomb.) (From M Ichimaru, T Ishimaru. A review of thirty years study of Hiroshima and Nagasaki atomic bomb survivors. II. Biological effects. D. Leukemia and related disorders. J Radiat Res 1975; 16 (Suppl.):89–96.)

(as in women treated with x-rays for acute postpartum mastitis), or over many months (as in luminous dial painters or women who received multiple fluoroscopic examinations of the chest in the treatment of pulmonary tuberculosis). The consistency of the dose-incidence relationship (Fig. 15-3) suggests that successive, small, widely spaced exposures are fully additive in their cumulative carcinogenic effects on the breast and that the in-

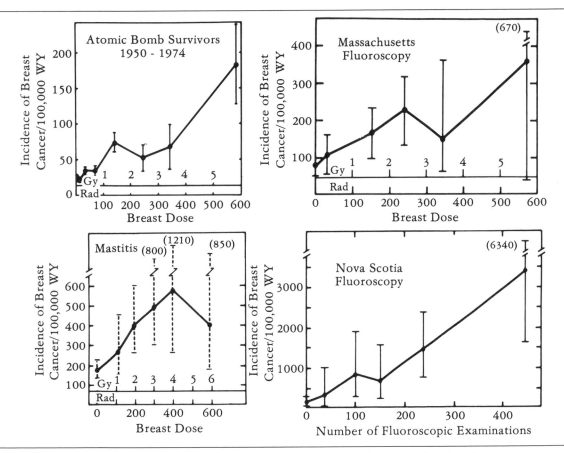

**Fig. 15-3.** Incidence of breast cancer in relation to dose in women exposed to atomic bomb radiation, women subjected to multiple fluoroscopic examinations of the chest in the treatment of pulmonary tuberculosis, and women given x-ray therapy to the breast for acute postpartum mastitis. (From JD Boice, Jr., et al. Risk of breast cancer following low-dose exposure. Radiology 1979; 131:589–97.)

cidence thus increases as a linear, nonthreshold function of the cumulative dose [6, 8].

Two additional lines of evidence for carcinogenic effects at low doses are (1) an increased incidence of thyroid cancer after 0.06 to 0.20 Gy x-irradiation to the thyroid gland in childhood and (2) an association between juvenile cancer and prenatal diagnostic x-irradiation [6, 8]. The latter has been interpreted to imply that exposure in utero to as little as 10 to 50 mGy may increase a child's risk of cancer by 40 to 50 percent [6, 8].

Other types of cancer also are increased in prevalence in irradiated populations (Table 15-6). The excess is generally dose-dependent, larger with high-LET radiation than with low-LET radiation, and of varying magnitude for a given dose, depending on the organ irradiated and the age at exposure (Table 15-6).

The total excess of all cancers combined approximates 2 to 10 cases per thousand persons per Sv per year, beginning 5 to 10 years after whole-body irradiation and continuing thereafter

**Table 15-6.** Estimated lifetime excess mortality from radiation-induced cancer (per million per mSv), by type of malignancy and age at whole-body irradiation

| | No. of fatal cancers by age at exposure | | | | |
| Type of malignancy | 25 yr | 35 yr | 45 yr | 55 yr | 65 yr |
| --- | --- | --- | --- | --- | --- |
| Leukemia | 35 | 55 | 90 | 145 | 170 |
| Respiratory system | 125 | 225 | 315 | 330 | 220 |
| Digestive system | 535 | 50 | 45 | 40 | 30 |
| Other | 355 | 230 | 120 | 45 | 15 |
| Total | 1050 | 560 | 570 | 560 | 435 |
| % of normal | 0.5 | 0.3 | 0.3 | 0.3 | 0.2 |

*Average for both sexes, values rounded.
Source: National Academy of Sciences/National Research Council. Committee on the Biological Effects of Ionizing Radiation. (BEIR V.) Health effects of ionizing radiation. Washington, D.C.: National Academy Press, 1990.

for the duration of life. The cumulative lifetime excess is thus estimated to approximate 800 additional cancers per thousand persons at risk per Sv, which corresponds to an increase of 40 to 50 percent per Sv in the average lifetime risk of cancer [6, 8].

## Comparative Magnitude of Radiation Risks

From the above risk estimates, the number of cancers attributable to occupational irradiation in radiation workers can be calculated to constitute less than 10 percent of the number expected to occur naturally in this population. Also, the average loss of life expectancy from all causes in radiation workers is estimated to be no greater than that in occupations (such as construction and transportation) that are generally considered to be relatively safe [7].

Nevertheless, since no amount of radiation is assumed to be entirely without risk, no dose in principle can be considered acceptable if it is readily avoidable. For this reason, the guiding rule in radiologic protection is the ALARA principle; that is, the dose should be kept *as low as reasonably achievable*.

## Radiation Protection

From the beginning of this century, increasing efforts have been made to prevent injury in radiation workers by limiting their occupational exposure. Initially, acute injuries were the main source of concern, and attempts were made to set "tolerance" doses, or threshold limit values (TLVs), to prevent such injuries. Gradually, however, it came to be suspected that genetic, carcinogenic, and teratogenic effects might have no threshold. Hence, the concept of a "tolerance" dose for the latter types of effects was eventually replaced by the concept of a "maximum permissible" dose, that is, a dose that was not intended to prevent stochastic effects altogether (since this would presumably be impossible without reducing the dose to zero) but that was intended to limit the frequency of such effects to levels that were acceptably low. At present, therefore, the system of protection for radiation workers involves two sets of dose limits; one of them is intended to prevent nonstochastic effects altogether, and the other is meant to limit the risks of stochastic effects to levels that are acceptably low [7].

To prevent the occurrence of nonstochastic, or deterministic, effects, the recommended annual dose equivalent limit has been set at 0.5 Sv (50 rem) for all organs other than the lens of the eye;

for the lens of the eye, the recommended annual dose equivalent limit has been set at 0.15 Sv (15 rem) [7]. To limit the risks of stochastic effects (genetic effects, carcinogenic effects, and teratogenic effects) to acceptable levels, the recommended dose equivalent limit for the whole body has been set at 50 mSv (5 rem) for any one year, and 2 mSv (2 rem) per year averaged over any 5-year period; the annual dose equivalent limits for individual organs have been weighted in such a way that the combined risks of stochastic effects resulting from irradiation of any combination of organs separately do not exceed the overall risk of stochastic effects resulting from irradiation of the body as a whole [7]. This system of dose limitation is intended to protect radiation workers completely against radiation-induced cataracts, impairment of fertility, depression of hemopoiesis, and other deterministic effects, and to keep their combined risks of radiation-induced cancers, serious genetic diseases, and teratogenic effects from exceeding 1 per 1,000 per year, a rate of fatal work-related injuries encountered in many industries that are generally regarded as acceptably safe [7].

To minimize the radiation exposure of workers without unduly sacrificing their efficiency requires careful design of the workplace and work procedures, thorough training and supervision of workers, implementation of a well-conceived radiation protection program, and systematic health physics oversight and monitoring (Fig. 15-4).

Also needed are careful provisions for dealing with radiation accidents, emergencies, and other contingencies; systematic recording and updating of each worker's exposures; thorough labeling of all radiation sources and exposure fields; appropriate interlocks to guard against inadvertent irradiation; and various other precautionary measures [7, 9–12].

General principles to be observed in every radiation protection program include the following [12, 13]:

1. A well-developed, well-rehearsed, and updated emergency preparedness plan should be in place, in order to enable prompt and effective response in the event of a malfunction, spill, or other radiation accident.
2. Appropriate use of shielding in facilities, equipment, and work clothing (apron, gloves, etc.).
3. Appropriate selection, installation, maintenance, and operation of all equipment.
4. Minimization of exposure time.
5. Maximization of distance between personnel and sources of radiation (the intensity of exposure decreases inversely with the square of the distance from the source).
6. Appropriate training and supervision of workers to accomplish routine tasks with minimal exposure and to cope safely with irregularities.

## Management of the Irradiated Worker

In any workplace where employees may be exposed accidentally to radiation or radioactive material, plans for coping with such contingencies must be made in advance. These require delineation of lines of authority for managing accidents, knowledge in the workplace of the local health care facilities capable of evaluating and treating radiation accident victims, plans for transporting radioactive victims, and an understanding by the workers of the hazards of radiation.

In managing a radiation accident victim, good medical judgment and first aid should come first. Hence, even if the victim has been heavily irradiated or contaminated, he or she must also be evaluated for other forms of injury, such as mechanical trauma, burns, and smoke inhalation. To guard against self-contamination, those handling or examining the victim should wear gloves, masks, and other protective clothing.

The following general principles also should be observed [9–13]:

### General Emergency Medical Procedures
1. Emergency diagnostic and therapeutic maneuvers to assure stability of airway, respiration,

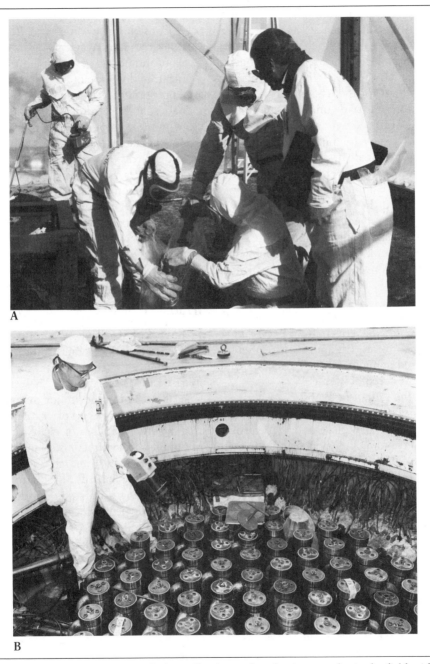

**Fig. 15-4.** A. Proper protection is necessary during collecting and packaging samples in the field with low-level radioactive contamination. B. Monitoring radiation levels atop a nuclear reactor. (Photographs courtesy of RL Kathren, Battelle Pacific Northwest Laboratory.)

circulation, and so forth, should be applied as necessary.

2. Appropriate transport of the victim should be summoned, and the attendants alerted to the effect that he or she has been irradiated or contaminated.

3. The appropriate medical facility should be notified to expect the victim and informed that he or she has been irradiated or contaminated.

4. Detailed records should be kept concerning all examinations, measurements, findings, procedures, personnel, and times involved.

### *Procedures for Radioactive Contamination*

1. Clothing should be removed promptly if contaminated, isolated in a plastic bag, and labeled to denote radioactivity.

2. Any contaminated parts of the body should be isolated with plastic or paper from the rest of the body and other surroundings, and monitored for radioactivity.

3. Contaminated parts of the body should be thoroughly rinsed, contaminated rinse water isolated as "radioactive waste," and the part monitored again.

4. Care should be taken to avoid abrasion of contaminated skin during rinsing in order to minimize hyperemia and further absorption of radioactivity.

5. To expedite elimination of any inhaled radioactivity, the victim should rinse the oral and nasal cavities by gargling and snorting water.

6. Secretions should be collected in plastic bags, labeled, and isolated for future examination.

7. The victim should be isolated from others who are not essential for emergency care.

8. Precautions should be taken to avoid contamination of other people, objects, and areas. For this purpose, the contaminated area should be sealed off as soon as possible.

## References

1. Lushbaugh CC, Fry SA, Ricks RC. Nuclear reactor accidents: Preparedness and consequences. Br J Radiol 1987; 60:1159–83.

2. National Council on Radiation Protection and Measurements (NCRP). The relative biological effectiveness of radiations of different quality. Bethesda, MD: National Council on Radiation Protection and Measurements, 1990. (NCRP report no. 104.)

3. National Council on Radiation Protection and Measurements (NCRP). Exposure of the U.S. population from occupational radiation. Bethesda, MD: National Council on Radiation Protection and Measurements, 1989. (NCRP report no. 101.)

4. International Commission on Radiological Protection (ICRP). Recommendations of the International Commission on Radiological Protection. Oxford: Pergamon, 1991. (ICRP publication 60, Annals of the ICRP, vol. 21, pp. 1–3).

5. Lloyd DC, Purrott RJ. Chromosome aberration analysis in radiological protection dosimetry. Radiat Prot Dosim 1981; 1:19–28.

6. National Academy of Sciences/National Research Council. Committee on the Biological Effects of Ionizing Radiation (BEIR V). Health effects of exposure to low levels of ionizing radiation. Washington, D.C.: National Academy Press, 1990.

7. International Commission on Radiological Protection (ICRP). Nonstochastic effects of radiation. Oxford: Pergamon, 1984. (ICRP publication 41, Annals of the ICRP, vol. 14, no. 3.)

8. United Nations Scientific Committee on the Effects of Atomic Radiation (UNSCEAR). Sources, effects and risks of ionizing radiation. Report to the General Assembly, with annexes. New York: United Nations, 1988.

9. National Council on Radiation Protection and Measurements (NCRP). Management of persons accidentally contaminated with radionuclides. Washington, D.C.: National Council on Radiation Protection and Measurements, 1980. (NCRP report no. 65.)

10. International Atomic Energy Agency (IAEA). What the general practitioner (MD) should know about medical handling of overexposed individuals. Vienna, Austria: International Atomic Energy Agency, 1986. (IAEA-TECDOC-366.)

11. Mettler FA, Kelsey CA, Ricks RC. Medical management of radiation accidents. Boca Raton, FL: CRC Press, 1990.

12. National Council on Radiation Protection and Measurements (NCRP). Operational radiation safety

program. Washington, D.C.: National Council on Radiation Protection and Measurements, 1978. (NCRP report no. 59.)

13. Kahn K, Ryan K, Sabo A, Boyce P. Ionizing radiation. In BS Levy, DH Wegman. eds. Occupational health. Boston: Little, Brown, 1983, pp. 189–206.

# Bibliography

International Commission on Radiological Protection (ICRP). Recommendations of the International Commission on Radiological Protection. Oxford: Pergamon, 1991. (ICRP publication 60, Annals of the ICRP, vol. 21, pp. 1–3.)

*A detailed summary and explanation of the Commission's recommendations for limiting the exposure of workers and the public to ionizing radiation.*

Lushbaugh CC, Fry SA, Ricks RC. Nuclear reactor accidents: Preparedness and consequences. Br J Radiol 1987; 60:1159–83.

*A review by recognized authorities on the causes, nature, and management of reactor accidents occurring in various countries between 1945 and 1987.*

National Academy of Sciences/National Research Council. Committee on the Biological Effects of Ionizing Radiation (BEIR V). Health effects of exposure to low levels of ionizing radiation. Washington, D.C.: National Academy Press, 1990.

*A comprehensive review of the biomedical effects of low-level irradiation, including estimates of the risks of genetic, carcinogenic, and teratogenic effects associated with occupational and environmental exposures.*

National Council on Radiation Protection and Measurements (NCRP). Exposure of the U.S. population from occupational radiation. Bethesda, MD: National Council on Radiation Protection and Measurements, 1989. (NCRP report no. 101.)

*A comprehensive review of the sources and levels of ionizing radiation to which the U.S. population is exposed.*

National Council on Radiation Protection and Measurements (NCRP). The relative biological effectiveness of radiations of different quality. Bethesda, MD: National Council on Radiation Protection and Measurements, 1990. (NCRP report no. 104.)

*A review of the extent to which the relative effectiveness of ionizing radiation for various types of biologic effects varies as a function of the linear energy transfer of the radiation.*

United Nations Scientific Committee on the Effects of Atomic Radiation (UNSCEAR). Sources, effects and risks of ionizing radiation. Report to the General Assembly, with annexes. New York: United Nations, 1988.

*A comprehensive review of the sources and levels of ionizing radiation to which the population is exposed, and of the associated risks of health effects. Included is a review of the Chernobyl accident and its consequences.*

# 16
# Noise and Hearing Impairment

Robert I. Davis and Roger P. Hamernik

Since the Industrial Revolution, the noise levels in most societies have increased continually to such an extent that exposure to excessively loud sound now constitutes a serious hazard to hearing, with profound impacts on the quality of life for the affected individual. Sound is ubiquitous. Excessive levels of noise are present in industrial and military work environments and permeate our social environments. The scope of the problem is large, with estimates of close to 8 million civilian workers in the United States exposed to potentially damaging levels of noise, and many more exposed to such levels in the military and outside of work. Thus, an understanding of the mechanisms of noise-induced hearing loss (NIHL) and the strategies for combating the hazards of exposure are essential to public health and occupational health professionals.

To protect hearing from excessive noise exposure, we are required to answer what appears to be a fundamentally simple question: "How much noise is too much?" However, the answer to this question has eluded researchers. The answer is problematic, because it transcends scientific methodology and requires that important political and economic decisions be made. In this chapter, we are concerned primarily with the consequences of excessive noise exposure on our ability to hear.

The ear at the periphery is composed of three major components—the external ear, the middle ear, and the cochlea—and centrally, the ascending and descending auditory pathways of the central nervous system. To understand how noise affects hearing, some knowledge of the function of these structures is necessary. Also, some familiarity with the science of acoustics is needed before a meaningful examination of the various approaches to developing noise exposure standards is possible.

## Sound as the Physical Stimulus— Some Definitions

There are two broad classes of noise: continuous and impulsive. A noise is continuous if, once initiated, it continues for a prolonged period of time. Since, in some respects, our scaling of time is relative to the event being studied, this definition is not very precise, but for an industrial exposure situation we might consider an eight-hour period as representing a continuous exposure. However, the typical workday exposure is invariably broken up by rest periods and lunch. Thus, in reality, the exposure is interrupted. Experimental data on the effects of interruption are, in general, lacking. Impulsive noise is generally considered to be a "relatively" short (in duration), often intense presentation, which can occur at regular intervals throughout a workday or only sporadically.

Various intermediate types of noise and various combinations of different types can be defined. In many industrial situations, impulsive noise components are superimposed on a background continuous noise. Current measurement practice is not designed to accurately assess such combination exposures and will usually underestimate considerably the hazard potential of impulse-continuous noise combinations. In practice, some standards for continuous noise currently exist, but standards for impulsive noise exposures are still evolving, and little consideration is given to the interaction between different classes of noise or other causes of trauma to the ear, such as vibration, drugs, or disease processes.

Standards for exposure to noise, as well as hearing conservation manuals, use a variety of specialized terms from the science of acoustics that are not generally familiar. Therefore, understanding of commonly used terms is necessary before one can interpret information or instructions associated with hearing conservation measures with confidence (see box).

Complex industrial noise is often characterized by the Fourier spectrum computed or measured in terms of octave bands; that is, we can measure the sound pressure level (SPL) of consecutive octave frequency bands to determine how the SPL is distributed across the range of frequencies of interest. Figure 16-1 illustrates two typical frequency spectrums for a metal stamping mill. The spectra are somewhat typical of industrial noises, with energy maxima in the 200- to 500-Hz region. Since the ear is differentially sensitive to sounds of different frequencies, such an analysis is an important step in the evaluation of the potential hazards of a noise environment. If the spectrum analysis shows that the energy of the noise in question is relatively uniformly distributed over a wide range of frequencies, the noise is called a broad band of noise. Prominent energy peaks in the spectrum in very narrow bands of frequencies may indicate the presence of pure tones or unusual concentrations of acoustic energy. In general, the more concentrated the acoustic energy is in the spectral domain, the greater the potential noise hazard is to the auditory system.

In addition to the variety of continuous noises, there is a large class of transient noises referred to as impulsive. Typically, these have high intensities and short durations (< 1 second). Both explosive

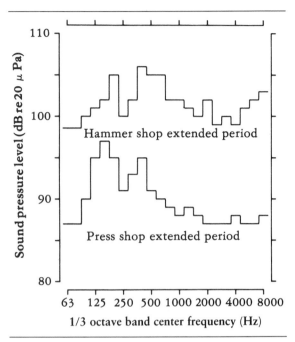

Fig. 16-1. An example of a $\frac{1}{3}$ octave band spectrum of the noise in a forging industry. (From W Taylor et al. J Acoust Soc Am 1984; 76:808.)

discharges, such as gunfire, and industrial impacts produced by intermittent metal-to-metal contact fall in this category. Such noises are common in industrial and military environments. Impulse noise exposures can, in general, be more hazardous than continuous noise exposures. Part of the reason for this is that, subjectively, we tend to underestimate the potential of an impulse for causing trauma because its transient nature makes it seem quieter than it truly is. Between the extremes presented above fall a myriad of intermediate types of noise.

When sound impinges on a surface, such as the walls of a room or the tympanic membrane, a part is reflected, a part is transmitted, and a part is absorbed by the surface. These properties of sound theoretically allow the engineer to control the sound environment: Suitable design of walls can contain the sound; suitable materials in the vicin-

## SOUND DEFINITIONS

*Sound*, or *noise*, is a fluctuation of the ambient pressure that propagates in the elastic media, air. This longitudinally propagating disturbance, or wave, is capable of exerting a fluctuating force (pressure × area) on any surface on which it impinges. Thus, the magnitude of the pressure change above and below atmospheric pressure can be used as a measure of the strength of the sound wave and is given in units of newtons per square meter ($N/m^2$), called *Pascals* (Pa). Because the ear is responsive to sound waves whose strength can cover a dynamic range on the order of more than $10^6$, it is advantageous to use a logarithmic scale to measure the strength of a sound wave. A range of $10^6$ on a linear scale converted into a logarithmic scale (Bel scale) is compressed into a range of 6 Bel units or a range of 60 units on a *decibel* (dB) scale. The dB scale is used in acoustical measurements where the strength of a sound wave can be defined in terms of a dB level. The *sound pressure level* (SPL) represents a ratio measure of the strength of the sound being measured relative to the reference pressure fluctuation. A sound wave that is twice as strong as the reference value produces a 6-dB increase in SPL over the reference value, which is still a very weak disturbance. The reference pressure is approximately equal to the smallest disturbance that the normal ear can just detect at its most sensitive frequency. If over time and space the disturbance of pressure follows a regular sine wave pattern, the sound is a *pure tone*. The rate at which the pressure fluctuations repeat in a sinusoidal fashion is called the *frequency* and is given in units of cycles per second, termed *Hertz* (Hz). Thus, a pure tone consists of a single frequency (f). The usual range of frequencies of interest in hearing science lies roughly between 20 and 20,000 Hz. The range of human

conversation is from about 300 to 3,000 Hz. The speed at which the wave propagates through the environment is called the *speed of sound*, c meters per second (m/s), and is uniquely determined by the thermodynamic properties of the media in which the wave is traveling. In air, at standard conditions, c = 343 m/s. Therefore, the spacial extent of the disturbance created by a pure tone f, called the *wave length* ($\lambda$), is given by $\lambda$ = c/f (meters); the duration of the disturbance in time, the period T, is given as T = l/f (sec). (This formula is nothing more complex than velocity × time = distance.) In most industrial situations, pure tones are uncommon and the noise usually consists of a relatively complex temporal pattern of pressure fluctuations. *Fourier analysis*, which can be applied to most noises likely to be encountered in practice, is a mathematical means of decomposing a complex wave form into a series of pure tones having specific amplitudes, frequencies, and temporal relations to each other (phase). Thus, the temporal pattern of sound (amplitude versus time), which we intuitively feel that we are sensing with our ears, can be transformed uniquely into the frequency and phase domain to obtain a different, but equivalent, physical description of the sound. Fourier analysis has a wide application in noise research. Different types of sound can be more precisely classified in the frequency domain: For example, an octave band of noise contains all frequencies lying between upper and lower frequency limits such that the upper frequency is equal to two times the lower frequency. An octave band is usually defined by its center frequency—that is, the geometric mean of the upper and lower frequencies. Thus, an octave band of noise with a center frequency of 1,000 Hz would have 710 and 1,400 Hz as the approximate lower and upper frequency limits.

ity of the sound source can absorb the sound energy and convert it into harmless heat energy; suitable design of machinery can reduce or eliminate the source of the noise. Although engineering solutions can be difficult and expensive to implement, they still need to be considered in many situations.

Under field conditions, sounds are usually measured with a portable sound level meter, which is capable of converting the forces generated by the pressure fluctuations acting on a sensitive microphone element into an electrical signal. The electronics of the meter process this signal to produce a single number representing a mean SPL in dB or dB(A), the weighted scale, which is discussed later. These meters can also be equipped with octave or ⅓ octave band analyzers to obtain the SPL in consecutive bands of frequencies.

## The Hearing Mechanism

Scientifically, much has been learned about the fundamental processes of hearing and how noise affects psychoacoustic performance, the basic physiology of the cochlea, and the morphology of the sensory elements of the cochlea [1, 2]. The need for the survival of the evolving species required that the sound-sensing organ be able to detect extremely low-level stimuli in the presence of various masking noises, such as the approach of a predator masked by the rustle of leaves. Under such pressures, the ear has evolved into an exquisitely sensitive mechanoelectric transducer, which converts airborne sound energy impinging on the external ear into a micromechanical wave motion in the cochlea and, in turn, into a series of ordered electrical discharges (action potentials) that are transmitted via the eighth cranial nerve into the brainstem for subsequent information processing in higher cortical centers. The ear was not designed for the types of contemporary noise environments to which it is being exposed.

The external ear and canal terminating at the tympanic membrane is the initial conducting pathway for sound entering the ear (Fig. 16-2A). Often modeled as a tube closed at one end, the external canal has resonance properties such that it can amplify certain regions of the environmental noise spectrum by more than 10 dB in the frequency range of approximately 2,000 to 4,000 Hz, thus increasing the potential of that noise for producing hearing loss [3].

The middle ear, as a sound transmission line, is bound laterally by the tympanic membrane and medially by the oval window. Between these two membranes are fastened the three smallest bones of the body, the ossicles: the malleus, the incus, and the stapes. These bones are suspended by several ligaments and are under limited muscular control. The two smallest muscles of the body, the tensor tympani and the stapedius, attach to the malleus and stapes, respectively. These muscles are under voluntary control in some individuals, but normally, contractions of these muscles are initiated by excessively loud sounds (the acoustic reflex). For sound to reach the fluid-filled cochlea, it must first be conducted through the middle ear—that is, from the air environment of the external canal into the liquid environment of the cochlea. Because of the different physical properties of air and water, the ability of airborne sound to penetrate into a fluid environment is severely limited and some form of mechanical advantage (amplification) is necessary. Without amplification, more than 99 percent of the acoustic energy incident on a water surface is reflected. The middle ear performs this amplification in a frequency-selective manner, being most efficient in the 500- to 5,000-Hz region of the sound spectrum and least efficient at the extremely low or high frequencies.

The contraction of the muscles of the middle ear stiffens the tympanic membrane and ossicular chain and thereby reduces the transmission of sound energy to the cochlea. This reduction in transmission is achieved by an increase in the input impedance to the cochlea and is itself a frequency-dependent phenomena. Since the effects of stiffness on the impedance are inversely related to frequency, the acoustic reflex affects middle-ear

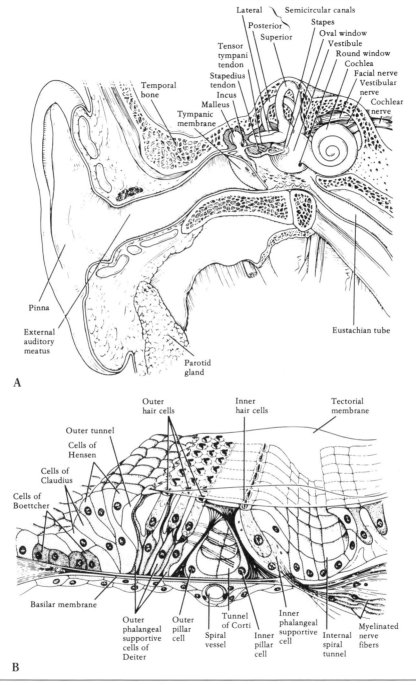

**Fig. 16-2.** A. Schematic representation of the relationships among the major anatomic components of the ear. (From LC Junqueira et al. Basic histology. San Mateo, CA: Lange, 1977.) B. A schematic of the organ of Corti illustrating the relation between sensory and supporting epithelia and the basilar membrane. (From WB Bloom, DW Fawcett. A textbook of histology. 10th ed. Philadelphia: Saunders, 1975.)

325

transmission most strongly at low frequencies. Contraction in response to loud sounds is initiated at sound pressure levels in the range of 70 to 100 dB above the hearing threshold.

A number of theories have been proposed concerning the functional role of the acoustic reflex. One popular theory contends that since the reflex is elicited by sound levels that are potentially damaging to the auditory system, the primary purpose of the reflex is the protection of the cochlea. However, this "protection theory" is weakened by the fact that the latency and the rapid adaptation of the reflex cause it to respond too slowly to sudden sounds, such as impact noises, and make it ineffective against steady, continuous noises. Although the greatest reduction in sound transmission (20–30 dB) occurs for low frequencies, the protection offered by the reflex appears to be a beneficial side effect of a more functional purpose. Since the reflex mainly attenuates low frequencies, and since most of an individual's physiologic noises as well as environmental noises are of a low-frequency nature, the reflex response, when activated, should reduce both internal and external noise environments, resulting in an improved signal-to-noise ratio and subsequent improvement of speech intelligibility in high noise level environments.

The transmission characteristics of the external ear and middle ear therefore alter the spectrum of sound that is ultimately received by the cochlea. Hence, a knowledge of the free-field spectrum (assigned to the source alone) is important as a first estimate of its potential for causing hearing damage. For example, the relative lack of sensitivity of the cochlea to low-frequency sounds has led to the development of the dB(A) scale of sound pressure measurement. This A scale, in essence, biases the measurement of the sound against the low-frequency end of the spectrum. In this sense, it is a scale that mirrors the ear's sensitivity and thus is frequently used for measurements of noise environments where the hazard to hearing is to be evaluated.

The final peripheral receptor of the sound stimulus is the organ of Corti, which lies within the cochlea (Fig. 16-2B). Recently described as the most complex of mechanical systems, it has about $10^6$ moving parts [4]. Packed into an organ the size of a housefly is a mechanical analysis system consisting of approximately 17,000 sensory cells orderly displayed on a membrane that possesses a mechanical frequency selectivity over a range of 20,000 Hz. The system at threshold is capable of detecting subangstrom level mechanical displacements with astonishing precision. Even more surprising, the cochlea performs this analysis over roughly a $10^6$ dynamic range.

The primary mechanical sensing elements of the cochlea are the sensory hair cells, grouped into inner and outer hair cells. The pattern of innervation to these two classes of sensory cells is quite different; the inner hair cells are primarily responsible for the afferent flow of information, whereas the outer hair cells possess predominantly efferent synapses. The sensory cells are arranged within a supporting matrix of epithelial cells that rest on the mechanically active basilar membrane. The entire complex is referred to as the organ of Corti. The cilia of the sensory cells are capped by an acellular membrane, the tectorial membrane, which has its own mechanical properties [5]. The arrangement of the sensory cells on the basilar membrane is tonotopic: The lowest portions of the membrane are most sensitive to high-frequency disturbances, whereas the uppermost portions are most sensitive to low frequencies. The tonotopic organization is maintained throughout the ascending auditory pathways. This organization of cells on the basilar membrane allows for the correlation between stimulus, or noise frequency, and the location of sensory cell lesions.

The cochlea is of particular concern because once damaged, its normal functioning cannot be completely regained. In a sense, the cochlea has two Achilles' heels: structural fragility and metabolic frailty. Excessive disturbances on the basilar membrane, caused by noise, can directly damage the cilia on the sensory cells and can alter the integrity of the tight cell junctions of the epithelial linings. The epithelial tight cell junctions within

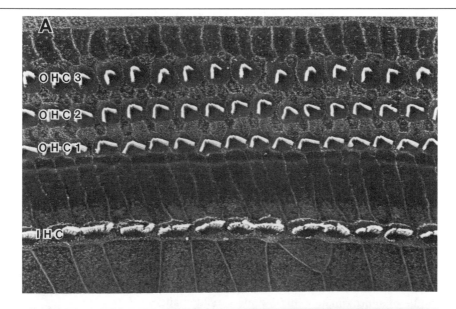

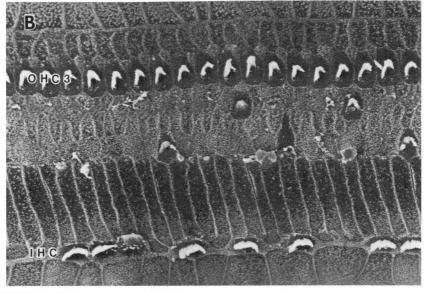

**Fig. 16-3.** A. A scanning electron micrograph of the surface of the organ of Corti. The W-shaped arrangement of the cilia on the outer hair cells (OHC) and the linear arrangement of the cilia on the inner hair cells (IHC) are easily distinguished. Noise-induced mechanical damage to these delicate cilia will result in abnormal function of this transducing sensory element. B. Scanning electron microscopic view of the surface of the organ of Corti, which has lost most of the first and second rows of OHCs and has scattered losses of inner hair cells. Compare this sparse population of sensory cells with the population in the normal-appearing organ of Corti in (A).

the cochlea confine and maintain unique fluid environments necessary for proper sensory cell function. Any change in these tight cell junctions can result in a change in the microhomeostasis of the organ of Corti. Such changes can lead to the ultimate loss of sensory cells. Also any changes that alter vascular physiology can lead to changes in the capillary beds of the cochlea (stria vascularis), which drive the metabolism of the cochlea. If these vessels are compromised, the normal functioning of the sensory cells can be altered or the cells permanently damaged. Typically, noise-induced lesions of the cochlea result in an irreplaceable loss of sensory cells (Fig. 16-3), changes in the capillary network, and a loss of first-order neurons of the spiral ganglion associated with the hair cells.

The auditory component of the eighth cranial nerve, which links the cochlea to the brainstem, consists of a bundle of approximately 30,000 myelinated afferent nerve fibers. Ninety-five percent of the afferent fibers innervate the inner hair cells, while a much smaller number of afferent fibers (about 5 percent) innervate the outer hair cells, which outnumber the inner hair cells by approximately 3 : 1. A smaller group of efferent fibers also enters the cochlea, terminating mostly on the outer hair cells. A series of nuclei beginning with the cochlear nucleus convey the coded cochlear signals through several brainstem nuclei, eventually to the temporal lobe of the cortex. Lesions of the sensory cells in the cochlea can result in changes in the ascending auditory pathways. Such central changes can have additional implications for what we hear or for the efficacy of prosthetic devices used to help correct hearing deficits.

## Behavioral and Audiologic Manifestations of Noise-Induced Hearing Loss

Sufficiently intense sounds have the potential of disrupting all parts of the peripheral and central auditory system. Noise can have direct mechanical effects on the middle ear, such as ossicular discontinuity, tympanic membrane perforation, or fistula of the oval window (Fig. 16-4), and on cochlear structures [1]. The outer hair cells are particularly vulnerable to the effects of excessive noise exposure, followed in vulnerability by the inner hair cells. The cochlea, once damaged, cannot be repaired; the subsequent loss of sensory cells and neural changes produces an auditory pathology that represents the morphologic substrate for the loss of hearing threshold, referred to as a noise-induced sensorineural hearing loss, or simply a noise-induced hearing loss (NIHL). A similar set of cochlear changes can be induced by lower levels of noise that continuously stress the metabolic processes of the cochlea. While these changes may initially produce a temporary loss of threshold, with repeated exposures they may lead to permanent changes [2].

Hearing loss resulting from noise exposure can be separated into three distinct categories: acoustic

**Fig. 16-4.** An example of a pig middle ear damaged by high levels of impulse noise. The tip of the manubrium of the malleus is broken (arrow), and there is a very large tear (dashed line) in the tympanic membrane.

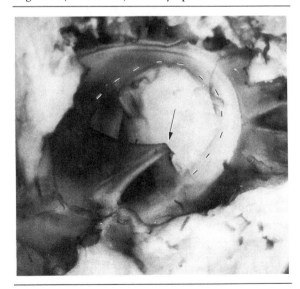

trauma, temporary threshold shift (TTS), and permanent threshold shift (PTS). A single, relatively intense noise exposure is referred to as an acoustic trauma and is usually followed by tinnitus and a change in hearing threshold. While hearing may improve slightly over time, if the exposure is sufficiently intense a PTS will result. One or both ears may be involved. Those who experience an acoustic trauma may also suffer from tympanic membrane perforation(s) and disarticulated or fractured ossicles. Such middle-ear disorders are more likely to appear, if at all, once the peak noise exposure level exceeds approximately 160 dB SPL. In general, however, any acute sound exposure that causes any of the following symptoms represents a hazard to the auditory system and could result in an acute acoustic trauma: immediate pain, a tickling sensation in the ears often occurring if the SPL exceeds approximately 120 dB, vertigo, tinnitus, hearing loss, or reduced communication skills.

Lower levels of noise (< 85 dB[A]) are potentially hazardous and may result in an NIHL if, following exposure, there is a transient shift in the threshold of hearing that recovers gradually (a TTS). While the onset of hearing loss in acute acoustic trauma is instantaneous, the onset and progression of NIHL is far more insidious since it accumulates, usually unnoticed, over a period of many years of exposure to noise on a daily basis. During the initial stages of NIHL, the temporary hearing loss recovers within a few hours or days following removal from the noise. However, if the exposure to this noise is repeated often enough, the hearing loss may not recover completely (that is, permanent sensorineural hearing impairment will begin).

The following is a typical case history of an individual with permanent NIHL:

A 48-year-old man had chief complaints of constant, high-pitched tinnitus and progressive hearing loss in both ears over the previous 2 years. He reported some difficulty hearing in quiet surroundings but noticed marked difficulty understanding speech in noisy environments. He did not report any previous serious illnesses, accidents, atypical drug use, or problems with his ears. For the past 8 years, he had worked in a noisy textile mill, where he said that he "occasionally" wore hearing protective devices. The patient had not been exposed to other hazardous noises off the job, such as gunfire or motorbikes.

The diagnosis of an NIHL comes under the domain of the audiologist, whose primary responsibility is the identification and measurement of hearing loss and the rehabilitation of those with hearing impairment. By measuring auditory thresholds in decibels (relative to a normal hearing level or 0 dB HL) for pure tones as a function of frequency, an audiogram (a frequency-intensity graph) is generated. *Hearing level (HL)* is a term used to designate an individual's hearing threshold at a given test frequency, referenced to an audiometric zero level. The audiogram will help answer the following questions: (1) Is there evidence of a hearing loss? (2) If so, what is the severity of the loss? (3) What is the nature of the loss (conductive, sensorineural, or mixed)? and (4) Can the use of a hearing aid(s) benefit the hearing-impaired individual? A typical normal audiogram and an audiogram from an individual with an NIHL are shown in Fig. 16-5.

Hearing loss induced by most industrial noise characteristically produces a bilateral symmetrical loss that is progressive in nature so long as the individual is continuously exposed to hazardous noise levels (Fig. 16-5). In the initial stages of development, the loss usually occurs at frequencies lying between 3,000 and 6,000 Hz [6]. The maximum loss is usually centered at 4,000 Hz. The audiometric configuration, therefore, is characterized by a downward slope with greater loss in the high-frequency region (3,000–6,000 Hz) than in the low- and mid-frequency regions (250–2,000 Hz). As the NIHL accumulates following further exposure, the 4,000-Hz loss increases in magnitude and the adjacent (higher and lower) frequen-

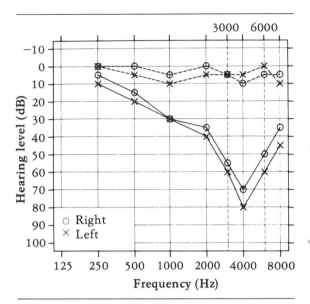

Fig. 16-5. An example of a typical audiogram from a normal individual (dashed lines) and an individual with a bilateral sensorineural hearing loss resulting from excessive noise exposure. Note the maximum loss at 4,000 Hz and the spread of loss to the lower frequencies.

cies also become increasingly affected. The progressive nature of NIHL may eventually result in a moderate to severe impairment across most of the usable hearing frequency range (250–8,000 Hz) unless preventive measures are taken to reduce the degree of hazard imposed by the noise.

Although the diagnosis of a permanent NIHL may be indicated by the audiometric configuration of the hearing loss (the 4,000-Hz notch), it would be premature to make a definitive diagnosis unless additional factors are considered, such as: (1) What is the duration, type, and time-weighted average of the individual's noise exposure? (2) What is the individual's hearing both before and after exposure? (3) What is the age and general health of the individual? (4) Are there any other disorders that may result in hearing impairment (such as middle-ear disorders, congenital factors, Ménière's disease, an eighth cranial nerve lesion, ototoxicity,

and presbycusis)? Consideration of these questions provides important information as to whether the cause and degree of impairment can be solely attributable to noise exposure. Two major diagnostic problems are distinguishing NIHL from hearing loss associated with presbycusis or ototoxic agents and determining the degree of impairment attributed to the aging process. A reported history of tinnitus or "muffled" hearing occurring immediately after any noise exposure or after leaving the work environment and a characteristic 4,000-Hz notch on the audiogram strongly suggest an occupational NIHL hearing loss. Complaints of vertigo are also common.

People usually do not report any difficulty in hearing until a hearing loss of more than 25 dB HL occurs at a frequency at or below 4,000 Hz. Difficulty in hearing the high-frequency sounds of speech (such as s, f, k, t, and sh) may provide the only clue to the individual of an NIHL. Performance on speech intelligibility tasks varies considerably depending on the magnitude of the loss and the affected frequencies [6]. If the hearing loss is confined to frequencies above 3,000 Hz, speech intelligibility measured in quiet surroundings is usually within normal limits. As the frequencies below 3,000 Hz become involved, intelligibility decreases in relation to the degree of impairment. Given that approximately 95 percent of the frequency components in speech lie between 300 and 3,000 Hz, it should not be surprising to find a deterioration in speech intelligibility performance once the NIHL extends into this range of frequencies. Also, individuals with sensorineural hearing loss, due either to noise exposure or other factors, usually have greater difficulty understanding speech against a competing background noise environment than in a quiet environment. This common complaint may be minor if the hearing loss is restricted to frequencies at or above 3,000 Hz but may present marked difficulty for those with losses below 3,000 Hz. Since the usual pattern of progressive NIHL is one in which the speech frequencies are affected last, it is important to identify

NIHL during its initial stages to help prevent future deterioration of hearing sensitivity and speech discrimination abilities.

Occupational health nurses and physicians involved in assessing and monitoring hearing status in hearing conservation programs should refer the worker to an audiologist if a significant change in hearing level ($\geq$ 10 dB at any frequency in either ear) is observed after the worker has had a minimum of 48 hours to recover from environmental noise exposure. Audiologic management of the individual with NIHL may include the use of hearing aids, aural rehabilitation, and assistive listening devices to help improve some of the communication dysfunction experienced in certain listening situations. What, if any, strategies are implemented depends largely on the severity of the communication handicap produced by the noise exposure and the listening needs of the individual.

The nature of hearing impairment is determined by conventional audiometric techniques (air conduction [AC] and bone conduction [BC] thresholds, impedance audiometry, speech discrimination, and site-of-lesion test procedures) [6]. Bone conduction audiometry is used in conjunction with air conduction audiometry to determine the nature of hearing impairment. In the former procedure, the stimulus is conducted directly to the cochlea by a source of vibration attached to the mastoid process of the temporal bone, thus bypassing the conventional route through the middle ear. "Normal" hearing is evident by an air-bone gap (the difference in dB between AC and BC thresholds of the same frequency) of 10 dB or less and a BC threshold less than 15 dB. If, for example, an air-bone gap of more than 10 dB is observed with normal BC threshold values, the loss is considered conductive (due to a defect of the sound-conducting mechanism: external auditory canal or middle ear). A sensorineural loss (a defect in the inner ear or auditory nerve) is characterized by similar, but elevated ($\geq$ 15 dB) AC and BC thresholds. If, on the other hand, there is an air-bone gap of 11 dB or more and BC thresholds are poorer than normal (> 15 dB), the nature of the loss is considered mixed (conductive and sensorineural). Consider the following examples:

| SUBJECT | AC THRESH-OLD (dB) | BC THRESH-OLD (dB) | AIR-BONE GAP (dB) | NATURE |
|---------|--------------------|--------------------|-------------------|--------|
| 1 | 40 | 10 | 30 | Conductive |
| 2 | 40 | 35 | 5 | Sensorineural |
| 3 | 40 | 25 | 15 | Mixed |

Each individual's AC threshold is the same, but their BC thresholds are different. Subject 1, for example, has a pure conductive hearing impairment since an air-bone gap (> 10 dB) is present with a normal BC threshold (< 15 dB). Subject 2 has a pure sensorineural impairment since there is no significant air-bone gap (< 10 dB), which rules out the presence of a conductive component, but an elevated BC threshold (35 dB HL). Subject 3 has a mixed impairment, given the presence of both an air-bone gap (> 10 dB) and an elevated BC threshold ($\geq$ 15). Although the use of threshold criteria is a valuable aid in determining the degree and nature of the loss, the audiologist will often use additional diagnostic test procedures to more accurately define the location of pathology within the auditory system. A normal audiometric pattern, however, does not necessarily indicate an absence of pathology to the auditory system (either peripherally or centrally in the nervous system).

## Otoacoustic Emissions

Otoacoustic emissions (OAEs) are sounds emitted by the cochlea in response to auditory stimulation [10]. They are the only noninvasive objective means of examining the active mechanical processes generated by the outer hair cells of the cochlea. Since the majority of permanent peripheral hearing impairments involve noise-induced, ototoxic, or hereditary hearing losses, which involve the sensory components of the cochlea, OAEs may complement or even supplement certain standard audiometric procedures in the assessment of cochlea functioning. Of the several types of OAEs identified, for example, spontaneous, evoked, and the difference intermodulation distortion product at the frequency of 2 $f_1$ to $f_2$, the distortion product emission (DPOAE) and transient evoked emission appear to have significant potential for evaluating hearing, particularly in the screening of hearing and threshold estimation in difficult-to-test individuals. DPOAEs are reduced or eliminated in ears with sensorineural hearing loss of various etiologies that affect cochlear function. Recent evidence also suggests that DPOAEs may eventually be applied to predict one's susceptibility to development of a permanent hearing loss resulting from exposure to excessively high noise levels in the work environment. The OAE methods are promising objective sensitive indicators of early signs and the progression of hearing impairments, including cases of NIHL.

## Hearing Conservation

Prevention of NIHL is the concern of workers and managers. In both industrial and nonindustrial noise environments, the control of NIHL is primarily through prevention, stressing a decrease in existing noise, a decrease in exposure noise levels, or both. No present medical therapy can restore the permanent changes in the inner ear (sensorineural hearing impairment) that have resulted from excessive noise exposure.

Occupational Safety and Health Administration (OSHA) regulations limit the occupational noise exposure according to duration of exposure and intensity of sound. A daily average exposure of 90 dBA over 8 hours is the current limit; however, the regulations also permit sounds of greater intensity for shorter periods. Workplaces in many industries sometimes exceed the 90-dBA OSHA limit: Noises associated with grinding, drilling, or stamping of metal to manufacture metal products

and machinery (Fig. 16-6), sawing of wood in lumber mills, printing machines in publishing and newspaper companies, air hoses in many industries, and looms in textile mills frequently approach or exceed the 90-dBA level. (See Chap. 6 for a discussion of noise control principles and measures.)

Federal law also mandates the institution of a hearing conservation program (HCP) if a noise exposure equals or exceeds a time-weighted average (TWA) of 85 dB(A) over an 8-hour period. Industries should, however, consider such programs if employees complain of either communication difficulty while working in the noise environment, tinnitus, or temporary hearing loss after leaving the working environment, even if the measured noise exposure is below a TWA of 85 dB(A).

As in the United States, many workers in Europe are being exposed to potentially harmful noise levels on a daily basis. Conservative estimates indicate that at least 7 million people (35 percent of the total industrial population) are exposed to noise of 85 dB(A) or greater.

For purposes of protecting the rights of the employer and the rights and hearing health of the employee, OSHA requires employers to obtain a baseline measurement of hearing (reference audiogram) within 6 months of an employee's first exposure to noise levels of at least 85 dB(A) for 8 hours a day [7]. An HCP should, therefore, include a preplacement hearing test and periodic repeat tests (air conduction thresholds at 500, 1,000, 2,000, 3,000, 4,000, and 6,000 Hz in each ear via binaural earphones). Periodic monitoring of hearing levels should also be carried out, preferably on Monday mornings or whenever the employee has had approximately 48 hours of limited noise exposure in order to recover.

The reference audiogram (1) detects the presence of existing hearing loss; (2) determines if cochlear injury due to noise exposure has occurred, by comparison to future tests; and (3) documents properly any claims that noise exposure was the main cause of an individual's hearing loss. If a significant change in hearing level is observed ($\geq 10$

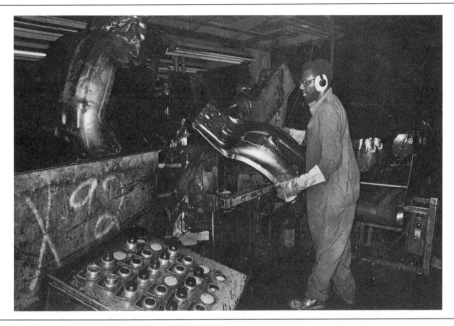

**Fig. 16-6.** Noise production in a stamping operation may be difficult to control at the source. (Photograph by Earl Dotter.)

dB) at any frequency in either ear, workplace managers, in order to prevent further hearing loss, should consider (1) providing and encouraging the use of ear protection devices, (2) reducing the noise level at the source(s), and (3) limiting the employee's exposure time or removing the employee from the noise environment. A complete audiologic and otologic evaluation should also be made to specify the nature of the hearing loss and the primary cause of its progression. Managers should be responsible for monitoring hearing levels by providing a retest 3 months after the reference audiogram or earlier if the employee reports a change in hearing or tinnitus. If no significant change is seen at this later time, periodic retests can be performed on an annual basis, or sooner if these symptoms occur.

Hearing tests conducted for industrial workers are usually performed by an audiologist, nurse, or audiometric technician using a calibrated puretone audiometer. The test environment and audiometer

must meet the criteria proposed by the American National Standards Institute [8]. Also, OSHA regulations specify that "audiometric tests shall be performed by a licensed or certified audiologist, otolaryngologist, or other physician, or by a technician who is certified by the Council of Accreditation in Occupational Hearing Conservation or by other technicians" [7]. Audiometric technicians are trained to perform only air conduction puretone tests. An example of the kind of information that might be required on an individual is shown in Fig. 16-7.

Medical management of an HCP is also highly desirable since diagnosis, prevention, and treatment of hearing loss are medical responsibilities. A physician, occupational health nurse, or audiologist should be responsible for (1) organizing and administering the hearing test program, (2) evaluating and validating hearing test records for compensation claims, (3) reporting inadequacies of noise control methods, and (4) providing ear pro-

| Time of test | | Date | Time and date of last exposure | Type of noise |
|---|---|---|---|---|
| Hour of day | Day of week | | | |
| 9:00 | Monday | 4/27/1987 | 5:00—4/24/1987 | Continuous TWA of 95 dB |

| Audiometer | Calibration | Date last calibrated | |
|---|---|---|---|
| MAICO MA-12 | ANSI—1969 | 1/20/1987 | |

HEARING THRESHOLD LEVEL

| Right ear | | | | | | Left ear | | | | | |
|---|---|---|---|---|---|---|---|---|---|---|---|
| 500 | 1,000 | 2,000 | 3,000 | 4,000 | 6,000 | 500 | 1,000 | 2,000 | 3,000 | 4,000 | 6,000 |
| 15 | 20 | 30 | 45 | 55 | 40 | 10 | 25 | 35 | 50 | 65 | 45 |

EAR PROTECTION

| Type plugs | Type muffs | Protection | |
|---|---|---|---|
| Neoprene inserts | None | 3 | 1. Satisfactory<br>2. Unsatisfactory<br>3. Questionable |

COMMENTS: Hearing levels have become progressively poorer from 500 to 4,000 Hz with some recovery at 6,000 Hz in each ear. These levels are approximately 10 dB poorer than those obtained one year ago at frequencies of 3,000 to 6,000 Hz in each ear. Recommend complete audiologic evaluation to determine nature of hearing loss and a reappraisal of adequacy of hearing protection currently used.

Fig. 16-7. Typical audiometric sheet used in hearing conservation programs.

tectors to employees and promoting attitudes that will benefit the program.

The success of an HCP depends on the cooperation of managers, workers, and others concerned with the health and safety of workers.

## Noise Standards

Much noise research has as its final objective the creation of a damage risk criterion (DRC) for human exposure to noise. As in all public health criteria, there are not only scientific questions that must be answered, but numerous social, economic, and legal considerations. In the scientific realm, we must first answer the question, "What do we want to protect?" Hearing is a multidimensional ability. "Do we protect hearing thresholds? Discrimination ability? The ability to understand speech? In quiet? In noise? Do we protect all aspects or only some? Which aspects and how much?" There is, as yet, no uniform agreement on such issues. Even the issue of how a hearing handicap is to be defined is unresolved. The most common, although debatable, approach is to protect against permanent threshold shifts and to accept some hearing loss as an inevitable compromise if that hearing loss is less than that considered to represent the beginning of a hearing handicap.

Currently, an average hearing level of 26 dB at 500, 1,000, and 2,000 Hz is taken as the onset of handicap, although this approach is not uniformly agreed on. At this point, social and legal issues begin to arise. A shift in the 26-dB fence upward represents a tremendous economic advantage to institutions that must compensate for handicap, but it may also represent a significant decrease in the quality of life for affected individuals. If the 26-dB fence is lowered 5 dB or if other frequencies are taken into consideration, the advantage goes to the affected individuals. Note that the higher frequencies are omitted from the above definition of handicap. Frequencies such as 4,000 Hz are usually the first and most affected frequencies in the audiogram of an individual exposed to noise (the classic 4,000-Hz dip or notch), and thus incorporating 4,000 Hz into the handicap definition would make it not only a more sensitive index (or liberal definition) but also a more expensive one for employers. The most common rationale for incorporating only 500, 1,000, and 2,000 Hz in the definition is that these frequencies contribute most toward understanding speech (in the quiet). Since handicap is equated with losses in ability to communicate, this group of frequencies has gained acceptance, although agreement is not unanimous.

Over the past 30 years, considerable efforts have been made by a number of government regulatory agencies to establish the permissible levels of noise that an individual may be exposed to during a working lifetime without developing NIHL. For a long time, the central argument focused around the efficacy of an 85-dB(A) versus a 90-dB(A) upper-limit criterion for an 8-hour workday. OSHA, for example, proposed keeping the allowable level of 90 dB(A), as recommended in the Walsh-Healey amendments, while the Environmental Protection Agency (EPA) suggested a reduction to 85 dB(A). The EPA criterion was established with the health and welfare effects of noise on humans in mind, with relatively less concern for the economic concerns of industry. OSHA, reluctant to comply with the EPA criterion, argued that only 2 percent of the population is at risk for NIHL under a 90-dB(A) standard, citing the American Academy of Ophthalmology and Otolaryngology–American Medical Association (AAOO-AMA) [9] low fence of a 26-dB average for frequencies 500, 1,000, and 2,000 Hz as the beginning of impairment. At present, the final OSHA rule, which became effective in 1983, maintains that a hearing conservation program must be introduced if a noise exposure equals or exceeds a time-weighted average (TWA) of 85 dB(A) over an 8-hour period. In addition, employers must provide hearing protection devices

to (1) workers exposed to an 8-hour TWA of 90 dB(A) and (2) those who have experienced a threshold shift of 10 dB or more from a baseline audiogram at the frequencies 2,000, 3,000, and 4,000 Hz—if exposed to an 8-hour TWA of 85 dB(A).

The determination of the acceptable noise exposure limits for less than an 8-hour exposure was also adapted from the Walsh-Healey Act. The "5 dB rule" was accepted; that is, 90 dB(A) of continuous noise exposure is equivalent to 4 hours of 95-dB(A) or 2 hours of 100-dB(A) exposure in an 8-hour day, with a maximum upper limit of 115 dB(A) for one-fourth of an hour or less. If the daily exposure is a mixture of different intensities, then a fractional method is specified for determining if the exposure exceeds the allowable limit. Impact noises are not to exceed 140 dB peak SPL, with no further specification of the parameters of the exposure, such as number of impulses or presentation rate.

# References

1. Hamernik RP, Henderson D, Salvi R. eds. New perspectives on noise-induced hearing loss. New York: Raven, 1982.
2. Lipscomb DM. ed. Noise and audiology. Baltimore: University Park, 1978.
3. Pickles JO. An introduction to the physiology of hearing. New York: Academic, 1982.
4. Hudspeth AJ. The cellular basis of hearing: The biophysics of hair cells. Science 1985; 230:745–52.
5. Zwislocki JJ. Sound analysis in the ear: A history of discoveries. Am Scientist 1981; 69:184–92.
6. Katz J. Handbook of clinical audiology. Baltimore: Williams & Wilkins, 1985.
7. Fed Register 48, March 8, 1983. (no. 46: 9738–85.)
8. American National Standards Institute. American National Standards Institute criteria for permissible ambient noise during audiometric testing. New York: Acoustical Society of America, 1977. (ANSI 53.1.)
9. AAOO guide for the evaluation of hearing impairment. Trans Am Acad Ophth and Otol 1959; 235–8; and American Council of Otolaryngology. Recommended, but not generally accepted alternative:

Guide for the evaluation of hearing handicap. JAMA 1979; 241:2055–9.
10. Brownell W. Outer hair cell electromotility and otoacoustic emissions. Ear Hear 1990; 11:82–92.

# Bibliography

Dancer AL, Henderson D, Salvi RJ, Hamernik RP. eds. Noise-induced hearing loss. St. Louis: Mosby–Year Book, 1992.
*An up-to-date collection of topics that focus on important basic science and applied issues of noise-induced hearing loss.*
Davis H, Silverman SR. eds. Hearing and deafness. New York: Holt, Rhinehart and Winston, 1970.
*An extensive review of hearing and hearing conservation, auditory disorders, diagnosis, and rehabilitation.*
Kryter KD. The effects of noise on man. New York: Academic, 1970.
*A comprehensive reference volume on virtually all aspects of the human psychophysical response to noise.*
Martin FN. ed. Medical audiology. New Jersey: Prentice Hall, 1981.
*Presents state-of-the-art information on the basic elements requisite to understanding medical conditions of the ear.*
Newby HA, Popelka GR. Audiology. New Jersey: Prentice Hall, 1985.
*Current treatment of basic and advanced hearing test procedures and hearing conservation.*
Northern JL. ed. Hearing disorders. Boston: Little, Brown, 1984.
*An orientation to the evaluation, manifestations, diagnosis, treatment, and management of hearing disorders.*
Salvi RJ, Henderson D, Hamernik RP, Colletti V. eds. Basic and applied aspects of noise-induced hearing loss. New York: Plenum, 1986.
*A reference manual that emphasizes the physiologic and anatomic aspects of noise-induced hearing loss.*

# 17
# Other Physical Hazards and Their Effects

Stephen Kales and Howard Hu

A welder is recently diagnosed as having a cataract. He notes to the physician that two other welders in his shop had developed cataracts over the last 5 years, and asks whether his work may have caused his condition.

A patient complains of loss of grip strength and sensation in both of her hands. During the examination, she tells her physician she operates a pneumatic chipper.

A joint labor-management committee seeks to decrease the number of heat-related illnesses among the company's construction workers during the heat of the summer. The head of the committee calls an occupational health professional for advice.

An electrical worker is planning a pregnancy, and asks her physician if she should plan on discontinuing work during her pregnancy because of the possible adverse effects of electromagnetic fields to which she is exposed at work.

In this chapter, several types of physical exposures and environments that may be hazardous to workers are discussed. These include *nonionizing radiation* (ultraviolet, visible light, infrared, microwave/radiofrequency, and laser radiation); *vibration*, including *ultrasound; atmospheric variations* (hot and cold environments and hyperbaric [compression/undersea] and hypobaric [high-altitude] environments); and *electric and magnetic fields*. Some of these have well-recognized health effects, but others are controversial and are still being studied.

## Nonionizing Radiation

*Nonionizing radiation* (see Chap. 15, Ionizing Radiation) refers to emissions from those parts of the electromagnetic spectrum where emitted photons generally have insufficient energy to produce ionization of atoms. These forms of radiation include microwaves, television and radio waves, visible light, and infrared and ultraviolet (UV) radiation, among others (Fig. 17-1). Laser radiation is an amplified form of nonionizing radiation.

All types of nonionizing radiation obey certain general laws of electromagnetic radiation. The equation that fundamentally characterizes electromagnetic radiation is

$$\lambda = c/f$$

where $\lambda$ = wavelength in meters, $c$ = velocity (usually the velocity of light, $3 \times 10^8$ meters per second), and $f$ = frequency in cycles per second.

Nonionizing radiation has other important characteristics shared by all forms of electromagnetic radiation: (1) It travels in straight lines and can be bent or focused, (2) the energy delivered is directly proportional to the frequency (and therefore inversely proportional to the wavelength), and (3) this energy occurs in small units called quanta.

When nonionizing radiation strikes matter, energy is absorbed. Nonionizing radiation is of lower frequency than ionizing radiation and, therefore, contains less energy. Instead of causing ionizations, this energy is usually transformed into heat,

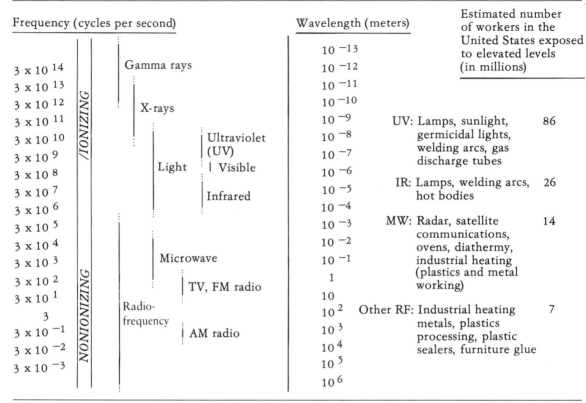

**Fig. 17-1.** The electromagnetic radiation spectrum. (From MM Key et al. Occupational diseases—a guide to their recognition. Cincinnati: NIOSH, 1977.)

which accounts for many of its important physiologic effects. Absorption in the UV and visible portions of the spectrum can also produce photochemical reactions or fluorescence; this occurrence depends on the absorption spectrum of the molecule that has been struck and the efficiency of the specific radiation wavelength in producing this effect.

### Ultraviolet Radiation

Ultraviolet radiation (UVR) is an invisible form of radiant energy produced naturally by the sun in a *low-intensity* form, and artificially by incandescent, fluorescent, and discharge types of light sources. The UVR radiation spectrum can be fur-

ther subdivided, based on wavelength, into UV-A ($4.0–3.2 \times 10^{-7}$ m, black light) and UV-B ($3.2–2.8 \times 10^{-7}$ m) radiation, which are the two principal radiations of sunlight; and UV-C ($2.8–2.0 \times 10^{-7}$ m) radiation, which is germicidal. In industrial work settings, *high-intensity* UVR exposure occurs primarily from exposure to arc welding. Other industrial sources include plasma torches, which are used in heavy industrial cutting processes; electric arc furnaces; germicidal and black-light lamps; and certain types of lasers. UVR light is also being used by some coal processing and refining companies to detect coal tar residues on the skin of workers and equipment (due to coal tar's fluorescence under UVR).

The skin and the eyes absorb UVR and are particularly vulnerable to injury, primarily due to UV-B radiation. The common sunburn is a well-known result of acute overexposure to solar UVR. Long-term, low-intensity UVR exposure from the sun is also responsible for a number of other skin conditions, including solar elastosis (wrinkling) and solar keratoses (premalignant lesions). It is also believed to be the major etiologic agent for the most common skin cancers, basal cell and squamous cell carcinoma (see Chap. 24). These effects are intensified in areas with greater solar UVR exposure (few clouds, equatorial location, or high altitude). On the other hand, the relationship between sunlight and malignant melanoma is more complex. In other words, melanoma risk does not appear to be determined by the cumulative dose of UVR. Intermittent, high-intensity, recreational sun exposure resulting in sunburn, especially in youth, appears to confer a greater risk for melanoma than continuous chronic exposure from an outdoor occupation [1]. Some epidemiologic studies have suggested that UVR in the form of fluorescent lighting can pose a slightly elevated risk for melanoma. The International Radiation Protection Association concluded that fluorescent light UVR did not pose a melanoma risk, but recent studies, including one that suggested moderately increased risks for men with increased cumulative exposure to fluorescent light UVR [2], indicate that further research is needed before this hypothesis can be completely dismissed.

Decreases in the earth's protective ozone layer due to chlorofluorocarbons (CFCs) have increased concern about the effects of UVR. Ozone losses will lead to increased UVR exposure and are expected to cause further increases in cataracts and basal cell and squamous cell skin cancer rates. The prospect of increased UVR also raises concern stemming from recent research suggesting that UVR can affect the immune system. UVR has been demonstrated to suppress certain aspects of cell-mediated immunity in mice. Langerhans cells (which activate T lymphocytes) are depleted in UV-irradiated human skin, and UVR is capable of reactivating both labial and genital herpes infections. UVR-related immunosuppression might provide a critical mechanism allowing the growth of skin cancers. The possibility that UVR-related immunosuppression may blunt cell-mediated immunity is particularly ominous for countries in which infectious diseases play a large role in morbidity and mortality.

Health effects of UVR can be potentiated by several photosensitizing agents; locally applied coal tar, as well as many plants containing furocoumarins and psoralens (such as figs, lemon and lime rinds, celery, and parsnips), are photosensitizers. When ingested, certain drugs (such as chlorpromazine, tolbutamide, and chlorpropamide) can increase susceptibility to UVR. Photosensitization can lead to an immediate sunburn-type effect upon exposure to a small dosage of radiant energy. Individuals vary in their susceptibility to this reaction, depending on their tendency to concentrate sufficient quantities of the photosensitizing agent in the skin.

Covering skin with hats and long sleeves when possible, and avoiding prolonged exposures, protects from the effects of low-intensity UVR. Benzophenone and anthranilate sunscreens absorb UVR and offer some protection to bare skin. Opaque sunscreens, such as titanium dioxide, offer the best protection and may be essential if photosensitization occurs.

Ultraviolet radiation from arc-welding[1] operations has not been associated with skin cancer, probably because these high-intensity exposures are of an acute, short-term nature, and operators usually wear protective clothing. High-intensity acute exposures, however, can result in eye damage. It most commonly occurs with exposure to arc welding, but can also result from exposure to direct or reflected radiation from UVR lamps, such as those used in laboratories as bactericidal agents.

[1]Arcs are high-temperature sources generated between electrodes; during the welding process, they appear as blinding flashes of light and emit UV radiation.

The end-result is conjunctivitis or keratitis (inflammation of the cornea), or both, a work-related condition commonly referred to as "ground-glass eyeball," "welder's flash," or "flash burn" (see Chap. 25). The welder or bystanders can be affected by just a brief moment of exposure to unprotected or underprotected eyes. Prevention requires the isolation of high-intensity UVR sources and the use of goggles and other shields with proper filters.

Long-term UV-B exposure is probably also a risk factor for the development of cortical cataracts [3].

Ultraviolet radiation also has an indirect impact on health through its ability to cause photochemical reactions. UVR, as encountered in welding operations, converts small amounts of oxygen and nitrogen into ozone and oxides of nitrogen, which are respiratory irritants (see Chap. 22). At certain wavelengths, UVR can also decompose solvent vapors into toxic gases such as perchlorethylene into hydrogen chloride and trichlorethylene into phosgene. Control of these hazards requires proper local exhaust ventilation and isolation of high-intensity UVR sources from solvent processes.

### Visible Radiation

Visible light plays an important role in determining working conditions. A considerable amount of literature in the field of ergonomics deals with the proper use of different lighting systems for different tasks. Inadequate lighting may cause ocular fatigue and discomfort and, more importantly, contribute to work accidents. Types of illumination may also play a role in ocular health (see Chap. 25).

### Infrared Radiation

An epidemiologic investigation on the prevalence of cataract included 209 workers over 50 years of age exposed to infrared (IR) radiation in the Swedish manual glass industry for 20 years or more, and 298 non–IR-exposed controls. The risk for an IR-exposed worker to have his or her vision reduced by cataract to 0.7 or less is 2.5 times as high as for nonexposed controls (95 percent confidence interval 1.4–4.4). The risk that he or she will have to be operated for cataract is 12 times as high (95 percent confidence interval 2.6–53) [4].

In industry, significant levels of IR are produced directly by lamp sources and indirectly by sources of heat. The primary effect of IR on biologic tissue is thermal; it can cause skin burns, although one is generally warned of IR exposure by the sensation of heat before skin burns can occur. The lens of the eye, however, is particularly vulnerable to damage because the lens has no heat sensors and a poor heat-dissipating mechanism. Cataracts may be produced by chronic IR exposure at levels far below those that cause skin burns (see Chap. 25). Glass blowers and furnace workers have been shown to have an increased incidence of all types of cataracts (particularly posterior cataracts) after chronic IR exposure for over 10 years. Other workers potentially at risk for harmful IR exposure include those involved in handling molten metal (such as foundry workers, blacksmiths, and solderers), oven operators, workers in the vicinity of baking and drying heat lamps, and movie projectionists.

Control of IR hazards requires shielding of the IR source and eye protection with IR filters. Increasing as much as possible the distance between workers and the IR source will reduce the intensity of the exposure.

### Microwave/Radiofrequency Radiation

Microwave/radiofrequency radiation (MW/RFR) encompasses a wide range of wavelengths used in radar, television, radio, and other telecommunications systems (see Fig. 17-1). They are also used in a variety of industrial operations, including the heating, welding, and melting of metals; the processing of wood and plastic (radiofrequency sealers); and the creation of high-temperature plasma. As many as 21 million workers in the U.S. may be exposed to MW/RFR, and its commercial use is expected to increase; thus, any health effect could have a very significant public health impact.

The heating effect of MW/RFR depends on the amount of energy absorbed from it, which, in turn, depends on the frequency of the radiation and the position, shape, and other properties of the exposed object. In general, detectable tissue heating requires relatively high-power MW/RFR, at power densities above 100 watts/m² (10 mW/cm²). This thermal mechanism is responsible for the recognized adverse health effects of MW/RFR, some of which have been reported in humans, such as cataract formation, testicular degeneration, and depressed sperm counts, focal areas of thermal necrosis, and, at extremely high intensities, death [5, 6].

Recognition of the thermal effects of MW/RFR led to the current federal exposure guidelines, which currently limit MW/RFR power to 10 mW/cm², as averaged over any 6-minute period.

Controversy exists as to whether adverse health effects can be caused by chronic exposure to MW/RFR at power densities *below* this standard. Some laboratory studies of animals have demonstrated that MW/RFR, at intensities that are too low to cause thermal effects, can cause biologic effects that are primarily of a neurologic and immunologic nature, such as alterations in electroencephalograms (EEGs) and behavior, and impairment of immune cell function [7]. At present, however, there is no clear evidence for nonthermal morbidity in humans, and no consensus that the nonthermal effects of MW/RFR can produce adverse health effects [5, 6]. Nevertheless, given the known potential for MW/RFR to cause thermal damage, a high priority must be given to establishing work guidelines, especially shielding and engineering controls, which will bring compliance to the existing standard, and to performing research on low levels of exposure.

Finally, microwaves and high-power radio waves have the potential to interact with medical implants, particularly cardiac pacemakers. Current pacemaker leads are shielded to prevent electromagnetic interference; however, although unlikely, disruption is conceivable. In occupationally exposed individuals, estimations of the exposure and subsequent possibility of interference should be made in consultation with the (pacemaker) manufacturer and a cardiologist. Interference due to microwave ovens is not thought to be a problem given the shielding of both modern pacemaker leads and microwave ovens [8].

### Laser Radiation

*Laser* is an acronym for Light Amplification by the Stimulated Emission of Radiation, a special category of human-made, nonionizing radiation. It is produced by forcing atoms of a particular gas media to emit a stream of photons that are monochromatic and in phase with each other. These photons are emitted at specific wavelengths that depend on the source medium. The many and increasing applications of laser radiation derive from its ability to concentrate a large amount of energy in a small cross-sectional area in a highly coherent and minimally divergent manner. Lasers of various types are widely used as reference lines in surveying, instrumentation, and alignments; as a heating agent in welding; as a cutting instrument in microelectronics and microsurgery; in communications; in holography; and in the military, where their application is expected to increase dramatically.

The eye, including the retina, lens, iris, and cornea, is extremely vulnerable to injury from laser radiation in the near-UVR, near-infrared, infrared, and visible-frequency ranges (see Chap. 25). Ocular damage can occur not only directly from intrabeam viewing, but also indirectly by exposure to diffuse reflections from a high-power laser. Lasers of wavelengths that fall outside the visible portion of the electromagnetic spectrum can be particularly hazardous, since exposure to the beam may not be readily apparent. Skin burns are caused by direct exposure to high-energy lasers.

Laser installations should be isolated wherever possible, and the laser beam should be terminated by a material that is nonreflective and fireproof. Special goggles can be helpful but must afford specific protection to the wavelength of laser being used. Care must be paid to minimizing diffuse reflected radiation that may not be visually detectable. Finally, proper worker education and a baseline eye examination must be included in the preventive program.

## Vibration

A 40-year-old man came to see his physician with a chief complaint of hand problems. About 12 years earlier, he started work as a copper stayer (metal smith) using a pneumatic hammer weighing 12¼ lb with a frequency of 2,300 vibrations a minute (38 Hz²). He wore a glove on his left hand. After he had been working for 2 years, he noticed that his fingers would go white starting with his left index finger, and along with this color change he noted a "pins and needles" sensation. Gradually, the right hand became involved and soon all his fingers on both hands were involved. His hands became very awkward to use and he began to have difficulty in buttoning his shirt. It often took 2 hours for normal sensation to return to his hands. At the start, the syndrome occurred only in winter, but after 4 years it occurred in summer as well. After over 6 years' work with the hammer, he had to give up this occupation because of these symptoms. He is now working as a laborer in the boiler shop [9].

*Vibration* refers to the mechanical oscillation of a surface around its reference point (see box, Chap. 6). Health hazards of interest generally stem from vibration at frequencies of 2 to 1,000 Hz. Occupational health effects of vibration stem from prolonged periods of contact between a worker and the vibrating surface. It has been estimated that 8 million workers in the United States are exposed to occupational vibration, either whole-body vibration or segmental vibration to a specific body part. Drivers of trucks, tractors, buses, and other vehicles, and certain heavy-equipment operators, are subject to chronic whole-body vibration (WBV) transmitted through the seat or floor of their work posts. This vibration is generally of lower frequency (2–100 Hz). Grinders and oper-

²1 Hz = 1 hertz = 1 cycle per second; 1 kHz = 1,000 Hz.

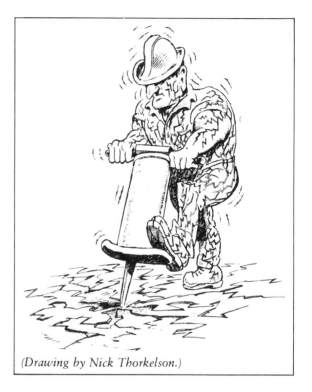

*(Drawing by Nick Thorkelson.)*

ators of chain saws, chipping hammers, and other pneumatic tools are exposed to segmental vibration, usually through the hands, that is of higher frequency (20–1,000 Hz).

### Whole-Body Vibration

Less is known about the chronic effects of low-frequency WBV than about segmental vibration. Several epidemiologic studies have suggested an association with changes in bone structure, gastrointestinal disturbances involving secretion and motility, prostatitis, and changes in nerve conduction velocity [10]. Vibration at the resonating frequency of the eyeballs (60–90 Hz) has been associated with disorders of vision. A growing body of evidence supports an association of WBV exposure to low back pain and degenerative changes of the spine among operators of various vehicles and equipment [11] and helicopter pilots [12]. While it is difficult to isolate the effects of WBV from confounders such as materials handling and posture, animal models lend biologic plausibility to this hypothesis. Thus, although definitive proof of causality is lacking, it would seem wise to limit exposure to whole-body vibration as much as possible.

## Segmental Vibration

Chronic exposure to segmental vibration at low frequencies of 20 to 40 Hz, such as is encountered with the operation of heavy pneumatic drills, has been associated with degenerative osteoarticular lesions in the elbows and shoulders. This is believed to represent a "wear and tear" process from repetitive impulse loading; however, epidemiologic proof of causality has so far been lacking.

At frequencies between 40 and 300 Hz, the use of vibratory hand tools (such as chain saws, grinders, hammers, and drills) has been well known to elicit Raynaud's phenomenon of occupational origin. Previously known as "vibration syndrome," "dead hand," "vibration white fingers," and "traumatic vasospastic disease," the phenomenon is now called the hand-arm vibration syndrome (HAVS). HAVS has three features: (1) an abnormal peripheral circulation marked by vasospastic attacks that cause finger blanching, (2) peripheral nerve motor sensory changes characterized by decreased hand sensation and dexterity, and (3) muscular abnormalities, which manifest as decreased grip strength [13]. A serious case of HAVS with frequent attacks can greatly interfere with a worker's performance and other activities. Moreover, many cases can progress to a chronic condition, with permanent disability.

Other factors besides vibration may also contribute to the development of HAVs. Work under cold conditions, as is commonly experienced by loggers working with chain saws, increases the risk of this condition. Another important aggravating factor is tobacco use. Nicotine acutely increases peripheral vasoconstriction, which may precipitate as an attack, while chronic use is associated with more advanced stages of the disease [14].

While it is commonly agreed upon that arterial vasospasm is the cause of blanching, the mechanisms by which vibration damages the neurovascular and muscular tissues of the hands remain unknown [15]. Early diagnosis is usually based on a history of typical symptoms, such as numbness or tingling of the fingers precipitated by exposure to vibration; these symptoms persist for progressively longer periods of time. Finger blanching is often the next symptom to occur with continued chronic exposure. Confirmation of the diagnosis and staging of disease severity have become increasingly reliant on objective vascular, neurologic, and muscular testing as well as the exclusion of other neuropathies [13].

Other potential effects of hand-arm vibration in this range include the carpal tunnel syndrome [16] and scleroderma especially when there is inhalation exposure to silica dust in addition to vibration [17].

Preventing these health effects requires minimizing exposure to segmental vibration and surveillance for early health effects. The National Institute for Occupational Safety and Health (NIOSH) has published a revised set of recommendations that includes (1) reduction in the intensity and duration of hand-arm vibration exposure; (2) exposure monitoring; (3) medical surveillance, including preplacement and periodic assessments of exposure history, possible vibration-related symptoms and signs, and discouraging tobacco use; (4) provisions for medical removal of symptomatic workers; (5) protective clothing against vibration and cold stress; and (6) worker training on the health hazards of vibration [18]. Once vibration-associated health problems begin to arise, exposure must be terminated. While some early vasospastic symptoms may reverse, neurologic and other features of HAVS may be irreversible [15].

No federal standard currently mandates limits on exposure to vibration, or the use of vibrating tools. Thus, workers, managers, and clinicians have crucial roles in the early recognition of segmental vibration–induced problems and the prevention of their progression.

### Ultrasound

The term *ultrasound* is used to describe mechanical vibrations at frequencies above the limit of human audibility (approximately 16 kHz[3]). These vibrations, like sound, are pressure waves and are unrelated to electromagnetic radiation. Ultrasound has many industrial and other uses, depending on the frequency of its generation. (With increasing frequency, ultrasound has a tendency to be absorbed by the transmitting medium and consequently has less penetrating ability.) Low-frequency (18–30 kHz), high-power ultrasound is used in industry for its penetrating and disruptive abilities to facilitate drilling, welding, and cleaning operations and to help in emulsifying liquids. It is also a component of noise generated by a variety of high-power engines. High-frequency (100–10,000 kHz) ultrasound has many analytical applications, and diagnostic ultrasound is increasingly used in many areas of medicine. No definitive evidence of any adverse effects of ultrasound on patients has been found [19].

Low-frequency ultrasound can cause a variety of health problems, either by its transmission through air or by bodily contact with the ultrasound generator or target, as when a worker immerses his/her hands in an ultrasound cleaning bath. A worker with such exposure may complain of headache, earache, vertigo, general discomfort, irritability, hypersensitivity to light, and hyperacusia (sensitivity to sound). Exposure through bodily contact with a source of ultrasound may eventually cause peripheral nervous system lesions, leading to autonomic polyneuritis or partial paralysis of the fingers or hands (see beginning of Vibration section).

High-frequency ultrasound may result in the same spectrum of problems; however, since high-frequency ultrasound is absorbed by air and poorly penetrating, excessive exposure is only ob-

[3]1 kHz = 1 kilohertz = $10^3$ cycles per second.

tained in cases of direct contact between the ultrasound generator and a part of the worker's body. Under these circumstances, the mechanism of harmful effects is similar to that of segmental vibration. Recent evidence has suggested a reduction of vibration perception in the fingers of ultrasonic therapists [20].

Protection from the harmful effects of ultrasound is primarily an engineering problem requiring insulation and isolation of the ultrasound process. Direct contact between workers and the ultrasound source should be minimized. Ear protective devices are also helpful. Workers with ultrasound exposure should undergo yearly audiometric and neurologic examinations.

## Atmospheric Variations

### Heat

A 24-year-old laborer was brought to the emergency room after collapsing during work. Several hours before, he had become extremely irritable and, for no apparent reason, had provoked arguments with several of his coworkers. He had been working on an incentive basis next to a blast furnace in a metals factory on a day when the temperature had not been more than 90°F, but the humidity exceeded 60 percent. Physical examination showed a stocky man who was totally unresponsive with hot, flushed, moist skin. He had dilated, equally sized pupils that were unresponsive to light. Fundi were normal. Rectal temperature was greater than 41°C (105.8°F), pulse rate was 160, blood pressure was 80/0 mm Hg, and respirations were deep at a rate of 30 per minute. Despite rapid cooling in an ice bath with decrease in core temperature and aggressive care in the intensive care unit, the patient suffered a series of grand mal seizures followed by marked metabolic acidosis, rhabdomyolysis, acute respiratory distress syndrome, and acute renal failure. Following emergency hemodialysis, the patient had another grand mal seizure followed by cardiac arrest, which was refractory to all attempts at resuscitation.

Heat is a potential physical hazard that can exist in almost any workplace, especially during summer. It is a particular hazard in tropical climates.

Hot industrial jobs requiring heavy work afford the greatest potential for problems because they add to the worker's heat load by generating more metabolic heat (Fig. 17-2). When a worker's physiologic capacity to compensate for thermal stress is exceeded, heat can lead to impaired performance, an increased risk of accidents, and clinical signs of heat illness.

Internal temperature is regulated within narrow limits, predominantly by sweat production and evaporation. To a lesser extent, temperature regulation is accomplished by (1) physiologic control of blood flow from muscles and other deep sites of heat production to the cooler surfaces of the body, where heat is dissipated by convective exchange with air, and (2) by evaporative cooling from the lungs, to a minor degree.

The relationship between heat loss or gain variables and internal heat production is described by a simple heat balance equation:

$$S = (M - W) \pm C \pm R - E$$

in which S = net amount of energy gained or lost as heat by the body, M = heat produced by metabolism, W = external work performed, C = heat transfer by convection and conduction, R = heat transfer by radiation, and E = body heat loss by evaporation (in kcal/hr). This formula can also be used to evaluate situations of extreme cold.

**Fig. 17-2.** Foundry workers with exposure to excessive heat at work. (Photograph by Earl Dotter.)

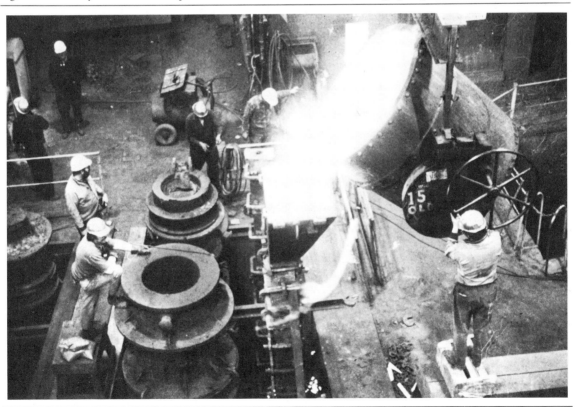

When homeostatic mechanisms are functioning properly, there will be no net gain or loss of heat (S = 0). Should S be greater than zero, heat imbalance occurs, leading to manifestations of heat stress. *Convection* refers to heat transfer between skin and the immediately surrounding air, assuming that air is being circulated. Its value is a function of the difference in temperature between skin and air, and the rate of air movement over the skin. *Conduction* refers to the transfer of heat from skin to a solid or liquid object resulting from direct contact. *Radiation* in this context refers to the radiative transfer of heat between surfaces of differing temperature, that is, the skin surface and the solid surroundings, such as an oven furnace or a cold floor.

The quantity (M − W) describes the total amount of body heat produced combining the gain from metabolic heat production and the loss due to external work effort. The C and R variables can be positive or negative because convection/conduction and radiation can occur in both directions. Ordinarily, with ambient temperature lower than surface body temperature (<95°F, or 35°C), convection and radiation promote transfer of body heat to the environment; however, if the environment is hotter than surface body temperature, radiation and convection can increase the body's heat load.

The heat loss/gain variables (C, R, and E) are influenced by environmental factors encountered in the workplace. In general, industrial heat exposures may be classified as either hot-dry or warm-moist. Hot-dry situations may prevail in a hot desert climate or near any furnace operation (such as is found in the metallurgical, glass, or ceramic industries), radiating high levels of heat. Heat absorption in these circumstances may overwhelm the cooling effect of sweat evaporation, leading to heat imbalance.

The most troublesome situation usually arises in warm-moist environments, as found in tropical climates, and in such industries as canning, textiles, laundering, and deep metal mining. High humidity and still air impede evaporative and convective cooling. Heat imbalance may occur despite an only moderate increase in ambient temperature; when this happens, thermal stress begins and can result in a variety of illnesses.

The mildest form of heat stress is discomfort. Prolonged exposure to a moderately hot climate may also cause irritability, lassitude, decrease in morale, increased anxiety, and inability to concentrate.

*Heat rash* (prickly heat) is common in warm-moist conditions due to inflammation in sweat glands plugged by skin swelling. Affected skin bears tiny red vesicles and, if sensitive, can actually impair sweating and greatly diminish the worker's ability to tolerate heat.

Heat rash can be treated with mild drying lotions, but it generally can be prevented by allowing the skin to dry in a cooler environment between heat exposures.

Prolonged exposure to heat may result in *heat cramps,* especially when there is profuse sweating and inadequate replacement of fluids and electrolytes. Heat cramps are alleviated by drinking electrolyte-containing liquids, such as juices.

As net retained body heat increases, *heat exhaustion* may occur, with pallor, lassitude, dizziness, syncope, profuse sweating, and clammy moist skin. An oral temperature reading may or may not reveal mild hyperthermia, whereas a rectal temperature is usually elevated (37.5–38.5°C, or 99.5–101.3°F). Heat exhaustion usually occurs in the setting of sustained exertion in hot conditions with dehydration from deficient water intake.

Finally, *heat stroke* can occur. This is a medical emergency that often is found in a setting of excessive physical exertion. In some cases, the central nervous system inappropriately shuts down perspiration leading to a loss of evaporative cooling; however, sweating may still be present in over half of exertional heat stroke cases [21]. Furthermore, heat stroke may occur even in a healthy, acclimatized person when heat loss becomes less than endogenous heat production. The uncontrolled accelerating rise in core temperature that follows is manifested by signs and symptoms that include dizziness, nausea, irritability, severe headache, hot dry skin, and a rectal temperature of 40.5°C (104.9°C) or higher. This often leads quickly to confusion, collapse, delirium, and coma. Cooling of the body must be started immediately if vital organ damage and death are to be averted. Workers who are not acclimatized (see below) are especially prone to heat stroke; other predisposing factors include obesity, recent alcohol intake, and chronic cardiovascular disease.

Workers with heat exhaustion or heat stroke must be removed to a cooler environment immediately. Heat exhaustion can be treated with oral rehydration or, if more severe, by the administration of intravenous saline fluids and observation. Heat stroke, however, must also be treated with immediate cooling. Methods include immersion in ice water, ice packs to the groin and axillae, and spraying with cooler water while the victim is fanned to speed evaporation. Cooling efforts should be slowed down and the patient observed once the temperature reaches 39°C (102°F) in order to avoid overcooling.

Monitoring a workplace environment for heat exposure is a task that involves measuring heat-modifying factors and assessing workloads. Occupational hygienists commonly use a measurement called the wet bulb globe temperature (WBGT) index, which takes into account convective and radiant heat transfer, humidity, and wind velocity. It is calculated by integrating the readings of three separate instruments that indicate the "dry" bulb temperature, the natural "wet" bulb temperature (which takes into account convective and evaporative cooling), and the "globe" temperature (which, through the use of a black copper sphere, registers heat transfer by radiation). The WBGT index has been used by NIOSH and the American Conference of Governmental Industrial Hygienists (ACGIH) as an indicator of heat stress in a recommended set of guidelines. These guidelines suggest maximally permissible standards of heat exposure, depending on the level of work performed in the hot environment [22, 23]. Even when these guidelines are followed, however, heat-related disorders may occur in exposed workers (Table 17-1).

Ideally, prevention of heat stress should be accomplished by isolating workers from hot environments through engineering design. However, as this is often not possible, heat stress is usually averted by a combination of engineering controls, work practice changes, use of personal protective clothing, and the education of those who work under conditions of excessive heat.

In addition to guidelines regarding heat exposure, NIOSH has made other recommendations concerning heat exposure, including (1) medical surveillance supervised by a physician and paid for by the employer for all workers exposed to heat stress circumstances above the "action" level, to include comprehensive history-taking, physical examinations, and overall assessment of a worker's ability to tolerate heat; (2) posting of warning signs in hazardous areas; (3) using protective clothing and equipment; and (4) providing information and training to workers. Workers should

Table 17-1. Permissible heat exposure threshold limit values (values are given in °C wet bulb globe temperature)

| | Workload | | |
|---|---|---|---|
| Work-rest regimen | Light | Moderate | Heavy |
| Continuous work | 30.0 | 26.7 | 25.0 |
| 75% Work 25% Rest, each hour | 30.6 | 28.0 | 25.9 |
| 50% Work 50% Rest, each hour | 31.4 | 29.4 | 27.9 |
| 25% Work 75% Rest, each hour | 32.2 | 31.1 | 30.0 |

Source: American Conference of Governmental Industrial Hygienists. Threshold limit values and biological exposure indices for 1985–86. Cincinnati: ACGIH, 1985: 69.

be trained to replace fluid losses systematically. During the course of a day's work in a hot environment, a worker may lose each hour up to 1 liter of fluid and electrolytes in sweat. This loss should be replaced by drinking fluids every 15 to 20 minutes, in greater amounts than are necessary to satisfy thirst, an inadequate stimulus for fluid replacement in stressful heat conditions. Other recommendations include (5) control of heat stress with engineering controls, and work and hygienic practices that specify time limits for working in hot environments, the use of a buddy system, provision of water, and other measures; and (6) maintaining and analyzing environmental and medical surveillance data.

One of the recommended work practices is an acclimatization program for new workers and for workers who have been absent from the job for longer than 9 days. Acclimatization is a process of adaptation that involves a stepwise adjustment to heat; it usually requires 1 week or more of progressively longer periods of exposure to the hot environment while working. Some workers may fail to acclimatize and consequently cannot work in such environments. Finding a short and easily administered screening test that can reliably predict heat intolerance is a research priority. NIOSH recommends (1) the reduction of peaks of physiologic strain during work; (2) the establishment of frequent, regular, short breaks for replacing water and electrolyte losses; and (3) preplacement and periodic medical examinations.

The recent finding that heat-acclimated workers lose less salt in sweat than previously thought, together with recognition of the high salt content in the average American diet and concern over exacerbating hypertension, has led experts to discourage the routine use of salt tablets to replace electrolyte losses. If salt replacement is required in a nonemergency situation, such as strenuous work on a hot dry day, adding extra salt to food is recommended. Workers on a low-sodium diet because of cardiovascular or other reasons require close medical supervision if working in a hot environment.

Decreasing heat stress can involve engineering measures such as devising heat shielding, or insulating and ventilating with cool, dehumidified air. Workers should be provided with a cooled rest area close to the workstation. Although clothing impedes the evaporation of sweat, it can reduce heat exposure in situations in which the ambient air temperature is higher than the skin temperature and the air is relatively dry, or when a worker is near a strong heat-radiating source. Some types of industrial heat exposure require protective equipment, such as gloves, aluminized reflective clothing, insulated and cooling jackets, and even self-contained air-conditioned suits.

### Cold

Cold stress is an environmental hazard that confronts cold-room workers, dry ice workers, liquefied gas workers, divers, and outdoor workers during cold weather. Other sources of cold exposure are the climates of the extreme Northern and Southern Hemispheres, and even poorly heated indoor workplaces during the winter in temperate zones. The body maintains thermal homeostasis in the face of a cold environment by decreasing skin heat loss through peripheral vasoconstriction and increasing metabolic heat production through shivering. Harmful effects of cold include frostbite, trench foot, chilblains, and general hypothermia, as described below.

*Frostbite* is actual freezing of tissue due to exposure to extreme cold or contact with extremely cold objects. Symptoms and signs range from erythema and slight pain to painless blistering, deep-seated ischemia, thrombosis, cyanosis, and gangrene. Windchill (loss of heat from exposure to wind) can play an important role in accelerating frostbite. Until a patient can receive definitive hospital treatment, it is imperative to protect the affected body part from trauma, including rubbing, to avoid rewarming if the possibility of refreezing exists. Emergency treatment includes warm-water immersion, elevation, debridement, analgesia, and tetanus prophylaxis. Long-term sequelae usually involve peripheral neurovascular changes.

*Trench foot* (immersion foot) is a condition that results from long, continuous exposure to damp and cold while remaining relatively immobile. It may involve not only the feet but the tip of the nose and ears as well; it typically occurs in a worker who has just experienced prolonged immersion in cold water or exposure to cold air. The clinical changes in affected tissue can progress from (1) an initial vasospastic, ischemic, hyperesthetic (oversensitive), pale phase; to a (2) later stage equivalent to a burn, with hyperemia, vasomotor paralysis, vesiculation, and edema; and (3) finally, to a gangrenous stage.

*General hypothermia* usually occurs in an individual who is subjected to prolonged cold exposure and physical exertion. When a person becomes wet, either from exposure or sweating, body heat is lost even faster. Most cases occur in air temperatures between $-1°C$ (30°F) and $+10°C$ (50°F); however, they can also occur in air temperatures as high as 18°C (64°F) or in water at 22°C (72°F), especially in the setting of fatigue. As exhaustion sets in, the vasoconstrictive protective mechanism becomes overwhelmed, resulting in sudden vasodilation and acute heat loss. Mental status changes, arrhythmias, coma, and death can ensue rapidly. Those at the extremes of age and those with certain conditions, such as hypothyroidism, adrenal insufficiency, and malnutrition are predisposed to hypothermia. The danger of hypothermia is also increased by the consumption of alcohol, phenothiazines, and other central nervous system (CNS) depressants. Management of hypothermia requires removal of the victim from the cold environment, removing any wet clothing, and specific warming measures. The method of warming depends on the degree of hypothermia. Most patients with mild hypothermia can be treated with passive rewarming (warm, dry clothes and blankets in a warm environment). More severe cases require active external warming (heating blankets) and active core rewarming including warmed oxygen, warmed intravenous fluids, and, in extreme cases, warmed dialysis fluids.

Finally, at temperatures below 15°C (59°F), the hands and fingers become insensitive long before these described cold injuries take place, thereby decreasing manual dexterity and increasing the risk of accidents. Many workers handle cold metal objects that can cause local freezing and metal-skin adhesions. The use of silk gloves makes it possible to handle cold metals up to $-40°C$ ($-40°F$) without freezing to them while retaining good manual dexterity.

In general, cold hazards are well recognized and preventable. Insulated clothing and protective barriers should be provided and workers should be able to take adequate breaks inside warm shelters, with warm beverages and dry clothing changes available. Pain in the extremities and severe shivering should be recognized as warning signs of cold injury and hypothermia. The additional cooling that occurs with increased wind speed (windchill) must also be taken into account when evaluating exposures.

### Hyperbaric Environments

In a handful of environments, including certain caisson[4] operations, underwater tunneling,[5] and diving, the ambient air pressure exceeds one atmosphere absolute (1 ATA), the atmospheric pressure found at sea level. These environments generally range from 2 to 5 ATA, although commercial divers often dive to depths greater than 100 meters at 11 ATA pressure (a 10-meter increase in depth below seawater adds 1 ATA pressure). In the United States, there are between 1.5 and 3 million certified divers, most of whom dive for recreation, with about 500 to 600 injuries and 75 to 100 deaths occurring each year.

---

[4]Caissons, tubular steel structures submerged in a river or sea bed or water-bearing ground, are used for construction or repair of bridges and piers, and excavation work. The pneumatic type of caisson has a closed top and is entered through an airlock; the bottom is open, allowing workers to excavate the ground, and water is excluded by the maintenance of a pressurized (hyperbaric) environment.

[5]In tunneling operations, compressed air is used to keep out water and to aid in supporting the structure.

The most common health problems stemming from working in a hyperbaric environment are caused by unequal distribution of pressure in tissue air spaces, incurred during compression (descent) or decompression (ascent). For example, when the eustachian tube becomes blocked as a result of inflammation or failure of a diver to clear the ears, descent compression causes negative middle-ear pressure with inward deformation of the tympanic membrane and possible rupture. Sinus cavities also experience pressure build-up. The lungs can become compressed in a breath-holding dive; conversely, if a diver with compressed air holds his or her breath during an ascent or during decompression in a chamber, the lungs can expand beyond their capacity, leading to rupture and pneumothorax, mediastinal emphysema, or even air embolism. Cerebral air embolism may resemble a stroke, but most commonly presents with stupor or loss of consciousness on surfacing. These symptoms in a diver should be treated as cerebral air embolism until proven otherwise (see below).

In addition to these mechanical hazards, workers in these environments encounter problems due to toxicity of the gas components of air at elevated partial pressures. At 4 ATA or greater, gaseous nitrogen induces a narcosis ("diver's high" or "rapture of the deep") marked by mood changes and euphoria. Oxygen inhalation at a high partial pressure can cause a toxic reaction with tingling, hallucination, confusion, nausea, vertigo, and sometimes seizures. These reactions can be avoided by limiting the depth of descent as well as limiting the proportion of oxygen in a compressed air mixture.

Another common problem arises when ascending too rapidly from a medium depth. As nitrogen becomes less soluble, bubbles are formed in blood and other tissues that impair circulation and lead to a variety of effects commonly known as decompression sickness (DCS). The same syndrome also may occur in high-altitude air flight when there is a loss of cabin pressure. DCS usually has a rapid onset, but may be delayed. Type I DCS, "the bends," is characterized by dull, throbbing joint pain and deep muscle or bone pain, generally occurring within four to six hours. Type II DCS is more severe and usually involves the CNS. Spinal cord lesions are most classic and can lead to paralysis. Recently, however, in a study of 23 patients with type II DCS, cerebral perfusion was also documented to be abnormal in every case [24]. Nitrogen bubbles in the pulmonary vasculature can cause cough and dyspnea and are known as the "chokes." Individuals with air embolism or DCS, or both, require oxygen therapy and immediate recompression (in a hyperbaric chamber) followed by prolonged decompression. Prolonged decompression is also the method of preventing the syndrome. A decompression rate of at least 20 minutes for each atmosphere (ATA) is recommended.

Most of these problems have been prevented through the use of decompression work practices. Procedures for medical surveillance and emergencies, involving divers and other workers in hyperbaric environments, are available in the literature [25].

Incompletely addressed hazards associated with compressed-air work include chronic exposure to hyperbaric environments with repeated decompressions. Workers so exposed have been found to have aseptic bone necrosis, mostly of the articular heads of long bones. The pathophysiology is believed to involve the occlusion of small-bore arteries by nitrogen bubbles, with platelet aggregates acting as microemboli during decompression. One follow-up study has suggested that this disease may progress even in the absence of further hyperbaric exposure [26]. Recent work from Norway has documented mild neuropsychological [27] and pulmonary function [28] abnormalities in commercial divers as compared with control subjects with no history of diving. It is possible that frequent hyperbaric exposures contribute independently to the risk of chronic pathology, even when one adheres to recommended decompression protocols.

Compressed-air workers should undergo routine examinations to try to identify aseptic bone necrosis as early as possible. Several experts recommend bone radiography at a frequency of every two or three years for workers who perform normal diving or compressed-air work and annually for workers regularly exposed to potential decompression sickness–provoking conditions. Bone scanning, though useful as a confirmatory diagnostic test, is not a more sensitive screening tool.

Finally, it is important to recognize an indirect hazard associated with hyperbaric environments: the potential contamination of compressed-air sources. Carbon monoxide is probably the most common contaminant of compressed air, particularly if a compressor is powered by a gasoline engine; other potential contaminants include carbon dioxide, oil vapor, and particulates.

### Hypobaric and Hypoxic (High-Altitude) Environments

A 41-year-old man was dead on arrival at the hospital. He had flown from 1,500 to 2,750 meters, and during the next few days had climbed to 4,270 meters, where he rapidly lost consciousness, dying 5 days after leaving 1,500 meters. Necropsy, about 5 hours after death, revealed severe cerebral edema, multiple petechial hemorrhages throughout the brain, bilateral pulmonary edema, bilateral bronchial pneumonia, dilatation and hypertrophy of the heart, and moderate arteriosclerosis of coronary arteries [29].

Workers, skiers, and mountain climbers in high-altitude regions, and pilots in unpressurized cabins, experience hypobaric (low-pressure) and hypoxic environments. At high altitudes, decreased pressure reduces the gradient for oxygen absorption, leading to a fall in arterial $pO_2$, despite the fact that the percentage of oxygen remains constant at 21 percent. Above 2,400 meters, arterial oxyhemoglobin saturation falls below 90 percent in most people. Illness associated with high altitude is rarely experienced below 2,000 meters; the incidence at 2,000 to 2,600 meters ranges from 1.4 to 25.0 percent, and it becomes even more common above 3,000 meters, especially in persons who venture to this altitude without taking time for acclimatization.

The most common health problem at high altitudes is *acute mountain sickness (AMS)*, an illness characterized by headache, nausea, vomiting, depression, and loss of appetite. Almost all people who undergo an abrupt altitude change by venturing into the mountains experience one of these symptoms to a degree within 24 hours; however, acclimatization usually occurs in a few days, and symptoms disappear over 4 to 6 days of exposure. The pathophysiology has been suggested to involve the imbalance occurring between the cerebral vasodilatation from hypoxia and the cerebral vasoconstriction from hypocarbia (a decrease in the partial pressure of carbon dioxide in the blood). Acclimatization with few symptoms is best achieved by slow ascent (350 m or 1,000 ft per day) and gradually progessive activity for several days. Some climbers who are required to reduce acclimatization time have lessened AMS symptoms by using acetazolamide, which results in a metabolic stimulus to increase the rate and depth of breathing. Dexamethasone is also effective as prophylaxis, and both drugs have been used to treat AMS when descent is not possible.

More serious is *high-altitude pulmonary edema (HAPE)*, which also strikes unacclimatized people, usually within 24 to 60 hours, and especially if they engage in vigorous activity soon after arrival at high altitude. Onset is usually insidious. Symptoms include shortness of breath, cough, weakness, tachycardia, and headache. This condition characteristically progresses to cough productive of bloody sputum, low-grade fever, and evidence of increasing pulmonary congestion, with rales and cyanosis. If the condition remains untreated, coma may ensue from hypoxia or cerebral edema (see below). The pathophysiology is unclear; clinical studies seem to suggest a process involving hypoxic vasoconstriction and pulmonary capillary leakage. It is treated ideally with descent to a lower altitude, rest, and administration of oxygen. Sometimes diuretics, positive pressure breathing, and nifedipine have been used when immediate descent has not been possible. Lack of recognition of this syndrome is probably most responsible for serious morbidity and mortality.

*Cerebral edema* is a rare, but often fatal, consequence of high altitude. The presence of neurologic signs and symptoms of headache, confusion, ataxia, and hallucinations in a person who has had an altitude change should make one suspect this diagnosis. Treatment, as in HAPE, centers on rapid descent and oxygen administration. Using dexamethasone in the same manner as for other forms of cerebral edema may be useful, but is not a substitute for immediate descent.

While most cases of acute high-altitude illness occur in persons visiting the mountains for recreation or work, nonacute forms are occasionally found in those living at high altitude for longer periods. Chronic mountain sickness was first recognized among certain natives of the Peruvian Andes. An analogous disease characterized by polycythemia, pulmonary hypertension, and right-heart enlargement has now been described in Tibet. It occurs almost exclusively among members of the Han population an average of 15 years after immigration to a high altitude, and is rare among the high-altitude natives. A subacute form with polycythemia, pleural effusion, right-sided congestive heart failure, and cardiomegaly has recently been recognized in a group of Indian soldiers stationed for about 11 weeks at 5,800 to 6,700 meters [30]. While chronic mountain sickness improves with transfer to a lower altitude, subacute disease resolves completely within several weeks of the move to low altitude.

Most cases of acute altitude-related illnesses can be prevented by slow acclimatization. The physiologic mechanism of acclimatization involves an increase in red blood cell production and hematocrit, increases in intraerythrocytic 2,3-diphosphoglycerate, or 2,3-DPG (leading to a favorable shift in the oxyhemoglobin dissociation curve), and mild hyperventilation. Exercise can be a part of this program, especially if heavy physical work is anticipated. The lack of a previous history of altitude-related illness while at high altitudes does not preclude the possibility of its occurrence later.

## Electric and Magnetic Fields

The ubiquitous use of electricity for a multitude of purposes has led to exposure of the general population and occupational groups to high-voltage electricity. While the hazards of electrocution and burns due to direct electrical exposure are well known, long-term effects, if any, due to exposure to electric and magnetic fields (E/MFs) associated with the use and transmission of electricity have not been determined.

An *electric field* exists around an electric particle. If an electric particle moves, as in an electric current, lines of electric force set up a *magnetic field,* whose lines of force are perpendicular to the particle's direction of movement. A variable electric field is always accompanied by a magnetic field; this interplay is often referred to as an *electromagnetic field.*

In general, workers who potentially sustain exposure to high-intensity E/MFs include those working near high-voltage electrical lines (Fig. 17-3), such as streetcar and subway drivers, power station operators, power and telephone line workers, and other groups of technicians and electrical workers, including electricians, movie projectionists, and welders.

Concern has been raised by several recent epidemiologic studies, which have suggested small, but inconsistent, increases in leukemia, brain cancer, and other cancers among occupational and residential groups exposed to higher levels of E/MFs [31, 32]. Criticism of the methodologies and interpretation of these studies has been intense. One of the most problematic aspects of these investigations is the tendency to find positive associations between cancer and surrogate exposure measurements, such as "electrical occupations" or wiring codes, but failure to find positive associations when actual field measurements of E/MF are

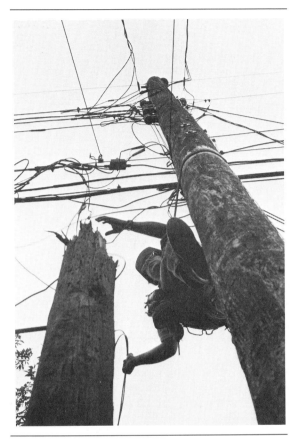

**Fig. 17-3.** Utility line workers exposed to high-voltage electrical lines are being studied for disease potentially induced by electromagnetic fields. They are at high risk for electrocution. (Photograph by Earl Dotter.)

made. Another serious concern is the possibility of publication bias against studies that do not support an association between E/MF exposure and cancer [31, 32].

While there is reason to believe that E/MFs may have an impact on health because endogenous electrical currents play crucial roles in physiologic processes, such as neural activity, tissue growth and repair, glandular secretion, and cell membrane function, the fields induced within the body by exposure are not large when compared to those generated by human cells [31]. While it has been dem-

onstrated that E/MFs can exert biologic effects, it is unclear what, if any, adverse health outcomes might be produced.

In addition to the lack of unequivocal epidemiologic evidence, there is no conclusive evidence from animal or in vitro studies that E/MFs are carcinogenic [32]. More basic scientific and epidemiologic research is required to determine whether E/MFs encountered in industry and the home pose a risk to health. Before future epidemiologic studies can generate meaningful results, more appropriate and precise exposure assessment metrics need to be established [31, 32].

## References

1. Elwood JM. Melanoma and sun exposure: Contrasts between intermittent and chronic exposure. World J Surg 1992; 16:157–65.
2. Walter SD, et al. The association of cutaneous malignant melanoma and fluorescent light exposure. Am J Epidemiol 1992; 135:749–62.
3. Cruickshanks KJ, Klein BEK, Klein R. Ultraviolet light exposure and lens opacities: The Beaver Dam Eye Study. Am J Public Health 1992; 82:1658–62.
4. Lydahl E, Philipson B. Infrared radiation and cataract. ii. Epidemiologic investigation of glass workers. Acta Ophthalmol 1984; 62:976–92.
5. Michaelson SM. Biological effects of radiofrequency radiation: Concepts and criteria. Health Physics 1991; 61:3–14.
6. Yost MG. Occupational health effects of nonionizing radiation. Occup Med State of the Art Rev 1992; 7:543–66.
7. Izmerov NF. Current problems of nonionizing radiation. Scand J Work Environ Health 1985; 11:223–7.
8. Whorton D, et al. Microwaves and pacemakers. J Occup Med 1992; 34:250.
9. Hunter D, McLaughlin AIG, Perry KM. Clinical effects of the use of pneumatic tools. Br J Ind Med 1945; 2:10.
10. Helmkamp JC, Talbott EO, Marsh GM. Whole body vibration—a critical review. Am Ind Hyg Assoc J 1984; 45:162–7.
11. Pope MH, Hansson TH. Vibration of the spine and low back pain. Clin Orthop 1992; 279:49–59.
12. Bongers PM, Hulshof CRJ, Dijkstra L, Boshuizen HC. Back pain and exposure to whole body vibra-

tion in helicopter pilots. Ergonomics 1990; 33:1007–26.

13. Wasserman DE, Taylor W. Lessons from hand-arm vibration syndrome research. Am J Ind Med 1991; 19:539–46.

14. Ekenvail L, Lindblad LE. Effect of tobacco use on vibration white finger disease. J Occup Med 1989; 31:13–16.

15. Taylor W, Pelmear PL. The hand-arm vibration syndrome: An update. Br J Ind Med 1990; 47:577–79.

16. Wieslander G, Norback D, Gothe CJ, Juhlin L. Carpal tunnel syndrome (CTS) and exposure to vibration, repetitive wrist movements, and heavy manual work: A case-referent study. Br J Ind Med 1989; 46:43–47.

17. Pelmear PL, Roos JO, Maehle WM. Occupational-induced scleroderma. JOM 1992; 34:20–5.

18. NIOSH. Criteria for a recommended standard: Occupational exposure to hand-arm vibration. U.S. Department of Health and Human Services (NIOSH) publication no. 89-106, 1989.

19. Ziskin MC, Petitti DB. Epidemiology of human exposure to ultrasound: A critical review. Ultrasound Med Biol 1988; 14:91–6.

20. Lundstrom R. Effects of local vibration transmitted from ultrasonic devices on vibrotactile perception in the hands of therapists. Ergonomics 1985; 28:793–803.

21. Knochel JP. Heat stroke and related heat stress disorders. DM 1989; 35:301–77.

22. NIOSH. Criteria for a recommended standard: Occupational exposure to hot environments (revised criteria). Department of Health and Human Services (NIOSH) publication no. 86-113, 1986.

23. American Conference of Governmental Industrial Hygienists. Threshold limit values and biological exposure indices for 1993–1994. Cincinnati: American Conference of Governmental Industrial Hygienists, 1993.

24. Adkisson GH, et al. Cerebral perfusion deficits in dysbaric illness. Lancet 1989; 2:119–22.

25. Downs GJ, Kindwall EP. Aseptic necrosis in caisson workers: A new set of decompression tables. Aviat Space Environ Med 1986; 57:569–74.

26. Van Blarcom ST, Czarnecki DJ, Fueredi GA, Wenzel MS. Does dysbaric osteonecrosis progress in the absence of further hyperbaric exposure? AJR 1990; 155:95–7.

27. Todnem K, Nyland H, Kambestad BK, Aarli JA. Influence of occupational diving upon the nervous system: An epidemiological study. Br J Ind Med 1990; 47:708–14.

28. Thorsen E, Segadal K, Kambestad B, Gulsvik A. Diver's lung function: Small airways disease? Br J Ind Med 1990; 47:519–23.

29. Houston CS, Dickinson J. Cerebral form of high-altitude illness. Lancet 1975; 2:758–61.

30. Anand IS, et al. Adult subacute mountain sickness—a syndrome of congestive heart failure in man at very high altitude. Lancet 1990; 335:561–65.

31. Thériault GP. Health effects of electromagnetic radiation on workers: Epidemiologic studies. Proceedings of the scientific workshop on the health effects of electric and magnetic fields on workers. In PJ Bierbaum, JM Peters. eds. Cincinnati: National Institute for Occupational Safety and Health, Department of Health and Human Services (NIOSH) publication no. 91-111.

32. Advisory Group on Non-Ionizing Radiation. Electromagnetic fields and the risk of cancer. Vol. 3, no. 1. Chilton, U.K.: National Radiological Protection Board, 1992.

## Bibliography

It is difficult to offer a general bibliography for this chapter given the wide assortment of hazards covered, their specific nature, and the rapid evolution of our understanding of many of these hazards. Reviews of specific topics that appear in the medical or environmental literature as well as technical monographs published by governmental agencies probably provide the best available overviews.

In general, much of the most up-to-date literature on clinical approaches to the physical environment hazard emergencies (i.e., heat, cold, and hyperbaric and hypobaric environments) can be found in the periodical *Environmental Emergencies.*

Other sources include the following:

Advisory Group on Non-Ionizing Radiation. Electromagnetic fields and the risk of cancer. Chilton, U.K.: National Radiological Protection Board, 1992.

NIOSH. Criteria for a recommended standard: Occupational exposure to hand-arm vibration. U.S. Department of Health and Human Services (NIOSH) publication no. 89-106, 1989.

Taylor W, Pelmear PL. The hand-arm vibration syndrome: An update. Br J Ind Med 1990; 47:577–79.

Yost MG. Occupational health effects of nonionizing radiation. Occup Med State of the Art Rev 1992; 7:543–66.

# 18
# Infectious Agents

Nelson M. Gantz

Work-related infectious diseases are caused by all categories of infectious agents. As with other types of disorders, the occupational history often provides the key clue to identifying the cause of a puzzling infectious disease.

Occupations associated with a risk of an infectious disease (Table 18-1) are divided into two categories: health care occupations, either with direct patient contact or laboratory exposure to infective material, and non–health care occupations, primarily those involving contact with animals or animal products, ground breaking or earth moving, or travel into endemic areas. Additional types of work-related infectious agents are prevalent in developing countries (see box). Table 18-2 presents the number of potentially work-related cases of selected infectious diseases in the U.S. reported to the Centers for Disease Control and Prevention (CDC) in 1992; it is not known how complete these data are or what percentage of these cases is actually work-related.

## Infectious Diseases in Health Care Workers

The hazards of hospital-acquired (nosocomial) infectious diseases have been well recognized since the mid-nineteenth century, when Semmelweiss discovered the cause of puerperal fever. The risk of nosocomial infection exists both for hospitalized patients and for workers involved in their care. (Table 18-3 lists some infectious agents that have

been transmitted from patients to health care workers.) Such problems exist not only for hospital workers but also for those in outpatient settings such as dentists' offices (Fig. 18-1). The risk of infection is also present for personnel working in, among other places, outpatient renal dialysis centers, laboratories where they have contact with blood, nursing homes, institutions for the retarded, and prisons.

### Hepatitis B

A 25-year-old intensive care unit nurse reported to the employee health service at her hospital. She complained of nausea, weakness, malaise, loss of appetite, dark urine, and jaundice of about 1 week's duration. She had not eaten any raw shellfish, never had a blood transfusion, did not know of any friends with hepatitis, and denied use of drugs. She recalled having been stuck with a needle 8 weeks before while caring for a patient who had a cardiac arrest, but she took no precautionary measures. Abnormal liver function tests and a positive blood test for hepatitis B surface antigen (HB$_s$Ag) confirmed the diagnosis of hepatitis B. Because of persistent vomiting and markedly abnormal liver function tests, she was hospitalized for 2 weeks. After this, she convalesced at home for 2 more weeks. She then thought she was ready to return to work. The cost of her illness, including hospital charges and lost wages, was approximately $9,000.

Viral hepatitis, type B (hepatitis B), is among the most frequently occurring work-related infectious diseases in the United States. It continues to be a major problem for physicians, nurses, dentists (es-

**Table 18-1.** Selected work-related infectious disease, by occupation

| Occupation | Selected work-related infectious diseases |
| --- | --- |
| Bulldozer operator | Coccidioidomycosis, histoplasmosis |
| Butcher | Anthrax, erysipeloid, tularemia |
| Cat and dog handler | Rochalimaea henselae, *Pasteurella multocida* cellulitis, rabies |
| Cave explorer | Rabies, histoplasmosis |
| Construction worker | Rocky Mountain spotted fever, coccidioidomycosis, histoplasmosis |
| Cook | Tularemia, salmonellosis, trichinosis |
| Cotton mill worker | Coccidioidomycosis |
| Dairy farmer | Milker's nodules, Q fever, brucellosis |
| Day care center worker | Hepatitis A, rubella, cytomegalovirus, other childhood infectious diseases |
| Delivery personnel | Rabies |
| Dentist | Hepatitis B, hepatitis C, AIDS |
| Ditch digger | Creeping eruption (cutaneous larva migrans), hookworm disease, ascariasis |
| Diver | Swimming pool granuloma (*Mycobacterium marinum*) |
| Dock worker | Leptospirosis, swimmer's itch (*Schistosoma* species) |
| Farmer | Rabies, anthrax, brucellosis, Rocky Mountain spotted fever, tetanus, plague, leptospirosis, tularemia, coccidioidomycosis, ascariasis, histoplasmosis, sporotrichosis, hookworm disease |
| Fisherman, fish handler | Erysipeloid, swimming pool granuloma |
| Florist | Sporotrichosis |
| Food-processing worker | Salmonellosis |
| Forestry worker | California encephalitis, Lyme disease, Rocky Mountain spotted fever, tularemia |
| Fur handler | Tularemia |
| Gardener | Sporotrichosis, creeping eruption (cutaneous larva migrans) |
| Geologist | Plague, California encephalitis |
| Granary and warehouse worker | Murine typhus (endemic) |
| Hide, goat hair, and wool handler | Q fever, anthrax, dermatophytoses |
| Hunter | Lyme disease, Rocky Mountain spotted fever, plague, tularemia, trichinosis |
| Laboratory worker | Hepatitis B, tuberculosis, salmonellosis |
| Livestock worker | Brucellosis, leptospirosis |
| Meatpacker/slaughterhouse (abattoir) worker | Brucellosis, leptospirosis, Q fever, salmonellosis |
| Mental retardation institute worker | Hepatitis A and B |
| Miner | Tuberculosis* |
| Nurse | Hepatitis B, rubella, tuberculosis, hepatitis C, AIDS, herpes simplex |
| Pet shop worker | *Pasteurella multocida* cellulitis, psittacosis, dermatophytoses |
| Physician | Hepatitis B, rubella, tuberculosis, hepatitis C, AIDS |
| Pigeon breeder | Psittacosis |
| Poultry handler | Newcastle disease, erysipeloid, psittacosis |
| Rancher | Lyme disease, rabies, Rocky Mountain spotted fever, Q fever, tetanus, plague, tularemia, trichinosis |

**Table 18-1 (continued).**

| Occupation | Selected work-related infectious diseases |
|---|---|
| Rendering plant worker | Brucellosis, Q fever |
| Sewer worker | Leptospirosis, hookworm disease, ascariasis |
| Shearer | Orf, tularemia |
| Shepherd | Anthrax, brucellosis, orf, plague |
| Soldier | Tularemia and other infectious diseases |
| Trapper | Leptospirosis, Lyme disease, tularemia, rabies, Rocky Mountain spotted fever |
| Veterinarian | Anthrax, brucellosis, erysipeloid, rabies, leptospirosis, *Pasteurella multocida* cellulitis, tularemia, salmonellosis, orf, psittacosis, Rochalimaea henselae |
| Wild animal handler | Rabies |
| Zoo worker | Psittacosis, tuberculosis |

*Silicotuberculosis (see Chap. 22) occurs among quarry workers, sandblasters, other silica processing workers, and workers in mining, metal foundries, and the ceramics industry.

---

## INFECTIOUS DISEASES IN DEVELOPING COUNTRIES

In developing countries, infectious diseases are highly prevalent. Some of these diseases are acquired in the workplace, from coworkers or other individuals, or from other sources in the work environment. Others result indirectly from work, such as sexually transmitted diseases that may be prevalent among male workers who have left their families and traditional cultural supports in a rural area to seek employment in a large city.

Specific categories of infectious diseases that may be occupational in origin, organized according to their usual mode of transmission, are as follows:

1. Vector-borne diseases, such as malaria, which can be acquired by working near mosquito breeding sites.
2. Water-borne and food-borne diseases, such as gastrointestinal disorders caused by *Salmonella*, *Shigella*, *Giardia lamblia*, and other organisms, which can be acquired at work, especially if workers have direct contact with water or food that has been contaminated by these or other microorganisms.
3. Sexually transmitted diseases, including AIDS, syphilis, gonorrhea, chlamydia, and other disorders, which can be transmitted at work. At high risk are commercial sex workers; at lower risk are clinical laboratory and health care workers.
4. Airborne diseases, which range from often benign viral respiratory infections to some more severe chronic respiratory infections, such as tuberculosis. Since HIV infection often leads to reactivation of latent infections with the tubercle bacillus, tuberculosis cases and deaths are increasing worldwide, including in developing countries.
5. Zoonoses, which include brucellosis, leptospirosis, anthrax, and rabies. These diseases are often prevalent in developing countries, especially in rural areas.

6. Other diseases, including viral hepatitis, type B (hepatitis B), which is highly prevalent in some developing countries.

## Bibliography

Benenson A. ed. Control of communicable disease in man. 15th ed., Washington, D.C.: American Public Health Association, 1990.

Levy BS, Choudhry AW. Endemic diseases. J Jeyaratnam. ed. Occupational health in developing countries. Oxford: Oxford University Press, 1992.

Table 18-2. Annual U.S. incidence (1992) of infectious diseases that are sometimes work-related*

| Disease | Number of reported cases |
| --- | --- |
| Anthrax | 1 |
| Brucellosis | 87 |
| Hepatitis, viral, type B | 14,751 |
| Leptospirosis | 51 |
| Lyme disease | 7,863 |
| Plague | 13 |
| Psittacosis | 86 |
| Rabies | 1 |
| Rocky Mountain spotted fever | 492 |
| Tetanus | 40 |
| Tuberculosis | 22,971 |
| Tularemia | 155 |
| Typhus fever, murine | 25–50 (estimate) |

*Actual number of cases that are work-related is unknown; data include both work- and non-work-related cases. Estimate not a reportable disease.
Source: Centers for Disease Control. MMWR 1993; 52 and 53:974.

pecially oral surgeons), and laboratory workers (particularly those who have direct contact with blood). Evidence of past hepatitis B virus (HBV) infection, based on the presence of antibody to $HB_sAg$ (anti-$HB_s$), is present in about 18 percent of physicians, over four times that reported for volunteer blood donors; rates are highest for pathologists and surgeons [1].

Blood is a major source of infective virus. Only minute amounts are required: One milliliter of blood from a chronic carrier diluted to $10^{-8}$ still retains infectivity. $HB_sAg$ is present not only in blood and blood products but also in saliva, semen, and feces; however, non-blood sources of infection are probably rare. The presence of $HB_sAg$ in serum correlates well, but not perfectly, with infectivity. (Infectivity is most highly correlated with $HB_eAg$.) All patients who are $HB_sAg$-positive, however, should be considered as potentially infectious.

Transmission of HBV may occur from an accidental percutaneous stick from a contaminated needle or other instrument. Infection may also develop after contaminated blood enters a break in the skin, splatters onto a mucous membrane, or is ingested, such as in a pipetting accident. Airborne transmission has not been reported.

Health care workers who are positive for $HB_sAg$ or anti-$HB_s$ often have had substantial contact with blood or blood products. Patient contact seems to be less important than direct contact with patients' blood. The incidence of hepatitis B infection for health care workers is increased in certain work areas, including hemodialysis units, hematology and oncology wards, blood banks and clinical laboratories (especially where personnel have contact with blood), operating rooms, dental offices and oral surgery suites, and wash areas for glassware and other equipment.

In the hospital, the major sources of HBV are patients with acute hepatitis B infection, patients with chronic liver disease, patients receiving chronic hemodialysis, immunosuppressed patients, parenteral drug abusers, and multiple blood transfusion recipients. In many hospitals, the

**Table 18-3.** Some infectious agents that are occupational risks for health care workers

| Virus | Bacteria | Others |
|---|---|---|
| Creutzfeldt-Jakob agent | *Bordetella* species | *Chlamydia psittaci* |
| Cytomegalovirus | *Campylobacter* species | *Coxiella burnetii* |
| Hepatitis B | *Corynebacterium diphtheriae* | *Cryptosporidium* species |
| Hepatitis C | *Mycobacterium tuberculosis* | *Mycoplasma* |
| Herpes simplex | *Neisseria meningitidis* | *pneumoniae* |
| Human immunodeficiency virus (HIV) | *Salmonella* species | *Sarcoptes scabiei* |
| Influenza | *Shigella* species | |
| Lassa fever | *Yersinia pestis* | |
| Measles | | |
| Mumps | | |
| Parainfluenza | | |
| Parvovirus B19 | | |
| Poliovirus | | |
| Respiratory syncytial virus | | |
| Rotavirus | | |
| Rubella | | |
| Rubeola | | |
| Varicella-zoster | | |

**Fig. 18-1.** Dentists and dental technicians require protection against pathogens in aerosols, blood, and saliva. (Photograph by Marvin Lewiton.)

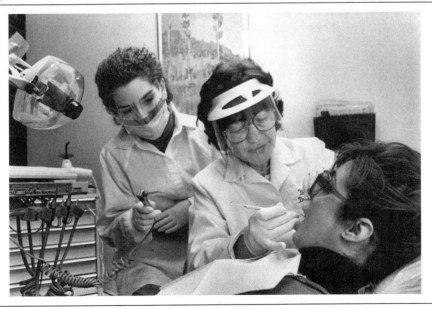

chronic hemodialysis unit is the highest risk area. Patients on chronic hemodialysis who become HB$_s$Ag-positive have up to a 60 percent chance of becoming chronic carriers. Other individuals at high risk of becoming chronic carriers are male homosexuals and residents of institutions for the retarded. Parenteral drug abusers have an HB$_s$Ag carrier rate of 1 to 5 percent, compared with a rate of 0.1 percent for volunteer blood donors [1].

Although certain features help distinguish hepatitis B from other forms of acute viral or toxic hepatitis, often they are not distinguishable clinically, and serologic studies are required for a specific diagnosis. Some patients are asymptomatic; others have malaise, fatigue, anorexia, nausea, vomiting, distaste for cigarettes, fever, abdominal pain, dark urine, light-colored stools, and other symptoms. Laboratory studies show abnormally high serum aminotransferases, such as serum glutamic-oxaloacetic transaminase (SGOT or AST) and serum glutamic-pyruvic transaminase (SGPT or ALT); often an increased serum bilirubin; and, in severe cases, a prolonged prothrombin time.

Hepatitis B surface antigen can be detected in the blood of a patient with hepatitis B usually 6 to 12 weeks after exposure and for about 1 to 6 weeks after onset of clinical illness. Of hepatitis B patients, 5 to 10 percent will become chronic carriers of HBV and serve as potential sources of infection for personnel. If a patient remains HB$_s$Ag-positive for 5 months, the probability of becoming a chronic carrier increases to 88 percent. Most chronic HB$_s$Ag carriers are asymptomatic; a subgroup of these carriers will have mild to moderate elevations in their liver function tests. Chronic active hepatitis will occur in 30 percent of chronic carriers and may result in cirrhosis.

***Prevention of Hepatitis B Infection.*** Prevention of infections with bloodborne pathogens, including HBV, is detailed in the Occupational Safety and Health Administration (OSHA) bloodborne pathogens standard (see chapter Appendix 2).

Recommendations for preventing hepatitis B in health care workers include immunization with hepatitis B vaccine as well as surveillance of staff in high-risk areas, employee education, appropriate sterilization and disinfection procedures, designation of a specific person responsible for safety, use of protective clothing and gloves, and avoidance of eating or smoking in laboratory work areas. (For an update on hepatitis B prevention, see MMWR 1990; 39 (no. RR-2):1–26.) Health care personnel should minimize their contact with potentially infectious patient secretions. Patients and staff in high-risk areas such as hemodialysis units can be screened for HB$_s$Ag and anti-HB$_s$. HB$_s$Ag-positive patients can be separated from HB$_s$Ag-negative patients and dialyzed by staff who have anti-HB$_s$ (or who are HB$_s$Ag positive). Personnel must carefully avoid needle sticks and contact of mucous membranes and skin with potentially contaminated blood or other secretions; wearing gloves is one means of achieving this. Use of the various new needleless devices for injections is another means of reducing needle-stick injuries (Fig. 18-2). All blood specimens should be handled as if potentially infectious. HBV-contaminated reusable equipment should be autoclaved before reuse, and HBV-contaminated disposable material should be disposed of in appropriate containers (Fig. 18-2). Syringe and other sharps manufacturers are focusing attention on proper design of these currently unsafe products.

Work practices should be consistent with the CDC guidelines on invasive procedures [2].

Hepatitis B immune globulin (HBIG) is recommended for prophylaxis within 1 week following either parenteral or mucosal contact with HB$_s$Ag-positive blood. Clinical hepatitis developed in 2 percent of HBIG recipients following a needle-stick exposure to HB$_s$Ag-positive blood compared with a rate of 8 percent in immune serum globulin recipients. The HB$_s$Ag and anti-HB$_s$ status of the exposed health care worker should be determined. If results of either test are positive, HBIG has no value and should not be given. If both tests are negative, HBIG should be given in two doses spaced 25 to 30 days apart.

Two types of hepatitis vaccines were developed

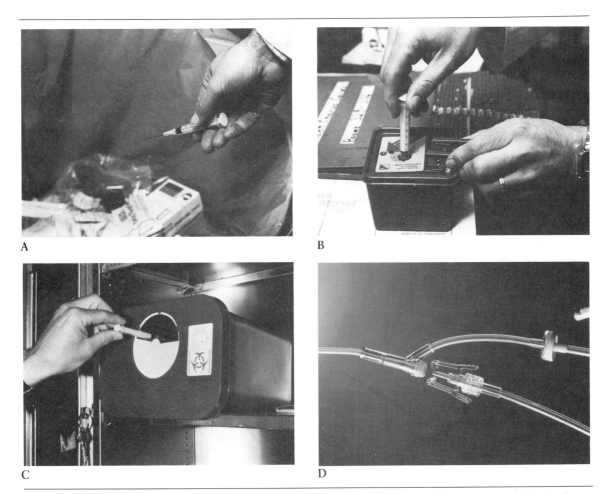

A

B

C

D

**Fig. 18-2.** Incorrect disposal of blood-contaminated needle in (A) a trash barrel and (B) a cutting device. C. Correct method of disposal. Proper disposal of needles is an important means of reducing the risk for hospital and other health care workers of hepatitis B and hepatitis C. (Photographs by Marilee Caliendo.) D. New needleless device for intravenous injection systems.

for prophylaxis. A plasma-derived vaccine, which consists of a suspension of $HB_sAg$ particles that have been inactivated and purified, was approved by the Food and Drug Administration in 1981. Although this vaccine was safe and efficacious, fear of receiving a product prepared from plasma in the era of acquired immunodeficiency syndrome (AIDS) somewhat limited its use by health care providers. In 1987 another vaccine became available that was prepared in baker's yeast using re-

combinant DNA technology. Two recombinant vaccines are available, Recombivax HB and Energix-B; the plasma-derived vaccine, Heptavax B, is no longer made. The vaccine induces a protective antibody (anti-$HB_s$). Three doses at 0, 1, and 6 months with hepatitis B vaccine are recommended. An alternate schedule using four doses of Energix-B vaccine given at 0, 1, 2, and 12 months has been approved for more rapid induction of immunity. The vaccines are administered intramuscularly in the deltoid and not the buttock. The vaccine has been studied in high-risk pre-exposure situations among male homosexuals and the staff of dialysis units. The results of the vaccine trials have been impressive, with efficacy rates from 71 to 92 percent. The vaccine has also been given in postexposure situations to sexual partners or spouses of those with hepatitis B and following needle-stick exposures. In the U.S., the three major target populations for the vaccine are individuals with occupational exposures, such as health care providers, all newborns, and those with sexual exposures. Target groups whose members, if susceptible, should receive hepatitis B vaccine are listed in the box.

In 1991 OSHA issued a regulation that hepatitis B vaccine be made available to all health care providers at risk (see chapter Appendix 2). This regulation and the availability of the new hepatitis vaccines made with recombinant DNA technology has increased vaccine usage. The duration of immunity and the necessity for booster doses of vaccine need to be defined. Antibody levels decline after 7 years, but persons may still be protected against clinical disease. (For recommendations on vaccine use, see MMWR 1990; 39 (no. RR-2): 1–26.)

The case of hepatitis B at the start of this section raises several questions concerning prevention of this disease: How should a needle stick be managed? When should HBIG be given? When (and should) this nurse return to work? If the needle has been in contact with a known individual ("donor"), then the $HB_sAg$ status of that person can be determined. If the donor is $HB_sAg$-positive or has a history of multiple blood transfusions and the worker is susceptible to hepatitis B (negative $HB_sAg$ and negative anti-$HB_s$), then the worker stuck by the needle is at risk of developing hepatitis B and should be given HBIG and hepatitis B vaccine. If the status of the "donor" is unknown and the worker is susceptible, then either HBIG or regular gamma globulin (immune serum globulin) can be given, plus hepatitis B vaccine. The nurse should be able to return to work when she is clin-

> ### GROUPS RECOMMENDED FOR HEPATITIS B VACCINE*
> 1. Persons whose work involves contact with blood or blood-contaminated body fluids such as health care and public safety workers
> 2. Clients and staff of institutions for the developmentally disabled
> 3. Hemodialysis patients
> 4. Sexually active homosexual men
> 5. Users of illicit injectable drugs
> 6. Patients with clotting disorders who receive clotting-factor concentrates
> 7. Household and sexual contacts of hepatitis B virus (HBV) carriers
> 8. Persons from countries of high HBV endemicity
> 9. Long-term inmates of correctional facilities
> 10. Sexually active heterosexual persons including sex workers
> 11. International travelers who plan to stay for more than six months in areas of high HBV endemicity, or short-term travelers who will have contact with blood, or sexual contact.
>
> *From Centers for Disease Control. Protection against viral hepatitis: Recommendations of the Immunization Practices Advisory Committee. MMWR 1990; 39(no. RR-2):14.

ically well, but if she remains $HB_sAg$-positive she should not draw blood from patients (or donate blood). Most importantly, however, had this nurse received hepatitis B vaccine, hepatitis B would not have developed. Measures should be taken to ensure that at-risk health care workers receive this effective vaccine. Immunization is the most important prevention measure for hepatitis B.

### Hepatitis A

Infection with hepatitis A virus is a risk for health care workers in institutions for the retarded where personal hygiene is poor and for certain animal caretakers, especially those with close exposure to chimpanzees. This virus is mainly transmitted by the fecal-oral route. Maximal viral shedding in the stool occurs during the 2-week period before onset of jaundice (and usually before diagnosis). Virus persists in the stool for about 7 to 15 days after the onset of jaundice [3]. There is no chronic carrier state of hepatitis A virus in the stool or blood.

Careful handwashing by health care personnel is probably the most important measure for preventing in-hospital spread of hepatitis A virus. Immune serum globulin (ISG) may be indicated for selected personnel working in institutions for the retarded within 1 to 2 weeks of contact with residents who have hepatitis A virus infection. Nonhuman primates, which may be a source of hepatitis A virus, should be quarantined for 2 months after importation. A vaccine to prevent hepatitis A is available in Europe and should be approved for use in the U.S. in the future.

### Delta Hepatitis

Delta hepatitis infection is caused by a unique RNA virus that requires $HB_sAg$ for its replication. Hepatitis caused by the delta agent occurs only in patients with a simultaneous hepatitis B infection or as a superinfection in a chronic $HB_sAg$ carrier. Diagnosis can be established by demonstrating the presence of either immunoglobulin M or G (IgM or IgG), delta antibody (anti-HD), or delta antigen in the serum. Delta infection occurs most often in intravenous drug addicts and patients with hemophilia. Nosocomial transmission of the delta agent among patients undergoing hemodialysis has been reported and the potential for acquisition of delta hepatitis by health care personnel exists. Clinically, delta agent can cause fulminant hepatitis and chronic carriage of delta agent may be found. Measures aimed at limiting the spread of hepatitis B should also limit the transmission of delta agent.

### Hepatitis C

Recent epidemiologic studies have clarified the natural history of this disease [4]. About 90 percent of transfusion-induced hepatitis cases are caused by hepatitis C virus (HCV) [5]. The risk of acquiring hepatitis following a transfusion has declined in recent years, and only about 6 percent of all cases of hepatitis are caused by a transfusion. Most cases of hepatitis C are related to drug use (42 percent) or are idiopathic (40 percent). Diagnosis relies on measuring antibody to HCV in the serum. The antibody to HCV is detectable 15 weeks after the onset of hepatitis and occasionally may be delayed as long as one year [6]. Tests to measure hepatitis C viral antigen are not yet available. Chronic liver disease due to hepatitis C is indicated by the presence of abnormal liver function tests and the persistence of hepatitis C antibody in the serum. Almost two-thirds of patients will become chronic carriers. The risk of acquiring HCV at work is only now being assessed. Rarely, disease in health care personnel has occurred following a needle stick, but the extent of this infection as an occupational hazard needs more research [7]. Dentists have an apparent increased risk of infection [8].

### Tuberculosis

A resurgence of tuberculosis has occurred in the U.S. in the 1990s secondary to the human immunodeficiency virus (HIV) epidemic, an increase in homelessness in the inner cities, and a change in immigration to this country [9]. This problem has been further complicated by the identification of strains of *Mycobacterium tuberculosis* that are resistant to the standard antituberculous agents—isoniazid, rifampin, and ethambutol. These multidrug-resistant tuberculous isolates (MDR-TB) have been responsible for both community and nosocomial cases. These developments have prompted the CDC to develop guidelines to attempt to control this serious problem. Studies are needed to address a number of issues, such as the efficacy of negative-pressure isolation rooms, the use of ultraviolet light germicidal irradiation, and the use of personal particulate respirators (see MMWR 1990; 39 (No. RR-17):1–29).

Transmission of tuberculosis (TB) from patients (often undiagnosed) to hospital workers and health care profession students remains a significant hazard. In one study TB was not initially suspected in one-half of the patients admitted with pulmonary TB, and in nearly one-third the diagnosis was not established by the time of discharge [10]. The diagnosis was often missed because of a low index of suspicion of this diagnosis by today's physicians, an atypical clinical or radiographic presentation in persons with HIV infection, and absence of tuberculin skin test positivity due to anergy. The incidence of tuberculin skin test positivity in U.S. physicians is at least twice the expected rate. Employees in nursing homes, mental health hospitals, and prisons are also at an increased risk of developing TB.

Prevention of TB in hospital employees requires that physicians have a high index of suspicion and institute respiratory isolation precautions pending confirmation of the diagnosis. Employees with nonreactive tuberculin skin tests should be screened with a tuberculin skin test once a year; tuberculin skin testing of exposed personnel is also indicated. Indications for isoniazid (INH) prophylaxis include household contacts of patients with active TB, recent converters, tuberculin reactors with an abnormal chest x-ray, special clinical situations such as patients who are tuberculin reactors on high-dose corticosteroids, and tuberculin reactors under 35 years of age. Isoniazid is also indicated for HIV-infected persons who are tuberculin skin test positive ($\geq 5$ mm induration), as well as for HIV-positive persons who are tuberculin skin test negative but who are at high risk for tuberculosis, such as intravenous drug abusers. Use of bacillus Calmette-Guérin (BCG) vaccination is not currently recommended for hospital personnel, since it would make skin testing less helpful in identifying tuberculin reactors. Fundamentals of tuberculosis infection control (Fig. 18-3) have been described by the CDC (see chapter Appendix 1).

### Rubella and Cytomegalovirus

*Rubella* infection may be transmitted from hospital employees to patients and from patients to sus-

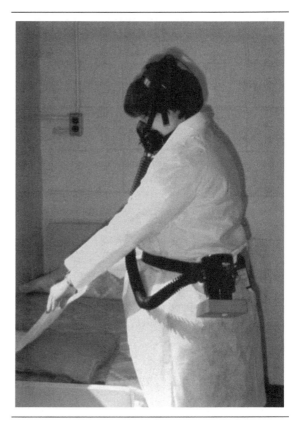

Fig. 18-3. Health care workers can be protected from TB by proper isolation of patients, use of enclosures, exhaust ventilation, and germicidal lamps. The last line of defense (illustrated) is the use of a powered air-purifying respirator. (Courtesy of NIOSH.)

ceptible personnel [11]. In one outbreak, 47 cases of rubella occurred among hospital personnel (a dietary worker was the suspected index case); this outbreak resulted in one pregnancy being terminated and 475 workdays being lost. The major hazard of rubella is infection in pregnant women, with the possibility of congenital rubella syndrome resulting in the offspring. Schoolteachers are also at an increased risk of acquiring rubella since they are likely to have contact with persons with the illness. About 15 percent of women in the childbearing age group are susceptible to rubella. Rubella vaccine is an effective means of preventing disease, and susceptible personnel should be immunized. Also, the trivalent mumps-measles-rubella (MMR) vaccine can be used. The vaccine is well tolerated and in the work setting results in minimal absenteeism. Pregnancy should be avoided for 3 months after vaccination.

*Cytomegalovirus (CMV)* is a potential threat for the developing fetus. Nurses who practice good personal hygiene are at no greater risk of acquiring this infection than their peers in the community [12]. In contrast, day care workers may be at an increased risk of acquiring CMV [13]. Cytomegalovirus is usually transmitted by sexual intercourse and via blood transfusions. Transmission of CMV appears to require prolonged intimate contact in the hospital. The use of gloves when handling potentially contaminated wastes as well as handwashing after each patient contact are the appropriate infection control measures to prevent acquisition of CMV.

## Measles
Since 1989 there has been a resurgence in cases of measles [14]. Ten cases acquired in the medical setting account for 3.5 percent of all reported cases. The source of the measles virus is usually a patient in whom the illness was not recognized during the prodromal stage, when a rash is absent. Almost one-third of cases in health care workers occur in those born before 1957, usually considered an immune group. In 1989 the Immunization Practices Advisory Committee issued new guidelines for hospital employees to provide proof of measles immunity or receive the measles vaccine [15].

## Parvovirus B19
Parvovirus B19 is a cause of several clinical problems including erythema infectiosum (also known as fifth disease), arthritis in adults, aplastic crisis, and fetal death in pregnancy. The virus has been detected in respiratory secretions and spread usually occurs by large particle aerosols or direct contact. Teachers and day care providers are at risk [16]. In the hospital, pregnant health care providers should not care for patients with a known parvovirus B19 infection. Since the infection in the index patient may not be recognized, use of universal precautions with the wearing of gloves and frequent handwashing is mandatory.

### Acquired Immunodeficiency Syndrome
Transmission of the AIDS agent, the human immunodeficiency virus, occurs only by sexual contact, by blood or blood products, and perinatally from an infected mother. Health care workers are at risk of acquiring HIV via exposure to patients' infected blood or body fluids. The greatest risk to medical personnel is percutaneous exposure, especially as a result of a needle-stick injury. The CDC estimates the risk of seroconversion to be 0.42 percent after a single percutaneous exposure. There is no evidence for transmission of this virus by casual contact, such as handshaking or face-to-face conversation. Although initial panic occurred among many health care workers assigned to care for patients with AIDS, these fears have proved excessive. To date, there have been 39 documented and 81 possible occupational transmissions of HIV among U.S. health care workers in which HIV-infected patients have been the source [17]. Most of the cases have been reported in nurses, laboratory technicians, and physicians. The majority of cases have occurred after a documented percutaneous injury and rarely after a mucous membrane or skin exposure. While cases have been seen in health care providers with no apparent risks, these individuals are being studied further. Lack of an adequate history is the likely explanation for HIV infection in those with an undetermined risk. The risk of a seroconversion to the AIDS virus following a needle-stick injury is estimated to be less than 1 percent, which is much lower than the risk (6–30 percent) of acquiring hepatitis B after a needle-stick injury [18]. Guidelines to prevent the transmission of HIV to health care workers have been developed. (See MMWR August 21, 1987; and MMWR 1991; 40 (no. RR-8):1–9. See chapter Appendix 2 for guidelines to prevent acquisition of HIV by a health care worker and recommendations to prevent the transmission

of HIV from an infected health care worker to a patient.)

Universal precautions and work practices designed to prevent transmission of hepatitis B are also effective against the bloodborne pathogens, such as HIV. Health care workers should take precautions to prevent needle-stick injuries and exercise care when handling blood, tissues, or mucosal surfaces of all patients. To reduce the risk of acquiring any bloodborne pathogen, such as HIV or hepatitis B and C viruses, the CDC has recommended that blood and bloody body fluids of *all* patients be considered as potentially infectious. These recommendations are known as universal precautions. To further reduce the risk of sharps injuries, safer products have been developed such as needleless systems. Guidelines have also been formulated for the management of occupational exposures to blood. Although the data of efficacy of zidovudine (AZT) are unavailable for postexposure prophylaxis, this drug is often given to health care providers after a critical exposure to blood from a patient with HIV. The CDC has published a statement on management of occupational exposure to HIV [19], and OSHA has published guidelines to prevent occupational exposure to bloodborne pathogens based on the CDC recommendations (see chapter Appendix 2).

While the health care and laboratory worker has a small risk of acquiring HIV, the risk of transmission from an infected health care provider to a patient during an invasive procedure is extremely low. In one dental practice in Florida, six patients acquired HIV infection presumably from an infected dentist. The mechanism of transmission is unknown. However, in 19,000 patients exposed to infected health care providers, no cases of HIV infection have occurred using retrospective investigations.

### Laboratory-Associated Infections

A 23-year-old hospital bacteriologist was admitted to the hospital with a 1-week history of chills, fever, headache, and diarrhea. She had a pulse of 80 beats per minute, temperature of 105°F, and a few macular areas on her abdomen. After blood cultures were obtained, she was given ampicillin and became afebrile. The blood cultures were positive for *Salmonella typhi*. The patient was diagnosed as having laboratory-acquired typhoid fever when further history revealed that she had been working with this organism 3 weeks earlier as part of a state laboratory proficiency-testing program. She admitted to smoking in the laboratory and occasionally eating her lunch there. The risk of infection from this organism can be reduced by immunizing laboratory personnel with typhoid vaccine as well as by enforcing basic laboratory safety procedures [20].

More than 6,000 cases of laboratory-associated infections and over 250 fatalities have been reported in the literature. The most frequently identified laboratory-associated infections are brucellosis, tuberculosis, tularemia, typhoid fever, hepatitis B, Venezuelan equine encephalitis, Q fever, coccidioidomycosis, dermatomycosis, lymphocytic choriomeningitis virus, and psittacosis. The Centers for Disease Control has classified infectious agents by risk hazard. Class 1 agents are the least hazardous; they include *Tinea capitis* (which causes ringworm of the scalp) and mumps virus. Class 4 agents pose the most risk and require the highest degree of containment; two examples are *Herpesvirus simiae* B and Lassa fever virus. Smallpox, a major threat to health care workers in the past, remains a concern for the few laboratory workers who still work with the virus.

Laboratory-acquired infections usually result from accidents. Syringes and needles, either as a result of self-inoculation or causing a spray, have been involved in 25 percent of these infections; another 25 percent are related to spilling or spraying the infectious material. Other accidents result from injuries due to broken glass or other sharp objects, aspirating material by mouth pipetting, and animal bites and scratches. The source of many laboratory-associated infections is obscure, although many of these are probably transmitted by aerosols. Air sampling techniques have shown that many laboratory procedures release organisms into the air.

Several approaches are available to prevent infection in laboratory personnel. Since inhalation of an infectious aerosol is assumed to be the major mode of transmission (although there are no data to support this contention), the use of biologic safety cabinets with filters and laminar air flow has been recommended to help protect against this hazard. Similarly, material being centrifuged should be put in tubes with sealable lids. Hand-pipetting devices should be used for pipetting infectious materials; mouth pipetting should always be avoided.

Extreme care is required in the use and disposal of needles and syringes to decrease this frequent source of accidental infection. Experimentally infected animals are another important source of infection, and attention should be given to the animal quarters to minimize airborne spread of infection (see the next section). In addition, measures must be employed to prevent animal biting and scratching accidents; vaccination to prevent rabies, tetanus, or plague may be indicated for persons at risk. Sera should be collected from employees and stored to be used diagnostically as acute-phase sera if an illness develops. Other measures to decrease the risk of infection include use of biohazard signs; limited access to laboratories; restrictions for pregnant employees working with cytomegalovirus, herpesvirus, and rubella virus; and educational programs for personnel regarding possible hazards and preventive measures. Laboratory safety must receive each employee's highest priority at all times.

Considerable interest has developed in the use of monoclonal antibodies for diagnosis as well as therapy of septic shock. Rat immunocytomas have been used in this work and the cell lines may be infected with various viruses. In one report, laboratory workers developed hemorrhagic fever from contact with rat cell lines infected with hantavirus. Prevention of these infections requires screening of the rats before their use.

## Infectious Diseases in Non–Health Care Workers

Most work-related infectious diseases among non-health care workers are zoonoses, diseases primarily of animals that are transmitted to humans. Al-though these diseases occur infrequently, they are occupational hazards for workers who have contact with animals, such as farmers, veterinarians, butchers, and slaughterhouse workers. Some zoonoses also can result from recreational exposures. Examples of these diseases are listed in Table 18-4.

### Bacterial Diseases

A sheep shearer became ill with fever and a headache. On examination he was found to have a 2-cm ulcerative skin lesion on his right hand and enlarged right epitrochlear and axillary lymph nodes. A Gram's stain of the skin ulcer drainage showed polymorphonuclear leukocytes but no organisms. Because of his occupation and the clinical presentation, tularemia was suspected. Isolation of the organism was not attempted because of the risk of creating an infectious aerosol in the bacteriology laboratory. The patient responded to oral tetracycline therapy and recovered in 10 days. The diagnosis of tularemia was later confirmed serologically by a fourfold rise in antibodies to tularemia agglutinins between the initial acute serum and convalescent serum.

Tularemia, like most other work-related bacterial diseases in non–health care workers, is an uncommon disease. However, the disease should be considered in the differential diagnosis of a patient with the appropriate work history who presents with a skin lesion and lymphadenopathy. Laboratory workers and others whose work requires repeated exposure to tularemia are candidates for tularemia vaccine.

Other work-related bacterial diseases that affect non–health care workers include anthrax, brucellosis, erysipeloid, leptospirosis, Lyme disease, *Pasteurella multocida* cellulitis, plague, nontyphoid salmonellosis, and swimming pool granuloma. Prevention of bacterial zoonoses is summarized in Table 18-4 and includes vaccination when available and use of protective clothing.

### Viral Diseases

Viral infections acquired occupationally by non–health care workers fall into two categories:

*Arthropod-borne:* Yellow fever; Colorado tick fever; and Venezuelan, California, St. Louis, and

**Table 18-4.** Examples of occupational zoonoses in the United States

| Disease | Clinical manifestations | Common animal sources | Mode of acquisition | Workers at risk | Prevention |
|---|---|---|---|---|---|
| BACTERIAL DISEASES | | | | | |
| Anthrax | Malignant pustule, regional lymphadenopathy, or pneumonia | Cattle, sheep, horses, goats (usually in form of imported animal products) | Direct contact of inhalation of spores, souring of hides | Farmers, butchers, veterinarians | Vaccination, identification of infected animals |
| Brucellosis | Fever, headache, profuse sweating, anorexia, arthralgias, fatigue | Cattle, pigs, goats, sheep, dogs | Direct contact, ingestion, or inhalation | Meat packers, livestock workers, rendering plant workers, veterinarians | Animal vaccines, protective clothing and gloves |
| Cat-scratch disease | Regional lymphadenopathy, fever, primary skin papule | Cats, dogs | Direct contact | Veterinarians, cat and dog handlers | Avoidance of cat scratches |
| Erysipeloid (not to be confused with the acute cellulitis erysipelas) | Localized purplish-red skin lesions | Fish, other wild and domestic animals | Direct contact (often after skin abrasions) | Fishermen, butchers, fish handlers, poultry handlers, veterinarians, homemakers | Gloves, handwashing |
| Leptospirosis | Chills, fever, myalgias, headache, hepatitis, conjunctival suffusion, skin rash | Rodents, dogs, cats, cattle, pigs, wild animals | Contact with urine-contaminated soil or water, or direct contact with infected animal | Veterinarians, farmers (of sugar and rice), sewer workers, trappers, slaughterhouse workers, dock workers | Animal vaccines, avoidance of contact with contaminated water, rat control |
| Lyme | Erythema chronicum migrans, Bell's palsy, heart block, arthritis | Mice, deer | Vectors of *B. burgdorferi* are various *Ixodes* ticks | Forestry workers, hunters, ranchers | Protective clothing, insect repellents |
| *Pasteurella multocida* cellulitis | Localized cellulitis (pain, swelling, and redness) | Cats and dogs (part of normal nasopharyngeal flora) | Animal bite | Veterinarians, pet shop workers | Prevention of animal bites |

| Disease | Symptoms | Reservoir | Transmission | Occupations at risk | Prevention |
|---|---|---|---|---|---|
| Plague | Chills, high fever, regional lymphadenopathy, septicemia, or pneumonia | Ground squirrels, rabbits, hares, prairie dogs, rats, mice, coyotes | Direct contact with infected animal, rat flea bite, or respiratory droplets of infected patients | Farmers, ranchers, hunters, geologists in Southwest and West | Rat and vector control, vaccination |
| Salmonellosis | Chills, fever, headache, diarrhea | Poultry, cows, horses, dogs, cats, turtles | Direct contact with infected animal or its feces, or ingestion of infected food | Veterinarians, cooks, food processing and abattoir workers | Vaccination for laboratory workers, improved food processing and preparation |
| Swimming pool granuloma | Skin ulceration | Fish (marine and freshwater) | Direct contact | Fishermen, tropical fish store workers, divers | Pool disinfection, gloves |
| Tularemia | Red skin, papule that becomes ulcer, regional lymphadenopathy, pneumonia, or conjunctivitis with chills and fever | Rabbits, hares, ticks | Direct contact with infected animal, ingestion, aerosolization, or tick bite | Trappers, fur handlers, ranchers, butchers, cooks | Vaccination, gloves, insect repellents |
| **VIRAL DISEASES** | | | | | |
| Encephalitis (for example, California encephalitis) | Lethargy, fever, headache, disorientation | Rodents, horses | Mosquito or tick bite | Agriculture and forestry workers, geologists, geographers, entomologists | Protective clothing, insect repellents |
| Rabies | Fever, headache, agitation, confusion, seizures, excessive salivation | Raccoons, dogs, cats, skunks, bats, foxes | Animal bite | Veterinarians, cave explorers, ranchers, trappers, farmers, wild animal handlers | Avoid animal bites, local wound care, pre- and postexposure immunization |
| **RICKETTSIAL DISEASE** | | | | | |
| Murine typhus (endemic typhus) | Headache, fever, skin rash, myalgias | Rats | Direct contact | Granary and warehouse workers | Rodent and vector control |
| **CHLAMYDIAL DISEASE** | | | | | |
| Psittacosis | Fever, headache, pneumonia | Parakeets, parrots, pigeons, turkeys | Inhalation of organism | Pet shop workers, pigeon breeders, zoo workers, veterinarians, poultry handlers | Tetracycline, chemoprophylaxis of fowl |

western and eastern equine encephalitis are in this group. A human vaccine is available only for yellow fever; other preventive measures involve use of protective clothing, insect repellents, and vector control programs.

*Non-arthropod-borne:* These diseases include rabies, orf, milker's nodules, and Newcastle disease. Orf is a skin disease caused by a poxvirus of sheep. Reddish-blue papules develop at sites of contact within 6 days of exposure to infected sheep; spontaneous recovery occurs. Milker's nodules is another viral skin disease transmitted to the hands of milkers from the udders of infected cows; the nodules resolve within 4 to 6 weeks. Newcastle disease virus, which causes pneumoencephalitis in fowl, may produce a self-limited conjunctivitis in exposed workers.

Rabies is a good example of a possibly work-related viral disease for which prevention is available. In recent years, particularly in the northeastern U.S., a marked increase has been seen in rabies cases in wild animals, such as raccoons. High-risk groups include veterinarians, animal handlers, and laboratory personnel who work with the virus. Of course, not all cases are work-related. Rabies prevention has been successful and has resulted in a decrease in the United States from an average of 22 cases per year from 1946 to 1950 to only 1 to 5 cases per year presently. Prevention of rabies includes local wound care, avoiding of animal bites, and immunization with vaccines or immune globulins. Persons at high risk of rabies should be immunized before exposure with multiple doses of human diploid-cell rabies vaccine. Postexposure prophylaxis with human rabies immune globulin (HRIG) and the human diploid rabies vaccine is also recommended. To prevent rabies, the public must be educated in ways to reduce the risk of exposure to wild animals in affected areas, and the need to keep current the rabies vaccination status of pet dogs and cats.

### Rickettsial Diseases

Rocky Mountain spotted fever (RMSF), Q fever, and murine typhus can be work-related. RMSF is a potential risk for workers exposed to ticks in endemic areas such as the South Atlantic states; disease may occur, for example, in foresters, hunters, and construction workers. Q fever occurs commonly in cattle, sheep, and goats; dairy farmers, ranchers, stockyard and slaughterhouse workers, and hide and wool handlers are at risk of inhaling the organism and aquiring pneumonia or hepatitis. Murine typhus occurs in persons working in rat-infested areas; granary and warehouse workers are at risk. (Most of the cases in the United States occur in Texas.)

### Chlamydial Disease

Psittacosis, which is caused by a strain of *Chlamydia psittaci* and usually takes the form of a pneumonia, is an occupational hazard for pet shop employees, pigeon breeders, zoo workers, and veterinarians. In addition, several outbreaks have been reported in turkey-processing plants [21].

### Parasitic Diseases

Some parasites are occupational hazards for non–health care workers in the United States; many more, not listed here, are hazards for workers in other countries. Schistosome dermatitis or "swimmer's itch" is an infrequent hazard for water workers, such as skin divers, lifeguards, clam diggers, and rice field workers. Workers who have direct contact with the soil, such as barefoot farmers, ditch diggers, sewer workers, and tea plantation workers, may infrequently develop hookworm disease, ascariasis, cutaneous larva migrans (creeping eruption), and visceral larva migrans. Mites, chiggers, and ticks that infest poultry and substances such as straw, dust, and grains may affect workers who handle them. Prevention of occupational parasitic diseases usually involves wearing protective clothing and shoes, health education, and measures to improve the standard of living.

### Fungal Infections

Workers involved in earth-moving jobs such as bulldozer operators are at risk of acquiring deep fungal infections. Infection usually results from inhalation of spore-containing dust in endemic areas. Occupational fungal infections include histoplasmosis, coccidioidomycosis, and sporotrichosis. Superficial fungal infections can also result from occupational exposures; for example, ringworm in dogs, cats, cattle, and other animals is common and therefore animal handlers are at increased risk. Superficial candidal infection may be a hazard for workers such as bakers whose hands are often wet.

Histoplasmosis is a well-recognized occupational pulmonary disease; the organism is found in certain soils, and its growth is stimulated by bat or bird guano. In the U.S., the peak incidence of disease is in the Ohio and Mississippi River Valleys. At great risk are cave explorers, bridge scrapers, excavators, bulldozer operators, and grave diggers. Earth-moving activities at sites of chicken coops or bird roosts in endemic areas such as Tennessee or Kentucky should be preceded by appropriate soil cultures for fungi. A 5% formalin solution sprayed on contaminated soil before earth-moving operations may be effective in preventing disease where a disease risk has been documented.

Coccidioidomycosis is caused by *Coccidioides immitis,* a fungus found in the soil in the Southwest. Infection is associated with earth-moving activities. Rarely, infection may be transmitted via inanimate objects (fomites) such as fruits, cotton, and vegetables containing spores that can become airborne. Archaeologists, geologists, bulldozer operators, and farm workers are at greatest risk. Prevention of naturally acquired disease is difficult at present, and workers involved in earth-moving activities should be aware of the risks. Before earth moving in an endemic area, one should consider obtaining soil cultures [22, 23].

Sporotrichosis infection usually results from traumatic inoculation of the organism into the skin. Sphagnum moss is often implicated as the source of the organism although timber and other plant material are potentially a risk. Florists, nursery workers, farmers, berry pickers, and horticulturists are at greatest risk. Spraying sphagnum moss with a fungicidal solution may help prevent infection.

## Influenza Control in the Workplace

Influenza outbreaks continue to occur. These outbreaks can be classified as pandemics, which occur every 30 to 40 years and have an associated very high excess mortality; epidemics, which occur more often with a lower excess mortality; and sporadic outbreaks, which occur most often and have the lowest associated excess mortality. The explanation for these outbreaks involves the unusual capability of the influenza viruses to undergo antigenic changes. These changes in the virus can be classified as antigenic shifts and antigenic drifts. Antigenic shifts result in major changes in one or both surface antigens, probably due to recombination of genetic material among different influenza viruses. Antigenic shifts are of great importance since the population generally lacks protective antibody against the new strain. Antigenic shifts can result in pandemics and epidemics. Antigen drift probably results from point mutations in the influenza virus genome leading to minor changes in the surface antigens. As a result of antigenic drift, persons will have some protection against the new influenza virus, but will still require the new influenza vaccine to achieve optimal protection for that year. Influenza viruses can be categorized as type A and type B viruses. Genetic recombination between the two types has not been demonstrated. Amantadine, a drug used for prophylaxis for persons who have yet to receive the influenza vaccine, is only effective against influenza A virus.

Influenza and other respiratory viruses are responsible for considerable morbidity and days lost from work for workers in both health care and non–health care settings. Hospital personnel may transmit influenza to elderly patients; those with underlying heart, lung, or metabolic diseases; or immunosuppressed patients, resulting in morbidity and mortality. Control measures include use of

## FEVER AND "FLU" MAY NOT BE INFECTIOUS*

Two work-related syndromes, metal fume fever and polymer fume fever, are characterized by fever and influenza-like symptoms but are non-infectious in origin.

Metal fume fever produces chills, increased sweating, nausea, weakness, headache, myalgias, and cough. It often begins with thirst and a metallic taste in the mouth. The white blood cell count is often elevated. Metal fume fever results from exposure to oxides of various metals, usually zinc, copper, or magnesium; aluminum, antimony, cadmium, copper, iron, manganese, nickel, selenium, silver, and tin have also been implicated. Welding, melting of copper and zinc in electric furnaces, and zinc smelting and galvanizing are work processes that have often been associated with this syndrome.

*For further information, see T Gordon, JM Fine. Metal fume fever. Occup Med State of the Art Rev 1993; 8:505–18; and DJ Shusterman. Polymer fume fever and other fluorocarbon pyrolysis-related syndromes. Occup Med State of the Art Rev 1993; 8:519–32.

Polymer fume fever is characterized by dry cough, tightness in the chest, a choking sensation, and shaking chills. It is caused by exposure to unknown breakdown products of fluorocarbons, which are among the substances formed when polytetrafluorethylene (PTFE, also known as Teflon or Fluon) is heated above 300°C. Since the first description of this syndrome in the 1950s, its control has been accomplished by preventing exposure to the heated fluorocarbon. In a workplace where there is PTFE exposure, however, cigarettes may become contaminated by PTFE on a worker's hands or in workplace air. Within the cigarette, PTFE is heated to temperatures high enough to convert it to substances that are strong respiratory irritants. Therefore, even when the fluorocarbon is not directly heated to sufficient temperature, if smoking is allowed at the workplace the classic syndrome may still occur.

Both syndromes often occur after a delay of several hours from initial exposure. Both syndromes resolve within 24 to 48 hours with as yet no known long-term sequelae.

---

antiviral compounds such as amantadine and influenza vaccines. Use of influenza vaccine in the work setting for health care personnel should be considered, depending on the recommendations of the Centers for Disease Control for that year.

There are relatively few industry-based influenza immunization programs. Target groups who should receive yearly influenza vaccine are outlined in the box.

## Traveling Patient

A number of resources are available for health care providers and travelers to prevent diseases related to travel. The best source is: Centers for Disease Control and Prevention, Atlanta, GA 30333; 404-

## TARGET GROUPS FOR INFLUENZA VACCINE

1. Persons $\geq$ 65 years of age
2. Residents of nursing homes and other chronic care facilities
3. Adults and children with chronic pulmonary or cardiovascular disease
4. Adults and children with chronic metabolic diseases (such as diabetes mellitus), renal disease, or hemoglobinopathies, or those who are immunosuppressed
5. Children and teenagers (6 months–18 years of age) receiving long-term aspirin therapy
6. Health care providers
7. Members of households with high-risk persons

629-3311 (workday); 404-629-2888 (after hours; emergency requests).

Malaria Branch: 404-488-4046
Malaria Prevention Hotline: 404-332-4555 (not available 24 hours)
Parasitic Diseases Drug Service: 404-629-3670
Rabies Branch: 404-629-3095
Travelers' Health Hotline: 404-332-4559

# References

1. Centers for Disease Control. Inactivated hepatitis B virus vaccine. MMWR 1982; 31:318.
2. Centers for Disease Control. Recommendations for preventing transmission of human immunodeficiency virus and hepatitis B virus to patients during exposure-prone invasive procedures. MMWR 1991; 40 (Suppl. no. RR-6).
3. Krugman S, Ward R, Giles JP. The natural history of infectious hepatitis. Am J Med 1962; 32:717–28.
4. Alter MJ, et al. The natural history of community-acquired hepatitis C in the United States. N Engl J Med 1992; 327:1899–1905.
5. Alter MJ, Purcell RH, Shih JW. Detection of antibody to hepatitis C virus in prospectively followed transfusion recipients with acute and chronic non-A, non-B hepatitis. N Engl J Med 1989; 321:1494–500.
6. Esteban JI, et al. Evaluation of antibodies to hepatitis C virus in a study of transfusion-associated hepatitis. N Engl J Med 1990; 323:1107–12.
7. Kiyosawa K, et al. Hepatitis C in hospital employees with needlestick injuries. Ann Intern Med 1991; 115:367.
8. Klein RS, Freeman K, Taylor PE, Stevens CE. Occupational risk for hepatitis C virus infection among New York City dentists. Lancet 1991; 338:1539–42.
9. Beck-Sagué C, et al. Hospital outbreak of multidrug-resistant *Mycobacterium tuberculosis* infections: Factors in transmission to staff and HIV-infected patients. JAMA 1992; 268:1280–6.
10. Counsell SR, Tan JS, Dittus RS. Unsuspected pulmonary tuberculosis in a community teaching hospital. Arch Intern Med 1989; 149:1274–78.
11. Polk BF, White JA, DeGirolami PC, Modlin JF. An outbreak of rubella among hospital personnel. N Engl J Med 1980; 303:541–5.
12. Balcarek KB, Bagley R, Cloud GA, Pass RF. Cytomegalovirus infection among employees of a children's hospital: No evidence for increased risk associated with patient care. JAMA 1990; 263:840–44.
13. Adler SP. Cytomegalovirus and child day care: Evidence for an increased infection rate among daycare workers. N Engl J Med 1989; 321:1290–6.
14. Atkinson WL, Markowitz LE, Adams NC, Seastrom GR. Transmission of measles in medical settings—United States, 1985–1989. Am J Med 1991; 91 (Suppl. 3B):320S.
15. Centers for Disease Control. Measles prevention: Recommendations of the Immunization Practices Advisory Committee (ACIP). MMWR 1989; 38(S-9):10.
16. Cartter ML, et al. Occupational risk factors for infection with parvovirus B19 among pregnant women. J Infect Dis 1991; 163:282–5.
17. Chamberland ME, et al. Health care workers with AIDS: National surveillance update. JAMA 1991; 266:3459–62.
18. Henderson DK, et al. Risk for occupational transmission of human immunodeficiency virus type 1 (HIV-1) associated with clinical exposures. Ann Intern Med 1990; 113:740–6.
19. Centers for Disease Control. Public Health Service statement on management of occupational exposure to human immunodeficiency virus, including considerations regarding zidovudine postexposure use. MMWR 1990; 39:(no. RR-1).
20. Holmes MB, et al. Acquisition of typhoid fever from proficiency-testing specimens. N Engl J Med 1980; 303:5I9.
21. Hedberg K, et al. An outbreak of psittacosis in Minnesota turkey industry workers; implications for modes of transmission and control. Am J Epidemiol 1989; 130:569–77.
22. DiSalvo AF. Mycotic morbidity—an occupational risk for mycologists. Mycopathologia 1987; 99:147–53.
23. Kohn GJ, Linné SR, Smith DM, Hoeprich PD. Acquisition of coccidioidomycosis at necropsy by inhalation of coccidioidal endospores. Diagn Microbiol Infect Dis 1992; 15:527–30.

# Bibliography

Acha PN, Szyfres B. Zoonoses and communicable diseases common to man and animals. 2nd ed. Washington, D.C.: Pan American Health Organization, 1991. *An excellent reference for further reading on zoonoses.*

Berenson AS. ed. Control of communicable diseases in man. 15th ed. Washington, D.C.: American Public Health Association, 1990.
*A very useful handbook on the prevention and control of communicable diseases.*

Centers for Disease Control and Prevention and National Institutes of Health. Biosafety in microbiological and biomedical laboratories. 3rd ed. Washington, D.C.: U.S. Department of Health and Human Services [publication no. (CDC) 93-8395], 1993.
*Safety guidelines for the laboratory.*

Geiseler PJ, Nelson KE, Crispen RG, Moses VK. Tuberculosis in physicians: A continuing problem. Am Rev Respir Dis 1986; 133:773.
*Risk still exists for medical students and physicians.*

Holmes GP, et al. B virum (*Herpesvirus simiae*) infection in humans: Epidemiologic investigation of a cluster. Ann Intern Med 1990; 112:833.
*B virus (Herpesvirus simiae)–infected persons who worked with monkeys at a research laboratory.*

Kelen GD, et al. Hepatitis B and hepatitis C in emergency department patients. N Engl J Med 1992; 326:1399.
*Twenty-four percent of patients were infected with hepatitis B virus, hepatitis C virus, or HIV-1, making use of universal precautions mandatory to prevent acquisition of these viruses.*

Occupational Safety and Health Administration. Occupational exposure to bloodborne pathogens: Final rule. 29 CFR 1010.1030. December 6, 1991.
*Regulations designed to protect employees from bloodborne or other infectious material.*

Patterson WB, et al. Occupational hazards to hospital personnel. Ann Intern Med 1985; 102:658.
*A review that emphasizes measures to prevent these problems.*

Sanford JP. Humans and animals: Increasing contacts, increasing infections. Hosp Pract 1990; 25:123.
*A review of zoonoses.*

---

APPENDIX 1

# Fundamentals of Tuberculosis Control*

An effective TB control program requires early detection, isolation, and treatment of persons with

---

*From Centers for Disease Control. Draft guidelines for preventing the transmission of tuberculosis in health-care facilities. MMWR 1990;39(No. RR-17).

active TB. The primary emphasis of the TB infection control plan should be the achievement of these three goals. In all health care facilities, particularly those in which persons who are at high risk for TB work or receive care, policies and procedures for TB control should be developed, periodically reviewed, and evaluated for effectiveness to determine the actions necessary to minimize the risk of TB transmission.

The control program should be based on a hierarchy of control measures. The first and most important level of the hierarchy is the use of administrative measures to reduce the risk of exposure to persons with infectious TB. This includes developing and implementing effective written policies and protocols to ensure the rapid detection, isolation, diagnostic evaluation, and treatment of persons likely to have TB, as well as implementing effective work practices by persons working in the health care facility.

The second level of the hierarchy is the use of engineering controls to prevent the spread and reduce the concentration of infectious droplet nuclei. This includes (1) direct source control using local exhaust ventilation, (2) control of air-flow direction to prevent contamination of air in areas adjacent to the infectious source, (3) dilution and removal of contaminated air via general ventilation, and (4) air cleaning via air filtration or ultraviolet germicidal irradiation (UVGI).

The first two approaches minimize the number of areas in the health care facility where exposure to infectious TB may occur, and reduce, but do not eliminate, the risk in those few areas (for example, TB isolation rooms and treatment rooms where cough-inducing procedures are performed) where exposure may still occur. Because persons entering isolation and treatment rooms may be exposed to *M. tuberculosis,* the third level of the hierarchy is the use of personal respiratory protective equipment in these and a few other situations of probable relatively higher risk.

Specific measures to reduce the risk of TB transmission include the following:

- Assigning supervisory responsibility for the design, implementation, and maintenance of the TB infection control program to specific persons in the health care facility
- Conducting a risk assessment to evaluate the risk of TB transmission in all parts of the health care facility, developing a written TB control program based on the risk assessment, and periodically repeating the risk assessment to evaluate the effectiveness of the TB infection control program
- Developing, implementing, and enforcing policies and protocols to ensure early detection of patients who may have infectious TB
- Providing prompt triage and appropriate management of patients who may have infectious TB in the outpatient setting
- Promptly initiating and maintaining TB isolation, diagnostic evaluation, and treatment for persons who may have infectious TB and who are admitted to the inpatient setting
- Developing, installing, maintaining, and evaluating ventilation and other engineering controls to reduce the potential for airborne exposure to *M. tuberculosis*
- Developing, implementing, maintaining, and evaluating a respiratory protection program
- Using appropriate precautions for cough-inducing procedures
- Educating and training (health care workers [HCWs]) about TB, effective methods for prevention of TB transmission, and the benefits of medical screening programs
- Developing and implementing a program for routine periodic screening of HCWs for active TB and TB infection
- Promptly evaluating possible episodes of transmission of TB in health care facilities, including purified protein derivative (PPD) skin test conversions of HCWs, clusters of cases in HCWs or patients, and contacts of TB patients who were not promptly detected and isolated
- Coordinating activities with the local public health department, emphasizing reporting and

adequate discharge follow-up, and ensuring continuation and completion of therapy

---

APPENDIX 2

# Fundamentals of HBV and HIV Infection Control

---

## OSHA Standard on Occupational Exposure to Bloodborne Pathogens

According to OSHA estimates, more than 5.6 million workers in health care and public safety occupations in the United States could be potentially exposed to the bloodborne pathogens, such as the human immunodeficiency virus (HIV) and the hepatitis B virus (HBV). Exposure of health care workers to bloodborne pathogens occurs most commonly by needle-stick injuries and also through contact with body fluids (including semen and vaginal secretions), mucous membranes, and nonintact skin of workers.

The OSHA bloodborne pathogens standard applies to all persons occupationally exposed[1] to blood or other potentially infectious materials. It helps to determine who has occupational exposure to bloodborne pathogens and how to reduce this exposure.

### Exposure Control Plan
The standard requires the employer to develop a written exposure control plan to include exposure determination, procedures for evaluating circumstances surrounding an exposure incident, and the schedule and method for implementing the standard. The plan must be reviewed, updated, and made accessible to employees. The exposure determination must be based on the definition of oc-

---

[1]Occupational exposure means reasonably anticipated skin, eye, mucous membrane, or parenteral contact with blood or other potentially infectious materials that may result from the performance of the employees' duties.

cupational exposure without regard to personal protective clothing and equipment. Separate consideration is given to groups in which all or only some of the employees have occupational exposure. All employees identified as exposed must be informed of the hazard.

### Information and Training

These must be provided at no cost to the employee, at the time of initial assignment, during working hours, and at least once a year thereafter. Trainers must be knowledgeable and the information provided must be appropriate in content and vocabulary to the educational level, literacy, and language of the audience, and must include information on obtaining the regulation; epidemiology, symptoms, and transmission; the exposure control plan; recognition of tasks that cause exposure; use and limitations of work practice and engineering controls, and personal protective equipment; hepatitis B vaccination; emergency procedures; reporting and following up on exposure incidents; and warning labels, signs, and color coding.

Additional training in standard microbiologic practices and techniques, practices and operations specific to the facility, and the proper handling of human pathogens or tissue cultures is required for employees who work in laboratories and production facilities where exposure to HIV and HBV might occur—before they start work.

### Hepatitis B Vaccination

At no cost, the employer must make hepatitis B vaccine available within 10 days of initial work assignment to all employees who have occupational exposure to blood or other potentially infectious materials and must provide a postexposure evaluation and follow-up to all employees who experience an exposure incident. Recommended booster doses must be provided.

### Universal Precautions

Universal precautions must be observed.

### Methods of Control

*Engineering and Work Practice Controls.* These types of controls are the primary methods used to prevent occupational transmission of HBV and HIV. Personal protective clothing and equipment are also necessary when occupational exposure to bloodborne pathogens remains even after instituting these controls. Engineering controls include use of self-sheathing needles, puncture-resistant disposal containers for contaminated sharp instruments, resuscitation bags, and ventilation devices. Work practice controls include restricting eating, drinking, smoking, applying cosmetics or lip balm, and handling contact lenses; prohibiting mouth pipetting; preventing the storage of food or drink in refrigerators or other places where blood or other potentially infectious materials are kept; providing and requiring the use of handwashing facilities; and routinely checking equipment and decontaminating it before servicing and shipping. Other work practice requirements include washing of hands when gloves are removed and as soon as possible after skin contact with blood or other potentially infectious materials occurs, and prohibition of recapping, removing, or bending needles, unless it is proved that no alternative is feasible, and then these tasks must be done by mechanical means. Shearing or breaking contaminated needles is not permitted.

*Personal Protective Equipment (PPE).* Personal protective equipment must be used if occupational exposure remains after engineering and work practice controls are instituted, or if these controls are not feasible. Such equipment includes gloves, gowns, laboratory coats, face shields or masks, and eye protection. Personal protective equipment is considered appropriate only if it does not permit blood or other potentially infectious materials to pass through or reach employees if torn, punctured, or contaminated, or if its ability to function as a barrier is compromised.

*Housekeeping.* The employer must develop and implement a cleaning schedule that includes appropriate methods of decontamination and tasks or procedures to be performed. It must be ensured that all equipment, work surfaces, covers, and reusable receptacles that have been, or could be, contaminated with blood or other potentially infectious materials are cleaned and decontaminated appropriately and immediately. Mechanical means should be used to pick up contaminated broken glassware. Regulated waste must be placed in closable labeled or color-coded containers constructed to prevent leakage. Handling of contaminated laundry must be limited and only with appropriate PPE. Wet contaminated laundry should be placed in leak-proof, labeled, or color-coded containers before being transported, and bagged at its location of use.

*Labeling.* Fluorescent orange or orange-red warning labels are required to be attached to containers of regulated waste, to refrigerators and freezers containing blood and other potentially infectious materials, and to other containers used to store, transport, or ship blood or other potentially infectious materials. The warning label must include the biohazard symbol and the word "BIOHAZARD" in a contrasting color, and it must be attached to each object by string, wire, adhesive, or other method to prevent loss or unintentional removal of the label.

*What to Do If an Exposure Incident Occurs.* The standard requires that the postexposure medical evaluation and follow-up be made available immediately for employees who have been exposed. At a minimum, the evaluation and follow-up must include documentation of routes and means of exposure, the source individual (unless infeasible or prohibited by law), and, with consent, testing of the source individual's blood as soon as possible for HIV and HBV infectivity.

*Recordkeeping.* Employers also must preserve and maintain for each employee an accurate record of occupational exposure and must include (and keep confidential) name and Social Security number, hepatitis B vaccination status and dates, examinations and medical testing results, and written opinions. Training records must be kept for three years.

*HIV and HBV Research Laboratories and Production Facilities.* Employers in research laboratories and production facilities engaged in the culture, production, concentration, experimentation, and manipulation of HIV and HBV must provide additional protections and services.

## Recommendations to prevent the acquisition of HIV by a health care worker from an infected patient.[2]

1. All health care workers should routinely use appropriate barrier precautions to prevent skin and mucous membrane exposure when contact with blood or other body fluids of any patient is anticipated. Gloves should be worn for touching blood and body fluids, mucous membranes, or nonintact skin of all patients, for handling items or surfaces soiled with blood or body fluids, and for performing venipuncture and other vascular access procedures. Gloves should be changed after contact with each patient. Masks and protective eyewear or face shields should be worn during procedures that are likely to generate droplets of blood or other body fluids to prevent exposure of mucous membranes of the mouth, nose, and eyes. Gowns or aprons should be worn during procedures that are likely to generate splashes of blood or other body fluids.

2. Hands and other skin surfaces should be washed immediately and thoroughly if contam-

[2]From MMWR 1987 36(Suppl. 2S):6S–7S.

inated with blood or other body fluids. Hands should be washed immediately after gloves are removed.

3. All health care workers should take precautions to prevent injuries caused by needles, scalpels, and other sharp instruments or devices during procedures; when cleaning used instruments; during disposal of used needles; and when handling sharp instruments after procedures. To prevent needle-stick injuries, needles should not be recapped, purposely bent or broken by hand, removed from disposable syringes, or otherwise manipulated by hand. After they are used, disposable syringes and needles, scalpel blades, and other sharp items should be placed in puncture-resistant containers for disposal; the puncture-resistant containers should be located as close as practical to the use area. Large-bore reusable needles should be placed in a puncture-resistant container for transport to the reprocessing area.

4. Although saliva has not been implicated in HIV transmission, to minimize the need for emergency mouth-to-mouth resuscitation, mouthpieces, resuscitation bags, or other ventilation devices should be available for use in areas in which the need for resuscitation is predictable.

5. Health care workers who have exudative lesions or weeping dermatitis should refrain from all direct patient care and from handling patient-care equipment until the condition resolves.

6. Pregnant health care workers are not known to be at greater risk of contracting HIV infection than health care workers who are not pregnant; however, if a health care worker develops HIV infection during pregnancy, the infant is at risk of infection resulting from perinatal transmission. Because of this risk, pregnant health care workers should be especially familiar with and strictly adhere to precautions to minimize the risk of HIV transmission.

7. All health care workers who participate in invasive procedures must routinely use appropriate barrier precautions to prevent skin and mucous membrane contact with blood and other body fluids of all patients. Gloves and surgical masks must be worn for all invasive procedures. Protective eyewear or face shields should be worn for procedures that commonly result in the generation of droplets, splashing of blood or other body fluids, or the generation of bone chips. Gowns or aprons made of materials that provide an effective barrier should be worn during invasive procedures that are likely to result in the splashing of blood or other body fluids. All health care workers who perform or assist in vaginal or cesarean deliveries should wear gloves and gowns when handling the placenta or the infant until blood and amniotic fluid have been removed from the infant's skin and should wear gloves during postdelivery care of the umbilical cord.

8. If a glove is torn or a needle-stick or other injury occurs, the glove should be removed and a new glove used as promptly as patient safety permits; the needle or instrument involved in the incident should also be removed from the sterile field.

## CDC recommendations to prevent transmission of HIV and hepatitis B virus to patients from health care workers infected with these viruses[3]

1. All health care workers (HCWs) should adhere to universal precautions, including the appropriate use of handwashing, protective barriers, and care in the use and disposal of needles and other sharp instruments. HCWs who have exudative lesions or weeping dermatitis should refrain from all direct patient care and from handling patient-care equipment and devices used in performing invasive procedures until the condition resolves. HCWs should also comply with

[3]From MMWR 1991; 40(Suppl. no. RR-8):5–6.

current guidelines for disinfection and sterilization of reusable devices used in invasive procedures.

2. Currently available data provide no basis for recommendations to restrict the practice of HCWs infected with HIV or HBV who perform invasive procedures not identified as exposure-prone, provided the infected HCWs practice recommended surgical or dental technique and comply with universal precautions and current recommendations for sterilization/disinfection.

3. Exposure-prone procedures should be identified by medical/surgical/dental organizations and institutions at which the procedures are performed.

4. HCWs who perform exposure-prone procedures should know their HIV antibody status. HCWs who perform exposure-prone procedures and who do not have serologic evidence of immunity to HBV from vaccination or from previous infection should know their $HB_sAg$

status and, if that is positive, should also know their $HB_eAg$ status.

5. HCWs who are infected with HIV or HBV (and are $HB_eAg$ positive) should not perform exposure-prone procedures unless they have sought counsel from an expert review panel and been advised under what circumstances, if any, they may continue to perform these procedures. Such circumstances would include notifying prospective patients of the HCW's seropositivity before they undergo exposure-prone invasive procedures.

6. Mandatory testing of HCWs for HIV antibody, $HB_sAg$, or $HB_eAg$ is not recommended. The current assessment of the risk that infected HCWs will transmit HIV or HBV to patients during exposure-prone procedures does not support the diversion of resources that would be required to implement mandatory testing programs. Compliance by HCWs with recommendations can be increased through education, training, and appropriate confidentiality safeguards.

# 19
# Occupational Stress

Dean B. Baker and Robert A. Karasek

A 54-year-old taxicab driver develops unstable angina after a 10-year history of hypertension and two episodes of bleeding duodenal ulcers. He does not drink alcohol or smoke cigarettes.

A 21-year-old video display terminal operator develops visual discomfort, headaches, backaches, irritability, and trouble sleeping.

A 46-year-old automobile assembly-line worker calls in sick at the start of the workweek for the fourth time in the past two months.

A 39-year-old investment banker with an exceptional record of achievement no longer seems able to complete projects on time. He reports feeling fatigue to the point where he has given up his regular recreational activities.

Each of these situations was related to stress at work. Consideration of stress in the evaluation, prevention, and treatment of potential occupational diseases substantially expands the range and complexity of the health care provider's task. Unlike other occupational hazards, which tend to be specific for tasks, stress is ubiquitous and, to a varying extent, is associated with all work. Instead of an unambiguous causal association between a single toxic agent and a limited range of health effects, there may be many causes of occupational stress that combine to contribute to a single effect or, conversely, a single "stressor" may manifest itself as many different effects. The health care provider must appreciate and be able to evaluate occupational stress as a complex process involving disequilibrium of integrated psychological and physiologic systems. Furthermore, because stress is affected by such factors as the nature of the work

process and perceptions of the individual worker, it is inherently a psychosocial phenomenon with organizational and economic ramifications. The health care provider may have little expertise and may be uncomfortable dealing with these factors.

Awareness of occupational stress is increasing in many countries as managers, workers, and health care providers have to address issues such as increased job pressure, insecurity, and feelings of powerlessness at work. There are indications that our modern mechanisms of production and international trade are contributing to an increase in stress risks throughout the world [1]. Some of these stress issues occur at the level of the individual's job, others have their source in increasingly complex organizational structures, and others operate at the level of the marketplace, even globally. The "free market" for labor, for example, means that any worker can be replaced at any time in the name of economic efficiency. Such a work environment provides a less stable basis for determining a person's major social role than has occurred in "less advanced" societies.

The exact magnitude of stress-related disorders is not known, although it is large. The National Council of Compensation Insurance reports that compensation claims for stress-related disorders are growing in number while virtually all other disabling work injuries are decreasing [2]. Stress contributes to the development of heart and cerebrovascular disease, hypertension, peptic ulcer and inflammatory bowel diseases, and musculoskeletal problems [3–6]. Evidence suggests that stress al-ters immune function, possibly facilitating the development of cancer [7, 8]. Anxiety, depression, neuroses, and alcohol and drug problems are associated with stress [9, 10]. These latter conditions contribute to the incidence of injuries, homicides, and suicides. Considered together, these disorders, which are affected by stress, are responsible for much mortality, morbidity, disability, and medical care utilization.

Although assessment of stress remains problematic, awareness of the role of stress in these conditions has increased during the past two decades. It is now generally recognized that stress plays an important role in the etiology of work-related disorders. The health care provider should be able to recognize stressful working conditions, to evaluate stress-related disorders, and to manage stress in the individual. We will discuss common usage of the term *stress* and its simple definitions, physical and mental processes that contribute to it, and integrated models of stress development.

## Definition of Stress

The term *stress* is used in a number of ways: as an environmental condition, as an appraisal of an environmental condition, as a response to an environmental condition, and as a form of relationship between environmental demands and a person's abilities to meet the demands [11]. In reality, there is no single agreed-upon definition of *stress,* so that it may be thought of as an umbrella term encompassing all of the definitions presented below. Many of the "definitions" of stress attempt to develop a general and unitary label for a complex phenomenon. They do not clarify how the process occurs, which must be resolved with the more complex conceptual mechanisms described in the following sections.

The first two uses of the term *stress* are found in the popular literature, where one reads that an environment is "full of stress" or that a person "experiences stress at work." The influence of this literature is demonstrated by studies of public be-

liefs about causes of heart attacks. The most frequently cited cause, ahead of accepted biologic risk factors, was "stress, worry, nervous tension, pressure." Unfortunately, these popular uses of *stress* are not specific enough to assist the health care provider in identifying and managing stress-related disorders.

The third use of *stress* as a response to an environmental condition is found widely in primary care medical literature and in the stress management literature. This definition is based on Selye's concept of stress as "the nonspecific response of the body to any demand made upon it" [12]. Within this paradigm, stress is a nonspecific neuroendocrine response related to the process of homeostasis. Stress can be either good (eustress) or bad (distress), depending on whether the adaptive response is overwhelmed and homeostasis is no longer achieved, although the level of stressor necessary to disturb homeostasis is not specified.

Another popular definition among clinical psychologists and stress managers is McGrath's definition of stress as "a (perceived) substantial imbalance between demand and response capability, under conditions where failure to meet demand has important (perceived) consequences" [13]. This definition differs from that of Selye in that stress is (1) a function of both the environment and the person; (2) a psychosocial, as well as biologic, phenomenon, linked to the perceptions of the individual; and (3) an undesirable phenomenon (this is what Selye would call "distress"; the constructive adaptation of workers to environmental challenges typically is not considered stress).

Both the "nonspecificity" of response in Selye and emphasis on personal capabilities and perceptions of the McGrath definition have obscured the need to identify environmental factors responsible for stress. Stress management programs based on these perspectives emphasize strategies to increase a person's adaptive resources, rather than to decrease causes of stress in the environment.

Despite ambiguity about the term *stress*, there is general agreement about related terms (see box). Thus, "stressors" interact with the individual to

## DEFINITIONS RELATED TO STRESS

*Stress*  A (perceived) substantial imbalance between demand and response capability, under conditions in which failure to meet demand has important (perceived) consequences [13]. The psychological or social environment is usually the locus of causes, and personal well-being or health is the locus of effects, with a linkage operating in a system-wide (nonspecific) manner. Alternatively, many clinicians define "stress" more generally as a rubric encompassing the sequence from stressors to stress reactions and long-term consequences.

*Stressor*  An environmental event or condition that results in stress.

*Stressful*  Pertaining to an environment that has many stressors.

*Strain*  Short-term physiological, psychological, or behavioral manifestations of stress.

*Modifier*  Individual characteristic or environmental factor that may act on each stage of the stress response to produce individual variation.

cause "strain" or short-term stress reactions. Unresolved stress reactions lead to stress-related disorders. "Modifiers" are factors that can act on each stage of the stress response to produce individual variation in the sequence from stressors to stress reactions to long-term consequences.

## Concepts of Occupational Stress Etiology and Mechanisms

### Development of Occupational Stress Models

Because of the complexity of the stress phenomenon, stress research has led to the development of a number of conceptual models of how occupational stress arises. The most common approach has been for investigators to provide an enumeration of environmental factors that are considered to be stressors. These factors include objective conditions, such as overtime, shiftwork, and unemployment, and subjective job attributes, such as overload, role conflict, and role ambiguity. Unfortunately, similar labels have commonly been used by different investigators in reference to different assessment instruments. Thus, for example, "role ambiguity" reported by one investigator may not be based on the same questions as "role ambiguity" reported by other investigators. This confusion over the definition of stressors has contributed to the inconsistent results reported in the stress research literature.

Other investigators have attempted to describe the essential characteristics of stressful work. An example is the list provided by Kasl [4]: (1) The stressful work condition tends to be chronic, rather than intermittent or self-limiting; (2) there is external pacing of work demands, such as those created by machines, payment mechanisms, or competition; (3) habituation or adaptation to the chronic situation is difficult and, instead, some form of vigilance or arousal must be maintained; (4) failure to meet demands leads to drastic consequences (regarding equipment, lives, and money); and (5) there is a "spillover" of the effect of the work role to other areas of functioning, such as family and leisure, so that daily impact of the demanding job situation becomes cumulative and health threatening, rather than being daily defused or eased. Kasl cites the jobs of air traffic controllers, sea pilots, and train dispatchers as prototypes.

These attempts at enumerating stressors or describing characteristics of stressful work have been useful in identifying components of the stress phenomenon, but they have not been able to clarify the etiologic dynamics of stress. Consequently, much research on occupational stress has been oriented toward developing integrated models of stress that are capable of identifying and predicting which characteristics of work are stressful. These models have evolved from earlier attempts at a stress theory from the field of cognitive psychology and from physiologic models of the stress response developed by Selye and others.

*Contributions to a Stress Model from Cognitive Psychology.* A central tenet of the cognitive stress models is that processes of perception and interpretation of the external world determine the development of psychological states in the individual, and ensuing risk for chronic disease. Analysis of psychological stress effects comes ·through the concept of mental workload. The cognitive psychological perspective defines workload on the basis of total information load that the worker is required to perceive and interpret while performing job tasks [14]. "Overload" and stress occur when this human information processing load is too large for the individual's information processing capabilities. These models emphasize the importance of information overloads, communication difficulties, and memory problems.

The cognitive psychological perspective tends to downplay the role of objective workplace stressors and emphasizes instead the importance of the individuals' interpretation of the situation. Psychologists such as Lazarus and Folkeman [15] have been central advocates of helping the individual "cognitively reinterpret" the situation in a way that is less threatening to reduce experienced stress. For example, if a worker is stressed about his or her supervisor's overbearing behavior, then this approach would suggest that the worker reinterpret the situation to understand that the supervisor is really not the problem, but the worker's faulty interpretation of the situation is problematic. While this approach might be appropriate where there is no possibility of modifying the environment, it could harm workers in situations in which the stressors are real and should be the target of change efforts.

Besides downplaying the role of objective stressors, the cognitive models do not take into account social and mental "demands" of work that do not translate into information loads, such as most time deadlines, conflict, and tasks that require much social organization or much concentration but little perception. The cognitive models also do not address the role of work "motivation" in psychological functioning and stress.

*Physiologic Stress Theories.* Fortunately, the areas omitted by the cognitive models were addressed by physiologic models of the stress response. The cognitive models tended to omit what were called "drives" in an earlier generation of psychology and the significant effects of social interactions. Also, there was no way to build motivation into the information processing model, and emotional responses, such as anxiety and depression, did not fit neatly. "Drives," emotional response, and response to social interactions are most affected by the limbic regions of the brain, not the cerebral cortex, which is associated with the processes described by cognitive psychology. Thus, a simplification of the physiologic stress response originating in the limbic system that appears to be relevant for the work environment focuses on two mechanisms: the adrenal medullary response involving epinephrine and norepinephrine, and the adrenal cortical response involving cortisol. These two mechanisms reflect distinct behavioral patterns for humans.

Cannon's [16] "fight-flight" response is most associated with stimulation of the adrenal medulla and epinephrine secretion. This pattern, occurring in conjunction with sympathetic arousal of the cardiovascular system, is an active response mode in which the organism is able to use metabolic energy to support both mental and physical exertion. While this response mechanism is a basic element in all animal behavioral repertoires, it is taxing in the short term, and long-term arousal of the psychoendocrine mechanisms can lead to difficulties of relaxation and a state of chronic overarousal. Adrenal medullary mechanisms reflect the importance of sustained arousal conditions, threats to security, time pressures for increased performance, and a range of workplace social situations, including authority challenges.

The adrenal cortical response, the second mode of stress response, is a response of defeat and withdrawal, possibly a situation in which the person faces stress with little control over it. Selye's stress research [12, 17] dealt with the adrenal cortical response of animals in a stressed, but passive, condition; that is, his animal subjects were restrained while they were stressed. Henry and Stephens [18] described this behavior as defeat or loss of social attachments, which leads to withdrawal and submissiveness in social interactions.

From the above research, one could infer that in the physiologic models, *stress* is a systemic concept referring to a disequilibrium of the system as a whole, in particular its control capabilities. Biologically occurring control systems include the nervous system, the cardiovascular system, and the psychoendocrine systems. All organisms must have control mechanisms to integrate the actions of separate subsystems. Psychosomatic diseases are regarded as disorders of regulations in which the process of attaining system equilibrium (homeostasis) is disturbed [18, 19].

### Integrated Occupational Stress Models Based on Human Behavior

There is a need to integrate the models of stress from cognitive psychology and physiology, taking into account the role of emotion and motivation. The integrated models have taken, as their point of departure, human behavior in complex environments, not brain functions. Behavioral models are almost always multidimensional in order to capture requisite complexity; thus, they offer richer models for understanding stressful job conditions. Two multidimensional, integrated models of occupational stress have received the greatest amount of attention among stress researchers in the United States during the past two decades: the person-environment fit model and the job demand-control model [20].

*Person-Environment (PE) Fit Model.* The PE fit model states that strain develops when there is a discrepancy (1) between the demands of the job and the abilities of the person to meet those demands (demand-ability dimension) or (2) between the motives of the person and the environmental supplies to satisfy the person's motives (motive-supply dimension) [9, 21]. Demands include workload and job complexity. Motives include factors

such as income, participation, and self-utilization. Supplies refer to whether the job, for example, provides sufficient income to satisfy the motives of the individual. The model distinguishes the *objective* environment and person from the *subjective* environment and person, where subjective refers to the perceptions of the individual. It assumes that strain arises due to poor fit between the subjective person and subjective environment. The emphasis of the PE fit model on subjective perceptions is consistent with the earlier cognitive model; the PE fit model, however, is enhanced by consideration of motivation. As with the cognitive model, the PE fit model does not acknowledge the role of objective workplace stressors other than their influence on a worker's perceptions.

According to this model, strain results from an excess in demands over abilities. On the motive-supply dimension, strain results from insufficient supplies for motives. However, unpredictability of strain outcomes when abilities exceed demands and when supplies exceed motives occurs because misfit on these dimensions may create misfit on other relevant dimensions.

A difficulty with the PE fit model is that it has demonstrated limited ability to predict what objective work conditions are likely to result in stress [11, 20]. The model states that stress may result from a misfit between the person and the environment in either direction of two possible dimensions, but the relationship between the dimensions of the model have not been clarified. Also, since interpretation of stressors is subjective, stress becomes a function primarily of individual perceptions. A strength of the model is its emphasis on the need for flexibility in job design and consideration of workers as individuals with varying abilities, motives, and perceptions.

*Job Demand-Control Model.* The demand-control model views strain as arising primarily from the characteristics of work, rather than from subjective perceptions of the individual worker. It states that strain arises as the result of an imbalance between demands and decision latitude (or control) in the workplace, where lack of control is seen as an environmental constraint on response capabilities [1, 22]. Decision latitude actually consists of two components that are usually highly correlated in job situations: personal control over decision making, and skill level and variety. Experimental research on psychological strain symptoms have demonstrated that psychologically demanding situations alone do not cause adverse reactions of being stressed. A major contingent factor determining the outcome is whether the individual has control over his or her actions in meeting the demands. In a sense, the demand-control model is consistent with McGrath's definition of stress as an imbalance between demand and response capability; however, the critical distinction is that the demand-control model recognizes that the essential characteristic of a stressful work environment is that it simultaneously places demands and creates environmental constraints on an individual's response capabilities. Thus, the stressful work environment per se creates the imbalance between demand and response that leads to strain.

The demand-control model characterizes jobs by their combination of demands and control (Fig. 19-1). Jobs with high demands and low control, such as those of waiters, video display terminal

Fig. 19-1. The demand-control model indicating the combined effects of job demands and decision latitude on strain (From DB Baker. The study of stress at work. Am Rev Public Health 1985; 6:367–81.)

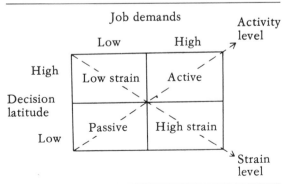

operators, and machine-paced assemblers, will result in strain (strain axis in Fig. 19-1). These characteristics typically are found in occupations with a high division of labor and deskilling of tasks. The model also hypothesizes that jobs in which psychological demands are accompanied by high control result in an active, motivation situation (activity axis in Fig. 19-1). This model is useful because it parsimoniously captures the two primary physiologic mechanisms described above. The adrenal medullary response has been shown to correspond to increased job demands, or possibly, increasingly active job situations, while increased adrenal cortical output is associated with decreased decision latitude, or possibly increased strain. For example, there is substantial evidence that workers with high-strain jobs report much higher levels of depression than other workers—and a depressed emotional state has often been associated with high levels of cortisol [1, 3].

Another advantage of the demand-control model is that it provides a second set of predictions that include other behavioral aspects relevant to long-term stress consequences: predictions about active behavior (that promotes learning) and passive behavior (that leads to long-term capability loss). As shown in Fig. 19-1, active behavior occurs when high demands are accompanied by high control, whereas passive behavior is promoted in situations in which both psychological demands and control are low. This learning model has been confirmed by Czickszentmihalyi [23], who associated the desirable "active" condition with "flow"—a positive feeling of demanding, but highly satisfying, competent performance. The negative learning in passive situations is generally confirmed by Seligman's research in learned helplessness, although that research was framed primarily within the cognitive psychological model [24].

The demand-control model can be expanded to connect environmental conditions and person-based perceptions by examining how the learning and strain processes can interact dynamically over time [1]. For example, over the long term, the active-passive behavior dimension of the model can interact with the strain dimension of the model in affecting the individual's ability to cope with strain. First, a high strain level may inhibit normal capacity to accept challenge and, thus, inhibit new learning. Decreased learning may, in turn, decrease coping resources and, thus, result in even greater strain. On the other hand, new learning may lead to the feeling of mastery or confidence. These feelings of mastery, in turn, can lead to reduced perceptions of events as stressful and increased coping success.

One omission of the demand-control model is the social behavior that plays such an important role in the operation of both human and animal limbic systems [18]; that is, the importance of social relations at the workplace is only indirectly included in the model. Research on the risk of stress-related illness using the demand-control model has been significantly augmented by considering the role of social support at the workplace. Much of the recent epidemiologic research on occupational stress and cardiovascular disease risk using the demand-control model has been done with an expanded version of the model that includes social support as an additional dimension [1, 5].

Studies using the demand-control model have demonstrated significant associations among job demands, decision latitude, and strain [1, 5, 25]. In general, investigators have concluded that decision latitude acts both as a modifier of demands and as an independent risk factor for strain. The amount of control over the job is now recognized as a decisive factor in the development of occupational stress [25]. Social support may also be an important modifier of this interaction. The demand-control model provides a conceptual framework for understanding the dynamics of the stress process. Research is under way to further test and refine this model. In the meantime, the health care provider is faced with the need to identify and manage stress-related disorders in individuals. Such practical matters necessitate that we return to a more pragmatic presentation of the stress process.

## Components of the Stress Process

Major components of the stress process include stressors, stress responses (strain) and long-term outcomes, and modifiers of the stress process (Table 19-1). The causal linkages among these com-

Table 19-1. Components of the stress process

Stressors
   Time demands, work schedule and pace—task demands, overtime, shiftwork, machine-pacing, piecework
   Psychosocial task structure—lack of control, skill underutilization, human-machine interface
   Physical conditions—unpleasant, threat of physical or toxic hazard, ergonomic hazards
   Organization—role ambiguity, role conflict, competition and rivalry
   Extra-organizational—community, job insecurity, career development, global economic
   Non-work sources—personal, family, community
Outcomes
   Physiologic:
      Short-term—catecholamines, cortisol, blood pressure increases
      Long-term—hypertension, heart disease, ulcers, asthma
   Psychological (cognitive and affective):
      Short-term—anxiety, dissatisfaction, mass psychogenic illness
      Long-term—depression, burnout, mental disorders
   Behavioral:
      Short-term—job (absenteeism, reduced productivity and participation), community (decreased friendships and participation), personal (excessive use of alcohol and drugs, smoking)
      Long-term—"learned helplessness"
Modifiers
   Individual—behavioral style and personal resources
   Social support—emotional, value or self-esteem, and informational

ponents are dynamic and complex. In a commonly cited University of Michigan model of the stress process [26], the causal pathway to disease development starts at *stressors*, moves to perceptions of stressors by workers that are *moderated* by individual characteristics and social situation, then moves to *short-term outcomes*, and eventually results in *chronic disease* and *long-term behavioral outcomes*. However, while this model has been useful in understanding the development of stress-related disease and while epidemiologic studies of large populations have been able to demonstrate some specificity in associations between stressors and stress responses, it is not possible to determine specific etiologic relationships between stressors and health effects for one individual or in a small group of workers. One cannot analytically separate the effects of many coexisting stressors when examining one or a few individuals. Thus, from a practical clinical perspective, the relationship between stressors and health outcomes is nonspecific.

### Stressors

Stressors can be divided into those relating to the individual's job, including the work schedule and pace, job content, and physical conditions; organizational factors such as role and organizational structure; and extra-organizational factors. The individual job stressors are often also called psychosocial job stressors.

***Time Demands, Work Schedule, and Pace.*** Time-related aspects of work demands are important (1) because the overall magnitude of demands per unit of time is an important aspect of the load, (2) because of the timing of demands in relation to the capabilities for activity mediated by a daily circadian cycle, and (3) because internal control over the timing of demands by the person appears to be important in determining capacity to cope with demands. Several studies have reported associations between working excessive hours or holding down more than one full-time job and coronary heart disease (CHD) morbidity and mortality [3,

27]. Lack of control over work hours exacerbates this stressor; required overtime has been associated with low job satisfaction and indices of poor mental health.

Substantial evidence indicates that the temporal scheduling of work can have a significant impact on physical, psychological, behavioral, and social well-being. Shift work exists when a facility has working periods other than the normal day shift. Workers may stay on fixed shifts or rotate through shifts. Rotating shift and permanent night work, in particular, has been linked to a variety of disturbances [28]. Major complaints include sleep disturbances, nervous troubles, and disturbances of the alimentary tract. Shift workers also have disruptions in their family and social lives.

An important factor is whether the work pace is controlled by the individual or is externally determined. Machine-pacing is when the pace of the operation and the work output are controlled to some extent by a source other than the operator. There are numerous varieties of pacing systems that require different amounts of cognitive and motor activity from the workers. In general, this work presents a deleterious combination of short interval demands with lack of control. It requires vigilance, yet it is monotonous and repetitive. As mentioned previously, research has indicated that machine-paced assembly-line work is highly stressful [9, 22, 29] (Fig. 19-2).

Piecework is when the worker's remuneration is based on the quantity of products produced. This system has been shown to induce stress responses similar to those of machine-pacing. Individuals who perform piecework may increase their work pace even to the point of discomfort. For example, one study found that when invoicing clerks were put on piecework, as opposed to their usual hourly rate, they doubled their work rate, but also increased their urinary epinephrine and norepinephrine levels by about one-third.

***Psychosocial Task Structure.*** Other psychosocial aspects of the worker's job have also been a central focus of stress research, particularly lack of control

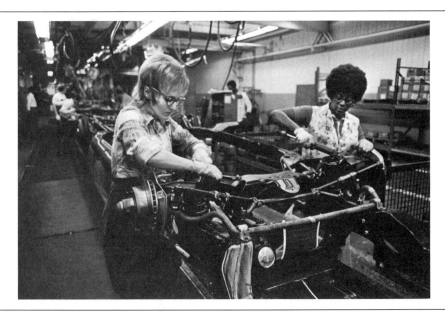

**Fig. 19-2.** Assembly-line workers have machine-paced jobs in a fractionated and dehumanizing work environment. (Photograph by Earl Dotter.)

by the worker and inability to use and develop new skills. These arise directly out of organizational decisions about allocation of decision authority to individuals and the division of labor into task specializations. Research based on the demand-control model has shown that the combination of high psychological demands and low decision latitude (low control and low ability to develop skills) leads to psychological and physiologic strain reactions [1, 5]. Table 19-2 describes the features of "good" and "bad" job characteristics, based on an understanding of the demand-control model of job content. Examples of high-demand task characteristics include having too much to do, time pressure or deadlines, or repetitious fast-cycle work flow. Low-decision latitude arises in tasks that are too narrow in content, lack stimulus variation, do not allow creativity or problem-solving, and do not have control over pace or work methods. Although these task characteristics are generally thought to relate only to industrial

assembly lines, modern office environments share many of them (Fig. 19-3).

Many complex task demands arise at the human-machine interface. Introduction of computer technologies in the work process, for example, can affect psychosocial work structure significantly, changing decision authority, skill use, and uncertainty.

Changes in social structure of the work organization may also be a source of stress. Transfers, demotions, and even promotions can be stressful. The potential for change to act as a stressor is affected by the predictability of the event and the control the individual or work group has over the transition process.

*Physical Conditions.* Unpleasant working conditions include improper lighting, excessive noise, inadequate workspace, depressing surroundings, and unsanitary conditions. Investigators have found a positive association between poor mental health

**Table 19-2.** Description of "good" and "bad" job characteristics based on demand-control model

| "Bad" or high-strain jobs | "Good" jobs |
|---|---|
| Psychological demands | |
| There are long periods under intense time pressures, with the threat of unemployment at the end, or there are long periods of boredom, but with the constant threat of crisis requiring huge efforts. There is great disorganization of work processes with no resources to facilitate order. | The job has routine demands mixed with a liberal element of new learning challenges, in a predictable manner. The magnitude of demands is mediated by interpersonal decision making between parties of relatively equal status. |
| Decision latitude: skill discretion | |
| Nothing is being learned, nothing is known of the product's destination. There is no hint of future development on the job. New technologies are difficult to understand, and knowledge is limited by secrecy requirements. | The job offers possibilities to make the maximum use of one's skill and provides further opportunities to increase skills on the job. New technologies are created to be effective tools in the workers' hands, extending their powers of production. |
| Decision latitude: autonomy | |
| The workers' minutest actions are prescribed and monitored by machine or by supervisors. There is no freedom to independently perform even the most basic tasks. New technologies restrict workers to rigid, unmodifiable information formats. | There is freedom from rigid "worker-as-child" factory discipline. Machine interfaces allow workers to assume control. Workers have influence over selection of work routines and work colleagues and can participate in long-term planning. It may be possible to work at home during flexible hours. |
| Social relations | |
| Workers are socially isolated from their colleagues. Random switching of positions prevents development of lasting relationships. Competition sets worker against worker. | Social contacts are encouraged as a basis for new learning and are augmented by new telecommunications technologies that allow contact when isolation was previously a necessity. New contacts multiply the possibilities for self-realization through collaboration. |

Source: Adapted from R Karasek, T Theorell. Healthy work—stress, productivity, and the reconstruction of working life. New York: Basic Books, 1992.

and unpleasant working conditions [4]. Investigators of complaints among office workers have found that uncomfortable workstations, crowding, and inadequate ventilation and temperature control are associated with stress responses.

Noise causes physiologic stress reactions at levels below that which leads to hearing loss. It is difficult to study the effect of noise per se since one cannot separate noise from an individual's interpretation of the sound. Nevertheless, it is clear that control over the source of noise can modify the stress response. A laboratory study showed that perception of ability to control noise eliminated the adverse effects of unpredictable high-intensity noise on task performance, even though none of the subjects ever actually used the dummy switch designated for turning off the noise [30] (see Chap. 16).

The threat of physical or toxic hazard can act as a stressor. Certain occupations are recognized to have increased risk of physical danger, such as police officers, mine workers, and firefighters.

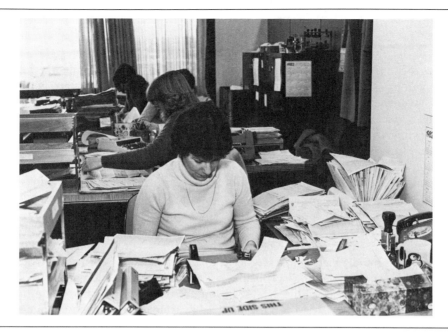

**Fig. 19-3.** Secretaries are among the most highly stressed workers. (Photograph by Marilee Caliendo.)

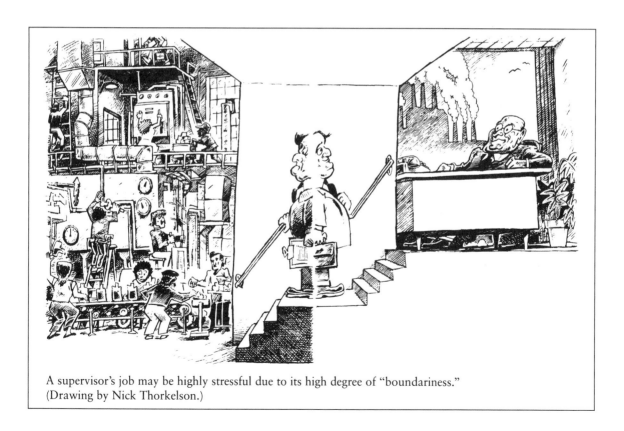

A supervisor's job may be highly stressful due to its high degree of "boundariness."
(Drawing by Nick Thorkelson.)

Chronic stress reaction among workers in these types of occupations is well recognized. More subtly, studies have revealed that among workers in the trade and service sectors, the potential for abuse or violence from clients is a significant source of stress. However, stress induced by the uncertainty of physical danger is substantially relieved if the worker feels adequately trained and equipped to cope with emergency situations.

Physically demanding tasks, such as meat trimming, when repetitive and fast paced, can lead to increased risk of acute injuries and repetitive trauma disorders. This rapidly increasing category of injuries, studied as work ergonomics, probably has both psychological stress and physical load risk factors.

For each of these work condition stressors, it appears that increased control over the condition ameliorates the stress response. Thus, the demand-control paradigm applies to physical conditions, as well as to job content.

*Organization.* Work is a social process that occurs within an organization. Major organizational stressors include role in the organization, organizational structure, and interpersonal relationships. Role ambiguity results from lack of clarity concerning the requirements of the job; the worker does not know the objectives, scope, and responsibilities of the job. Studies have indicated that between 35 and 60 percent of workers are affected by role ambiguity [31]. This stressor may lead to job dissatisfaction, feelings of tension, and lowered self-confidence. Role conflict occurs when conflicting demands are made on the worker by different groups in the organization or when the worker is required to do work that he or she dislikes or believes to be outside of the requirements of the job. One survey indicated that 48 percent of workers in the United States are affected by role conflict [31].

Large organizations with a "flat" structure (relatively few job levels) are associated with greater job dissatisfaction, absenteeism, and accidents. Jobs at the boundaries of organizations have in-

creased stress. For example, the job of the supervisor, who is at the interface between union and management, could be considered a boundary job. Elevated rates of peptic ulcer disease and, in some industries, of heart disease have been demonstrated for supervisors.

Competition and rivalry are sources of stress for many workers. Poor work relationships are "those which include low trust, low supportiveness, and low interest in listening to and trying to deal with problems that confront the organizational member" [32]. Conflict tends to occur when inadequate information is provided to designate responsibilities, job roles, and the means of carrying them out. Poor interpersonal relationships can have a debilitating effect not only on individuals but also on the organization.

*Extra-Organizational Stressors.* Extra-organizational stressors are factors that are related to work, but extend beyond the specific job or organization. These stressors include factors related to commuting, career security and advancement, unemployment, and issues of job security in relation to the global economy and free market.

An evaluation of work stress must consider sources of stress related to preparing for and going to and from work. In many cities, commuting can be arduous, and even dangerous, taking as long as three hours a day. Among shift workers, public transportation may not be provided during late evening and nights.

Several conditions associated with career development or job future (lack of job security, underpromotion, overpromotion, and fear of job obsolescence) have been related to adverse behavioral problems, psychological effects, and poor physical health. Lack of job security is a primary stressor for many workers. Evaluation of career as a stressor must consider anticipated changes associated with the stage of the worker's career. Lack of change may be a stressor if it represents thwarted ambition or "inadequate forward mechanisms"— that is, personal recognition, promotion, or financial return. Retirement can be a stressor. It is an anticipated change that is modified by the extent that the worker requires work for self-image and has potential for constructive activity outside of work. Stress reactions may begin long before retirement.

Unemployment may have dramatic effects on stress-related illness, not only on those who become unemployed, but also on those who remain working. Brenner and Mooney [33] observed that increasing unemployment is usually followed by increased cardiovascular mortality, often with a time lag of three years. Recently a Swedish group made a similar observation [34]. Most of the association between unemployment and cardiovascular mortality occurred during the same year. Dramatic effects of unemployment on mental health [34], cortisol levels [35], and immune function [36] have been observed. The effects are particularly damaging for young unemployed people, who may develop excessive alcohol consumption as well as psychosomatic symptoms that normally exist only in middle-aged people [37].

*The Global Economy.* Recent evidence from a series of case studies examined by the International Labour Organization (ILO) suggests that modern mechanisms of production and international trade may be contributing to an increase in stress risks throughout the world [38]. These case studies showed that most of the stress prevention programs had been undertaken in mass production or commodity production in private industries involved in international competition, including some in less developed countries. Another category of cases occurred in large-scale public bureaucracies, particularly those with restricting budgets. Both of these situations are increasingly common in the global market.

In current economic theory, a global market implies profitability for an almost unlimited specialization of labor, that is, reduced job skill breadth and authority and, thus, low decision latitude. With a global market, a large producer could achieve economies of scale and undercut the competition from other countries. Division of labor increases labor's productivity for mass distributed goods. Indeed, there is actually now excess capacity of production in the world in many major industries, such as in production of ships, steel, automobiles, petrochemicals, computer chips, home electronics, textiles, and clothing [39].

Global interdependence and production overcapacity, however, are leading to increasing job insecurity for workers around the world with competition for jobs by one country's workers against those of another country. The possibilities for global market transactions has exploded with the advent of computer-based international market transactions. Now, the instantaneous communication of price and quantity information around the world by rapidly expanding computer-based, satellite-dependent information systems means that a customer or competitor is only a phone call or a keystroke away. This situation can mean insecurity for everyone from stock broker, to corporate manager, to manufacturing worker. This macrolevel competition represents an abstract force for most of the participants in this "game," which is very different from normal biologic competition. Phenomena of this type can create a profound feeling of insecurity in all levels of operation as well as equally strong feelings of powerlessness and lack of control.

*Non-Work Stressors.* Finally, sources of stress other than work must be considered in an evaluation of the stress process. The boundary between work and non-work stressors is not distinct. They clearly interact in causing stress responses. Personal, family, and community factors can be stressors. Non-work stresses are not reviewed in this chapter.

### Adverse Health Outcomes

Stress responses can be divided into short-term reactions and long-term consequences. Long-term consequences develop following chronic unresolved short-term reactions or "strain." Most investigators consider three major categories of stress responses: physiologic, psychological, and behavioral. Effects on the organization should also be considered.

The multifactorial relationship between work stress and health outcomes has engendered some confusion among health professionals. Many practitioners mix up the concept of psychosocial factors as etiologic agents with the notion of work-related mental health. One should be clear that *psychosocial factors*, such as stress, may cause both psychological and physiologic disorders. On the other hand, work-related *psychological disorders* may be caused by both psychosocial factors and toxic chemical exposures. Intoxication due to acute solvent exposure and mood disturbances due to chronic mercury exposure are examples of the latter.

*Physiologic.* Work-related stressors have been shown to induce a variety of short-term physiologic reactions. Much of this work derives from Cannon's [16] and Selye's [12, 17] previously described physiologic stress theories. A classic example is a study that demonstrated that serum cholesterol increases and blood coagulation accelerates among tax accountants as tax deadlines approach [40].

Substantial advances in understanding have occurred in recent years as telemetry and biochemical measurement techniques have evolved [3]. Bioelectric measures of stress reactions include heart rate and rhythm, electromyogram results, and galvanic skin response. Increases in galvanic skin response were found to be a sensitive index to behavioral changes related to boredom, fatigue, and monotony. Biochemical measures include catecholamines, corticosteroids (such as cortisol), cholesterol, uric acid, free fatty acids, glucose, thyroxine, and growth hormone. Measurement of metabolites of the catecholamines and corticosteroids in the blood and urine has received much attention in the past few years. It is now possible to demonstrate short-term physiologic responses to work stressors. The significance of these short-term responses for chronic health outcomes re-

mains to be determined, although such a relationship makes intuitive sense.

The chronic pathophysiologic effects of stress are generally considered within the rubric of psychosomatic disorders. Depending on one's perspective, this category may be as narrow as including only headache and gastritis or may encompass such diseases as hypertension, cardiovascular disease, ulcers, asthma, and musculoskeletal disorders. Unfortunately, the label *psychosomatic* has developed the deprecating connotation of being "not real," and it probably should be avoided. Some researchers have suggested replacing the term *psychosomatic* with *psychophysiologic*. In any case, the association between work stress and this group of health outcomes is strongly suggestive, but difficult to prove in cause-effect terms.

Much research has focused on the potential effect of stress on CHD [1, 4, 5, 41]. However, methodologic limitations (for example, lack of measurement instruments, uncertainty about the objectivity of reports about the psychosocial environment, potential for bias due to job selection, and potential confounding by traditional cardiovascular risk factors) have made it difficult to quantify the contribution of stress. Studies during the past decade based on the demand-control model have shown significant associations between high-strain (high-demand, low-control) occupations and subsequent development of angina pectoris and myocardial infarction, after analytically controlling for other potential risk factors such as age, smoking, education, and obesity [1, 5]. Figure 19-4 shows associations between a mortality-validated indicator of CHD for a random national sample of Swedish men according to the demand-control model [42]. The frequencies of illness are significantly higher for high-demand and low decision latitude conditions. The associations persist when controlled in multivariate logistic regression analysis for age, other demographic factors, smoking, and obesity. The standardized odds ratio is approximately 1.5, only moderately less than the 1.7 range found for cholesterol and its

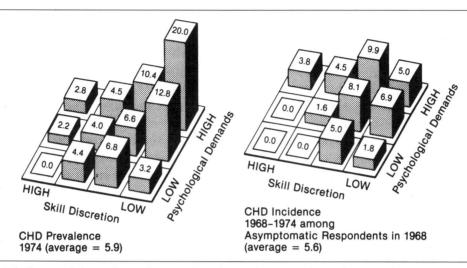

**Fig. 19-4.** Job characteristics and prevalence and incidence of coronary heart disease indicator among Swedish men. Number on vertical bar is percentage in each job category with indicator (two of four symptoms: ache in chest, trouble breathing, hypertension, heart weakness. (From RA Karasek et al. Job decision latitude, job demands, and cardiovascular disease: A prospective study of Swedish men. Am J Public Health 1981; 71:694–705.)

fractions. Other studies have concluded that 25 to 33 percent of CHD risk could be attributed to psychosocial job conditions [41]. More precision in these estimates should come in a new generation of research that specifically tests for psychosocial occupational risks.

*Psychological.* A large body of research has demonstrated the association between job stress and adverse short-term psychological effects, including anxiety, situational depression, and job dissatisfaction [10, 11]. Association with chronic mental illness is not as well documented. Nevertheless, data from workers' compensation claims indicate that psychological disorders due to chronic occupational stress are a major health problem [10]. During the past decade, workers' compensation systems in many jurisdictions in the United States have provided compensation for "gradual mental stress," which is stress that arises during the normal course of employment and is not limited to cases of psychological disorders that follow specific, identifiable traumatic events. According to a study conducted in the early 1980s by the National Council on Compensation Insurance, claims for "gradual mental stress" accounted for about 11 percent of all occupational disease claims [2, 10].

Causes of depression and job dissatisfaction follow the predictions of the demand-control model. Among blue-collar workers, major stressors are lack of job complexity, role ambiguity, and job insecurity. Particularly among clerical and service workers, low self-esteem arises out of lack of respect from supervisors. For white-collar workers, major stressors are responsibility for people, high job complexity, and high and variable workload.

*Behavioral.* Short-term behavioral responses to stress include deleterious personal behaviors, such as escapist drinking of alcohol and increased usage of tobacco and drugs. Quantitative workload has been directly associated with cigarette smoking and an inability to quit smoking. It also has been related to escapist drinking, absenteeism, low work motivation, lowered self-esteem, and lack of interest in contributing suggestions to management.

The work organization also is affected. Deleterious personal behaviors, such as absenteeism, alcoholism, and accidents, have a negative impact on the organization. Stress decreases productivity through reduced output, production delays, and poor quality of work, which leads to lost time, equipment breakdown, and wasted material. Poor morale can lead to labor unrest, excessive number of grievances, sabotage, and increased turnover. Thus, both the individual and the organization suffer from manifestations of job stress.

The long-term behavioral manifestations of job stress include what Seligman has referred to as *learned helplessness* [24, 27]. In essence, the individual gives up on the possibility of controlling his or her own destiny, which leads to escapism and passive behavior. Studies based on the demand-control model have shown that workers with little control at work eventually become passive at home and in their community, with decreased participation in union, recreation, social, and religious activities [22].

*Specific Stress-Related Disorders.* For the effects just described, job stress is one of multiple factors in the etiology of the conditions. For some disorders, stress is recognized as the primary etiologic agent. Examples include burnout, post-traumatic stress disorder, and mass psychogenic illness.

*Burnout* is a phenomenon that has been recognized mostly in professional settings, although it can affect any worker [43]. It may occur after years of high-quality performance. The individual suddenly seems unable to perform his or her work. Behavioral manifestations include decreased efficiency and initiative, diminished interest in work, and an inability to maintain work performance. Symptoms characterizing the syndrome are fatigue, intestinal disturbances, sleeplessness, depression, and shortness of breath. Other symptoms include irritability, decrease in frustration tolerance, blunting of affect, suspiciousness, feelings of helplessness, and increased risk-taking.

There is a tendency to self-medicate with tranquilizers, narcotics, and alcohol, all of which may lead to addiction. When away from the job, the individual is unable to relax and often reports giving up recreation and social contacts.

Actually burnout does not emerge spontaneously; it progresses in stages beginning during the initial stages of employment. Because burnout-prone individuals often start out as enthusiastic overachievers, the organization tends to heap more and more responsibilities on them. Failure to recognize the connection between constant over-achievement and burnout and to exercise proper preventive measures can lead to an exhausted workforce whose achievement, desire, and creative talents are defunct [43].

*Post-traumatic stress disorder (PTSD)* is a specific anxiety disorder that occurs following a stressful or traumatic event [44]. The disorder may occur among workers who have had occupational toxic exposure or injury. Any situation that evokes feelings of intense fear, helplessness, loss of control, or annihilation may precipitate the disorder. The trauma may be massive and discrete like an accident or may be comprised of episodes of exposure to a dangerous chemical or work process. The cardinal feature is repeated reexperiencing of the traumatic event. Typically, any stimulus that resembles the initial event will evoke the reexperience of the event. Patients may believe that they are allergic to everything. Other symptoms include emotional blunting, detachment from others, sleep disturbances, and trouble concentrating. The recurrent symptoms and anxiety experienced by individuals with PTSD may be disabling. It is important to recognize the psychological effect of the initial trauma in order to avoid costly, unnecessary, and sometimes reinforcing medical diagnostic evaluations.

*Mass psychogenic illness* is the label applied to apparent group anxiety reactions in industrial establishments [45, 46] (see also Chap. 26). A number of workers simultaneously become ill at the worksite. As rumors of the illness spread through the plant, worker anxiety and general confusion may escalate to such an extent that it becomes necessary to close the facility. The outbreak usually is triggered by a physical stimulus, such as an odor, that the workers believe to be harmful. Specific symptoms vary among incidents, but typically they consist mainly of somatic complaints, such as headache, nausea, and chills. Studies have indicated that these outbreaks tend to occur among industrial workers who experience substantial underlying psychosocial stressors and physical strain. Many investigators have reported that high stress in the workplace is a key feature in outbreaks of mass psychogenic illness. The triggering event is the last straw that exhausts the adaptive resources of the individuals and organization.

Evaluation of these outbreaks is difficult because specific complaints often have resolved by the time an investigative team can reach the site. Brodsky [46] stated that the following characteristics can help distinguish mass psychogenic illness from illness due to physical causes: No laboratory or physical findings identify a specific organic cause; there is evidence of specific physical or psychological stressors; affected individuals are mostly women or persons of lower socioeconomic status in the workplace; symptoms that are usually associated with hyperventilation are prominent; there is apparent transmission among the workers by audiovisual cues—that is, affected persons generally can see or hear each other; there is a rapid spread of the illness followed by rapid remission of symptoms; and there is generally benign morbidity among most workers. Unfortunately, since none of these characteristics is definitive, substantial judgment is required of the health care professional in evaluating these situations. Another complication is that following some outbreaks of mass psychogenic illness a few of the affected individuals may develop chronic symptoms, including the condition known as multiple chemical sensitivity syndrome (see discussion of low-level exposures in Chap. 3). It can be difficult to determine the causal association between the outbreak and the individual's subsequent illness, and to disentangle the contribution of workplace stressors and individual

susceptibility. Ultimately, treatment involves demonstrating that the triggering event does not represent an ongoing risk and reducing the level of underlying stressors.

### Modifiers

The association between stressors and stress responses is modified by characteristics of the individual and environment. This notion is intrinsic to all models of psychosocial stress. Stressors, individual characteristics, and social environment are specific instances of the generally recognized public health triad: agent, host, and environment.

*Individual.* Individual characteristics that affect vulnerability to stressors include degrees of emotional stability, conformity (versus inner-directedness), rigidity (versus flexibility), achievement orientation, and also behavioral style. A behavioral style that has received much attention as a risk factor for CHD is the type A coronary-prone behavior, characterized by a sense of competitiveness, time urgency, and overcommitment [47]. Despite substantial research since Friedman and Rosenman originated the concept two decades ago, no one has been able to identify and reliably measure the precise aspects of the type A behavior pattern that lead to CHD. Some research findings have suggested that interaction between job stressors and type A characteristics may lead to increased risk for CHD, but the evidence is not convincing [48, 49].

An unfortunate side effect of the research on the type A behavior pattern is that it has tended to focus attention on individual vulnerability rather than on environmental stressors. In fact, occupational stress does not affect an identifiable subpopulation of vulnerable individuals. Thus, the primary prevention strategy should be the identification and reduction of environmental stressors, and not the treatment or removal of possibly vulnerable individuals.

*Environment.* Many investigators have concluded that the most important factor ameliorating the stress response is social support, including emotional, informational, and instrumental support. Informational support depends on the clarity and effectiveness of communication patterns in the organization. Instrumental support includes such factors as having adequate instructions and tools to complete the task. A large amount of research has demonstrated that social support can reduce the adverse health effects of stress [4, 25, 50]. Some investigators have even recommended that social support be added to the demand-control model of stress as a key third dimension of the stress model [1]. There has been disagreement, however, about whether the primary effect of social support is to modify or *buffer* the effect of stressors or whether social support has a direct effect in reducing stress [1, 51]. Regardless of whether social support directly reduces stress or acts as a modifier of the effect of stressors, a prime strategy of stress management is to encourage and develop supportive networks on the job [1, 25].

## Management of Stress

The phrase *stress management* typically denotes worksite programs that address employee stress; however, management of work stress should occur in multiple settings, including the medical office or clinic. A comprehensive approach should encompass assessment, treatment, and prevention of stress in the individual worker, family, and organization. This effort requires the expertise of a multidisciplinary team of professionals working in a variety of settings. Stress management should be considered in this broader sense. Table 19-3 provides an overview of stress management approaches.

### Principles

While any effort to reduce stress will have some beneficial effect, certain strategies are more likely to lead to long-term success. Programs should view prevention and control of stress as a shared

**Table 19-3.** Approaches to the prevention and control of stress

Treat the individual:
  Medical treatment—hypertension, backache, depression
  Counseling services
  Employee assistance programs—alcohol, drugs
Reduce individual vulnerability:
  Counseling—individual, group programs
  Training programs—relaxation, meditation, biofeedback
  General support—exercise programs, recreational activities
Treat the organization:
  Diagnosis—attitude surveys, rap sessions
  Develop flexible and responsive management style
  Improve internal communications
Reduce organizational stress:
  Variable work schedules
  Job restructuring—enlargement, enrichment, increased control
  Supervisor training and management development

Source: Adapted from JJ Warshaw. Managing stress. In LW Krinsky, SN Kieffer, PA Carone, SF Yolles. eds. Stress and productivity. New York: Human Sciences Press, 1984, pp. 15–30.

responsibility between the health care provider and employer. In the past, program approaches have covered the range from "stress is a personal problem" to superpaternalism [52]. Neither extreme has achieved lasting success. Rather, programs should develop a balance between requiring some responsibility for self-help and providing a variety of support mechanisms. All parties should work together to identify and control stressors.

Effective control of stress requires an appreciation of the dynamic, multifactorial nature of stress. Programs should take an ecological systems approach that recognizes the inherent interrelationship of physical, biologic, chemical, psychological, and social factors in the determination of health status. In particular, it is inappropriate to dichotomize etiologic factors into "toxic" or "psychosocial" and relegate the latter to a secondary level of consideration. One must be aware that potential stressors range from the micro-environment of the individual workstation to the broad socioeconomic context of the work organization. Assessment requires parallel consideration of multiple stressors since it is unlikely that any one stressor would be a sufficient etiologic agent. Assessment of interaction between factors is even more critical than for other workplace exposures. Since stress is a dynamic process, stress management must be a continuous cycle of assessment, intervention (treatment and prevention), and evaluation of the intervention. Control of stress requires ongoing feedback from the individual and organization.

Long-term prevention strategies should be based on an understanding of the etiology of stress. The PE fit model suggests that every job must be designed to supply rewards at the same time it presents demands. The balance between motives-supplies and demands-abilities may be particular for each individual worker. Thus job requirements and stress management efforts should be flexible and individualized. The demand-control model demonstrates that the fundamental sources of imbalance between the person and work environment are environmental constraints on the worker. Ultimately, primary prevention strategies must be directed toward modification of stressors in the environment, and, in particular, increasing the control workers have over their work environment.

A statement of principles for control of stress based on these precepts is worth noting. The National Institute for Occupational Safety and Health (NIOSH) has proposed a strategy for the prevention of work-related psychological disorders that recommends four categories of action: (1) job design to improve working conditions; (2) surveillance of psychological disorders and risk factors; (3) information dissemination, education, and training; and (4) enrichment of psychological health services for workers [10] (Table 19-4). This strategy acknowledges the interplay of work and non-work factors in the etiology of psychological

**Table 19-4.** NIOSH recommendations for job design

Work schedule—Work schedules should be compatible with demands and responsibilities outside of the job. When schedules involve rotating shifts, the rate of rotation should be stable and predictable.

Workload—Demands should be commensurate with the capabilities and resources of individuals. Provisions should be made to allow recovery from demanding tasks or for increased job control under such circumstances.

Content—Jobs should be designed to provide meaning, stimulation, and an opportunity to use skills.

Participation and control—Individuals should be given the opportunity to have input on decisions or actions that affect their jobs and the performance of their tasks.

Work roles—Roles and responsibilities at work should be well defined. Job duties need to be clearly explained, and conflicts in terms of job expectations should be avoided.

Social environment—Jobs should provide opportunities for personal interaction both for purposes of emotional support and for actual help as needed in accomplishing assigned tasks.

Job future—Ambiguity should not exist in matters of job security and opportunities for career development.

Source: Adapted from S Sauter, LR Murphy, JJ Hurrell Jr. Prevention of work-related psychological disorders: A national strategy proposed by the National Institute for Occupational Safety and Health. Am Psychol 1990; 45:1146–58.

disorders. Consequently, it not only focuses on understanding and controlling job factors, but also on the promotion of workplace health services that could remedy worker's psychological disorders whether or not they are occupationally related. The NIOSH strategy can guide managers and health care providers in controlling work stress.

### Assessment

The initial step in the prevention and control of stress is an assessment of potential stressors, stress reactions, and modifiers. For many factors, there are no indicators that can be measured by purely objective methods, which may not be needed. Subjective indicators are indispensable for identifying components of the stress process. Objective and subjective indicators can be used simultaneously.

*Measuring Stressors.* Evaluation of physical and chemical agents should include environmental measurement and toxicologic assessment together with an assessment of psychosocial impact. Knowledge of workplace exposures is an important aid in the interpretation of psychosocial stressors. Questionnaires or interviews should be used to determine whether or not workers perceive the existence of and to what extent they are concerned about their effects.

Analysis of the work environment should include monitoring of tasks and work organization. Sources of information other than the workers themselves can be used after these indicators have been demonstrated to reliably predict stressors. Examples include objective descriptions of job structure (such as overtime, shiftwork, and machine-pacing), task analysis, and organizational structure. Since perceptions of workers must be taken into account, the assessment should include a questionnaire survey of workers or interviews with them about their perceptions. Structured questionnaires are available to assess task and organizational characteristics. A job content questionnaire (JCQ) based on the demand-control model has been developed and validated [53].

The JCQ was designed to measure the "content" of a respondent's work task in a general manner that is applicable to all jobs and jobholders. Primary scales based on defined combinations of questions are used to measure the demand-control model of stress, but other aspects of work and the worker, such as physical workload, job insecurity, and social interaction on the job, can be assessed. The instrument comes in sets of questions of several different lengths, ranging upward from the minimum "core" of 27 questions and the recommended standard instrument of 49 questions. Ap-

proximately 60 percent of the questions were derived from the U.S. Department of Labor's Quality of Work Surveys of 1969, 1972, and 1977. Use of these questions has allowed the generation of nationally standardized scales for comparison with small study populations.

*Measuring Stress Reactions and Health Outcomes.* Practical assessment of the effects of stress must be based on diagnostic skills already familiar to the health care provider. Many of the more specific and reliable stress diagnostic instruments developed in recent years remain too expensive or time consuming to be of practical use outside of the research setting. Examples include measurement of urinary metabolites of catecholamines, galvanic skin response, or assessment of mental health status using extensive structured-interview instruments [3, 54]. The health care provider may have to make a diagnosis based on the results of several nonspecific, but accessible, indicators, rather than by relying on the results of one definitive test.

A minimal assessment should include the following observations: (1) complaints of "distress"— symptoms and motivation related to work conditions; (2) emotional reactions—anxiety, depression, and other reactions; (3) cognitive function and work performance—psychometric testing and performance evaluations at work; (4) behavioral changes—such as sleep disturbances and drug and alcohol use; (5) physiologic function—such as heart rate, blood pressure, and serum cholesterol; and (6) symptoms and diseases that may be due to stress. One also should consider behavioral characteristics that may affect susceptibility or resistance and the worker's family, community, and cultural environment.

*Diagnosis.* The large number and complexity of factors involved in the stress process virtually preclude exhaustive documentation of each factor utilizing definitive instruments. There is no simple, yet comprehensive, instrument for measuring stressors and stress reactions. Consequently, the health care provider must inventory the range of factors discussed above and ultimately make a judgment as to the likelihood that the identified stressors were responsible for the observed stress reactions. This judgment must take into consideration the presence of potential occupational and nonoccupational stressors; physical, psychological, and behavioral health status (consistency with known patterns of stress reactions); presence of other accepted risk factors for observed health conditions; individual characteristics and social factors that may affect vulnerability to stress; and presence of similar health conditions among coworkers.

### Stress Treatment and Prevention for the Individual

Control of stress involves treatment for individuals already suffering from stress, identification and secondary prevention for individuals who demonstrate early stress reactions, and primary prevention through reducing individual vulnerability and increasing social support. Treatment of clinically apparent stress effects follows the traditional medical model, for example, treatment of hypertension, depression, or excessive use of alcohol. At the same time, it is necessary to reduce exposure to stressors and increase individual resistance in order to prevent future sequelae.

Reducing individual vulnerability to stress can be done by health care providers or through group counseling, courses, and workshops. Common denominators of successful programs include training in self-awareness and problem analysis so that the individual is better able to detect signs of increasing stress and to identify the stressors that may be producing it. Another common denominator is training in assertiveness so that the individual can become more active in controlling stressors. When the stress is clearly related to work organization, it is important for workers to understand the contribution of the environment. A professional can help workers realize that other workers in similar situations also have similar neg-

ative reactions. This realization can help workers overcome self-imposed blame for their psychosocial distress, recognizing that stress is not due to personal weakness. Also important are techniques, such as meditation, relaxation programs, exercise programs, and biofeedback, that will reduce personally experienced stress to more tolerable levels [51]. The following components for teaching individual control of stress have been recommended (adapted from [43]):

1. Increasing awareness of particular stressors that cause distress
2. Teaching how to avoid unnecessary stressors
3. Teaching the skills to react more positively to unavoidable stressors
4. Demonstrating and providing practice in techniques to reduce the physical and psychological effects of stress
5. Pointing out how to minimize dysfunctional coping responses and maximize those that tend to help achieve personal equilibrium, for example, dealing with the problem head-on but with a constructive attitude and rethinking the problem carefully to see new possible solutions

These approaches have been implemented most widely for white-collar workers, although principles apply to blue-collar workers as well. Teaching styles and materials may need to be adapted for educational level and past experience.

### Control of Stress at the Workplace and Through Work Reorganization

Two kinds of programs exist: those that support stress reduction as a part of a health-promotion program and those that contribute to healthy work reorganization in order to reduce stress problems at the source. A 1985 survey by the U.S. Public Health Service revealed that nearly two-thirds of private worksites with 50 or more employees were supporting at least one health-promotion activity. More than one-fourth of these worksites had stress management programs, and the number of such programs has increased since then. Many health care providers will likely be asked to assist employers or unions in the development and implementation of these programs.

The health care provider may be asked to make a recommendation on which program should be implemented. One expert states that it does not really matter, because all of the approaches will work, to some extent, for some time for some people [51]. Significant differences exist among programs, however. The development of stress programs focused on health promotion is less sensitive and less demanding, but much less effective, at eliminating problems at their source than are work reorganization programs.

A three-step process for implementing a work reorganization program focused on stress management has been suggested [51]:

1. Use a stress diagnostic test, such as a worker attitude survey, that can provide information on stress levels and sources. However, an attitude survey that does not report results and is not followed by demonstrable actions to address problems that are uncovered may be counterproductive.
2. Once assessments of stress have defined problem areas, leading managers should become involved in relieving worker stress and instituting and supporting corrective and preventive programs. Interventions may include developing variable work schedules, job restructuring (enlargement, rotation, and enrichment), supervisor training, management development, changing management style, improving internal communications, and encouraging organizational development. Some stress managers state that the most important strategy is to increase social support through the organization of cohesive work groups, development of improved communication patterns, and provision of recreational facilities for employees. Workers' participation in analyzing problems and in planning programs can be an important contributor to success.

3. There should be an evaluation of the program. Follow-up surveys permit comparison with baseline conditions.

Work reorganization programs can be a set of learning experiences for managers, workers, and health care providers. Negative experiences should be avoided. For example, if a significant program starts, begins to raise expectations, and then is terminated before achieving results, it can leave a feeling of powerlessness behind that will inhibit further attempts at change. Adequate resources for the change process should be allocated in advance. Each workplace must be treated as if it were a living system with a growth potential and with vulnerabilities to change processes that are too demanding. Each organization has its own personality; it operates in a context of the industry, community, and society of which it is a part. Long-term success requires a true commitment of the organization to do something about stress and allocate resources to make this possible. The alternative may be resources unnecessarily expended on health care costs.

Recent international studies have shown that a key factor is that the work reorganization program must be based on a commitment to enhance the participation of employees and, thus, their decision latitude and control in job content and organizational issues. In 1991 the ILO commissioned 20 case studies of stress prevention programs in workplaces of nine developed and developing countries [55]. At these workplaces, employers and workers had attempted to address stress problems at their source by modifying the work situation rather than by attending to stress symptoms after the fact. Approximately 90 percent of the studies reported some evidence of success, indicating that elimination of stress due to work organization can succeed, and, in particular, that programs that engage workers in a participatory change process can succeed [38] (Table 19-5).

For a participatory process to occur, a feeling of trust must be created among lower-status employees that information they share openly about their

**Table 19-5.** Program type and success rate in work organization change—summary of International Labour Organization case studies

| Scope of work reorganization | Average score (scale: 0–8) |
| --- | --- |
| Person-based coping enhancement programs—expert guided (5 cases) | 0.6 |
| Task and work organization restructuring—expert guided (3 cases) | 3.0 |
| Task and work organization restructuring—worker participation process (3 cases) | 6.0 |
| Large-scale work reorganization—expert guided (5 cases) | 5.4 |
| Large-scale work environment focus—worker participation process (3 cases) | 4.3 |

Source: Adapted from RA Karasek. Stress prevention through work organization. A summary of 19 international case studies. In Conditions of work digest, preventing stress at work, vol. 11(2). Geneva: ILO, 1992.

feelings of job stress, and their ideas for work environment change, are protected from reprisals by management. For trust to develop, broad institutional support should be mobilized even if the program is at the departmental level. A joint labor-management program, which may create the trust necessary for open communication, is associated with program success.

Successful programs appear to combine multiple intervention approaches covering both individually focused and environmentally focused activity, often in an ordered sequence. For example, stress education is often a first step, followed by group discussions of the problems and action-planning sessions, and later by discussion of technical and economic resource issues. This process starts at the stress response in discussions generating awareness of the personal meaning of stress, moves to analysis of the task situation, and finally focuses on the level of work organization. The platform of raised awareness is necessary to gain support for job design and organizational issues. The sequence also has some power: Even when the original program design focuses on person-based change, environmental issues are likely to arise in the discussion if group members are from the same work situation.

The basic process observed in the ILO case studies involved expanding workers' awareness and then providing them with tools for active problem-solving. This approach gives workers new understanding of the linkages between people and envi-

ronments. Three types of activities are observed at each level: Workers gain new awareness in areas such as stress, task organization, and work system issues; workers evolve for themselves new vocabularies of explanations to build action plans with the help of overviews; and workers develop an improved understanding of limits and possible solutions based on work systems. Israel and associates described one such process in a large United States auto-manufacturing plant as "a series of overlapping phases in which movement from one phase to the next was triggered by the consolidation of accumulated learning into revised understandings of problems, problem contexts, and intervention possibilities" [56].

One German example [57] of an ILO work redesign process involves the "health circle"—a concept similar to the popular management-initiated "quality circle," but initiated at the joint request of employees to focus on issues of employee health. While it begins by examining the same detailed job factors that quality circles often review—and also maintains attention to productivity—the focus on health and well-being leads to significantly more involvement by employees and solutions that have broader impact on the work environment than quality circles typically have.

A key feature of organizational intervention is to encourage an active process of joint labor and management participation that can lead to better understanding of potential stressors and the possibilities for job redesign, changes in organizational function, and increases in buffering factors, such as social support to reduce the level and effects of work-related stress.

# References

1. Karasek R, Theorell T. Healthy work—stress, productivity, and the reconstruction of working life. New York: Basic Books, 1992.
2. National Council of Compensation Insurance. Emotional stress in the workplace—new legal rights in the eighties. New York: NCCI, 1985.
3. Sharit J, Salvendy G. Occupational stress: Review and reappraisal. Hum Factors 1982; 24:129–62.
4. Kasl SV. Stress and health. Ann Rev Public Health 1984; 5:319–41.
5. Baker D, Schnall P, Landsbergis P. Epidemiologic research on the association between occupational stress and cardiovascular disease. In S Araki. ed.: Behavioral medicine: An integrated biobehavioral approach to health and illness. New York: Elsevier, 1992, pp. 115–22.
6. Murphy LR. Job dimensions associated with severe disability due to cardiovascular disease. J Clin Epidemiol 1991; 44:155–66.
7. Fox BH. Psychosocial factors and the immune system in human cancer. In R Adler. ed. Psychoneuroimmunology. New York: Academic, 1981, pp. 103–57.
8. Baker GHB. Psychological factors and immunity. J Psychosom Res 1987; 31:1–10.
9. Caplan RD, et al. Job demands and worker health. Washington, D.C.: NIOSH (publication no. 75-160), 1977.
10. Sauter S, Murphy LR, Hurrell JJ Jr. Prevention of work-related psychological disorders: A national strategy proposed by the National Institute for Occupational Safety and Health. Am Psychol 1990; 45:1146–58.
11. Kasl SV. Epidemiological contributions to the study of work stress. In CL Cooper, R Payne. eds. Stress at work. Chichester: Wiley, 1978.
12. Selye H. The stress concept: Past, present and future. In CL Cooper. ed. Stress research issues for the eighties. Chichester: Wiley, 1983, pp. 1–20.
13. McGrath JE. A conceptual formulation for research on stress. In JE McGrath. ed. Social and psychological factors in stress. New York: Holt, Rinehart, & Winston, 1970, pp. 22–40.
14. Saunders M, McCormick E. Human factors in engineering design. 7th ed. New York: McGraw-Hill, 1992.
15. Lazarus R, Folkeman S. Stress appraisal and coping. New York: Springer, 1984.
16. Cannon WB. Stresses and strains of homeostasis. Am J Med Sci 1935; 189:1–14.
17. Selye H. A syndrome produced by diverse noxious agents. Nature 1936; 138:32.
18. Henry JP, Stephens PM. Stress, health, and the social environment: A sociobiological approach to medicine. New York: Springer, 1977.
19. Weiner H. Psychobiology of human disease. New York: American Elsevier, 1977.
20. Baker DB. The study of stress at work. Ann Rev Public Health 1985; 6:367–81.
21. French JR Jr, Caplan RD, Van Harrison R. The mechanisms of job stress and strain. Chichester: Wiley, 1982.
22. Karasek RA. Socialization and job strain: The implications of two related psychosocial mechanisms for job design. In B Gardell, G Johansson. eds. Working life. London: Wiley, 1981.
23. Czickszentmihalyi M. Beyond boredom and anxiety. San Francisco: Josey-Bass, 1975.
24. Seligman ME. Helplessness: On depression, development and death. San Francisco: W.H. Freeman, 1975.
25. Sauter S, Hurrell JJ Jr, Cooper CL. Job control and worker health. Chichester: Wiley, 1990.
26. Katz D, Kahn R. The social psychology of organizations. 2nd ed. New York: Wiley, 1978.
27. Gardell B. Scandinavian research on stress in working life. Intl J Health Serv 1982; 12:31–41.
28. Scott AJ. ed. Shiftwork. Occup Med 1990; 5:165–428.
29. Salvendy G, Smith AJ. Machine pacing and occupational stress. London: Taylor and Francis, 1981.
30. Kryter KD. Non-auditory effects of environmental noise. Am J Public Health 1972; 62:389–98.
31. LaDou J. Occupational stress. In C Zenz. ed. Developments in occupational medicine. Chicago: Year Book, 1980, pp. 197–210.
32. French JR Jr, Caplan RD. Organizational stress and individual strain. In AJ Manow. ed. The failure of success. New York: AMACOM, 1973.
33. Brenner MH, Mooney A. Relation of economic change to Swedish health and social well-being. Soc Sci Med 1987; 25:183–95.
34. Starrin B, et al. Societal changes, ill health and mortality: Sweden during the years 1963–1983; a macro-epidemiological study (Swedish). Research report no. 13, Department of Community Medicine, County of Varmland, Karlstad, Sweden, 1988.
35. Brenner S-O, Levi L. Long-term unemployment amoung women in Sweden. Soc Sci Med 1987; 25:153–61.

36. Arnetz B, et al. Immune function in unemployed women. Psychosom Med 1987; 49:3–12.

37. Hammarstrom A, Janlert U, Theorell T. Youth unemployment and ill health: Results from a two-year follow-up study. Soc Sci Med 1988; 26:1025–33.

38. Karasek R. Stress prevention through work reorganization: A summary of 19 international case studies. In Conditions of work digest, preventing stress at work, vol. 11(2). Geneva: ILO, 1992.

39. Wall Street Journal. Glutted markets; a global overcapacity hurts many industries; no easy cure seen. March 9, 1987.

40. Friedman MD, Rosenman RD, Carrol V. Changes in serum cholesterol and blood clotting time in men subjected to cyclic variation of occupational stress. Circulation 1958; 17:852–61.

41. Karasek RA, et al. Job characteristics in relation to the prevalence of myocardial infarction in the U.S. Health Examination Survey (HES) and the Health and Nutrition Examination Survey (NHANES). Am J Public Health 1988; 78:910–18.

42. Karasek RA, et al. Job decision latitude, job demands, and cardiovascular disease: A prospective study of Swedish men. Am J Public Health 1981; 71:694–705.

43. Fielding JF. Corporate health management. Reading, MA: Addison-Wesley, 1984, pp 309–331.

44. Schottenfeld RS, Cullen MR. Occupation-induced posttraumatic stress disorder. Am J Psychiatry 1985; 142:198–202.

45. Colligan MJ, Murphy LR. Mass psychogenic illness in organizations: An overview. J Occup Psychol 1979; 52:77.

46. Brodsky CM. The psychiatric epidemic in the workplace. Occup Med 1988; 3:653–62.

47. Rosenman RH, Brand RJ, Sholtz RI, Friedman M. Multivariate prediction of coronary heart disease during 8.5-year follow-up in the western collaborative group study. Am J Cardiol 1976; 37:903–10.

48. Ivancevich JM, Matteson MJ, Preston C. Occupational stress, type A behavior and physical well-being. Acad Manag J 1982; 25:373–91.

49. Ganster DC. Type A behavior and occupational stress. J Organiz Behav Manag 1986; 8:61–84.

50. LaRocco JM, House JS, French JR Jr. Social support, occupational stress, and health. J Health Soc Behav 1980; 21:202–18.

51. Warshaw JJ. Managing stress. In LW Krinsky, SN Kieffer, PA Carone, SF Yolles. eds. Stress and productivity. New York: Human Sciences Press, 1984, pp. 15–30.

52. Ganster DC, Fusilier MR, Mays BT. Role of social support in the experience of stress at work. J Appl Psychol 1986; 71:102–10.

53. Karasek RA, with Pieper C, Schwartz J. Job content questionnaire and user's guide, version 1.5. Lowell (Boston), University of Massachusetts Lowell, Department of Work Environment, 1993.

54. Kalimo R. Assessment of occupational stress. In M Kaovonen, MI Mikheev. eds. Epidemiology of occupational health. Copenhagen: WHO Regional Publications (European series no. 20), 1986, pp. 231–50.

55. International Labour Office. Conditions of work digest, preventing stress at work, vol. 11(2). Geneva: ILO, 1992.

56. Israel B, Schuman S, Hugentobler M, House J. A participatory action research approach to reducing occupational stress in the United States. In Conditions of work digest, preventing stress at work, vol. 11(2). Geneva: ILO, 1992.

57. Kuhn K. Health circles for foremen at Volkswagen (Germany). In Conditions of work digest, preventing stress at work, vol. 11(2). Geneva: ILO, 1992.

## Bibliography

*Addison-Wesley Series on Occupational Stress.* This series of monographs, each written by an expert in the field, is oriented toward a general audience. Each book stands on its own as a review of an aspect of the stress phenomenon. The following titles are examples:

House JS. Work stress and social support. Reading, MA: Addison-Wesley, 1981.
   *Clear presentation on the role and importance of social support.*

Levi L. Preventing work stress. Reading, MA: Addison-Wesley, 1981.
   *Principles to prevent work stress as seen from the perspective of a leading researcher in Sweden; it discusses the relationship between work stress and social policy.*

Warshaw LJ. Managing stress. Reading, MA: Addison-Wesley, 1979.
   *This monograph provides an introduction to the principles and practice of stress management by a recognized expert.*

*Wiley Series on Studies in Occupational Stress.* This is another series of monographs on occupational stress. These monographs tend to be more technical than the Addison-Wesley series, but still provide an excellent source of material. Selected titles include:

Beech HR, Burns LE, Sheffield BF. A behavioural approach to the management of stress. Chichester: Wiley, 1981.

Cooper CL, Payne R. eds. Stress at work. Chichester: Wiley, 1978.

*A collection of chapters reviewing research on work stress and role of person, environment, and person-environment fit.*

Cooper CL, Payne R. eds. Current concerns in occupational stress. Chichester: Wiley, 1980.

Cooper CL. Stress research: Issues for the eighties. Chichester: Wiley, 1983.

*A collection of chapters by leading researchers covering topics such as the relationship between cancer and stress, type A behavior, and the person-environment fit. A chapter by Selye reviews his initial conceptualization of the stress phenomenon.*

International Labour Office. Conditions of work digest, preventing stress at work, vol. 11(2). ILO: Geneva, 1992.

*This is a unique compendium of resources for practitioners and researchers who want to reduce worker stress through work reorganization. It includes an introductory overview of the occupational stress problems, 19 case studies of preventive change from nine countries, a summary analysis of the case studies, and a very useful review of visual aids, articles, and books in the stress prevention (through work environmental change) field.*

Karasek R, Theorell T. Healthy work—stress, productivity, and the reconstruction of working life. New York: Basic Books, 1990.

*This book combines explanations of stress development in the work process via the demand-control model (first half) with a proposal for work reorganization that could reduce psychosocial health risks (second half). The model is presented at the task level, by occupation, at the psychophysiologic level, and in epidemiologic studies. A psychosocial, skill-based productivity model, congruent with healthy work goals, is used to guide the book's second-half discussion through joint health and productivity topics: intervention processes, organizational issues, occupational strategies, and global economic challenges.*

Sauter S, Hurrell J Jr, Cooper CL. Job control and worker health. Chichester: Wiley, 1990.

# 20
# Shiftwork

Torbjorn Akerstedt and Anders Knutsson

A 22-year-old man came to an occupational health clinic complaining of gastrointestinal symptoms and sleep disturbances. He was currently employed at a paper mill and for 3 years he had been working on a three-shift schedule that included night shifts. The work schedule was a rotating shift schedule where the shifts changed at 0600, 1400, and 2200 hours in the following sequence:

|       | WEEK 1   | WEEK 2    | WEEK 3    | WEEK 4    | WEEK 5   |
|-------|----------|-----------|-----------|-----------|----------|
| Mon   | Night    | Morning   | Day off   | Afternoon | Day off  |
| Tues  | Night    | Morning   | Day off   | Afternoon | Day off  |
| Wed   | Night    | Day off   | Morning   | Afternoon | Day off  |
| Thurs | Night    | Afternoon | Morning   | Day off   | Day off  |
| Fri   | Day off  | Afternoon | Morning   | Night     | Day off  |
| Sat   | Day off  | Afternoon | Morning   | Night     | Day off  |
| Sun   | Day off  | Morning   | Day off   | Night     | Day off  |

He had previously been well with no history of sleep complaints or gastrointestinal problems. For the past 6 to 12 months he had experienced increasing disturbance in his sleep, especially after night shifts, when, on average, he could sleep only 1 to 2 hours. He felt excessively tired at the end of his workday and on his days off. He had also experienced epigastric pain, heartburn, and diarrhea. These problems had all developed insidiously over the past 6 months. He did not smoke or drink alcohol. He liked his work and his fellow workers. He lived with a female partner in a house of his own in a small, calm village 25 miles from the paper mill where he was employed. At home he was not disturbed by noise during sleep. His physical examination was normal except for a tender epigastrium. He had no anemia. A month later he was transferred to day work and 2 months later his sleep problems and gastrointestinal disturbances had disappeared, without any drug treatment.

This case illustrates the two most common disorders associated with shiftwork: disturbed sleep and wakefulness. Other major effects are increased accident risks, gastrointestinal disorders, and cardiovascular disease (see below for details). The central problem in shiftwork disorders is that the work hours force the individual to adopt temporal patterns of biologic and social functioning that are at odds with those of the day-oriented environment. Night work, in particular, presents a problem.

Before continuing along these lines we must, however, have a look at the term *shiftwork*. It is an imprecise concept, but usually refers to a work-hour system in which employee work schedules are organized to extend the period of production beyond the conventional daytime third of the 24-hour cycle. Shiftwork is generally organized into one of four major types: day work, permanently displaced work hours, rotating shiftwork, and roster work.

*Day work* involves work periods that fall between approximately 7:00 AM and 7:00 PM. *Permanently displaced* work hours require the individual to work either a morning shift (approximately 6:00 AM to 2:00 PM), an afternoon shift (approximately 2:00 PM to 10:00 PM), or a night shift (approximately 10:00 PM to 5:00 AM). *Rotating shiftwork* involves alternation between shifts, either all three (three-shift work) or two of them (two-shift work). The latter usually involves the morning plus the afternoon shift. Three-shift is often subdivided according to the number of teams that are used to cover the 24 hours, usually three to six teams. *Roster work* is similar to rotating shiftwork but may be less regular, more flexible, and less geared to specific teams. In contrast to the other types of shiftwork, roster work is not used in manufacturing industry but rather in service-oriented occupations, such as transport, health care, and law enforcement. In most industrialized countries approximately one-third of the population has some form of "non–day work" (shiftwork) and between 5 and 10 percent have shiftwork that includes night work.

The remainder of the chapter is organized into two sections: a short introduction discussion of circadian rhythms and sleep since these concepts are necessary for the understanding of shiftwork problems, followed by a presentation of the major health problems in shiftwork, their mechanisms and possible countermeasures.

## Circadian Rhythmicity and Sleep

Practically all physiologic and psychological functions describe a rhythmic behavior during a 24-hour period; that is, the function level oscillates between high and low values with a periodicity of 24 hours (hence the term *circadian*: circa dies = about 1 day). The parameters used to describe a rhythm are those of a sine function, that is, the amplitude (difference between the maximum and the minimum), the acrophase (or "phase" = the time of the maximum), and the period length (time between two successive peaks—under normal conditions, 24 hours).

The circadian rhythm of rectal temperature and cortisol during 64 hours of continuous activity and two-hourly intake of food and drink is illustrated in Fig. 20-1. Note the regularity of the pattern. Even though the basic circadian pattern is the same for most functions, the timing differs greatly. Thus, the hormone cortisol has its peak early in the morning, body temperature peaks in the late afternoon, and the pineal hormone melatonin

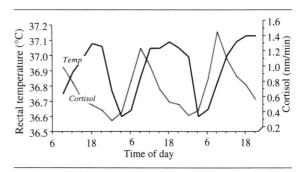

**Fig. 20-1.** Rectal temperature and urinary cortisol during 64 hours of continuous activity. N = 12.

peaks at night. On the whole, however, most rhythms peak during the daytime.

It is generally considered that the clock structures reside in the suprachiasmatic nuclei of the hypothalamus. These structures receive neural input from the retina, which presumably is used to adjust the timing of the clock. This may affect not only the phase of the rhythm but also the spontaneous period length. The latter is not 24 hours but just above 25 hours. If a human is deprived of the normal time cues ("synchronizers" or "Zeitgebers"), as, for example, light, he or she will start to live on a 25.2-hour day/night schedule [1].

An important aspect of circadian rhythms is their pattern of adjustment to shifted synchronizers. Since the spontaneous circadian period is 1 to 2 hours longer than that of the astronomical day (24 hours) [2], it will be very easy to go to bed 1 to 2 hours later than normal and rise 1 to 2 hours later. This will simply phase-delay the rhythm by 1 to 2 hours. In contrast, it is much more difficult to accomplish a phase advance, since this means going to bed 1 hour earlier, reducing the period length to 23 hours, 2 hours less than the spontaneous period. The major influence causing adjustment seems to be light. With proper timing of light circadian rhythms may be completely phase shifted [3].

For the shiftworker it appears that full adjustment never occurs to the night shift, not even in permanent night workers. At best the adjustment is partial, but frequently only marginal [2].

Sleep is quantified via a combination of the electroencephalogram (EEG), the electro-oculogram (EOG), and the electromyogram. Sleep normally encompasses six stages: stage 0 is wakefulness; stage 1 is transitory between wakefulness and sleep, accounting for only a small part of total sleep; stage 2 constitutes the basic feature of sleep, accounting often for 50 percent of sleep; stage 3 is a transitory stage between stages 2 and 4 and makes up only a minor amount of total sleep; stage 4 represents deep sleep and constitutes 20 percent of total sleep (stages 3 and 4 are often considered together and referred to as "slow-wave sleep" [SWS] since it is characterized by low-frequency and high-amplitude EEG activity); and finally, stage REM (traditionally given no stage number) involves dreaming and makes up about 25 percent of sleep.

The function of sleep is not completely understood. However, it seems that the normal (6–9 hours) amount of sleep is essential for the ability to sustain waking activity in the short run and life itself in the long run. The minimum amount of sleep necessary for reasonable daytime functioning seems to be around 6.5 hours over the long run. In the short run—day to day—sleep reductions from 8 to 6 hours have only marginal effects. Reductions as large as 3 hours begin to show effects on behavior, whereas total sleep loss during one night will result in very clear reductions in performance capacity. Three nights of sleep loss will result in almost complete inability to carry out normal tasks that involve perception, thinking, and decision making.

## Shiftwork Effects on Health and Well-Being

### Sleep

The dominant health problem reported by shiftworkers is disturbed sleep and wakefulness. At least three-fourths of the shiftworking population is affected [4].

Electroencephalographic studies of rotating shiftworkers and similar groups have shown that day sleep is 1 to 4 hours shorter than night sleep [5–7]. The shortening is due to the fact that sleep is terminated after only 4 to 6 hours without the individual being able to return to sleep. The sleep loss is primarily taken out of stage 2 sleep ("basic" sleep) and stage REM sleep (dream sleep). Stages 3 and 4 ("deep" sleep) do not seem to be affected. Furthermore, the time taken to fall asleep (sleep latency) is usually shorter. Also, night sleep before a morning shift is reduced but the termination is through artificial means and the awakening is usually difficult and unpleasant. It should be emphasized that the level of sleep disturbances in shiftworkers is comparable to that seen in insomniacs.

Interestingly, day sleep does not seem to improve much across a series of night shifts [8, 9]. It appears, however, that night workers sleep slightly better (longer) than rotating workers on the night shift [10].

The long-term effects of shiftwork on sleep are rather poorly understood. However, the amount of sleep/wake and related disturbances in present-day workers has been shown to be positively related to their previous experience of night work [11], and former shiftworkers with different clinical sleep/wake disturbances have been found in a sleep clinic population [12].

One reason for the disturbed daytime sleep may be the higher noise level during the day. On the other hand, sleep after a night shift is also shown to be dramatically shortened under optimal laboratory conditions. Thus noise does not seem to be the major cause of disturbed day sleep. A stronger influence is exerted by the circadian rhythm. Figure 20-2 shows that the more sleep is postponed from the evening toward noon on the next day, the more truncated it becomes (plotted at bedtime), and when noon is reached the trend reverts. Thus, sleep during the morning hours is strongly interfered with, despite the sizable sleep loss that, log-

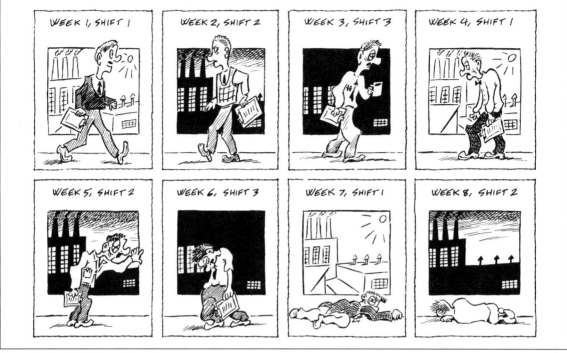

(Drawing by Nick Thorkelson.)

ically, should enhance the ability to maintain sleep. The same data are shown plotted at rising, yielding more accurate information on when maximal interference of sleep occurs. Similar observations have been made in subjects who can select their own preferred sleep/wake pattern under conditions of long-term isolation from time cues.

It should also be emphasized that homeostatic influences control sleep. For example, the expected

**Fig. 20-2.** Sleep at different times of day.

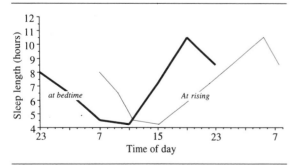

4 to 5 hours of daytime sleep, after a night spent awake, will be reduced to only 2 hours if a normal night sleep precedes it, and at least 3.5 hours if a 2-hour nap is allowed. Thus, the time of sleep termination depends on the balance between the circadian and homeostatic influences.

### Alertness, Performance, and Safety

Night-oriented shiftworkers complain as much of fatigue and sleepiness as they do about disturbed sleep [4]. The sleepiness is particularly severe on the night shift, hardly appears at all on the afternoon shift, and is intermediate on the morning shift. The maximum is reached toward the early morning (5:00 to 7:00 AM). Frequently incidents of falling asleep occur during the night shift. At least two-thirds of the respondents report that they have experienced involuntary sleep during night work.

Ambulatory EEG recordings verify that incidents of actual sleep occur during night work [7].

Figure 20-3 shows an example from an ambulatory recording of a process operator. This subject falls asleep twice during the night shift. Remarkably, most workers seem unaware of the fact that they fall asleep. This suggests an inability to judge one's true level of sleepiness.

Other groups, such as train engineers or truck drivers, show clear EEG signs of falling-asleep incidents while driving at night [13, 14]. These occur toward the second half of the night and appear as repeated bursts of alpha and theta EEG activity, together with closed eyes and slow undulating eye movements. As a rule the bursts are short (1–15 seconds) but frequent, and seem to reflect the letdowns in the effort to fend off sleep proper. Approximately one-fourth of the subjects recorded show the EEG/EOG patterns of fighting with sleep. This is clearly a larger proportion than what is found in the subjective reports of falling-asleep episodes.

As may be expected, sleepiness on the night shift is reflected in performance. One of the classic studies demonstrating this showed that errors in meter readings over a period of 20 years in a gas works had a pronounced peak on the night shift [15] (Fig. 20-4). There was also a secondary peak during the afternoon. Similarly, it has been demonstrated that telephone operators connected calls considerably slower at night [16], and that train drivers failed to operate their alerting safety device more often

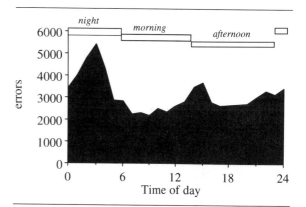

Fig. 20-4. Meter reading errors in three-shift workers. Illustration of sleepiness model.

at night than during the day [17]. Most other studies of performance have used laboratory tests and demonstrated, for example, reduced reaction time or poorer mental arithmetic on the night shift. It is noteworthy that flight simulation studies have shown that the ability to "fly" a simulator at night may decrease to a level corresponding to that after moderate alcohol consumption (0.05% blood alcohol) [18]. Differences have been noted between types of night shiftwork; for example, reaction time performance among night shift nurses has been demonstrated to be better in permanent than in rotating shiftworkers [19].

If sleepiness is severe enough, interaction with the environment will cease. When this coincides with a critical need for action an accident may ensue. Such potential performance lapses due to night work sleepiness were seen in several of the train engineers referred to earlier [13]. The transport area is, in fact, where most of the available accident data on night shift sleepiness have been obtained; for example, single-vehicle accidents have, by far, the greatest probability of occurring at night [20].

From conventional industrial operations very little relevant data are available, but an interesting analysis has been presented by the Association of Professional Sleep Societies' Committee on Catastrophes, Sleep and Public Policy [21]. Their con-

Fig. 20-3. Sleep stages for 24-hour ambulatory recording of three-shift worker in connection with a night shift.

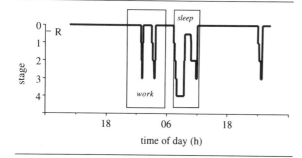

sensus report notes that the nuclear plant melt-down at Chernobyl occurred at 1:35 AM and was due to human error (apparently related to work scheduling). Similarly, the Three Mile Island reactor accident occurred between 4:00 and 6:00 AM and was due not only to the stuck valve that caused a loss of coolant water but, equally importantly, to the failure to recognize this event leading to the near meltdown of the reactor. The committee noted that similar incidents, although with the ultimate stage being prevented, occurred in 1985 at the David Beese reactor in Ohio and at the Rancho Seco reactor in California. Finally, the committee also reported that the NASA Challenger space shuttle disaster stemmed from errors in judgment made in the early-morning hours by people who had insufficient sleep (through partial night work) for days before the launch. Yet, in all of these accidents the technical problems have been given practically all official attention. The aspects of human factors, in particular night work, still await serious consideration.

The two obvious major sources of night shift sleepiness are circadian rhythmicity and homeostasis (sleep loss). Their effects may be difficult to separate in field studies but they are clearly discernible in laboratory sleep deprivation studies. Alertness falls rapidly after awakening but gradually levels out as wakefulness is extended. The circadian influence appears as a sine-shaped effect superimposed on this exponential fall in alertness. These two components may be easily separated, as illustrated in Fig. 20-5.

A "three-process" model of alertness regulation has been described, including derivation of the two functions represented in Fig. 20-5 [22]. *Process C* represents sleepiness due to circadian influences and has the general sinusoidal form indicated below. *Process S* is an exponential function of the time since awakening. Maximum alertness is reached on awakening, then falls rapidly, but levels out and gradually approaches an asymptote. At sleep onset process S is reversed (now called S') and recovery occurs as an exponential function. Recovery initially increases at a very rapid rate but

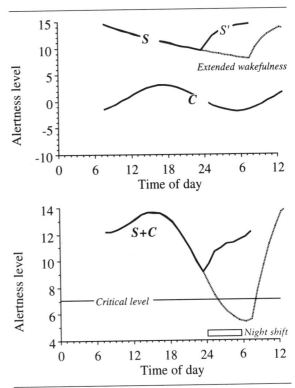

Fig. 20-5. Illustration of the three-process model of alertness regulation (see text).

subsequently levels off toward an upper asymptote. A third component exists that involves sleep inertia, but it is not relevant to the present discussion.

The estimate alertness (or sleepiness) is expressed as the arithmetic sum of the functions above. The lower part of the figure illustrates the extension of wakefulness that occurs with the first night shift. Much of the night shift is worked below the critical level since it occurs at the circadian trough of alertness and after a long period of waking.

### Other Effects on Health and Well-Being

*Gastrointestinal Complaints.* These complaints are more common among night shiftworkers than among day workers. A review of reports from among 34,047 persons with day work or shift-work found ulcers occurring in 0.3 to 0.7 percent of day workers, in 5 percent of workers with morning and afternoon shifts, in 2.5 to 15 percent of persons with rotating shifts involving night shifts, and in 10 to 30 percent of ex-shiftworkers [23]. Other gastrointestinal disorders, including gastritis, duodenitis, and dysfunction of digestion, are more common in shiftworkers than in day workers [24].

The pathophysiologic mechanism underlying gastrointestinal disease in shiftworkers is unclear, but one possible explanation is that intestinal enzymes and intestinal mobility are not synchronized with the sleep/wake pattern. Intestinal enzymes are secreted with circadian rhythmicity, and shiftworkers' intake of food is irregular compared with intestinal function.

Another contributing factor to gastrointestinal diseases might be the association between shiftwork and smoking. A number of studies have reported that smoking is more common among shiftworkers [23].

Studies concerned with alcohol consumption comparing day workers and shiftworkers have produced conflicting results, probably due to differences in local cultural habits [25–27]. One study, which used g-glutamyltransferase as a marker of alcohol intake, did not indicate that the shiftworkers had a higher intake of alcohol than the day workers [25].

*Cardiovascular Disease.* A number of studies have reported a higher incidence of cardiovascular disease, especially coronary heart disease, in male shiftworkers than in men who work days [28]. One study of 504 paper mill workers followed for 15 years found a dose-response relationship between years of shiftwork and incidence of coronary heart disease in the exposure interval of 1 to 20 years of shiftwork [29]. As with gastrointestinal disease, a high prevalence of smoking among shiftworkers might contribute to the increased risk of coronary heart disease, but smoking alone cannot explain the observed excess risk [25].

*Mortality.* The mortality of shift and day workers has been studied among 8,603 male manual workers in England and Wales between 1956 and 1968 [30]. Using figures available in the report, estimates of standardized mortality ratios (SMR) for deaths from all causes were 97, 101, and 119 for day, shift, and ex-shiftworkers, respectively. Although the differences were not statistically significant, the same study also showed significantly increased incidence of neoplastic disease in shiftworkers (SMR 116).

*Sickness Absence.* Absences due to illness are often used as a measure of occupational health risks. However, sickness leave is influenced by many factors not related to illness alone and cannot be considered as a reliable measure of true morbidity. Studies on sickness absence in day and shiftworkers have revealed conflicting results and there is no evidence that shiftworkers have more sickness absence than do day workers.

*Pregnancy.* Only a few studies have addressed the issue of pregnancy outcome in shiftworkers. In one, laboratory employees who were operating on shiftwork during pregnancy had a significantly increased risk of miscarriage (a relative risk of 3.2) [31], while a study of hospital employees also demonstrated a significantly increased risk of miscarriage for shiftwork (a relative risk of 1.4) [32]. Lower birth weight of infants of mothers who worked irregular hours has been reported [32, 33], although no teratogenic risk was associated with shiftwork [33].

*Social Activity.* One of the major effects of shiftwork is the interference of work hours with various social activities. The direct time conflict that results from shiftwork reduces the amount of time available to spend with family and friends or in various forms of recreation or voluntary activities. In addition, the alternating pattern of work hours and their anticipated interference may make participation in regular activities less worthwhile, resulting in passivity. Friends might also find the availability of a shiftworker too complicated by the shiftwork patterns, and therefore refrain from contacts. The result is often social isolation and a reduced capacity to fulfill the various social roles expected by society. Note, however, that being free from work during daytime carries certain advantages. The variable work hours also provide a means for solving problems of child care for working couples.

## Factors That Affect Adjustment

Which aspects of shiftwork are the most problematic? Which are most conducive to well-being? The following discussion addresses the characteristics of shift systems and of individuals in order to explore how possible guidelines for countermeasures may be derived.

### Shift System Characteristics

From the preceding sections it should be evident that the major problem of shiftwork is the night shift. As long as a night shift is involved in the work schedule, the problems of adjustment will persist. In comparison, other shift system characteristics will be of minor importance.

*Number of Night Shifts.* Aside from the night shift per se, an important shift system characteristic is the number of night shifts in a row. Most studies indicate that the circadian system and sleep do not adjust (improve) much across a series of night shifts. Not even in permanent night workers is an improvement seen. Thus, one should expect a long series of night shifts (>4) to be particularly taxing. For example, it has been found that rated alertness and general well-being in three-shift workers improved when a 2- to 3-day rotation was substituted for the old 7-day rotation. On the whole, the advantage with rapid rotation is that the taxing night shift is not permitted to exert its influence for more than a limited period of time. On the other hand, if it is of major importance that performance capacity remains high during the night it

would appear that a solution with permanent night shifts is preferable to rotating shifts that include the night shift. Permanent night shifts could be combined with other work teams that are assigned to a two-shift system with morning and afternoon shifts only.

*Direction of Rotation.* Another important aspect of the shift schedule may be the direction of rotation. Since the "true" period of the human sleep/wake cycle averages 25 hours, and since it can be adjusted by environmental time cues only within 1 to 2 hours of the "true" period, delays in phase are easier to accomplish than advances in phase. For the rotating shiftworker this implies that schedules that rotate clockwise (morning-afternoon-night) should be preferred to those that rotate counterclockwise. There have been, however, very few practical tests of this theory, particularly in relation to sleepiness. Still, it was demonstrated that a change from counterclockwise to clockwise rotation, together with a change from 7-day to 21-day rotation, improved production and well-being in three-shift workers [34]. Another study found that a change in the same direction among police officers following a rapidly (1 day) rotating shift schedule reduced blood pressure and improved well-being [35]. It appears that similar effects may be obtained simply by having the night shift moved from the start to the end of the shift cycle.

*Length of Workshift.* The length of a workshift is another parameter that one would expect to have an influence on sleepiness. In one field experiment 2-hourly ratings demonstrated that, as expected, a 12-hour night shift produced higher ratings of fatigue than an 8-hour night shift. In spite of this the 12-hour shift was preferred by the employees because of the extra day off involved [36]. In another study, it was shown that there was a U-shaped relationship between hours driven and accidents for truck drivers. After an initial "warm-up" period with higher accident rates, accident risk was low, but then increased again toward 11 hours of driving [20]. These results tend to support a common sense notion of fatigue/sleepiness being a function of the time worked. Current economic demands on families may exacerbate this problem if the days freed by long hours of off-shift time are used for holding a second job. There is a clear trend both in the International Labour Organization and the European Community to limit night work hours to 8 and to prohibit overtime work for (night) shiftworkers [37].

### Individual Differences and Strategies

Health problems in shiftworkers usually increase with age [4, 39]. The problems also increase with increasing exposure to shiftwork [40–42]. Being a morning-type person (or "lark") as compared with an evening-type (or "owl") is associated with poorer adjustment to shiftwork [41]. Similarly, rigidity of sleep patterns is associated with difficulties in shiftwork [41, 42]. Another factor that will exacerbate night work sleepiness is sleep pathology such as that associated with, for example, sleep apnea.

Gender is not in itself necessarily related to shiftwork tolerance. On the other hand the extra load of household work may put many women at a disadvantage since they are often the primary caretakers of the home.

Interestingly, good physical conditioning may facilitate accommodation to shiftwork. In one study of three-shift workers an improvement in physical fitness through a training program resulted in greatly reduced ratings of overall fatigue [43].

A number of diseases have been considered incompatible with shiftwork, for example, diabetes and ulcer. There is, however, very little evidence that such diseases will be exacerbated with shiftwork.

## Prevention Measures

The discussion above can be summarized in a number of possible countermeasures presented in Table 20-1. The most important individual countermeasure is sleep hygiene: Sleep in a dark, cool,

**Table 20-1.** Measures to Counter Effects of Shiftwork

Avoid night work

The direction of rotation should be clockwise

The speed of rotation should be rapid (2-3 days on each shift)

Permanent night work might be optimal under certain conditions

Night shifts should be placed at the end of the shift cycle

Rest days must be interspersed in the shift cycle

Free time between shifts should not be less than 16 hours

The duration of the night shift should not exceed 8 hours

Schedule naps during the night shift

Shiftworkers above the age of 45 should have a right to transfer to day work

sound-insulated bedroom; use ear plugs; inform family and friends about the sleep schedule; shut off the telephone during sleep hours; and hang a "do not disturb" sign on the door.

Another important countermeasure is strategic sleeping. In connection with night shiftwork the sleep period should lie between 2:00 and 9:00 PM. This would mean starting the night shift fairly refreshed from sleep with only the circadian trough to combat. Since sleep at the suggested hours may not be socially feasible, the next best alternative is to have a moderate morning sleep and then add a two-hour nap in the evening. This "split sleep" should provide a solid base of alertness for the subsequent night shift.

Very little is known about optimal food intake strategies in connection with shiftwork. Common sense suggests, however, that one should avoid intake of major meals during the night shift.

Sleeping pills may improve daytime sleep but should be avoided over the long run. New methods have been suggested for phase shifting the circadian system, such as bright light exposure or intake of the pineal hormone, melatonin. As yet, however, these methods are merely research topics.

# References

1. Wever RA. The circadian system of man. Results of experiments under temporal isolation. New York: Springer, 1979.
2. Akerstedt T. Adjustment of physiological circadian rhythms and the sleep-wake cycle to shift work. In TH Monk, S Folkard. eds. Hours of work. Chichester: Wiley, 1985, pp. 185–98.
3. Czeisler CA, et al. Exposure to bright light and darkness to treat physiologic maladaptation to night work. N Engl J Med 1990; 322:1253–59.
4. Akerstedt T. Sleepiness as a consequence of shift work. Sleep 1988; 11:17–34.
5. Matsumoto K. Sleep patterns in hospital night nurses due to shift work: An EEG study. Waking and Sleeping 1978; 2:169–73.
6. Tilley AJ, Wilkinson RT, Drud M. Night and day shifts compared in terms of the quality and quantity of sleep recorded in the home and performance measured at work: A pilot study. In A Reinberg, N Vieux, P Andlauer. eds. Night and shift work. Biological and social aspects. Oxford: Pergamon, 1981, pp. 187–96.
7. Torsvall L, Akerstedt T, Gillander K, Knutsson A. Sleep on the night shift: 24 hour EEG monitoring of spontaneous sleep/wake behavior. Psychophysiology 1989; 26:352–58.
8. Foret J, Benoit O. Shiftwork: The level of adjustment to schedule reversal assessed by a sleep study. Waking and Sleeping 1978; 2:107–12.
9. Dahlgren K. Adjustment of circadian rhythms and EEG sleep functions to day and night sleep among permanent night workers and rotating shift workers. Psychophysiology 1981; 18:381–91.
10. Tepas DL, Mahan RP. The many meanings of sleep. Work and Stress 1989; 3:93–102.
11. Guilleminault C, Czeisler S, Coleman R, Miles L. Circadian rhythm disturbances and sleep disorders in shift workers. In PA Buser, WA Cobb, T Okuma. eds. Kyoto Symposia (EEG Suppl. 36). Amsterdam: Elsevier, 1982, pp. 709–14.
12. Dumont M, Montplaisir J, Infante-Rivard C. Insomnia symptoms in nurses with former permanent nightwork experience. In WP Koella, F Obal, H Schulz, P Visser. eds. Sleep '86. Stuttgart: Gustav Fischer Verlag, 1988, pp. 405–6.
13. Torsvall L, Akerstedt T. Sleepiness on the job: Continuously measured EEG changes in train drivers. Electroencephalogr Clin Neurophysiol 1987; 66: 502–11.
14. Keoklund G, Akerstedt T. Sleepiness in long distance truck driving: An ambulatory EEG study of night driving. Ergonomics 1993; 36:1007–17.
15. Bjerner B, Holm A, Swensson A. Diurnal variation of mental performance. A study of three-shift workers. Br J Ind Med 1955; 12:103–10.
16. Brown RC. The day and night performance of teleprinter switchboard operators. Occup Psychol 1949; 23:121–6.
17. Hildebrandt G, Rohmert W, Rutenfranz J. 12 and 24 hour rhythms in error frequency of locomotive drivers and the influence of tiredness. Int J Chronobiol 1974; 2:175–80.
18. Klein DE, Bruner H, Holtman H. Circadian rhythm of pilot's efficiency, and effects of multiple time zone travel. Aerosp Med 1970; 41:125–32.
19. Wilkinson RT. How fast should the night shift rotate? Ergonomics 1992; 35:1425–46.
20. Hamelin P. Lorry driver's time habits in work and their involvement in traffic accidents. Ergonomics 1987; 30:1323–33.
21. Mitler MM, et al. Catastrophes, sleep and public policy. Consensus report. Sleep 1988; 11:100–9.
22. Folkard S, Akerstedt T. A three process model of the regulation of alertness and sleepiness. In R Ogilvie, R Broughton. eds. Sleep, arousal and performance: Problems and promises. Boston: Birkhauser, 1991, pp. 11–26.
23. Angersbach D, et al. A retrospective cohort study comparing complaints and disease in day and shift workers. Int Arch Occup Environ Health 1980; 45:127–40.
24. Koller M. Health risks related to shift work. Int Arch Occup Environ Health 1983; 53:59–75.
25. Knutsson A. Shift work and coronary heart disease. Scand J Soc Med 1989; 544:1–36.
26. Smith MJ, Colligan MJ, Tasto DL. Health and safety consequences of shift work in the food-processing industry. Ergonomics 1982; 25:133–44.
27. Romon M, Nuttens MC, Fievet C. Increased triglyceride levels in shift workers. Am J Med 1992; 93:259–62.
28. Kristensen TS. Cardiovascular diseases and the work environment. Scand J Work Environ Health 1989; 15:165–79.
29. Knutsson A, Akerstedt T, Jonsson BG, Orth-Gomer K. Increased risk of ischemic heart disease in shift workers. Lancet 1986; 2:86–92.
30. Taylor PJ, Pocock SJ. Mortality of shift and day workers 1956–68. Br J Ind Med 1972; 29:201–7.
31. Axelsson G, Lutz C, Rylander R. Exposure to solvents and outcome of pregnancy in university laboratory employees. Br J Ind Med 1984; 41:305–12.
32. Axelsson G, Rylander R. Outcome of pregnancy in relation to irregular and inconvenient work schedules. Br J Ind Med 1989; 46:306–12.
33. Nurminen T. Shift work, fetal development and

course of pregnancy. Scand J Work Environ Health 1989; 15:395–403.

34. Czeisler CA, Moore-Ede MC, Coleman RM. Rotating shift work schedules that disrupt sleep are improved by applying circadian principles. Science 1982; 217:460–3.

35. Orth-Gomer K. Intervention on coronary risk factors by adapting a shift work schedule to biological rhythmicity. Psychosom Med 1983; 45:407–15.

36. Rosa RR, Colligan MJ. Extended workdays: Effects of 8-hour and 12-hour rotating shift schedules on performance, subjective alertness, sleep patterns, and psychosocial variables. Work and Stress 1989; 3:21–32.

37. Kogi K, Thurman JE. Trends in approaches to night and shiftwork and new international standards. Ergonomics 1993; 36:3–13.

38. Akerstedt T, Gillberg M. The circadian variation of experimentally displaced sleep. Sleep 1981; 4:159–69.

39. Foret J, Bensimon B, Benoit O, Vieux N. Quality of sleep as a function of age and shift work. In A Reinberg, N Vieux, P Andlauer. eds. Night and shift work: Biological and social aspects. Oxford: Pergamon, 1981, pp. 149–54.

40. Dumont M, Montpaisir J, Infant-Rivard C. Past experience of nightwork and present quality of life. Sleep Res 1987; 16:40.

41. Folkard S, Monk TH, Lobban MC. Towards a predictive test of adjustment to shift work. Ergonomics 1979; 22:79–91.

42. Costa G, Lievore F, Casaletti G, Gaffuri E. Circadian characteristics influencing interindividual differences in tolerance and adjustment to shift work. Ergonomics 1989; 32:373–85.

43. Harma ML, et al. The effect of physical fitness intervention on adaptation to shiftwork. In M Haider, M Koller, R Cervinka. eds. Night and shift work: Long-term effects and their prevention. Frankfurt am Main: Peter Lang, 1986, pp. 221–8.

## Bibliography

Folkard S, Monk TH. Hours of work. Chichester and New York: Wiley, 1985.
*This book is a carefully selected series of articles designed to address how to best design work hours to meet human needs as well as production goals. The first half of the book reviews aspects of circadian rhythms and sleep as well as non–24-hour rhythms. The remainder of the book considers practical aspects of the effects of normal and abnormal work hours.*

Moore-Ede M. The twenty-four hour society. Reading, MA: Addison-Wesley, 1993.
*This book summarizes the scientific findings on sleep/wake cycles, alertness, and fatigue, illustrating their effects and discussing ways in which one can protect against them. Discussion includes redesign of work schedules, management of information flow, and how to design jobs and work environments to take account of circadian needs.*

Office of Technology Development. Biological rhythms: Implications for the worker. U.S. Congress, Office of Technology Assessment. OTA-BA-463. Washington, D.C.: U.S. Government Printing Office, 1991.
*As one of a series of reports on "New Developments in Neurosciences," this monograph discusses the scientific basis of biologic rhythms and the roles they play in regulating physiologic and cognitive functions. The majority of the monograph is devoted to discussing the effects of nonstandard work hours on health, performance, and safety of workers.*

# 21

# Building-Related Factors: An Evolving Concern

Kathleen Kreiss

This chapter deals with a less well-defined series of exposures than those of the previous chapters in this section. It focuses mainly on low-level exposures (see Chap. 3) to (1) factors that can cause well-recognized respiratory and other disorders (see Chap. 22), and (2) other factors that epidemiologists, industrial hygienists, and others are working to understand. The content of this chapter relates to other chapters on toxic chemicals (Chap. 13) and stress (Chap. 19), for example. It also relates mainly to office workers, whose problems are also covered elsewhere in this book, for example, in the chapters on ergonomics (Chap. 8) and women (Chap. 32).

## Sick Building Syndrome

Since the 1970s office workers in North America and Europe have commonly complained of mucous membrane irritation, fatigue, and headache when working in specific buildings, with improvement within minutes to an hour of leaving the building. This constellation of symptoms, with tight temporal association to building occupancy, is called sick building syndrome. It is the most frequent of the building-associated health complaints in industrialized countries, which also include diseases caused by infection, hypersensitivity, and specific toxins. Researchers have estimated that as high as 30 percent of office workers report symptoms attributed to poor air quality, and workers in buildings not known to have indoor air-quality

problems have many complaints attributed to the indoor work environment.

Despite the impacts on productivity and employee morale when many of a building's workers have a high prevalence of sick building syndrome, little progress has been made in understanding the causes of this syndrome. Early investigations of this phenomenon sometimes concluded that symptoms were caused by mass psychogenic illness (see Chap. 26), since no specific contaminants were measured in concentrations that could account for symptoms. However, the endemic nature of complaints in specific buildings and the consistency of complaints from workers in sealed buildings across the world did not satisfy diagnostic criteria for mass psychogenic illness. Fortunately, such attribution to psychological cause is no longer common or acceptable, although work stress is associated with reporting of symptoms among occupants of specific buildings. Occupants of buildings with high levels of complaints are often angry and fearful, since they have often encountered resistance of managers to investigation, inconclusive results, or ineffectual remediation for a syndrome whose scientific cause remains elusive.

The recognition of building-related complaints by public health authorities in the United States followed an energy crisis in which ventilation standards were lowered to 5 ft$^3$ of outdoor air per person per minute. This observation led to the hypothesis that the new building-related symptoms were attributable to lower rates of ventilation in relation to indoor contaminant sources. Little evidence exists, in either cross-sectional or experimental studies, that ventilation rates are related to sick building syndrome prevalence, except possibly at very low ventilation rates below the now-current standard of 20 ft³ per person per minute. Indoor air-quality consultants commonly measure carbon dioxide levels in buildings with high complaint rates. However, human occupants, who are the source of increased concentrations of carbon dioxide in indoor air as compared to outdoor air, are not the likely source of contaminants that would explain sick building syndrome. Carbon dioxide measurements simply reflect ventilation effectiveness in relation to human occupancy.

The most interesting work on causes of sick building syndrome comes from epidemiologic studies of occupants of buildings selected without regard to known indoor air-quality complaints. These cross-sectional studies suggest that certain building features and occupant characteristics are related to sick building syndrome prevalence. The variation in prevalence of building-related complaints among buildings suggests remediable causes. Occupants of buildings with air conditioning have been shown to have higher rates of building-related symptoms than occupants of naturally ventilated buildings or buildings with mechanical ventilation that does not alter air temperature or humidity. This observation and other work suggest that the ventilation system itself may be the source of poor air quality in some buildings. However, measurable parameters do not yet exist that correlate with symptom rates. Other environmental correlates of sick building syndrome include carpeting, high occupancy load, and video display terminal use. Personal factors associated with building-related symptoms in many cross-sectional studies include female gender, job stress or dissatisfaction, and allergies.

The health care provider with the challenge of responding to indoor air-quality complaints must proceed without the benefit of scientific understanding of what may be a multifactorial syndrome. No single measurement establishes whether air quality is adequate or inadequate, and the ac-

ceptability of indoor air quality rests with the occupants and not a laboratory. In the difficult situation of indoor air-quality complaints, a multidisciplinary approach will allow attention to design and maintenance of air-conditioning systems, exclusion of obvious contaminant sources in the occupied space, and reassurance of occupants that sick building syndrome is a self-limited condition. Indoor air-quality investigations customarily assess the ventilation in relation to occupant load by measuring carbon dioxide, suggest remediation of ventilation system maintenance and cleanliness deficiencies, and examine smoking policies. On the multidisciplinary team alongside industrial hygienists and ventilation engineers, the health care provider has an important role to exclude the possibility of less common, but more medically serious, building-related diseases that nearly always occur with a background of sick building syndrome complaints among other workers.

### Case of Building-Related Asthma

A 48-year-old social services eligibility technician began working in the implicated office building in October 1986 with a history of previous sinus symptoms and 15 pack-years of cigarette smoking, having been an ex-smoker for 10 years. She had insidious onset of dry cough in January 1987, which was diagnosed as asthma in March. Skin prick tests were negative to aeroallergens, and she was referred to an occupational medicine clinic in August 1987 because she noted deterioration during the workday and recovery in the evenings and on weekends, when she did not require inhaled bronchodilators. Her asthma had become much worse when she manipulated dusty records while her desk was being moved. She performed peak-flow measurements with a mini-Wright peak flowmeter, which showed reproducible, striking air-flow limitation shortly after entering the building, with partial recovery during lunch breaks outside the building and full recovery on weekends (Fig. 21-1). Methacholine challenge testing on September 30 and November 2, 1987, before and after a 16-day vacation, showed provocative concentrations ($PC_{20}$) of 0.29 and 0.47 mg/ml, respectively, for a 20 percent decrement in forced expiratory volume in 1 second (normal $PC_{20} > 15$ mg/ml). Although she had notified her employer, her relocation to another building was de-

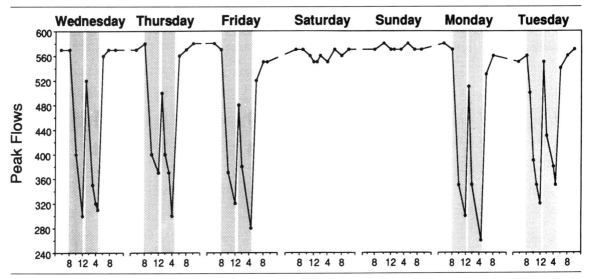

**Fig. 21-1.** Peak-expiratory flow measurements by time and day in a case of building-related asthma, Denver, Colorado, 1988.

layed until late February 1988, after her third course of prednisone treatment. She had resolution of her work-related air-flow limitation (documented by peak-flow measurements), her symptoms, and her need for asthma medications. Her $PC_{20}$ normalized to above 25 mg/ml in early May 1988.

In mid-February 1989 she was moved back to the original building into a set of offices that shared no ventilation system with the offices that she had previously occupied. She had increasing symptoms and airflow limitation over the following 6 weeks, once again requiring daily medication. Her $PC_{20}$ fell to 0.22 by March 28, 1989. She was medically restricted from the implicated building on April 10, 1989, with resolution of her work-related decrements in peak flows, decreased medication requirements, and increased $PC_{20}$ (to 5.19 mg/ml on June 23, 1989). She has had no further difficulty with clinical asthma since leaving the building. Coincident with her asthma in the building, she noted an eczematous skin rash, which improved considerably but did not fully resolve when she worked away from the implicated building.

This building was built into an earthen bank, and workers reported musty odors and visible mold growth on the interior wall that abutted the bank. *Aspergillus* species of fungi were detected in the interior air but not in simultaneous measurements of outdoor air, suggesting amplification and dissemination of this bioaerosol indoors. The presumed source of the woman's asthma was fungal bioaerosols associated with moisture coming in from the earthen bank.

Building-related asthma is infrequently recognized by physicians, but can lead to chronic irreversible illness, unlike sick building syndrome. Early recognition and removal from the building, as in this woman's case, can result in cure of asthma. Permanent asthma can result when recognition of occupational etiology is delayed and asthma becomes severe before the patient leaves the implicated exposure. Such sentinel cases of asthma imply risk for other workers. In this case, public health investigation following two sentinel cases showed that coworkers had nearly five times the prevalence of physician-diagnosed asthma with onset or exacerbation since building occupancy compared to workers in a social service agency [1].

Building-related asthma occurs in water-damaged buildings and in relation to microbially contaminated humidifiers or biocides used in them. The biologic aerosols containing mold spores and perhaps bacteria are thought to be the sensitizing agents. Characterization of bioaerosols is difficult, since few laboratories have expertise in identifying saprophytic fungi, in contrast to fungi that cause human infection. Despite the difficulty in characterizing the exposure, the history and peak-flow measurements can be valuable in documenting the occupational nature of building-related asthma. Cases of building-related asthma may occur alongside of cases of hypersensitivity pneumonitis in water-damaged buildings.

### Case of Building-Related Hypersensitivity Pneumonitis

A 46-year-old pediatrician had been followed by an allergist for 10 years for upper respiratory and chest complaints after moving into an office suite. At first, he complained of sinus drainage and a sore feeling in his nose and throat. Over the years, he had developed achiness in his chest associated with fever, productive cough, chest tightness, wheezing, fatigue to exhaustion, and shortness of breath on exertion. His forced vital capacity (FVC) fell within 3 years of building occupancy, consistent with a restrictive pattern. He had been treated with nasal cromolyn, inhaled steroids, bronchodilators, theophylline, antibiotics, and intermittent oral corticosteroids, without receiving a diagnosis. A year before his referral to an occupational medicine specialist, he had noted exacerbation in his chest symptoms and wheezing when he returned to his office suite after a week away from work. He then began to suspect an office-related cause to his symptoms, with increased cough, chest tightness, and achiness when he entered his suite, and resolution over hours after leaving and improvement on weekends. He noted a musty smell and fungal discoloration of wall board in the suite bathroom, which resulted from leaking pipes.

Upon referral, he was found to have basilar rales, bronchial hyperreactivity on histamine challenge test, and reduced exercise tolerance with excessive respiratory rate at rest and excessive minute ventilation for oxygen consumption. The chest x-ray was normal, but a high-resolution computed axial tomography (CT) scan showed fine centrilobular nodules. Bronchoalveolar lavage showed a lymphocytic alveolitis compatible with hypersensitivity pneumonitis, and a transbronchial lung biopsy showed a mild patchy lymphocytic interstitial pneumonitis. His symptoms resolved with prednisone and removal from the office suite.

However, 2 months later chest aching, exertional shortness of breath, sick fatigue, and chilly feelings recurred within 45 minutes of using a musty restaurant bathroom that had been recurrently water damaged from roof leaks. He had a prolonged recovery time, requiring systemic steroids for 7 months. A year after this acute exacerbation, he again had a recurrence of chest symptoms, within hours of handling medical records from his previous office suite that had become wet when a hot water heater broke in his basement. Again he required months of prednisone use and felt that he had fully recovered his health only a year after this last exposure.

This case of building-related hypersensitivity pneumonitis is typical in the medical delay in suspecting and diagnosing a building-related etiology for symptoms. Few physicians are aware that office settings can be associated with diseases related to organic antigens. In contrast to building-related asthma, however, there are many published case reports and epidemic investigations of hypersensitivity pneumonitis and humidifier fever. Typically, persons with hypersensitivity lung diseases may not be able to reoccupy a building in which they were sensitized to biologic aerosols from contaminated humidifiers, ventilation systems, or water-damaged materials on which fungal growth occurred. Even after remediation of the conditions that led to sensitization and disease, low levels of exposure can trigger recurrent symptoms. Since hypersensitivity pneumonitis can lead to irreversible lung fibrosis after recurrent acute episodes or prolonged exposure, early recognition is the best means of preventing progression by restricting cases from the implicated building. Remediation can prevent cases in coworkers who are not yet sensitized. Occupational health practitioners can encourage specialists to proceed with diagnostic tests before the classic late-stage abnormalities are present, such as abnormal chest x-rays. The history of this pediatrician suggests that he was sensitized to an antigen that was not unique to his water-damaged office setting.

Cases of hypersensitivity pneumonitis often have systemic symptoms of myalgias, fever, and profound fatigue. These symptoms are not usually present in asthma, although both diseases commonly share chest symptoms such as cough, chest tightness, and wheezing. In contrast to asthma and hypersensitivity pneumonitis, sick building syndrome alone is not accompanied by chest symptoms. When indoor air-quality complaints exist, health care providers should ensure, in addition to the more common complaints of mucous membrane irritation, headache, and fatigue, that building-related asthma and hypersensitivity pneumonitis are not occurring. The occurrence of building-related chest disease dictates evaluation for sources of fungal growth and means of dissemination from water damage or from the ventilation system. Chest disease also requires more aggressive medical restriction from the building in order to prevent chronic disease.

Many patients report that they have building-related nose and sinus symptoms. It is likely that allergic rhinosinusitis can occur, in a way analogous to the response of airways and lung tissue to building-related antigen exposure. Little research has been done on this common clinical complaint to epidemiologically document its occurrence, to distinguish it from mucous membrane complaints in sick building syndrome, or to link it to exposures in implicated buildings.

## Building-Related Infection

In 1976, 182 cases of a mysterious pneumonia occurred among members of the American Legion attending a convention in Philadelphia. After months of laboratory investigation, a newly discovered bacterial organism, *Legionella pneumophila*, was found responsible. We now know that this common environmental organism frequently grows in warm waters of building cooling towers in the absence of vigorous attempts to eradicate it. When contaminated cooling tower mists are entrained in air intakes of large buildings, cases of infection with the organism (legionnellosis) can occur. Outbreaks have also been recognized as a result of contaminated industrial water sprays, hospital shower heads, and hot tubs.

In addition to pneumonia, *Legionella* organisms have been associated with another building-related disease called Pontiac fever, which is characterized by fever, chills, headache, and myalgia. This disease was first described in 1968, in a building-related epidemic of 144 cases in a county health department in Michigan. The attack rate was nearly 100 percent, with an average incubation of 36 hours.

In addition to infections that cannot be spread to other people, such as *Legionella* pneumonia, building ventilation characteristics are important to the spread of infections that can be passed on to other people, such as viral respiratory infection. A study in the United States Army showed that febrile acute respiratory disease occurred more frequently among basic trainees living in energy-efficient army barracks than in trainees living in old "leaky" barracks [2]. Other airborne infections, such as tuberculosis, varicella, and measles, may be affected by ventilation rates. The control of tuberculosis infection in hospital workers, prisons, and shelters is a major concern, for which ventilation and air disinfection techniques are being investigated.

## Building-Related Complaints Due to Specific Toxins

Health professionals responding to building-related complaints must also consider specific exposures or toxins as a possible explanation. This is particularly important when complaints differ from those of sick building syndrome or occur in epidemic, rather than endemic, fashion. For example, complaints of headache and nausea dictate consideration of carbon monoxide poisoning, which can occur when air intakes entrain fumes from loading docks, parking garages, or boiler stack emissions. Building-related itching without rash can occur with fibrous glass exposure, which can result when air duct lining is entrained in the airstream entering the occupied space. Epidemic coughing, dry throat, and eye irritation can result from detergent residues following the misapplication of carpet cleaning products. In instances of building-related complaints associated with specific exposures, a careful evaluation of types of symptoms, their prevalence, and their temporal onset may point investigators to the cause and to remediation resources.

Environmental tobacco smoke may contribute to the irritant symptoms of sick building syndrome. In many buildings, environmental tobacco smoke is circulated throughout the building as air is recirculated, with modest dilution from outdoor air ventilation. In buildings with indoor air-quality complaints, restriction of smoking to areas with separate exhaust ventilation may result in improved air quality for the remainder of the building.

Sometimes building-related exposures do not lead to occupant symptoms, but nonetheless pose a health risk. For example, radon gas emitted from building materials and infiltrating buildings from soil and water poses increased risk of cancer. Similarly, asbestos in insulation and some building materials in older buildings poses a risk of cancer and lung disease if it is disturbed during occupant activities or renovation. Occupational health specialists and other health care providers are often called to help communicate risks of such exposures to building occupants or the public during removal of asbestos from older buildings.

## References

1. Hoffman RE, Wood RC, Kreiss K. Building-related asthma in Denver office workers. Am J Public Health 1993; 83:89–93.
2. Brundage JF, et al. Building-associated risk of febrile acute respiratory diseases in army trainees. JAMA 1988; 259:2108–12.

## Bibliography

Kreiss K. The epidemiology of building-related complaints and illness. In JE Cone, MJ Hodgson. Problem buildings: Building-associated illness and the sick building syndrome. Occup Med State of the Art Rev 1989; 4:575–592.
*A more comprehensive review of the literature pertinent to building-related complaints, with exhaustive references.*
Kreiss K, Hodgson MJ. Building-associated epidemics. In PJ Walsh, CS Dudney, ED Copenhaver. eds. Indoor air quality. Boca Raton, FL: CRC Press, 1984, pp. 87–108.
*Contains a tabular listing of early literature on building-related hypersensitivity pneumonitis outbreaks and case reports for those faced with such a problem.*
Mendell MJ. Nonspecific symptoms in office workers: A review and summary of the epidemiologic literature. Indoor Air 1993; 3:227–236.
*Describes the conclusions about risk factors for sick building syndrome that can be drawn from the literature through the lenses of methodologic strength of design and consistency of findings among investigations.*
Mendell MJ, Smith AH. Consistent pattern of elevated symptoms in air-conditioned office buildings: A reanalysis of epidemiologic studies. Am J Public Health 1990; 80:1193–1199.
*A useful paper that allows some sense to be made of the seemingly disparate epidemiologic findings of studies looking for building-related and personal risk factors for sick building syndrome.*

# IV
# Occupational Disorders by System

# 22

# Respiratory Disorders

David C. Christiani and David H. Wegman

A 60-year-old man, a sandblaster for 23 years, was hospitalized for the third time in the past 4 months for shortness of breath (SOB). Three years ago he began having respiratory problems, first mild SOB and increased heart rate when walking in snow and climbing steps and with heavy exertion at work. These symptoms increased moderately over the next several months. He was seen by the company physician, who told him that he had "bad lungs" but gave him no treatment. Two years ago he sought therapy at a community hospital due to increasing SOB while walking at normal speed on the level ground for one to two blocks. He was hospitalized. Resting room-air arterial blood gases were $PaO_2 = 87$ and $PaCO_2 = 31$. A chest x-ray showed multiple interstitial nodules without evidence of hilar disease. Pulmonary function tests revealed a reduced forced vital capacity (73% of predicted) with a normal diffusing capacity. Tuberculosis smear, culture, and cytology of bronchial washings were negative. The patient was sent home without therapy. He was told not to return to work; he has not worked since.

Seven months ago, he developed a cough occasionally productive of clear to grayish, thin sputum. Three more hospital admissions for increasing SOB occurred with no new findings reported. Since the last hospitalization 1 month ago, he has been on oxygen continuously and stays in bed most of the day. He has also had dysuria and some trouble initiating his urinary stream, which seems to make his SOB worse.

The patient had smoked one pack of cigarettes per day for 5 years until he quit 20 years ago. He has no history of asthma, pneumonia, surgery, or allergies.

Occupational history revealed a 23-year period of operating a sandblasting machine located in a basement room (20 × 40 ft). Dust escaped continuously through crevices of the sandblasting unit; every time the patient opened the door to remove and install a piece to be blasted, much fine dust escaped. The windows were closed; there was an exhaust fan in the wall that did not seem to help. A room fan, installed to circulate the air in the room, was often out of order. The patient wore a helmet with a cloth apron on the bottom, covering his shoulders, and, when the room was especially dusty, a compressed air supply.

Physical examination revealed a thin man in moderate respiratory distress, sitting hunched over, gasping for breath, with grunting expirations. The pulse was 110, respiratory rate 40, blood pressure 110/80, and temperature 98°F. Pulmonary and cardiac examinations were normal, except for a systolic ejection murmur and an increased second heart sound over the pulmonic area. His extremities revealed clubbed fingernails and cyanosis. The rest of the examination was normal. Resting room-air arterial blood gases were $PaO_2 = 39$ and $PaCO_2 = 38$. Chest x-ray showed diffuse interstitial small rounded densities throughout both lung fields with hilar fullness. These were judged to be "q"-sized with a 2/2 profusion in all lung fields, using the International Labour Organization (ILO) nomenclature for chest x-rays. The diagnosis of silicosis was made. He remained completely disabled and died 3 months later.[1]

This case is characteristic of severe occupational respiratory disease, in this instance, pneumoconiosis. Workplace exposure responsible for such chronic disabling lung disease occurs gradually over long periods of time; initially, exposures do not result in any obvious acute symptoms, but

[1]Case courtesy of Stephen Hessl, Daniel Hryhorczuk, and Peter Orris, Section on Occupational Medicine, Cook County Hospital, Chicago.

427

once symptoms do appear, in many instances little can be done beyond making the worker comfortable. Unless discovered very early in their course, most work-related respiratory diseases are not curable; it is for this reason that disease prevention is so important.

Occupational lung disease is recorded in accounts of ancient history. Case reports exist in the writings of Hippocrates, and evidence of silicosis is present in pictographs from Egypt. Yet today some of those chronic diseases are still an important problem for workers. Recently, attempts have been made to quantify the prevalence and incidence of occupational respiratory disease, but few data exist for estimates of its actual magnitude. Estimates suggest that less than 5 percent of chronic occupational respiratory disease is correctly identified as associated with work.

Pneumoconiosis and occupational asthma are two work-related respiratory diseases that are often not correctly diagnosed. For example, approximately 5 percent of Americans suffer from what physicians diagnose as asthma, but a much larger proportion of people report either having asthma or episodes of wheezing; physicians who see workers who report wheezing should determine if a work-related bronchoconstrictive response is occurring.

## Evaluation of Individuals

Evaluation of pulmonary response to toxic exposures is important because work-related respiratory disease is frequently a contributory cause—and commonly a primary cause—of pulmonary disability. Complete evaluations can generally be performed effectively in a physician's office.

The clinical evaluation of pulmonary disease includes a minimum of four elements: (1) a complete history including occupational and environmental exposures, a cigarette-smoking history, and a careful review of respiratory symptoms; (2) a physical examination with special attention to breath sounds; (3) a chest x-ray with appropriate atten-

tion to parenchymal and pleural opacities; and (4) pulmonary function tests.

### History
Review of symptoms should include questions on chronic cough, chronic sputum production, shortness of breath (dyspnea) on exertion when compared with peers or usual level of activity, wheezing unrelated to respiratory infections, chest tightness, chest pain, and reports of allergic or asthmatic responses to work or non-work environments. For example, one peculiar characteristic of several types of occupational asthma and of pulmonary edema is that the symptoms may peak in intensity approximately 8 to 16 hours after exposure has ended. The symptoms will often occur at night as shortness of breath or cough. In assessing acute airway disease, one should question the patient about the principal symptoms: chest tightness, wheezing, dyspnea, and cough. A formal survey questionnaire, the American Thoracic Society (ATS) respiratory symptom questionnaire, for systematic respiratory effect studies is available [1]. (See Chap. 3 for information on the occupational history.)

### Physical Examination
The physical examination is helpful when abnormal. The most remarkable finding in most patients with occupational lung diseases is the relative absence of physical signs; however, certain conditions are associated with physical signs and the presence or absence of such abnormalities should be noted.

Auscultation can reveal important diagnostic clues. Fine rales at the bases, often at end inspiration, are more common in asbestosis than in other interstitial lung diseases. Wheezes and their relationship to exposure are helpful in evaluating a suspected case of work-related asthma. A pleural rub can occur with pleural reaction due to acute, chronic, or long-distant asbestos exposure.

Clubbing of the digits occurs rarely in relatively advanced lung diseases including asbestosis and therefore usually appears after other evidence of the disease has become apparent. This finding is nonspecific and cannot be used as a reliable clinical indication for asbestosis. It does not usually occur in other mineral pneumoconioses or in hypersensitivity pneumonitis. The most common nonoccupational causes of clubbing are bronchogenic carcinoma and idiopathic pulmonary fibrosis.

Examination of the heart is important since left ventricular failure can present as dyspnea alone, and right ventricular failure may indicate severe lung disease.

### Chest X-ray

A chest x-ray should be taken and, in addition to a standard interpretation, it should, if possible, be interpreted according to the ILO classification for pneumoconiosis by a trained reader [2] (Fig. 22-1). Although this classification is only now beginning to be used in radiology departments, it serves an important function in the general x-ray interpretation. The standard technique permits semiquantitative interpretation of x-rays to identify early evidence and progression of parenchymal and pleural disease; it focuses on size, shape, concentration, and distribution of small parenchymal opacities as well as distribution and extent of pleural thickening or calcification. For example, rounded opacities in the upper lung fields are generally associated with silicosis, whereas linear (irregular) opacities in the lower lung fields are usually associated with asbestosis (Figs. 22-2 and 22-3). It is important to note that deviations from these patterns are not uncommon; that is, both silicosis and coal workers' pneumoconiosis can be associated with irregular opacities. Moreover, workers exposed to mixed dusts, for example, silica and asbestos, can present with mixed rounded and irregular opacities in any or all lung fields. The ILO system has the distinct advantage of a standardized set of comparison x-ray films, which can be used to classify x-rays at one point in time or to follow an individual or a population for change over time. Even though chest x-rays present evidence of abnormality, they do not provide information on disability or impairment and do not necessarily correlate well with pulmonary function test findings. An individual with severe obstructive disease may show little evidence of it on chest x-ray. In contrast, an individual exposed chronically to iron oxide or tin oxide may show a dramatically abnormal chest x-ray (Fig. 22-4), but iron or tin oxide in the lung causes little, if any, pulmonary inflammatory reaction or lung function abnormality.

### Pulmonary Function Tests

A critical element in determining respiratory status is an evaluation of pulmonary function. In a well-equipped pulmonary function laboratory, spirometry, lung volume determinations, gas exchange analyses, and exercise testing can be performed with relative ease. In a physician's office, only the spirometry is readily and inexpensively performed; it does, however, provide a surprising amount of information. Pulmonary function tests, required for medical surveillance by some Occupational Safety and Health Administration (OSHA) standards, are commonly used and are easy to perform, reliable, and reproducible. Most lung disease may yield abnormal results or accelerated declines within the "normal" ranges before onset of clinical symptoms, especially if individuals are followed at regular 1- to 3-year intervals. Although the tests may demonstrate several patterns of abnormalities, they are not capable of determining etiology by themselves. The hospital-based tests (lung volume determinations, gas exchange analyses, exercise tests, and bronchial challenge tests) can contribute to a refined diagnostic evaluation once an abnormality is suspected.

The basic tests of ventilatory function can be obtained with a simple portable spirometer. Test results are derived from the forced expiratory curve (Fig. 22-5). Many types of equipment are currently being marketed to provide these tests, yet several have been inadequately standardized and are either insufficiently or overly sensitive. The National Institute for Occupational Safety and Health (NIOSH) and the ATS have evaluated spi-

**I.   Size and Shape of Small Opacities**

| | ROUNDED OPACITIES | | | IRREGULAR OPACITIES |
|---|---|---|---|---|
| p | ≤ 1.5 mm diameter | | s | fine linear opacities > 1.5 mm width |
| q | 1.6 - 3.0 mm diameter | | t | medium opacities 1.6 - 3.0 mm width |
| r | 3.1 - 10.0 mm diameter | | u | coarse, blotchy opacities 3.1 - 10.0 mm width |

· Size recorded by two letters to distinguish single type from mixed type. For example, q/q
if only q opacities are present, but q/t if q opacities predominate but t are also present

**II.   Concentration (Profusion) and Distribution**

### SMALL OPACITIES

| | Major Categories | Minor Divisions | | | Distribution· | |
|---|---|---|---|---|---|---|
| 0 | Small Opacities Absent or Less than Category I Normal Lung Markings Visible | 0/- | 0/0 | 0/1 | RU | LU |
| 1 | Small Opacities Present but Few Normal Lung Markings Usually Visible | 1/0 | 1/1 | 1/2 | RM | LM |
| 2 | Small Opacities Numerous Normal Lung Markings Partially Obscured | 2/1 | 2/2 | 2/3 | RL | LL |
| 3 | Small Opacities Very Numerous Normal Lung Markings Totally Obscured | 3/2 | 3/3 | 3/+ | | |

### LARGE OPACITIES

| A | One or More Opacities with Greatest Summed Diameter 1 - 5 cm |
|---|---|
| B | One or More Opacities Larger or More than Category A. Total Area < Equivalent of Right Upper Zone |
| C | One or More Opacities. Total Area Exceeds Equivalent of Right Upper Zone |

· Recorded by dividing lungs into 3 regions per side and checking all regions containing the designated small opacities

**III.   Pleural Thickening**

| | WIDTH· | | EXTENT· | | CALCIFICATION· |
|---|---|---|---|---|---|
| a | Maximum Up to 5 mm | 1 | Up to 1/4 Lateral Wall | 1 | One or Several Regions Summed Diameter ≤ 2 cm |
| b | Maximum 5 - 10 mm | 2 | 1/4 - 1/2 Lateral Wall | 2 | One or Several Regions Summed Diameter 2 - 10 cm |
| c | Maximum > 10 mm | 3 | Exceeds 1/2 Lateral Wall | 3 | One or Several Regions Summed Diameter > 10 cm |

· **Width** estimated only if seen in profile. **Extent** estimated as maximum length of thickening (profile or face on).
**Calcification** site (diaphragm, wall, other) and extent are noted separately for two sides.

**Fig. 22-1.** Schematic of ILO classification system for chest x-rays. In addition to these scores, the reader is guided in scoring technical quality of the x-ray (good, acceptable, poor, unacceptable) and in identifying other relevant features (for example, bullae, cancer, abnormal cardiac size, emphysema, fractured rib, pneumothorax, tuberculosis).

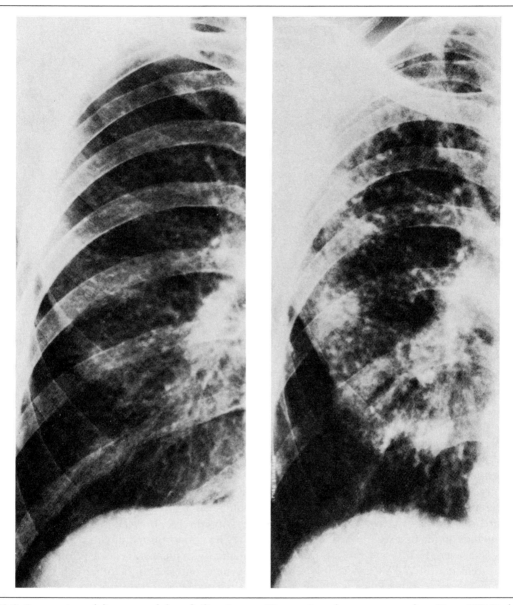

**Fig. 22-2.** Progression of discrete nodules of silicosis over 10 years in a slate quarry worker. (From WR Parkes. Occupational lung disorders. 2nd ed. London: Butterworths, 1982.)

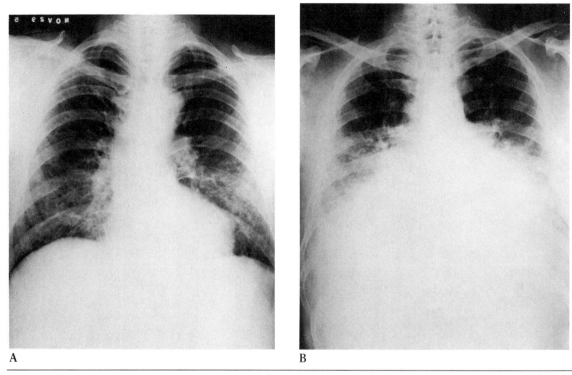

A                                          B

**Fig. 22-3.** Chest x-ray showing early (A) and advanced (B) fibrosis in asbestosis, especially in lower lung fields.

rometers and can provide information on which ones are most reliable and accurate [3]. Although many measures are possible from the forced expiratory curve, the simplest and generally the most useful ones for evaluating work-related respiratory disease are forced vital capacity (FVC), forced expiratory volume in the first second of a forced vital capacity maneuver (FEV$_1$), and the ratio of these two measurements (FEV$_1$/FVC). A simple scheme for the interpretation of these tests is shown in Table 22-1 and Fig. 22-5. Results are compared to Knudson's expected values, derived from a normal population of nonsmoking adults, and are expressed as a percentage of the expected value.

No reliable race-specific expected values are available; OSHA recommends multiplying Knudson's values by 0.85 for African-Americans. Criteria for the proper performance and evaluation of

spirometry are based on ATS recommendations [4, 5].

Pneumoconioses, such as silicosis and asbestosis, are considered restrictive diseases because lung volume is reduced. In the absence of significant airways disease, flow rates will be maintained and may be above normal due to decreased lung compliance with increased elastic recoil. Coal workers' pneumoconiosis, on the other hand, is more often associated with an obstructive pattern, with decreased air flow and normal or increased lung volumes. Also, occupational asthma is considered an obstructive disease because there is obstruction of air flow without reduction in lung volume. Of course, with multiple environmental exposures (including tobacco smoking), a mixed condition is frequently present, and precise pattern discrimination is not possible. Moreover, some mineral

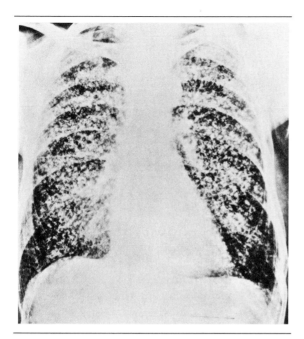

**Fig. 22-4.** Chest x-ray demonstrating stannosis, the benign pneumoconiosis due to the inhalation of tin oxide, in a man who worked as a furnace charger in a smelting works for 42 years. (From WR Parkes, Occupational lung disorders. 2nd ed. London: Butterworths, 1982.)

dusts, such as asbestos and coal, have been shown to cause abnormalities both of the airways and the interstitium. Nevertheless, the basic distribution of ventilatory function abnormalities (see Table 22-1) is useful in considering the general characteristics of work-related respiratory disease.

## Evaluation of Groups

If the physician is able to examine several workers from the same work environment, careful attention should be directed toward evaluation of the grouped results in addition to those of each individual. For an individual, emphasis is on the work history and collection of information to explain specific symptoms and signs. It should be recognized, however, that absence of basilar rales does not exclude asbestosis, wheezes do not necessarily diagnose occupational asthma, opacities on chest x-ray do not specify their pathology, and pulmonary function tests may be falsely considered "normal" because of the wide variation in standard populations. In fact, it may not be until a group of coworkers is evaluated that pulmonary disease can be recognized as associated with work. Group

**Fig. 22-5.** Spirographic results in normal and disease states. (Adapted from JA Nadel. Pulmonary function testing. Basics of RD [American Thoracic Society] 1973; 1:2.)

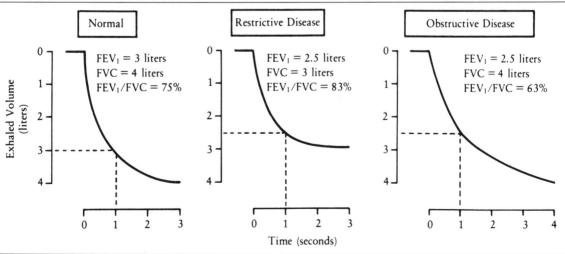

**Table 22-1.** Spirometry interpretation

| Type of response | Percent predicted[a] | | FEV$_1$/FVC % | Response to inhaled bronchodilators |
|---|---|---|---|---|
| | FEV$_1$ | FVC | | |
| Normal | ≥80% | ≥80% | ≥75% | — |
| Obstructive | <80% | ≥80%[b] | <75% | ± |
| Restrictive | ≥80% | <80% | ≥75% | — |
| Mixed | <80% | <80% | <75% | ± |

[a]Predicted FEV$_1$ and FVC based on RJ Knudson et al. Changes in the normal maximal expiratory flow volume curve with growth and aging. Am Rev Respir Dis 1983;127:725.
[b]Severe obstruction can result in reduction of FVC also.

evaluations have the benefit that results can be subdivided according to duration of work or types of exposure. Chest x-ray findings, pulmonary function tests, and symptom histories can be examined by subgroups to evaluate previously unrecognized work effects (see examples in Chap. 5). Furthermore, the average value of a group of tests has less variability than an individual test result. For example, measurements of FEV$_1$ and FVC in individuals that vary between 80 and 120 percent of the population standards are still considered normal; a group of 10 or 20 actively working individuals, however, should have a mean result much closer to the standard values (100 percent). If the difference is as little as 10 percent lower (that is, 90 percent of the predicted value), then an adverse health effect in that population should be seriously considered.

Comparisons to baselines should be performed whenever possible to permit evaluation of change over time in individuals or a group compared to a known—not a predicted—value. Accelerated decrements in lung function, accelerated development of respiratory tract symptoms, or recognition of subtle chest x-ray abnormalities are far more significant when the comparison is based on earlier examinations rather than on expected population experience. These evaluations can be made effectively and completely in a physician's office. Any worker potentially exposed to respiratory hazards at work should have a baseline ventilatory function test included in the medical record.

The major types of respiratory response to external agents discussed in this chapter are summarized in Table 22-2. Occupational lung cancer and work-related infectious diseases of the respiratory tract are discussed in Chaps. 14 and 18, respectively.

## Acute Irritant Responses

Irritation in the upper respiratory tract, in contrast to the mid- or lower tract, is frequently associated with work-related symptoms. Acute symptoms are often due to regional inflammation, which a patient perceives as irritation. With nasal and paranasal sinus irritation, there is congestion that can result in violent frontal headache, nasal obstruction, runny nose, sneezing, and occasionally nosebleed. Throat inflammation is commonly reported as a dry cough. Laryngeal inflammation can cause hoarseness and, if severe, may result in laryngeal spasms associated with glottal edema, presenting dramatic symptoms: anxiety, shortness of breath, and cyanosis.

In the mid-respiratory tract, the acute reaction is characteristically bronchospasm. The extreme case is asthma, which is histologically distinguished by a thickened basement membrane, increased number of goblet cells with secretions, mucus plugging, and increased smooth muscle at preterminal bronchioles. Asthma associated with work is being recognized with increasing fre-

**Table 22-2.** Major types of occupational pulmonary disease

| Pathophysiologic process | Occupational disease example | Clinical history | Physical examination | Chest x-ray | Pulmonary function pattern |
|---|---|---|---|---|---|
| Fibrosis | Silicosis | Dyspnea on exertion, shortness of breath | Clubbing, cyanosis | Nodules | Restrictive or mixed obstructive and restrictive DLCO normal or decreased |
| | Asbestosis | Dyspnea on exertion, shortness of breath | Clubbing, cyanosis, rales | Linear densities, pleural plaques, calcifications | |
| Reversible airway obstruction (asthma) | Byssinosis, isocyanate asthma | Cough, wheeze, chest tightness, shortness of breath, asthma attacks | Respiratory rate $\uparrow$, wheeze | Usually normal | Normal or obstructive with bronchodilator improvement Normal or high DLCO |
| Emphysema | Cadmium poisoning (chronic) | Cough, sputum, dyspnea | Respiratory rate $\uparrow$ $\uparrow$ expiratory phase | Hyperaeration bullae | Obstructive low DLCO |
| Granulomas | Beryllium disease | Cough, weight loss, shortness of breath | Respiratory rate $\uparrow$ | Small nodules | Usually restrictive with low DLCO |
| Pulmonary edema | Smoke inhalation | Frothy, bloody sputum production | Coarse, bubbly rales | Hazy, diffuse air-space disease | Usually restrictive with decreased DLCO, hypoxemia at rest |

DLCO = diffusing capacity; $\uparrow$ = increased.

quency; precipitating agents include isocyanates, detergent enzymes, and Western red cedar dust (Table 22-3). In addition to asthma caused by exposure to agents listed in this table, many irritant substances not usually associated with asthma can produce bronchial hyperreactivity when high levels of exposure have occurred. Single high-dose exposure and episodic low-dose exposure to irritants such as ammonia or chlorine can result in nonspecific bronchial reactivity, referred to by some authors as reactive airways dysfunction syndrome (RADS) or irritant asthma, which may persist for months to years or may never fully resolve.

The conditions deriving from acute irritation of the deep respiratory tract are pulmonary edema and pneumonitis. With pulmonary edema there is extravasation of fluid and cells from the pulmonary capillary bed into the alveoli. Primary pulmonary edema is due to direct toxic action on the capillary walls. For example, exposure to ozone and oxides of nitrogen is common in industrial settings; both agents can cause pulmonary edema either acutely (when a trapped worker cannot escape exposure), or in a more delayed fashion when overexposures are not too high. Pneumonitis, on the other hand, is an inflammation of the lung pa-

**Table 22-3.** Selected causes of occupational asthma*

| Agents | Jobs |
| --- | --- |
| High molecular weight compounds | |
|   Animal products: dander, excreta, serum, secretions | Animal handlers, laboratory workers, veterinarians |
|   Plants: grain, dust, flour, tobacco, tea, hops | Grain handlers, tea workers, bakers, and workers in natural oil manufacturing and in tobacco and food processing |
|   Enzymes: *Bacillus subtilis*, pancreatic extracts, papain, trypsin, fungal amylase | Bakers and workers in the detergent, pharmaceutical, and plastic industries |
|   Vegetable: gum acacia, gum tragacanth | Printers and gum-manufacturing workers |
|   Other: crab, prawn | Crab and prawn processors |
| Low molecular weight compounds | |
|   Diisocyanates: toluene diisocyanate (TDI), methylene-diphenyldiisocyanate (MDI) | Polyurethane industry workers, plastics workers, workers using varnish, and foundry workers |
|   Anhydrides: phthallic and trimellitic anhydrides | Epoxy resin and plastics workers |
|   Wood dust: oak, mahogany, California redwood, Western red cedar | Carpenters, sawmill workers, and furniture makers |
|   Metals: platinum, nickel, chromium, cobalt, vanadium, tungsten carbide | Platinum and nickel-refining workers and hard-metal workers |
|   Soldering fluxes | Solderers |
|   Drugs: penicillin, methyldopa, tetracyclines, cephalosporins, psyllium | Pharmaceutical and health care industry workers |
|   Other organic chemicals: urea formaldehyde, dyes, formalin, azodicarbonamide, hexachlorophene, ethylene diamine, dimethyl ethanolamine, polyvinyl chloride pyrolysates | Workers in chemical, plastic, and rubber industries; hospitals; laboratories; foam insulation manufacture; food wrapping; and spray painting |

*Mechanism believed to be immunoglobulin E–mediated for high molecular weight compounds and some low molecular weight compounds. The immunologic mechanism for asthma from many low molecular weight substances remains undefined.
Source: Adapted from M Chan-Yeung, S Lam. Occupational asthma. Am Rev Respir Dis 1986; 133:686–703.

renchyma in which cellular infiltration rather than fluid extravasation predominates. Beryllium, cadmium, and chemicals such as isocyanates can cause acute pneumonitis.

### Factors Involved in Toxicity

The most widespread causes of acute responses are irritant gases. Water is a major constituent of the respiratory tract lining, and solubility of these gases in water is the most significant factor influencing their site of action. Gases with high solubility act on the upper respiratory tract within seconds. For example, fatal epiglottic edema has been associated with irritants of high solubility, such as ammonia, hydrogen chloride, and hydrogen fluoride. The moderately soluble gases act on both the upper and lower respiratory tract within minutes. Chlorine gas, fluorine gas, and sulfur dioxide are irritants of this type, producing upper respiratory irritation as well as symptoms of bronchoconstriction. The low-solubility irritants are most insidious; they penetrate to the deep portions of the respiratory tract and act predominantly on the alveoli 6 to 24 hours after exposure. Because of the considerable delay in onset of symptoms, large doses can be delivered without any irritant symptoms to serve as warnings. Pulmonary edema is the major effect of overexposures to materials such as ozone, oxides of nitrogen, and phosgene.

Other factors influencing the site of action of an irritant gas are intensity and duration of exposure. The amount of exposure depends not only on air concentrations but also on work effort: A worker with a sedentary job who is exposed to a given concentration of a respiratory irritant will receive a much lower dose than one with an active job that requires rapid breathing and a high minute ventilation (tidal volume × respiratory rate).

A final element that influences the site of action is interaction—both synergism and antagonism. Sulfur dioxide and particulates of water are synergistic; they combine to deliver a sulfuric acid–like vapor to the respiratory tract. Ammonia and sulfur dioxide, however, are antagonistic and to-gether produce less response than either can individually. The presence of a carrier such as an aerosol may increase the effect of an irritant gas: Sulfur dioxide may cause a moderate effect and a sodium chloride aerosol no effect on the respiratory tract, whereas animal studies indicate that the two combined may result in a marked effect because the aerosol delivers the sulfur dioxide more deeply into the lung.

### Highly Soluble Irritants

Primary examples of highly soluble irritants are (1) ammonia, used as a soil fertilizer, in the manufacture of dyes, chemicals, plastics, and explosives; in tanning leather; and as a household cleaner; (2) hydrogen chloride, used in chemical manufacturing, electroplating, and metal pickling; and (3) hydrogen fluoride, used predominantly for etching and polishing of glass, as a chemical catalyst in the manufacture of plastics, as an insecticide, and for removal of sand from metal castings in foundry operations.

The primary physical effects of highly water-soluble irritants are first the odor and then eye and nose irritation; throat irritation is slightly less frequent. In high doses, the respiratory rate can increase and bronchospasm can occur. Lower respiratory tract effects, however, do not occur unless the individual is severely overexposed or trapped in the environment. The irritant effects are powerful and generally provide adequate warning to prevent overexposure of individuals free to escape from exposure. The history and physical examination are the most important parts of irritant exposure evaluation. Reflex bronchoconstriction may be evident on pulmonary function tests shortly after exposure. Chest x-rays are not helpful unless pulmonary edema is present.

Management of reactions to these irritants is immediate removal of the worker and, if breathing is labored or hypoxemia is present, provision of oxygen. If severe exposure or unconsciousness occurs, observation in a hospital for development of pulmonary edema is advisable.

Prevention of exposures relies on proper industrial hygiene practices with local exhaust ventilation as an essential component. Respirators should only be relied on as a temporary control measure in an emergency, but, if routine respirator use is required to prevent adverse effects from overexposures, then workers must be trained in their proper use and maintenance.

A 25-year-old man came to the emergency room with acid burns. Before taking a job as an electroplater 5 weeks before admission, he was in perfect health. On the first day at this job, itching developed. Subsequently, sores developed, which healed with scars at sites of splashes of workplace chemicals. After 4 days on this job, he had a runny nose, throat irritation, and a productive cough. He also noted some shortness of breath at work.

His work involved dipping metal parts into tanks containing chrome solutions and acid. He wore a disposable paper respirator, rubber gloves, and an apron, but no eye protection. Although heavy fumes were present in the 60 × 20 × 14 ft room, no ventilation was provided. Apparently, none of the other eight workers in the room had similar medical problems.

Past history revealed three prior hospitalizations for pneumonia but not asthma or allergies. He smoked about four cigarettes per day.

From age 16 to 18, he worked as a sheet-metal punch-press operator for a tool and die company. From age 18, he worked as a drip-pan cleaner for a soup company. He was a student in an auto mechanics school from age 19 to 21. From age 23 to 24, he occasionally worked as a gas station attendant.

Physical examination was normal, except for multiple areas of round, irregularly shaped, depigmented 1-mm atrophic scars on both forearms and exposed areas of anterior thorax and face; a 4-mm, rounded, punched-out ulcer, with a thickened, indurated, undermined border and an erythematous base on his left cheek; an erythematous pharynx; and bilateral conjunctivitis. There was no perforation of the nasal septum. Patch tests with dichromate, nickel, and cobalt were all negative, as was chest x-ray.

The diagnoses were irritation of the upper respiratory tract and an irritant contact dermatitis, both due to chromic acid mist. His symptoms resolved with removal from exposure. Periodic medical surveillance was advised to provide early diagnosis of a possible malignancy of the nasal passages for which he may be at risk as a result of the chromium exposure.[2]

Many small electroplating firms have no local ventilation over open vats of chromic and other acids. Frequently a high level of chrome or other metals in the fumes is liberated as metal parts that are being plated are immersed. Chrome and chromic acid mist are local irritants and chromates (hexavalent forms especially) are considered to be carcinogens, although it is not known whether electroplaters have a special cancer risk.

### Moderately Soluble Irritants

The moderately soluble irritants commonly encountered in industrial settings are chlorine, fluorine, and sulfur dioxide. Chlorine is widely used in the chemical industry to synthesize various chlorinated hydrocarbons, whereas outside the chemical industry its major use is in water purification and as a bleach in the paper industry. Fluorine is used in the conversion of uranium tetrafluoride to uranium hexafluorides, in the development of fluorocarbons, and as an oxidizing agent. Fluoride is used in the electrolytic manufacture of aluminum, as a flux in smelting operations, in coatings of welding rods, and as an additive to drinking water. Sulfur dioxide is commonly used as a disinfectant, a fumigant, and a bleach for wood pulp, and is formed as a by-product of coal burning, smelter processes, and the paper industry.

These irritants, like the highly soluble ones, initially cause mucous membrane irritation, often manifested by a persistent cough. Acute symptoms are usually of short duration. Low levels of continuous exposures, which are better tolerated than exposures to highly soluble irritants, may cause obstructive respiratory disease.

[2]Case courtesy of Stephen Hessl, Daniel Hryhorczuk, and Peter Orris, Section of Occupational Medicine, Cook County Hospital, Chicago.

In addition to causing respiratory symptoms, these irritants lead to other health problems. Chlorine gas contributes to corrosion of the teeth, while fluorine is a significant cause of chemical skin burns. Chronic exposure to fluoride is associated with increased bone density, cartilage calcification, discoloration of teeth in the young, and possibly rheumatologic syndromes. Sulfur dioxide, in particular, is associated with bronchospasm, especially in asthmatics, with some epidemiologic studies suggesting a possible role in chronic obstructive pulmonary disease.

Again, the history and physical examination are most important in evaluating an industrial case. Management and prevention are similar to those for highly soluble irritants. Pulmonary function tests, especially the $FEV_1$, are indicated in surveillance programs for workers with chronic exposure.

### Irritants of Low Solubility

Usually the effects of irritants with low solubility are mild throat irritation and occasionally headache. Much more significant is pulmonary edema, which manifests itself 6 to 24 hours after exposure, preceded by symptoms of bronchospasm (chest tightness and wheezing) (Fig. 22-6). Ozone and oxides of nitrogen are the two low-soluble irritants most commonly encountered. Both occur in welding fumes and therefore are found in many work environments. Ozone is used as a disinfectant; as a bleach in the food, textile, and pulp and paper industries; and as an oxidizing agent. Oxides of nitrogen are used in chemical and fertilizer

Fig. 22-6. Chest x-rays in a copper miner. A. Twenty-four hours after overexposure to oxides of nitrogen. Pulmonary edema is evident. B. One week after exposure, showing resolution of pulmonary edema. (Courtesy of Benjamin G. Ferris, M.D.)

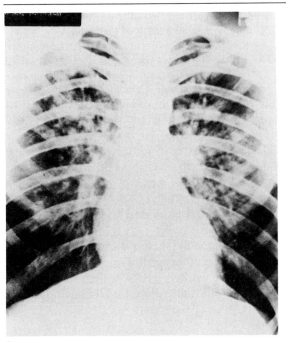

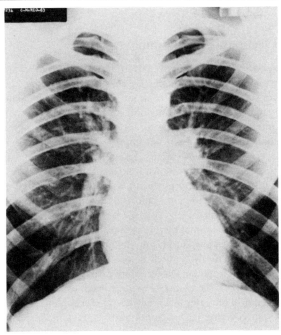

A

B

manufacture and in metal processing and cleaning operations.

Chronic exposure to oxides of nitrogen may result in bronchiolitis obliterans. In addition to the history, the physical examination, and the acute obstructive defect evident on pulmonary function tests, the chest x-ray can be examined for evidence of early pulmonary edema and the appearance of bronchiolitis obliterans. A specific syndrome associated with oxides of nitrogen is silo filler's disease, which results from exposures to this gas in the upper chambers of grain silos, where it forms in the anaerobic fermentation of green silage. The brownish color of nitrogen dioxide is an important warning sign for farmers. Numerous instances of acute overexposures and death have resulted from inadequately ventilated silos.

Although management and prevention are similar to that for highly soluble irritants, overnight observation is frequently necessary when excess exposures have occurred due to the insidious onset of pulmonary edema.

## Occupational Asthma

An 18-year-old woman arrived at an emergency room complaining of SOB. Eight weeks previously, she had consulted her physician about daytime wheezing and cough productive of white phlegm. She was treated with antibiotics and an expectorant and remained at home for 3 days with significant improvement. A week later, a cough and SOB again developed. Again she was treated with antibiotics, an expectorant, and bed rest with significant improvement. She had an exacerbation of coughing, SOB, and cyanosis of her fingertips the day before her visit.

Her occupational history revealed that she had begun working at a tool supply and manufacturing company 9 weeks previously, a week before her symptoms began. Her usual job there was grinding carbide-steel drill bits. In her work she used one of four machines that sharpened drill bits. Her machine generated much metal dust, often covering the machines and her face, hands, and clothes. There was no exhaust system to draw dust away from her breathing zone, and no respiratory protection was provided.

After being treated the first time 8 weeks previously, she was temporarily assigned to cleaning drill bits in a solvent bath. On this job she felt lightheaded but had no difficulty breathing. After a long holiday weekend, she was again assigned to drill-bit grinding and after several hours a cough developed. The next day the cough increased and SOB developed, prompting a second visit to her physician. When she improved from that episode, she returned to work again and experienced exacerbation of coughing and SOB. This prompted her emergency room visit.

Past medical history revealed occasional seasonal rhinitis as a child but no asthma, eczema, or other allergies. She had no family history of allergies or asthma.

Physical examination revealed a pulse rate of 128 and a respiratory rate of 40. She had cyanosis of the lips and fingertips. Chest examination revealed diffuse bilateral wheezes and use of accessory muscles for breathing.

Arterial blood gases on room air at rest revealed a $PaO_2$ of 39. Spirometry showed normal forced vital capacity but markedly abnormal $FEV_1$ (53 percent of predicted). Chest x-ray was normal. White blood cell count was 11,200, with 10 percent eosinophils.

She was treated with oxygen, bronchodilators, and steroids. She improved clinically; by the second day, her $FEV_1$ improved to 82 percent of predicted.

A later call by her physician to the state occupational safety and health agency revealed that carbide-steel bit alloys contain nickel, cobalt, chromium, vanadium, molybdenum, and tungsten. Grinding such bits can produce cobalt and tungsten carbide dusts, which are recognized pulmonary sensitizers.[3]

The diagnosis in this case was occupational asthma. No specific agent was proved responsible, but the presence of tungsten carbide and cobalt dusts suggests probable agents. Since changing jobs, she has felt well and has not had further bronchospasm.

Many occupational asthma cases are not seen by physicians or other health care providers, probably because workers recognize the association between exposure and asthma and thus avoid further contact.

[3]Case courtesy of James Keogh, School of Medicine, University of Maryland, Baltimore (unpublished curriculum materials).

Individual responses may be so clear and occur so early in a new job that those workers who respond adversely may leave quite soon after being hired. Thus, in population surveys very few workers may be identified with immediate sensitivity because most of those who had experienced adverse effects had already left the job to avoid the asthma-producing exposure. A wide variety of materials and circumstances have been shown to cause occupational asthma (see Table 22-3).

### Diagnosis of Occupational Asthma

Diagnosis of occupational asthma depends greatly on the occupational history. Major or minor constituents of substances as well as accidental by-products can incite attacks. Many individuals who suffer occupational asthma have a history of atopy, especially when the exposure is to high molecular weight compounds. However, those without such a history may become sensitized after exposure to specific environmental agents such as diisocyanates. Suspicion of this diagnosis should be aroused even when a worker has had no previous history of asthma. Often the worker will report wheezing, chest tightness, or severe cough developing in the evening or at night with recovery overnight or over a weekend away from work. However, if exposure and its effects have been prolonged, the symptoms may persist at home or over the weekend. Specific questioning about nocturnal symptoms may elicit responses otherwise not volunteered. The physical examination of an acutely ill worker will reveal wheezing and rhonchi.

A particularly useful test for bronchoconstriction of occupational origin is the $FEV_1$ before and after a work shift. A drop of 300 ml or 10 percent or more of $FEV_1$ (measured as the mean of the two best of three acceptable curves each time) between the beginning and end of the first shift of the workweek suggests a work-related effect. (It should be noted that an acute drop in $FEV_1$ as large as 1.8 liters has been measured without the worker reporting symptoms.) Serial measurements of peak flow (for example, four times per day) on and off workdays with a simple, inexpensive peak flowmeter can be extremely valuable in detecting work-associated declines in air flow [6]. Peak-flow monitoring has also become a mainstay of asthma management. Excessive eosinophils in the sputum or blood may distinguish asthma from bronchitis. Reliance should not be placed on skin tests for diagnosing allergic reactions since skin and bronchial responses do not always correlate well. Specific bronchoprovocation with suspected offending agents is usually not needed for diagnosis and can be dangerous. However, nonspecific bronchoprovocation testing with methacholine, histamine, or cold air may be necessary to confirm reversible airways disease. Since virtually any chemical substance can precipitate an asthma attack, health professionals should rely heavily on the patient's medical and work histories even in the absence of a documented association between a given exposure and asthma.

Acute care of those with attacks of occupational asthma is the same as for any case of asthma. Long-term management, however, almost always requires removal from exposure, since after sensitization even very low levels of exposure can trigger an asthmatic response. Close monitoring of symptoms and lung function should be maintained for an individual who must continue exposure to a suspected offending agent.

## Hypersensitivity Pneumonitis

Hypersensitivity pneumonitis refers to reactions associated with the most picturesque of all occupational disease names (Table 22-4). This response results from organic materials, commonly fungi or thermophilic bacteria, that are present in a surprising variety of settings. In contrast to asthma, this response is more focused in the lung parenchyma (respiratory bronchioles and alveoli). Characteristics of this kind of reaction are antibodies (precipitins) present in serum and the collection of lymphocytes in pulmonary infiltrates. Activation of pulmonary macrophages with an increased number of T lymphocytes and probably a change

**Table 22-4.** Examples of hypersensitivity pneumonitis

| Disease | Antigenic material | Antigen |
|---|---|---|
| Farmer's lung | Moldy hay or grain | |
| Bagassosis | Moldy sugar cane | |
| Mushroom worker's lung | Mushroom compost | Thermophilic actinomycetes |
| Humidifier fever | Dust from contaminated air conditioners or furnaces | |
| Maple bark disease | Moldy maple bark | *Cryptostroma* species |
| Sequoiosis | Redwood dust | *Graphium* species, Pallurlaria |
| Bird breeder's lung | Avian droppings or feathers | Avian proteins |
| Pituitary snuff user's lung | Pituitary powder | Bovine or porcine proteins |
| Suberosis | Moldy cork dust | *Penicillium* species |
| Paprika splitter's lung | Paprika dust | *Mucor stolonifer* |
| Malt worker's lung | Malt dust | *Aspergillus clavatus* or *A. fumigatus* |
| Fishmeal worker's lung | Fishmeal | Fishmeal dust |
| Miller's lung | Infested wheat flour | *Sitophilus granarius* (wheat weevil) |
| Furrier's lung | Animal pelts | Animal fur dust |
| Coffee worker's lung | Coffee beans | Coffee bean dust |
| Chemical worker's lung | Urethane foam and finish | Isocyanates (TDI, HDI), anhydrides |

in their function appear to be the underlying cellular mechanisms. The end-result can be fibrosis, yet the responses are much less dose-dependent than those for primary fibrosis due to inorganic dusts. Once hypersensitivity is established, small doses may trigger episodes of alveolitis. It should be emphasized that this disease is a complex inflammatory response often to bacterial or fungal material, not an infection or a true allergic response. Therefore, the commonly used clinical term *hypersensitivity pneumonitis* is actually inaccurate. Current research has focused on developing terminology for this condition that more accurately reflects pulmonary reactions to organic dust constituents.

The worker suffering hypersensitivity pneumonitis will experience shortness of breath and nonproductive cough. In contrast to asthma, wheezing is not a prominent component. In acute episodes, the sudden onset of the respiratory symptoms along with fever and chills is dramatic. Physical examination may show rapid breathing and fine basilar rales. Pulmonary function tests can show

marked reduction in lung volumes consistent with restrictive disease. The $FEV_1$ is reduced, but in proportion to the decreases in FVC and total lung capacity; generally, there is a normal or increased $FEV_1/FVC$ ratio. Arterial blood gas measurements show an increased alveolar-arterial oxygen difference $[D(A-a)O_2]$ and a reduced diffusing capacity (DLCO). Chest x-ray can be quite helpful in the acute episodes in revealing patchy infiltrates or a diffuse fine micronodular shadowing.

If the individual is removed from exposure, symptoms and signs generally disappear in 1 to 2 weeks. If repeated exposures are experienced, especially at levels low enough to result in only mild symptoms, a more chronic disease may ensue. The worker may be unaware of the work association, as the low-level effects may appear symptomatically like a persistent respiratory "flu." Over a period of months, however, the gradual onset of dyspnea develops, which can be accompanied by weight loss and lethargy. The physical examination is similar to that in the acute episode, although the patient may appear less acutely ill and may demonstrate finger clubbing. Chest x-ray, however, is more suggestive of chronic interstitial fibrosis, and the pulmonary function tests show a restrictive defect. The disease may progress to severe dyspnea and the end-result resembles, even histologically, chronic interstitial fibrosis of unknown etiology. Sometimes an asymptomatic patient without an episode of acute pneumonitis in the past will develop interstitial fibrosis.

Prevention rests on removal from exposure. This can be more readily accomplished than with asthma since environmental controls can focus on the elimination of conditions that foster bacterial or fungal growth. Process changes may also be necessary to prevent antigen production, and local exhaust ventilation rather than respiratory protective equipment should be relied on.

## Byssinosis and Other Diseases of Vegetable Dusts

Some types of airway constriction are believed not to be immunologic in origin but due to direct toxic effect on the airways. This has been referred to as pharmacologic bronchoconstriction, although for byssinosis, the pathogenesis is still poorly understood.

Byssinosis (meaning "white thread" in Greek) is associated with exposure to cotton, hemp, and flax processing. It has been popularly called "brown lung" (a misnomer since the lungs are not brown), an analogy to the popular term "black lung" used to describe the lung diseases of coal miners.

Byssinosis has been shown to develop in response to dust exposure in cotton processing. It is especially prevalent among cotton workers in the initial, very dusty operations where bales are broken open, blown (to separate fibers from impurities), and carded (to arrange the fibers into parallel threads). A lower rate of disease occurs in workers in the spinning, winding, and twisting areas, where dust levels are lower. The lowest prevalence rate of

byssinosis has been found among weavers, who experience the lowest dust exposure. Processing of cloth is practically free of cotton dust, as in the manufacture of denim, which is washed during dyeing before thread is spun. Byssinosis has also been described in other than textile sectors where cotton is processed, such as cottonseed oil mills, the cotton waste utilization industry, and the garnetting or bedding and batting industry. The same syndrome has been shown to occur in workers exposed in processing soft hemp, flax, and (probably) sisal.

Byssinosis is characterized by shortness of breath and chest tightness. These symptoms are most prominent on the first day of the workweek or after being away from the factory over an extended period of time ("Monday morning tightness"). No previous exposure is necessary for symptoms to develop.

Symptoms are often associated with changes in pulmonary function. One characteristic of the acute pulmonary response to cotton dust exposure is a drop in the $FEV_1$ during the Monday work shift or the first day back at work after at least a 2-day layoff. Since workers do not normally lose lung function during a workday, an acute loss of 10 percent or 300 ml or more (whichever is greater) in an individual, or 3 percent or 75 ml (whichever is greater) in a group of 20 or greater, can be considered significant enough to require further investigation. Over time, cotton dust workers have an accelerated decrement in $FEV_1$ consistent with fixed air-flow obstruction and chronic obstructive lung disease. Diagnosis is based mainly on symptoms; no characteristic examination or chest x-ray findings are associated with byssinosis. Therefore, the patient should be questioned systematically about symptoms.

It is assumed that progression of disease occurs if duration of exposure to dust levels is sufficiently high and prolonged. Mild byssinosis probably is reversible if exposure ceases, but long-standing disease is irreversible. Individuals with severe byssinosis are rarely seen in an industrial survey since they are too disabled to be working. Byssinosis seems more severe when it is associated with chronic bronchitis. The end stage of the disease is fixed airway obstruction with hyperinflation and air trapping. Cigarette smokers are at increased risk of irreversible byssinosis.

Much research has been done on possible etiologic mechanisms and effects. Extracts of cotton bract have been shown to release pharmacologic mediators, such as histamine, as well as prostaglandins. From recent studies it seems likely that the mechanism of byssinosis involves stimulation of the same inflammatory receptors by endotoxin and by cotton dust. Gram-negative bacterial endotoxin contaminates cotton fiber, and aqueous extracts of endotoxin have produced acute symptoms and lung function declines.

Two other respiratory conditions associated with work in the cotton industry are:

Mill fever: This self-limited condition usually happens on first exposure to a cotton dust environment. It lasts for 2 to 3 days and has no known sequelae. It is characterized by headache, malaise, and fever. A flu-like illness, it has symptoms similar to those of metal fume fever and polymer fume fever. Gin mill fever is probably related to gram-negative bacterial material in mill dust; it usually afflicts workers only once, except that after prolonged absence from a mill, re-exposure may trigger another attack (see box on p. 372).

Weaver's cough: Weavers have suffered outbreaks of acute respiratory illness characterized by a dry cough, although their dust exposure is comparatively low. It may result from sizing material or from mildewed yarn that is sometimes found in high-humidity weaving rooms.

## Chronic Respiratory Tract Responses

### Pneumoconiosis

Pulmonary fibrosis is the most readily recognized work-related chronic pulmonary reaction. This condition, which varies according to inciting agent, intensity, and duration of exposure, is generally referred to as a pneumoconiosis. It is usually due to an inorganic dust or coal that must be of respirable size ($<5 \mu$) to reach terminal bronchioles and alveoli; dust of this size is not visible and therefore its presence may not be recognized by a worker. There are two basic types of fibrosis: localized and nodular, usually peribronchial, fibrosis (such as silicosis) and diffuse interstitial fibrosis (such as asbestosis). The clinical features of all the pneumoconioses are similar: initial nonproductive cough, shortness of breath of increasing severity, and, in the later stages, productive cough, distant breath sounds, and signs of right heart failure. Although it is not commonly known, the pneumoconioses are quite often associated with obstructive airways effects caused by the same agents.

### Silica-Related Disease

Crystalline silica ($SiO_2$) is a major component of the earth's crust. Therefore, exposure occurs in a wide variety of settings: mining, quarrying, and stone cutting (see Fig. 6-4); foundry operations; ceramics and vitreous enameling; and in fillers for paints and rubber.

Estimates of the prevalence of silicosis in the United States vary, ranging from 30,000 to 100,000 current cases. No distinct clinical features can be cited beyond the ones listed above, but there is distinct pathology. Silicosis occurs more frequently in the upper than the lower lobes, with nodules varying in size from invisible to the naked eye to 6 mm in diameter. In severe cases, nodules aggregate and become fibrotic masses several centimeters in diameter. Nodules are firm and intact with a whorled pattern and rarely cavitate (Fig. 22-7). Microscopically, the nodules are hyalinized, with a well-organized circular pattern of fibers within a cellular capsule. The amount of fibrosis appears proportional to the free silica content and to the duration of exposure. One notable characteristic of this disease is that fibrosis progresses even after removal from exposure. Except in acute silicosis, symptoms generally do not occur until af-

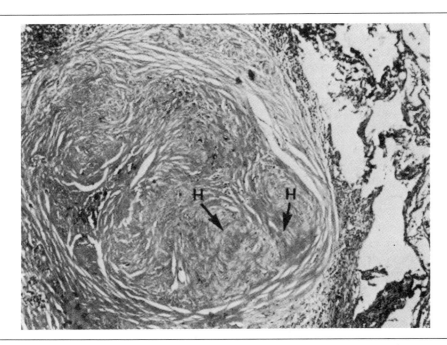

**Fig. 22-7.** Microscopic section of a typical silicotic nodule showing the concentric ("onion skin") arrangement of collagen fibers, some of which are hyalinized (H); lack of dust pigmentation; and the cellularity of the periphery. The lesion is clearly demarcated from adjacent lung tissue, which is substantially normal. (From WR Parkes. Occupational lung disorders. 2nd ed. London: Butterworths, 1982.)

ter 10 to 20 years of exposure. Evidence of pathologic response to silica exposure exists well before symptoms occur.

Evaluation of workers exposed to silica includes lung function tests (which may show either reduced FVC or total lung capacity as well as mixed obstructive and restrictive patterns), a chest x-ray (which may appear more abnormal than the lung function tests), and determination of (a reduced) hemoglobin oxygen saturation on exercise. As the disease progresses, there is decreased oxygen saturation and reduced total lung capacity. The x-ray shows rounded opacities, localized initially to the upper lung fields (see Fig. 22-2). The size and distribution of these opacities will increase over time, and "egg shell" calcification of hilar lymph nodes occurs in a minority of cases.

Chronic silicosis is classified either as simple or complicated, although there is a continuum be-

tween these two forms of the disease. The simple form is noted on the chest film by the presence of multiple small, round opacities, usually in the upper zones. The concentrations of these opacities are used in classifying simple silicosis (categories 1 to 3)[2]. Although simple silicosis alone is not a common cause of disability, it can contribute to disability as well as progress to complicated silicosis. In progressive massive fibrosis (PMF), several of the simple nodules appear to aggregate and produce larger conglomerate lesions, which enlarge and encroach on the vascular bed and airways (ILO categories A, B, C). The extent of lung function impairment appears directly related to the radiographic size of the lesions and is most severe in categories B and C.

An important complication of silicosis is tuberculosis, which persists today as an added hazard peculiar to this pneumoconiosis. The association between silicosis and pulmonary tuberculosis has been known for decades. More recent publications also show an increased incidence of tuberculosis among workers in the mining, quarrying, and tunneling industries, and steel and iron foundries. There is some epidemiologic evidence that workers exposed to silica are at increased risk of tuberculosis even in the absence of radiographic evidence for silicosis. Infection with atypical mycobacteria (for example, *M. kansasii, M. avium-intracellulare*) can also occur and is related to the geographic distribution of these organisms. Treatment of such cases may require more vigorous drug treatment than tuberculosis without silicosis. To date, no interaction of silicosis has been shown with cigarette smoke effects.

Prevention of silicosis focuses on reduction of exposure through wet processes, isolation of dusty work, and local exhaust ventilation. Annual tuberculosis screening by purified protein derivative (PPD) or, if the PPD is positive, chest x-ray is essential in silica-exposed workers.

Acute silicosis, a distinct entity, is a devastating disease. It is due to extraordinarily high exposures to small silica particles (1–2 μ). These exposures currently occur in abrasive sandblasting and in the production and use of ground silica. Symptoms include shortness of breath progressing rapidly over a few weeks, weight loss, productive cough, and sometimes pleuritic pain. Diminished resonance on percussion of the chest and also rales on auscultation can be found. Lung function tests will show a marked restrictive defect, with impressive decrement in total lung capacity. The x-ray has a diffuse ground-glass or miliary tuberculosis-like appearance, rather than the classic nodular silicosis. The pathology in this disease shows a widespread fibrosis, with diffuse interstitial rather than nodular macroscopic appearance, and microscopic appearance and chemical constituency resembling pulmonary alveolar proteinosis, but with double refractile particles of silica lying free within the alveolar exudate. Disease onset usually occurs 6 months to 2 years after initial exposure. Acute silicosis is often fatal, generally within 1 year.

Diatomaceous earth is an amorphous silica material mined predominantly in the western United States. It is used as a filler in paints and plastics, as a heat and sound insulator, as a filter for water and wine, and as an abrasive. In contrast to the various forms of crystalline silica, amorphous silica has relatively low pathogenicity. However, some processes using diatomaceous earth include heating (calcining) it to remove organic material. This heating process can produce up to 60 percent crystalline silica as cristobalite, which is highly fibrogenic. Exposure to this form of diatomaceous earth, therefore, must be treated the same as exposure to crystalline silica described above.

### Silicate-Related Diseases, Including Asbestosis

Silica appears in a wide variety of minerals in different combined forms known as silicates. Many of these silicates (such as asbestos, kaolin, and talc) also cause pneumoconiosis, but the forms they produce have features distinct from those of silicosis. Asbestos is the most widespread and best known of the silicates and is responsible for asbestosis as well as several types of cancers (see Chap. 14).

*Asbestos* appears in nature in four major types (chyrsotile, crocidolite, amosite, and anthophyllite) with relatively similar chronic respiratory reactions. All four types are characterized by their being fibrous and are indestructible at temperatures as high as 800°C. Use and production of these materials have greatly increased in the past century; more than 3 million tons of asbestos are produced in the world annually. Over 30 million tons have been used in construction and manufacture in the U.S. alone. It is used in a variety of applications: asbestos cement products (tiles, roofing, and drain pipes), floor tile, insulation and fireproofing (in construction and ship building), textiles (for heat resistance), asbestos paper (in insulating and gaskets), and friction materials (brake linings and clutch pads). Probably the most hazardous current exposures occur in repair and demolition of buildings and ships and in a variety of maintenance jobs in which exposures may be unsuspected by the workers (Fig. 22-8). Currently in the U.S., the construction industry is the major source of asbestos exposure to workers, mainly from asbestos products in place.

As with silicosis, the predominant symptoms of asbestosis are cough and SOB (the latter may be more severe than the appearance of the chest x-ray would indicate). Although not common, pleuritic pain or chest tightness may occur, and these are more frequent than in other pneumoconioses. In 20 percent of those affected, basilar rales are present, and pleural rubs and pleural effusions can occur. Pleural effusion in a person with a history of asbestos exposure even many years earlier should be considered evidence of mesothelioma until proven otherwise.

Pathologically, the macroscopic appearance of the lung is a small, pale, firm, and rubbery-like organ with a fibrotic adherent pleura. The cut surface shows patchy to widespread fibrosis and the lower lobes are more frequently affected than the upper. Microscopic appearance shows interstitial fibrosis. Chest x-ray shows widespread irregular (linear) opacities more common in the lower lung fields (see Fig. 22-3), in contrast to the round opacities seen in silicosis, which occur first in the upper lung fields.

A great deal of attention has focused on asbestos (or ferruginous) bodies in sputum and lung tissue. These are dumbbell-shaped bodies from 20 to 150 $\mu$ in width that appear to be fibers covered by a mucopolysaccharide layer. Iron pigment (from hemoglobin breakdown) gives them a golden-brown appearance. They are not diagnostic of asbestos-related disease, but when present even in small numbers in sputum or tissue sections, they indicate substantial (for example, occupational) exposure to airborne fibers. While it is true that most urban dwellers in the industrialized world have a measurable asbestos burden, the actual concentrations of asbestos bodies in the nonoccupationally (or paraoccupationally) exposed population are orders of magnitude lower than in those with known direct or indirect exposures. Pathology studies have shown that in the "background" population of urban dwellers, one would have to search 50 to 100 sections of lung to find a single asbestos body, whereas persons with even the earliest asbestosis have asbestos bodies in nearly every section, and persons with more severe asbestosis have scores of asbestos bodies per section. Asbestos bodies may also be found in other parts of the body besides the lungs, forming round fibers transported by lung lymphatics into the circulation.

A particular feature of asbestos exposure, unlike the other pneumoconioses, is the frequent presence of asbestos-induced circumscribed pleural fibrosis known as pleural plaques, which are sometimes the only evidence of exposure. These plaques, which can calcify, may be bilateral, and are located more commonly in the parietal pleura. In fact, the evidence for prior asbestos exposure or the explanation of abnormal pulmonary function tests may sometimes be found because of the calcified pleural plaques seen on chest x-ray (Fig. 22-9).

Pleural plaques are one manifestation of the rather marked pleural reaction to asbestos fibers. Other such evidence seen on the chest x-ray is "shaggy"-appearing cardiac or diaphragmatic border. An early nonspecific sign is a blunted costophrenic angle. Diffuse pleural thickening also occurs, probably less commonly than the more specific pleural plaques. Asbestos-induced diffuse visceral pleural fibrosis may also occur and may impair lung function. Advanced pleural fibrosis may act like a cuirass, severely constricting breathing and leading to respiratory failure.

The evaluation of a worker suspected of having asbestosis includes determination of whether there has been a history of exposure; a physical examination to ascertain if rales are present; a chest x-ray, which may show irregular linear opacities and a variety of pleural reactions; and pulmonary function tests, which may show evidence of an interstitial type of abnormality—that is, restrictive disease and diminished diffusing capacity. In addition, the peribronchiolar fibrosis may have an obstructive component. Hence, in both nonsmok-

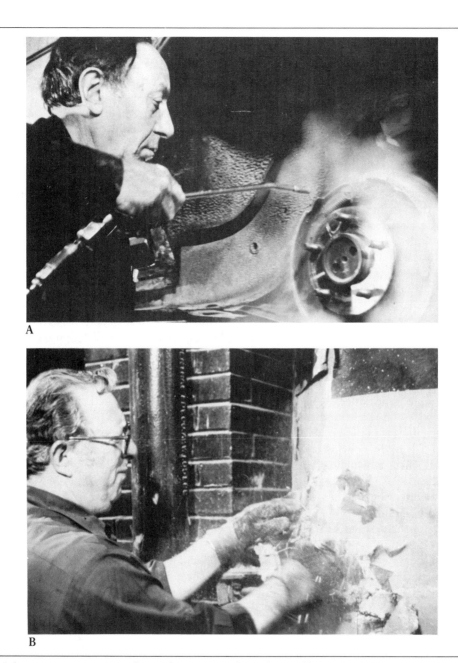

**Fig. 22-8.** Asbestos exposures. A. Brake mechanic exposed to asbestos fibers while using compressed air to clean brake drum. B. Boilermaker exposed to asbestos fibers while repairing insulation. Improper protection is illustrated. In both instances, local exhaust ventilation or personal protective equipment should be vigorously employed. (Photographs by Nicolas Kaufman.)

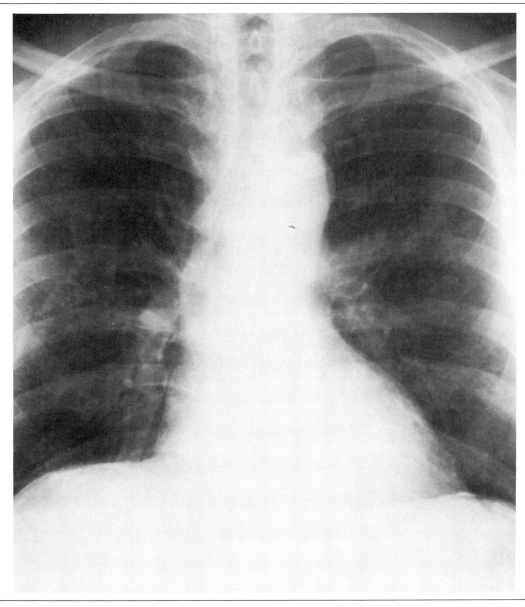

**Fig. 22-9.** Asbestos exposure is suggested by the presence of calcified pleural plaques seen in this anteroposterior chest x-ray, particularly on the right diaphragmatic border. (Courtesy of L Christine Oliver, MD)

ers and smokers with asbestosis (as with all pneumoconioses), a mixed restrictive-obstructive pattern may be seen.

Asbestosis, like silicosis, may progress after removal from exposure. Asbestos exposure even without asbestosis carries with it the added risk of cancers of the lung, pleura and peritoneum (mesotheliomas), gastrointestinal tract, and other organs (see Chap. 14). Prevention focuses on substitution with materials such as fibrous glass, use of wet processes to reduce dust generation, and local exhaust ventilation to capture the dust that is generated. Exposed patients who smoke should be advised to stop smoking for the rest of their lives.

*Talc* is a hydrated magnesium silicate that occurs in a variety of forms in nature. The two major types are nonfibrous and fibrous. The nonfibrous forms, such as those found in Vermont, are free of both crystalline silica and fibrous asbestos tremolite; the fibrous forms, such as those found in New York State, can contain up to 70 percent fibrous material, including amphibole forms of asbestos. Talc exposures occur mainly during its use as an additive to paints and as a lubricant in the rubber industry, especially in inner tubes. Current evidence suggests that high doses of nonfibrous talc or moderate doses of fibrous talc accumulated over a long time will result in chronic respiratory disease known as talcosis, with the same symptoms as other pneumoconioses.

Pathologically, the macroscopic appearance of the lung is of poorly structured nodules, unlike the firm nodules of silicosis and the diffuse fibrosis of asbestosis. The microscopic appearance consists of ill-defined nodules with some diffuse interstitial fibrosis. Evaluation of persons exposed to talc includes pulmonary function tests and a chest x-ray. The chest x-ray could show both nodular and linear opacities and also pleural plaques. The possibility of a cancer risk associated with fibrous talc exposure has been addressed in several studies. Early reports found an increased risk of lung cancer in New York State talc miners, and follow-up of this group confirmed a fourfold increase in risk.

*Kaolin* (China clay) is a hydrated aluminum silicate found in the United States (in a band from Georgia to Missouri), India, and China. It is used in ceramics; as a filler in paper, rubber, paint, and plastic products; and as a mild soap abrasive. Kaolin is not particularly hazardous in the mining processes since it is generally a wet ore and mined by jet-water mining techniques.

The pneumoconiosis resulting from chronic exposures to kaolin dust produces no unique clinical features. Pathologically, the macroscopic appearance is of immature silicotic nodules, although conglomerate nodules may appear. Pleural involvement occurs only if the lung is massively involved. The microscopic appearance shows nodules with randomly distributed collagen.

### Coal Workers' Pneumoconiosis
In the United States until the 1960s, coal workers' respiratory disease was considered a variant of silicosis and was often known as anthracosilicosis. Now it is clear that coal workers' pneumoconiosis (CWP) is an etiologically distinct entity, which both coal dust and pure carbon can induce. CWP exists both in simple and complicated forms; the latter, known as progressive massive fibrosis (PMF), is the most severe form of the disease. Although exposure to coal dust occurs most commonly in underground mines, there is some exposure in handling and transportation of coal above ground as well. Significant exposure also occurs in the trimming or leveling of coal in ships when preparing material for transport.

Simple CWP, especially ILO profusion category 3 (on a scale of 1 to 3), increases the likelihood for future development of the complicated form, which is generally agreed to be a disabling condition. Simple CWP is not clearly a disabling condition; however, the prevalence of small irregular opacities is linked to reduced lung function. The diagnosis of simple CWP has, to date, relied primarily on the chest x-ray, which shows nodular opacities of less than 1 cm (mostly <3 mm) in diameter. PMF, in contrast, is seen on chest x-ray as the development of conglomerations of these small opacities to a size of greater than 1 cm in diameter.

In the early stages CWP is asymptomatic. The initial symptoms are breathlessness on exertion with progressive reduction in exercise tolerance. As nodular conglomeration begins and PMF is diagnosed, symptoms become more severe with marked exertional dyspnea, severe disability, or total incapacity. There is general agreement that PMF leads to premature disability and death. No such agreement, however, exists presently for the impact of simple CWP of grade 2 or less.

Coal mine dust also independently contributes to the disability observed in coal workers through the production of chronic bronchitis, airways obstruction, and emphysema. The bronchitis and pulmonary function loss are dose-related to coal dust in both smokers and nonsmokers.

Pathologically, simple CWP appears as soft, black indurated nodules. Microscopic observations show dust in and around macrophages near respiratory bronchioles. Nodules show random collagen distribution and the lung shows centrilobular emphysema. Chest x-ray shows widely distributed small, round opacities.

In PMF, the large conglomerate masses have variable shape and do not respect the architecture of the lung. The surfaces are hard, rubbery, and black, and cavitation often occurs (Fig. 22-10). Copious, black sputum is often produced. Microscopically, the appearance is not distinct from the simple nodules. Chest x-ray shows large conglomerate opacities (Fig. 22-11). A separate condition called Caplan's syndrome, or rheumatoid CWP, is PMF accompanied by rheumatoid arthritis. There is a different pathologic appearance: alternate black and gray-white bands of material in the conglomerate masses. The conglomerate masses frequently cavitate or calcify. It is not known whether PMF accompanied by rheumatoid arthritis has a different clinical course.

Although evaluation for CWP is the same as for the other pneumoconioses, a particular feature affecting evaluation is the federal Mine Safety and

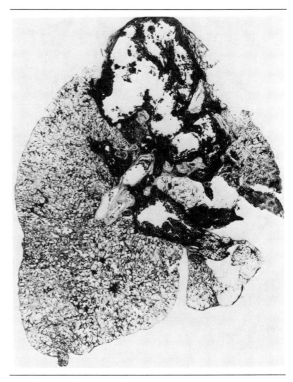

Fig. 22-10. Gough section of lung of coal worker with 18 years of mining experience completed 20 years before death. It shows cavitation as well as centrilobular emphysema, which was present in both lungs. (Courtesy of JC Wagner, MRC Pneumoconiosis Unit, Llandough Hospital, Penarth, Wales.)

Health Act of 1977, which prescribes what types of abnormalities make .an individual eligible for disability benefits. Since these are subject to continuous revision, consultation with the Mine Safety and Health Administration in the U.S. Department of Labor is advisable.

### Miscellaneous Inorganic Dusts

*Hard Metals.* The term *hard metal disease* (HMD) refers to the diffuse interstitial pulmonary fibrosis that results from overexposure to cobalt-containing dusts present in work environments where hard metals are manufactured or used. "Hard met-

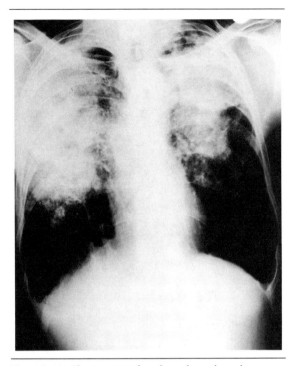

**Fig. 22-11.** Chest x-ray of coal worker whose lung section appears in Fig. 22-10. It was taken two weeks before his death. The appearance is classic for progressive massive fibrosis (PMF) with larger conglomerate masses in both lung fields. (Courtesy of JC Wagner.)

als" consist of very fine metal carbide particles (most commonly tungsten carbide) that are cemented in a metal binder (most commonly cobalt). Exposures occur where hard metals are produced and where they are used to manufacture tools. The majority of tool manufacturing and reconditioning occurs outside of plants producing hard metal, resulting in environments less well designed to protect against excess exposures.

Symptoms of HMD are often nonspecific until the development of progressive dyspnea, which may occur after long-term cobalt exposure or after short-term, high-level exposure. Chest x-ray shows diffuse or patchy infiltrates. Pulmonary function tests show restrictive or mixed restrictive-obstructive defects. Since cobalt exposure can also

result in asthma, reversible air-flow obstruction may complicate the picture of interstitial fibrosis or occur in the absence of fibrosis (see previous section, Occupational Asthma). Since the presenting symptoms and signs are nonspecific, a careful history is essential and lung biopsy may be necessary. Early or mild forms of fibrosis may be reversible on removal from exposure, but recovery is not certain and relatively severe cases may continue to worsen after exposure ceases.

Little is known about the occurrence of HMD in the U.S. About 30,000 workers are currently exposed to tungsten carbide and are therefore at risk. Some epidemiologic surveys suggest that between 1 and 10 percent of those exposed have x-ray changes consistent with HMD, with 1 to 2 percent of this group being symptomatic.

Prevention of HMD is accomplished by suppressing or eliminating dust in cemented tungsten carbide manufacturing facilities and in sites where tungsten carbide tools are ground. Medical surveillance consisting of history, chest x-ray, and spirometry should be done yearly on those exposed.

*Fibrous Glass and Related Products.* These products, referred to as synthetic vitreous fibers (SVF) and also known as manmade vitreous fibers (MMVF), have been used for insulation purposes for over 60 years. Recently, they have played an important role as an asbestos substitute. SVF are amorphous silicates with a length-diameter ratio of greater than 3 : 1. They are made mainly from rock, slag, glass, or kaolin clay and can be divided into three main groups: mineral wool, fiber glass, and ceramic fiber.

Synthetic vitreous fibers can induce skin and upper respiratory tract irritant responses. There have been few case reports of pulmonary disease due to SVF exposure. Prevalence studies of chest x-ray findings, respiratory symptoms, and lung function in exposed workers have generally been negative. However, limited studies of workers exposed to fine diameter fibers have revealed evidence of irregular opacities consistent with pneumoconiosis. No abnormalities in lung function were reported in these studies. There is growing concern about the possible carcinogenicity of these very fine fibers. The International Agency for Research on Cancer (IARC) has classified glass wool, rock wool, slag wool, and ceramic fiber as possibly carcinogenic to humans and continuous glass fiber as not classifiable as to human carcinogenicity. Epidemiologic studies have suggested some chronic pulmonary effects, including lung cancer, associated with SVF exposures, but a number of studies are still in progress and longer-term follow-up is necessary. Long-term studies of employment in industries using the respirable sizes of SVF are now being performed.

Individual exposures to iron dusts, particularly those resulting from steel-grinding operations, welding, or foundry work, are common. The only clinical effect of pure iron oxide exposure is a reddish-brown coloring of the sputum. Lung function tests on individuals show no clinical abnormality, while the chest x-ray shows many small (0.5–2.0 mm) opacities without confluence (as with stannosis; see Fig. 22-4). Lung sections show macrophages laden with iron dust but without fibrosis or cellular reaction. With removal from further iron oxide dust exposure, the x-ray abnormalities slowly resolve. Similar results can be seen in exposures to tin, barium, and antimony.

### Chronic Bronchitis

Probably the most common of the chronic responses of the respiratory tract is chronic bronchitis, which results from excessive mucus production in the bronchi. Diagnosis is made strictly on clinical grounds. *Chronic bronchitis* is a formally defined term, which must meet criteria of the ATS: recurrent productive cough occurring four to six times a day at least 4 days of the week, for at least 3 months during the year, for at least 2 years. The definition of simple bronchitis ("the production of phlegm on most days for as much as 3 months out of the year") can be used to distinguish those with

probably important symptoms from those without. The excess mucus production associated with bronchitis is often, but not invariably, associated with air-flow obstruction. Chronic bronchitis is not a unique occupational pulmonary response; it is frequently superimposed on other respiratory diseases due to occupational toxins and most often cigarette smoke. Occupational toxins that can cause chronic bronchitis include mineral dusts and fumes (such as from coal, fibrous glass, asbestos, metals, and oils), organic dusts (such as ozone and oxides of nitrogen), plastic compounds (such as phenolics and isocyanates), acids, and smoke (such as experienced in firefighting).

### Emphysema

Emphysema is a chronic response that depends more specifically on a pathologic description: It is the enlargement of air spaces distal to terminal (nonrespiratory) bronchioles, which includes destruction of the alveolar walls and results in air trapping. Occupational examples of this response are not well studied, but evidence suggests that fixed airway obstruction is the end stage of disease due to chronic coal dust or chronic cadmium exposure.

### Granulomatous Disease

Granuloma formation is another type of chronic response not commonly described as work-related. In a granuloma many cells responding to an inciting agent become surrounded by bundles of collagen. The foreign-body granuloma in the skin is an analogous kind of tissue reaction. The best occupational example of pulmonary granulomas is chronic beryllium disease; workers who make metal alloys containing beryllium are exposed when dust control is poor. The disease appears as a restrictive pneumoconiosis although the pulmonary reaction is out of proportion to the amount of metal dust in the lungs. It is very similar to sarcoid and can be impossible to distinguish without measuring tissue levels (in lung and lymph nodes) of beryllium. Recently, a more specific test became available: measurement of the lymphocyte blast transformation test (LTT) on peripheral or lavaged lymphocytes. The development of the LTT, which is available at a few academic centers, has been useful in the early diagnosis of beryllium disease. Longitudinal studies will be helpful in clarifying whether positive blood LTT predicts the future development of disease in beryllium-exposed workers.

## References

1. Ferris BG. Epidemiology standardization project. Am Rev Respir Dis 1978; 118:1–120 (Part 2 of 2).
2. International Labour Organization. Guidelines for the use of the ILO international classification of pneumoconioses. Geneva: International Labour Office, 1980. Occupational Safety and Health Series 22, rev. 80.
3. Enright PL, Hyatt RE. Office spirometry: A practical guide to the selection and use of spirometers. Philadelphia: Lea & Febiger, 1987.
4. American Thoracic Society. Lung function testing. Selection of reference values and interpretation strategies. Official statement of the American Thoracic Society. Am Rev Respir Dis 1991; 188:1208–18.
5. European Respiratory Society Official Statement. Standardized lung function testing: Lung volumes and forced ventilatory flows, 1993 update; Report Working Party. Standardization of lung function tests. Eur Respir J 1993; 6 (Suppl. 16).
6. National Asthma Education Program. Guidelines for diagnosis and management of asthma. Publication no. 91-3042, U.S. Health and Human Services, Public Health Service, National Institutes of Health, August 1991.

## Bibliography

Bernstein IL, Chan-Yeung M, Malo J-L, Bernstein D. Asthma in the workplace. New York: Marcel Dekker, 1993.

*This is an excellent summary of the many issues in the rapidly evolving understanding of occupational asthma. The book includes a comprehensive look at the nature of etiologic agents, the range and types of asthmatic responses, the different approaches to identifying asthma as resulting from workplace exposures, and the various methods used to identify and track individuals who are at risk or have experienced occupational asthma attacks.*

Merchant JA, Boehlecke BA, Taylor GT. Occupational respiratory diseases. Washington, D.C.: U.S. Government Printing Office, 1986. (DHHS [NIOSH] publication no. 86-102.)

*An inexpensive and well-written review of many of the major occupational respiratory conditions. Includes useful chapters on methods of study and evaluation of occupational respiratory disease, including environmental sampling, radiology, pulmonary function, and laboratory studies.*

Occupational Medicine: State of the Arts Reviews:

Beckett WS, Bascom R. eds. Occupational lung disease. Occup Med, State of the Art Rev, 1992; 7(3).

Eisen EA. ed. Spirometry. Occup Med, State of the Art Rev, 1993; 8(2).

Harber P, Balmes JR. eds. Prevention of pulmonary disease in the workplace. Occup Med, State of the Art Rev, 1991; 6(1).

Rosenstock L. ed. Occupational pulmonary disease. Occup Med, State of the Art Rev, 1987; 2(2).

*These four volumes in the State of the Art Review series provide an excellent compendium of up-to-date articles addressing a variety of clinical and research issues in the recognition, screening, management, and prevention of occupational respiratory disorders.*

Parkes WR. Occupational lung disorders. 3rd ed. London: Butterworths, 1992.

*Excellent, detailed summary of occupational respiratory disease. Includes clinical and pathologic details. Some terminology is British but this does not cause a significant problem. Best used as a reference.*

Rom WN. ed. Environmental and occupational medicine. 2nd ed. Boston: Little, Brown, 1992.

*Excellent general reference text with strong chapters on occupational lung diseases.*

# 23

# Musculoskeletal Disorders

Gunnar B. J. Andersson, Lawrence J. Fine, and Barbara A. Silverstein

Work-related musculoskeletal disorders commonly involve the back, cervical spine, and upper extremities. Understanding of these problems has developed rapidly during the past decade. The two sections of this chapter provide an overview of these problems and a framework for recognizing and preventing them.

## Low Back Pain

Gunnar B. J. Andersson

A 30-year-old married auto mechanic had occasional pain in the lower back for at least 5 years. Early one morning at work, he bent forward and to the side to pick up a tire. He experienced sudden back discomfort. He continued to work, but, as the day went on, his back symptoms increased progressively. Toward the end of the day, he was unable to bend, was in much discomfort, and had to leave work. He rested in bed and improved slightly, but was unable to return to work the next day. After 3 days his pain subsided, and he returned to work, but he found that he had persistent discomfort and stiffness.

Two weeks later he bent over again and the back pain returned, this time with radiation into the left thigh. He was unable to finish the workday, went home again, and called his family physician. The doctor advised him to remain in bed for 2 weeks and to take aspirin and a muscle relaxant. After 2 weeks of rest, the mechanic still had persistent pain. He was referred to an orthopedic surgeon, who found no evidence of neurologic impairment; there was tenderness over his lower lumbar spine

and sacroiliac area, and his straight-leg raising was mildly limited. The range of motion of the spine was severely limited. The orthopedist indicated that the mechanic's pain might be related to a disc herniation, and recommended continued medication and a structured exercise program.

A week passed. The pain subsided and the patient started exercises, but could not tolerate them. He returned to the orthopedist, who took an x-ray and found no abnormalities; again, he was advised to continue resting. After another week had passed, he was able to walk about for short periods, but had difficulty sitting, bending, and lifting and required much time lying in bed. Six weeks had now elapsed since the mechanic had stopped working; he returned to work improved, but not feeling back to normal. The mechanic remained in relative comfort until 6 months later, when he again experienced the sudden onset of low back pain. Again he could not work, and again he sought the advice of the orthopedist and was put to bed for 2 weeks. A month later he could tolerate some activity during the day, but was unable to return to work. A second month passed; the mechanic then returned to work but could not work the entire day, and was unable to resume his former job; bending, twisting, and lifting were not possible. He asked the orthopedist for a statement of disability and was given one, but he was informed by his supervisor that he could not keep even the available job if he did not work a normal day. He took a medical absence for another 3 weeks. His financial situation worsened. He was receiving disability pay, but many of the payments were overdue. He was very depressed. His wife was irritated with his grouchiness and lack of interest in sex. The patient sought advice from his family physician, who said that he really did not know what he could do for him and referred him back to the orthopedist, who again found no neurologic abnormalities but thought that surgery might be indicated. First, however, the orthopedist wanted magnetic resonance imaging (MRI) to be performed. The MRI showed evidence of disc degeneration at L5, but no herniation or spinal stenosis. A small central bulge was reported. The patient continued conservative care. He consulted with a lawyer regarding his work and compensation. He became increasingly disgusted and depressed. He was asked by the orthopedist to see a psychiatrist.

This case is not unusual, and the story unfortunately often continues. Work-related back problems are common and sometimes lead to persistent or recurrent pain with complex medical, psychological, occupational, and legal implications. Treatment is variable and sometimes inappropriate. As pain persists, the psychological component becomes more significant.

## Magnitude and Cost

Low back pain is one of the oldest occupational health problems in history. In 1713 Bernardino Ramazzini, the "founder" of occupational medicine, referred to "certain violent and irregular motions and unnatural postures of the body by which the internal structure" is impaired. Ramazzini examined the harmful effects of unusual physical activity, such as the sciatica caused by constantly turning the potter's wheel, lumbago from sitting, and hernias among porters and bearers of heavy loads. Before Ramazzini, physicians in ancient Egypt used leg-moving exercises to diagnose sciatica, then already recognized as being connected with vertebral problems.

In addition to being one of the oldest occupational health problems, low back pain is one of the

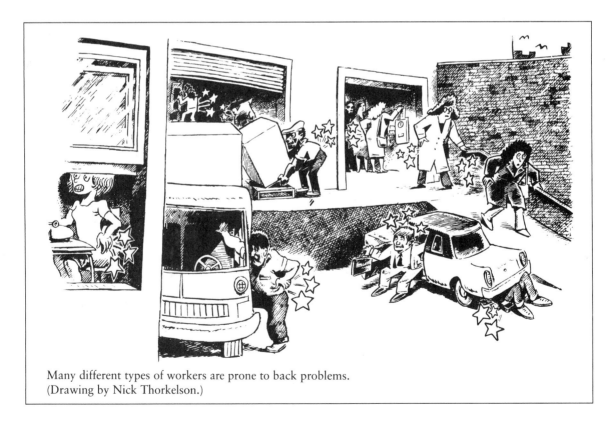

Many different types of workers are prone to back problems. (Drawing by Nick Thorkelson.)

most common. Approximately 80 percent of workers will experience low back pain sometime during their active working life. At any given moment, 10 to 15 percent of the adult population of the United States experiences low back pain [1, 2]. Approximately 11 percent of Americans report low back impairment, or a reduced ability to function. Every year, about 2 percent of the employed population lose time from work because of low back pain, and approximately half of these people receive compensation for lost wages. Lost time from low back pain averages 4 hours per worker per year, and among medical reasons for work absence, it is second only to upper respiratory infections.

Low back pain is clearly the most costly occupational health problem. More than $16 billion is spent each year on the treatment and compensation of low back pain in the United States [1]. The total cost for the back problem has been estimated to be as high as $50 to $80 billion [3]. However, back pain expenses are not equally distributed; they are highly biased toward the more expensive cases—25 percent of low back pain cases account for about 90 percent of the expenses. Most cases are relatively inexpensive. Psychological impairments accompany many of the more expensive cases, either preceding or in response to the physical disability. Therefore, in cases of chronic low back pain, one must address both the medical and the psychological aspects.

## Pathophysiology

Pain in the lumbosacral spine can result from inflammatory, degenerative, neoplastic, gynecologic, traumatic, metabolic, and other types of disorders. However, the great majority of low back pain (LBP) is nonspecific and of unknown cause. Many theories regarding the origin of nonspecific low back pain have been proposed, but so far no one has been able to prove how and where the pain arises.

The intervertebral disc as a source of low back pain has attracted much attention for mainly two reasons. Discs herniate and the herniated nucleus pulposus (HNP) is such an obvious, dramatic, and reputed cause of back pain and sciatica that most workers have heard about or know someone with this diagnosis. Furthermore, most workers know that a herniated disc may require surgical treatment with variable results. The second reason for the attention to the disc is that it degenerates, and that the degenerative process is readily visible on MRI, and can often be seen on radiographs and computed tomographic (CT) scans as well.

The significant focus on the disc as a source of back pain is unwarranted. In reality, herniated discs are responsible for only a minor share of the back problems, estimated at between 1 and 5 percent. A herniated disc is a specific clinical entity characterized by sciatica, and usually accompanied or preceded by low back pain. Physical examination often reveals the presence of one or more objective neurologic changes, such as reflex asymmetry, sensory change in the distribution of a nerve root, or muscle weakness. Additionally, the clinical diagnosis requires the presence of a positive nerve root tension test, of which the straight-leg raising test is most commonly used. Less than 1 percent of patients who have lumbar disc herniations will have a massive extrusion of nuclear material sufficient to interfere with nerve control of bladder and bowel function. Although not common, this effect of disc extrusion, called cauda equina syndrome, is a true surgical emergency, since failure to decompress the lesion may result in permanent loss of bladder and bowel control. Most patients who meet the clinical criteria for HNP will recover spontaneously from acute symptoms and have minimal residual functional or work capacity impairment.

Disc degeneration is not synonymous with back pain and, indeed, is common in people without low back pain. Disc degeneration may, however, predispose to herniations and to other clinical changes, such as "spinal instability" and spinal stenosis. All human spines degenerate with time. Most autopsy specimens show the onset of gross and microscopic evidence of intervertebral disc degeneration by the third decade of life. These pathologic changes are accompanied by alterations in the chemical composition of the disc, such as decrease in water content, increase in collagen, and decrease in proteoglycans. The onset of changes occurs earlier in life in men and occurs most commonly in the L4–5 and L5–S1 discs.

Radiographic changes indicative of disc degenerations, such as disc space narrowing and spinal osteophytes, lag behind the histologic and chemical events. The prevalence of these degenerative changes is the same in patients with and without low back pain. It is important to recognize that the presence of a narrowed intervertebral disc is not correlated with the risk for, or the presence of, a disc herniation, and it does not provide an explanation of the patient's pain in most cases. This issue is of even greater importance in the interpretation of imaging studies such as CT scans and MRI studies. The presence of disc bulging is equally common in those with and without a history of back pain. Furthermore, 20 to 30 percent of asymptomatic patients even have evidence of disc herniation on these structural examinations, emphasizing the need to carefully correlate the patient's symptoms and signs with imaging studies. A positive image without appropriate clinical symptoms and signs is insufficient to make a clinical diagnosis.

Back sprains and strains are probably the most common causes of occupational low back pain. A strain is defined as a muscle disruption caused by indirect trauma, such as excessive stretch or tension. Sprains are actually specific to ligaments, but the terms *sprain* and *strain* are loosely interchanged. There is currently no available method to specifically diagnose a sprain or strain injury, complicating the management of these injuries, which are usually diagnosed by excluding other possible causes of pain. Animal studies have shown that strains heal rapidly and that the healing process, after the first few days, is positively influenced by

controlled activation (smooth movements within the normal range of the affected joint). The previously common recommendation of prolonged rest has been abandoned.

Other spinal diagnoses of relevance to occupational low back pain include spinal stenosis, spinal instability, facet syndrome, internal disc disruption, and spondylolysis/spondylolisthesis. (A brief description of those entities is provided here; for detailed description, please refer to [3] and [4] at the end of this chapter.)

Spinal stenosis is defined as a narrowing of the spinal canal or nerve root foraminae, or both. Diffuse narrowing of the spinal canal (central spinal stenosis) may be due to many causes, but most commonly the stenosis results from degeneration with posterior osteophytes projecting into the spinal canal, hypertrophy of the articular facets, and buckling of the ligamentum flavum. Neurogenic claudication is a common symptom, as is pain on extension relieved by flexion. Reflex, motor, and sensory changes are often completely absent. Unlike lumbar disc herniations, positive nerve root tension signs, such as the straight-leg raising test, are often negative.

A subgroup of patients with spinal stenosis have predominantly lateral recess (nerve root canal) stenosis, which is often caused by a combination of facet hypertrophy and disc bulge, which reduces the space available at the affected disc level(s) and compromises the nerve root. These patients may present with disc hernia-like symptoms. It is important to recognize the relationship between spinal stenosis and disc herniations. When the spinal canal and lateral nerve root canals are narrowed, a relatively small disc herniation can produce clinically significant symptoms, such as sciatica, which would not have occurred if the canal had been of adequate dimensions. Thus, the preexistence of the spinal stenosis can contribute to the development of symptoms caused by a disc herniation.

Spinal instability is an uncertain clinical entity characterized by recurrent episodes of low back pain or sciatica, or both, triggered by minor mechanical overloads. For definite diagnosis, a shift in the alignment of vertebrae observed on flexion/extension radiographs or other provocation radiographs is required. A special case of spinal instability includes the gross instabilities caused by fractures, tumors, and infections. In these patients, flexion-extension radiographs are usually not necessary for diagnosis and can, in fact, be harmful, causing damage to the nerve structures.

Facet syndrome or facet osteoarthritis can contribute to back pain. Its role has been de-emphasized in recent years, however, because it does not appear possible to classify the "facet syndrome" clinically with any certainty. Furthermore, specific treatment aimed at the facet joints has been largely unsuccessful.

Internal disc disruption is another syndrome in which the classification remains uncertain. Injections into the disc with contrast media (discography) should reproduce the patient's pain, and also demonstrate disruption of the disc architecture. Although internal disc disruption probably exists, it should be considered a rare cause of occupational low back pain.

Spondylolysis (a defect in the neural arch) and spondylolisthesis (a forward displacement of one vertebra relative to the underlying vertebra or sacrum) occur most commonly at the L5–S1 level, developing during adolescence with little further risk of slippage in adulthood. It is generally believed to be a fatigue fracture of the neural arch, occurring at a specific region (the pars interarticularis), which fails to heal. Workers with spondylolysis are no more at risk for back pain than those without, while spondylolisthesis may render the worker somewhat more susceptible to low back pain. This is particularly the case when the olisthesis is grade 2 or greater—that is, the slip is greater than 25 percent of the vertebra below.

A variety of classification systems have been developed for low back pain. The most comprehensive system is based on symptoms and was developed by the Quebec Study Group [5]. Table 23-1 outlines the system, which is applicable to all anatomic regions of the human spine and is recommended for general use to provide a standard way to report low back pain.

Category 1 represents most patients with low back disorders. Pain is typically aggravated by mechanical factors such as activity, worsening over the course of the day and relieved by rest. Commonly used diagnoses for this patient group include low back strain or sprain. Category 2, in which the pain radiates to the proximal leg, is consistent with pain from structures that derive their innervation from the posterior primary rami, such as muscle, facet joints, ligaments, and bone. Category 3, in which pain radiates distally into the leg(s) may arise from structures innervated by the posterior primary rami. Category 4 patients have neurologic signs, such as a positive nerve root tension sign, loss (or reduction) of reflex, sensation, or motor power. In the instance of a monoradiculopathy, a lumbar disc herniation is a likely diagnosis. Category 5 includes other causes of nerve root and cauda equina compression. Included in this category are obvious spinal fractures that compromise the spinal canal. Category 6 defines the cause of pain through imaging or electrodiagnostic techniques. Category 7 specifically refers to the most common cause of polyradiculopathy and claudication, spinal stenosis. Categories 8 and 9 include patients who have undergone one or more surgical interventions. The separation of the postoperative period into 1 to 6 months and greater than 6 months is important because most patients with simple disc operations should have recovered and returned to work within 6 months of the intervention. Similarly, the separation of category 9 into 9.1 (asymptomatic) and 9.2 (symptomatic) has important implications for both causation and prognosis for long-term recovery. Category 10 (chronic pain syndrome) includes primarily patients for whom an anatomic cause is not identified.

Table 23-1 also demonstrates two other important means for classifying low back disorders: duration of symptoms and working status. The Quebec Study Group states that acute symptoms are 7 days or less, subacute 7 days to 7 weeks, and

**Table 23-1.** Classification of low back disorders

| Classification | Symptoms | Duration of symptoms from onset | Working status at time of evaluation |
|---|---|---|---|
| 1 | Pain without radiation | | |
| 2 | Pain + radiation to extremity, proximally | a (<7 days) | W (working) |
| 3 | Pain + radiation to extremity, distally | b (7 days–7 weeks) | I (idle) |
| 4 | Pain + radiation to upper/ lower limb, neurologic signs | c (>7 weeks) | |
| 5 | Presumptive compression of a spinal nerve root on a simple roentgenogram (i.e., spinal instability or fracture) | | |
| 6 | Compression of a spinal nerve root confirmed by specific imaging techniques (i.e., CT, myelography, or MRI) Other diagnostic techniques (e.g., electromyography, venography) | | |
| 7 | Spinal stenosis | | |
| 8 | Postsurgical status, 1–6 months after intervention | | |
| 9 | Postsurgical status, >6 months after intervention 9.1 Asymptomatic 9.2 Symptomatic | | |
| 10 | Chronic pain syndrome | | W (working) |
| 11 | Other diagnoses | | I (idle) |

Source: From WO Spitzer, et al. Scientific approach to the assessment and management of activity-related spinal disorders: A monograph for clinicians. Report of the Quebec Task Force on Spinal Disorders. Spine 1987; 12 (Suppl. 7):S1–S59. Used by permission.

chronic more than 7 weeks, a convenient division that reflects the normal recovery of patients with back pain. Work status is also important because of its influence on prognosis.

## Diagnosis

The cornerstones of diagnosis are the history and physical examination [3, 4]. In most patients, this is the only evaluation necessary. Patients with re-current or chronic symptoms, as well as those with more severe back pain of an unrelenting nature and those with neurologic deficits, may require imaging, electrodiagnostic, or laboratory studies. The use of these tests should be based on specific indications derived from the history and physical examination, and the results must be correlated to the history and physical examination. Patients with more chronic symptoms sometimes also need a psychological evaluation.

The history should contain information about

present and previous symptoms, significant other medical diseases, and use of medications. The onset of the symptoms should be explored in detail, including significant trauma. Pain is the most important symptom. Its pattern should be determined, as well as its intensity, site, and radiation, and factors that accentuate and relieve it. The time of day when pain is most severe should be ascertained. Worsening through the day suggests mechanical low back pain, which is the most common pattern. Pain on arising in the morning with improvement during the day suggests an inflammatory condition. Pain that is most severe at night and awakens the patient is a sign of possible malignancy or infection. Pain distribution is critical in correctly classifying patients, particularly when pain radiates down the leg.

Neurologic symptoms should be identified, including sensory changes such as numbness and tingling, subjective sense of lower-extremity weakness, and changes in bladder and bowel control or sexual function. Loss of ability to initiate voiding and urinary or fecal incontinence are symptoms of a cauda equina syndrome that must be further evaluated with urgency. Progressive weakness and "foot drop" are other symptoms requiring further evaluation.

The physical examination consists of inspection, palpation, range of motion measurements, and neurologic tests. Body movements, gait, and standing posture will indicate the severity of symptoms as well as allow an estimate of functional limitations. The range of flexion-extension, lateral bending, and axial rotation are observed and measured. Examination of the lower extremities is used to determine the presence or absence of any significant joint deformities and to assess neurologic function. Hip motion should also be evaluated. Knee (quadriceps) and ankle (Achilles) reflexes should be obtained in the sitting or supine positions, or both. The knee reflex can be affected by an L4 root compression; the ankle reflex is primarily mediated by the S1 nerve root. Nonspecific loss of sensation must be differentiated from well-defined dermatomal loss. Motor function is also grossly

evaluated. Strength of the extensor hallucis longus is typically affected by an L5 nerve root compression.

The evaluation of nerve root tension signs is important. The straight-leg raising (SLR) test is the test most commonly used. It is positive when sciatica (posterior leg pain) is reproduced. The degree of elevation at which the symptoms occur is recorded.

At the completion of the history and physical examination, a general formulation can be made of the patient's low back problem, including decisions regarding the need for further diagnostic tests and an initial therapeutic plan.

For most patients, further diagnostic studies are not required. Additional evaluation of the patient depends on symptom response to treatment and the severity of any remaining symptoms. The diagnostic tests under consideration for patients with back conditions fall into two categories; those performed to detect physiologic abnormalities, and those to detect anatomic abnormality and provide anatomic definition. Tests of physiologic dysfunction include laboratory tests, bone scans, and electrodiagnostic studies (EMG). Anatomic tests include x-rays and other imaging studies (CT, MRI, and myelography). In select cases a psychological evaluation may also be required.

Radiographs are commonly used, but have limited value as a screening tool. Degenerative changes are nonspecific and often unrelated to the patient's pain. A variety of other imaging techniques, as indicated above, are now available to assess patients who fulfill criteria for their use. These tests allow assessment of the anatomy of the spinal canal and its contents. These tests should not be used routinely in patients with low back pain, but only when indicated, based on the patient's history and physical examination. In other words, these tests are used to confirm a clinical suspicion. The basic principle is that anatomic images are only as valid as their correlation with clinical signs and symptoms. This is important because imaging abnormalities are common in individuals who have never had low back symptoms or sciatica. Further, in addition to clinically significant abnormalities, a number of other findings of questionable or unknown importance are commonly observed. These include disc bulging and disc degeneration, which are both nonspecific. Other diagnostic tests are more rarely indicated [5].

## Risk Factors—High-Risk Jobs

It is difficult to determine the relationship between occupational factors and low back pain because (1) low back pain is not easily defined and classified; (2) sickness absence and other disability data are influenced not only by pain, but also by physical and psychological work factors, social factors, and insurance systems; (3) there is a poor relationship between tissue injury and disability; (4) the healthy worker effect influences data; and (5) exposure is difficult to determine. The retrospective assessment of exposure in most studies limits casual interpretation.

The seven most frequently discussed factors are listed in Table 23-2 [2, 6]. The six physical work factors have been experimentally associated with the development of injuries in spinal tissues. The seventh, psychological and psychosocial work factors, is probably more related to back disability than to an actual back injury.

There is presently an enormous body of data implicating heavy work in increasing the risk of back pain, sciatica, and disc herniations. Most investigators are using sickness absence and injury re-

Table 23-2. Occupational factors associated with an increased risk of low back pain

Heavy physical work
Static work postures
Frequent bending and twisting
Lifting, pushing, and pulling
Repetitive work
Vibrations
Psychological and psychosocial factors

ports as their sources, and thus, reflect not only back pain, but also disability caused by back pain. However, some studies are based on questionnaires, interviews, and even disc hernia operations. Several countries report similar data. One study, using occupational safety and health data from the United States, found significantly higher rates of back sprain/strain among workers in heavy industries and in physically demanding occupations [7]. These data were confirmed by others studying other populations [2, 8]. Others related injury rates to predicted spine compression forces in 55 industrial jobs. Back pain was twice as common if the predicted disc compression was above 6,800 newtons (1,500 lb) [9].

Static work postures include primarily long-term sitting, which appears to increase the risk of low back pain and, in combination with driving, increases the risk of disc herniation [2, 10–12]. Frequent bending and twisting are usually associated with lifting when reported as causes of back injuries. However, one study found low back pain to be associated with asymmetrical postures in a car assembly plant even when lifting was not performed [13].

Lifting is a well-known triggering event for back pain [2, 14–17]. One study compared workers performing heavy manual lifting to sedentary workers; the odds ratio (OR) was 8 [18]. Insurance company data indicate that a worker is three times more susceptible to compensable low back pain if exposed to excessive manual handling [19]. Associations between prevalence of low back pain and lifting were also established by others [15–17, 20]. Another study found that disc herniations were more frequent among subjects who had to lift, particularly when lifting was performed in bent and twisted postures (OR = 6) [21]. Repetitive work increases sickness absence in general and, as some evidence supports, disability caused by low back pain.

Low back pain is more frequent in vehicle drivers than in control subjects, implicating vibrations (perhaps in combination with the sitting posture).

One study found truck drivers to have a fourfold increased risk of disc herniations, while simple car commuting increased the risk by a factor of two [22]. Other studies also indicate an increased risk of low back pain with vibration [2]. Another study found that the risk of being hospitalized for herniated nucleus pulposus in Finland was particularly high for professional motor vehicle drivers [23]. Studies of vehicle drivers have disclosed that radiographic changes occur over time [2].

Psychological and psychosocial work factors have received increasing attention because of the effect on low back disability. Monotony has been identified as a risk factor for back pain [15], as has poor work satisfaction [14, 15]. Investigators concluded, based on the "Boeing study," that psychological work factors were more important than physical factors as risk indicators of filing workers' compensation claims for low back pain [14, 24].

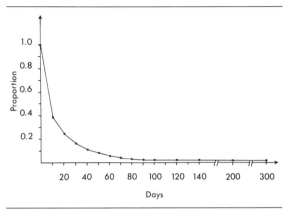

Fig. 23-1. The recovery rate after a back injury is rapid (Andersson GBJ, Svensson H-O, Oden A: The intensity of work recovery in low back pain. Spine 8, 880-884, 1983). The figure shows the proportion of people who were absent from work at different times after first reporting sick.

## Management

The management of patients with low back problems has undergone major changes over the last decade or so [3, 4]. In general, patients recover from an acute episode in days to a few weeks and require little treatment [5] (Fig. 23-1). When symptoms continue, physical activation has replaced recommendations of rest, which were often used in the past.

Early treatment should include (1) information about back pain and its excellent prognosis; (2) help with control of symptoms, including medication and advice on activity; and (3) a reassessment plan. Many patients are concerned about a back problem when it first arises, and have misconceptions about its natural history and effect on their future lives. This fear can be eliminated by appropriate information. Symptom control is typically achieved by medication, but manipulation can also have beneficial effects in the acute stages of the problem. Analgesics and nonsteroidal anti-in-

flammatory medications (NSAIDs) are the medications that are used most frequently. Muscle relaxants can cause drowsiness and appear to be no more effective than NSAIDs.

Activity advice is critical. Some degree of activity restriction is often necessary to reduce symptom severity. This can often be accomplished by modifying work activities and work postures, while allowing the patient to continue working. Bed rest should only be advised in more severe cases, and then for no more than 2 to 3 days [25]. Early return to work is critical to prevent prolonged disability and should be emphasized as being part of the recovery process. Activity recommendations (restrictions) may include limitation on lifting, twisting, and bending, and on the duration of sitting, standing, and walking [3]. Restrictions should only be in place for a short period. The beneficial natural history should allow unrestricted evaluation after a few to several weeks.

Many treatment alternatives have been and continue to be needed in the treatment of acute low back pain. Few have been rigorously studied for treatment effect [5, 26]. There is no evidence that physical therapy modalities influence the natural history of recovery, although the patient may sometimes feel temporary relief. The medical literature also does not support benefits of using transcutaneous electrical nerve stimulation (TENS), corsets, traction, acupuncture, or biofeedback in treatment of acute low back pain. Corset use may allow the patient to return to physical activities, such as lifting earlier, but does not affect long-term results. Back schools provide an efficient method of education and can be an excellent adjunct, particularly when the patient is treated in a busy clinical setting (see below). Manipulation appears to hasten recovery in patients with acute low back pain without radiculopathy, when used during the first 4 weeks of symptoms.

Surgery is almost never indicated in the first 4 to 6 weeks, but should then be considered in patients with severe persistent sciatica that has not responded to conservative treatment and where findings on clinical examination and confirmatory diagnostic tests indicate nerve root compromise [27]. Simple disc surgery does not prevent return to physically demanding jobs.

## Prognosis

Nonspecific low back pain is a self-limiting disorder that resolves rapidly in over 90 percent of cases. Approximately 40 percent of the patients will recover within 1 week, 80 percent within 3 weeks, and 90 percent within 6 weeks, regardless of treatment. The rate of recurrence, however, is very high—estimates range up to 90 percent. A British study indicates that the probability of low back pain is almost four times greater in individuals who have had previous episodes of low back pain [28]. A Swedish study found that industrial workers who have a first-time episode of low back pain have a 28 percent chance of a new episode during the next year.

At the onset of low back pain, it is difficult to predict which patients will require longer than 6 weeks to recover. A specific diagnosis, prior injury, and psychological impairment have all been correlated with longer recovery times. Sciatica (posterior leg pain) has a slower recovery than low back pain. If workers have been off the job for longer than 6 months, it is estimated that there is only a 50 percent possibility of ever returning to productive employment; over 1 year, only 25 percent; and over 2 years, almost none [29]. The last decade has witnessed the development of comprehensive treatment programs that have improved on these data using different types of pain treatment and activation programs, but prognosis after long work absence still remains poor [30].

Early return to work is now considered an important part of the therapy. However, there are many reasons why patients do not go back to work. The obstacles to early return to work are several. These include (1) patient motivation, (2) illness behavior (conscious or unconscious exaggeration of symptoms), (3) the problem of identifying and providing modified work, (4) the unwillingness by employers to accept workers back unless they are fully recovered (despite evidence that accepting a partially recovered worker may be less costly and more effective in promoting recovery than continued disability), (5) difficulties imposed by rigid work rules, (6) inappropriate treatment by practitioners or prolonged use of ineffective treatment, and (7) legal advice to accept a "lump sum" settlement instead of a rehabilitation program designed to return the person to work. The physician should be aware of these situations and recognize their relative importance in each case of low back pain.

## Prevention and Control

Preventing work-related low back pain is a complex challenge. Low back pain prevention in work settings is best accomplished by a combination of measures that are listed in Table 23-3. Only a combination of measures can prevent low back pain, although some measures are more effective

**Table 23-3.** Prevention of low back pain

Job design (ergonomics)
    Mechanical aids
    Optimum work level
    Good workplace layout
    Sit/stand workstations
    Appropriate packaging
Job placement (selection)
    Careful history
    Thorough physical examination
    No routine x-rays
    Strength testing
    Job-rating programs
Training and education
    Training workers
        Biomechanics of body movement (safe lifting)
        Strength and fitness
        Back schools
    Training managers
        Response to low back pain
        Early return to work
        Ergonomic principles of job design
    Training labor union representatives
        Early return to work
        Flexible work rules
        Reasonable referrals
    Training health care providers
        Appropriate medication
        Prudent use of x-rays
        Limited bed rest
        Early return to work (with restrictions, if
           necessary)

than others and therefore should be implemented first.

Low back pain can be controlled by reducing the probability of the initial episode, reducing the severity of the symptoms, reducing the length of disability, and reducing the chance of recurrence.

It is estimated that good ergonomic design of the job can reduce up to one-third of compensable low back pain in industry [20]. Not only can good job design reduce the probability of initial and recurring episodes, it will also allow the worker with moderate symptoms to stay on the job longer and permit the disabled worker to return to the job

sooner. Good ergonomic design reduces the worker's exposure to the risk factors of low back pain through the following:

1. Mechanical aids (powered or manual) to assist with heavy weights and forces (Figs. 23-2 and 23-3)
2. Optimum work level to reduce unnecessary bending and stretching (Fig. 23-4)
3. Good workplace layout to reduce unnecessary twisting and reaching (Fig. 23-5)

**Fig. 23-2.** Load positioners offer the ability to counterbalance the weight of a load, enabling the operator to position it accurately. They are particularly applicable to loading and unloading heavy pieces into machines. They use air pressure to balance the weight but still require the operator to move the piece in the direction needed, giving the operator more actual control and greater speed than with an electric chain hoist. (From Liberty Mutual Insurance Company.)

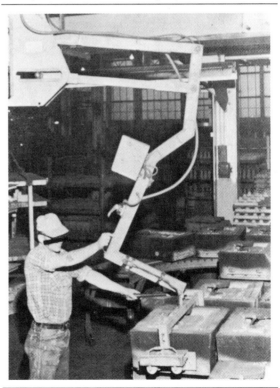

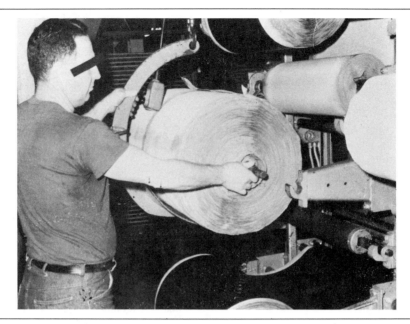

**Fig. 23-3.** Overhead hoists/lifting attachments. Overhead hoists with specially designed lifting attachments to fit the objects being handled eliminate the awkward manual handling tasks. This C-shaped attachment allows quick and easy placement of heavy rolls on a tire building machine. (From Liberty Mutual Insurance Company.)

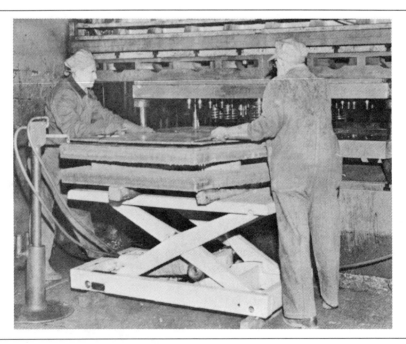

**Fig. 23-4.** Scissors lift. Hydraulic scissor lifts have a variety of uses in industry to position the work piece so that a minimum of effort can be used to perform the operation. Workers can place the work piece at the proper height to convert lifting and lowering tasks to carries or pushes. (From Liberty Mutual Insurance Company.)

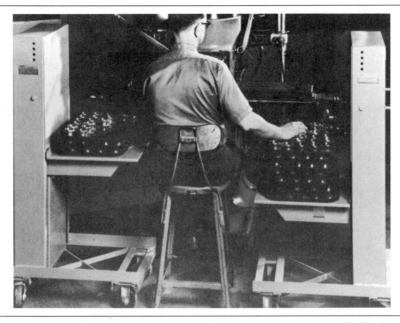

**Fig. 23-5.** Work dispensers are self-leveling devices designed to keep parts at a particular height, eliminating the need to bend over to pick up or release an item. Models are available to utilize trays or pans, as well as for bulk-dispensing of small parts. The dispensers are portable and can be wheeled from station to station, eliminating the need to lift, carry, and lower trays as well as individual parts. (From Liberty Mutual Insurance Company.)

4. Sit/stand workstations to reduce prolonged sitting and standing
5. Appropriate packaging to match object weights with human capabilities
6. Good work organization to reduce repetitive high loading and fatigue
7. Good chairs to support the back properly

The National Institute for Occupational Safety and Health (NIOSH) has provided guidelines for evaluating and designing manual lifting tasks [31]. Guidelines for other manual-handling tasks, such as pushing, pulling, or carrying, have also been developed [32].

In recent years, considerable attention and hope have been placed on the use of "lifting belts" as a means to reduce back injuries from lifting. Currently, there are insufficient data on the use of these belts to make recommendations on a scientific basis. The mechanical effect of the belts is un-

clear, but from spinal loading it appears to be minor. Recent information suggests that an initial beneficial effect on number of back injury claims filed may occur, but the data remain preliminary. As we understand today, there are no direct negative effects of belt use, although long-term effects on trunk muscles have been discussed as a possible disadvantage.

Although job design may be applicable to many manufacturing operations, other jobs are difficult to design and control, such as firefighting, police work, and certain construction and delivery operations. These jobs require greater dependence on preplacement testing and selection of workers [3, 30, 33]. In the past the preplacement medical examination was used in many industries, especially since the enactment of workers' compensation laws. The introduction of the Americans with Disabilities Act (ADA) has, to a degree, changed the screening process. Preemployment examinations are no longer acceptable, while preplacement examinations continue to be used to determine whether the worker is capable of performing the job. However, it has been estimated that, with careful history taking and a thorough examination, about 7 or 8 percent of young individuals prone to future back problems might be identified. The identification rate would be substantially higher with applicants in older age groups, where the findings of disease are more frequent and more obvious.

Many authorities feel that the medical history is the most important part of the medical examination in identifying workers who are susceptible to future low back pain [33]. Knowing that the worker has had previous low back pain is significant, because after an initial episode of back pain, the probability of additional episodes of low back pain is four times greater [28].

Routine x-rays of the lumbar spine have often, but mistakenly, been part of the preplacement medical examination, since the preponderance of evidence indicates that the small yield does not justify the radiation exposure or increased cost. According to guidelines issued by the American College of Occupational and Environmental Medicine, lumbar spine x-ray examinations should not be used as a risk assessment procedure for back problems, but only as a special diagnostic procedure used by the physician when there are appropriate indications [3]. Such indications include recurrent episodes of back pain and suspicion of an underlying congenital defect, or rheumatologic, neoplastic, or infectious etiology.

Several studies have demonstrated the relationship between strength/fitness and the incidence of low back pain [9, 30, 34]. Studies of isometric strength testing have shown that the probability of a musculoskeletal disorder is up to three times greater when job-lifting requirements approach or exceed the worker's isometric strength capability [9]. A Danish study revealed that men who experienced low back pain for the first time had lower isometric endurance of the back muscles when measured up to 1 year before the episode [34]. In women, however, the lower endurance had no predictive value. Although isometric strength testing may be an effective selection technique, it should only be used for jobs that are difficult to design or control and for which a careful ergonomic evaluation has been made [3]. Strength testing should never be used as a substitute for good job design. Furthermore, it should only be used when the job has been thoroughly analyzed so that the test truly reflects the demands of the work. Strength testing, using a general protocol does not appear to be effective in preventing back injury reports [14]. Several attempts have been made to develop dynamic lifting tests, since dynamic lifting represents a better simulation of the actual lifting task. Unfortunately, there have been no studies showing the effectiveness of dynamic strength testing as a preplacement technique for reducing the incidence and severity of musculoskeletal disorders.

Job-rating programs are structured attempts to evaluate the job as well as the worker, and then to obtain a good match between the two. These programs not only screen out applicants who lack the physical capacity to perform critical job tasks, but also find suitable work for people of varying abilities. However, these programs have not been proven to reduce the occurrence of low back pain.

Training and education are the oldest and most commonly used approaches for reducing low back pain in industry [3, 30]. Safety and personnel departments have typically used education and training to instruct employees in proper methods and work procedures. For example, training the worker in the biomechanics of safe lifting has been a part of safety programs in industry for over 50 years. However, according to NIOSH, the value of training programs in safe lifting is open to question because there have been no controlled studies showing consequent decreases in rates of manual-handling accidents or back injuries [31]. A major problem is compliance; even after training, most workers do not lift correctly because it is a more difficult way to lift. Greater compliance with training results from workers who have (or have had) low back pain. Exercises to increase strength and fitness have been a part of low back pain treatment programs for many years, but only recently have strength and fitness programs been advocated in industry to reduce or prevent the onset of low back pain.

The back school is an attempt to educate the worker in all aspects of back care; it represents a much more comprehensive approach to back care that includes the previous topics of safe lifting, strength, and physical fitness. The original concept of the back school was to educate patients who were already suffering (or had recently suffered) from low back pain; that is, it was a form of treatment. A more recent use of the back school is to educate workers on how to prevent low back pain. Controlled studies have demonstrated the effectiveness of a low back school when used as treatment for patients [35]. However, no controlled study has been reported showing the effectiveness of a low back school as a preventive technique for workers.

Training managers is as important as training workers, both for primary and tertiary prevention. Long-term disability is associated with adversary situations, litigation, hospitalization, and lack of follow-up and concern. Many of these situations can be alleviated by training foremen, supervisors, and upper-level managers in appropriate responses to low back pain. Also important is providing modified, alternative, or part-time work as a means of returning the worker to the job as quickly as possible.

A program in which management was trained in the positive acceptance of reporting back pain has been described [36, 37]. An atmosphere was created in which workers were encouraged to report all episodes of low back pain—even minor episodes—to the company clinic. Immediate and conservative in-house treatment, including worker education, was provided by the company nurse. Attempts were made to keep the worker on the job, often with modified duties or a redesigned job. If necessary, referrals were made to the company physician, who closely monitored treatment and progress. Over a 3-year period, annual workers' compensation costs for low back pain claims were reduced from over $200,000 to less than $20,000. Although this was not a controlled study, the results were impressive.

In addition to training managers, efforts to incorporate union leaders into prevention efforts are important. Early return to work should be encouraged, especially where management cooperation is necessary to achieve this goal. Early return to work is an important part of the treatment of low back pain. Unions can often assist in the recovery of their members by allowing early return to work through flexible work rules and referrals to clinicians and lawyers who likely will not unnecessarily prolong the disability.

Company medical personnel should be trained in the benefits of early intervention, conservative treatment, patient follow-up, and job placement techniques. Both physicians and nurses should be familiar with recent literature that objectively evaluates various types of treatment for low back pain. Medical personnel should also become familiar with the physical demands of jobs performed in the company in order to adequately place injured workers—and new employees.

The effectiveness of a standardized approach to the diagnosis and treatment of low back pain in industry has been demonstrated [30, 38]. This approach was used to monitor the course and treatment for employees with low back pain. If there was any disagreement between the investigators (who were orthopedic surgeons) and the treating physician, they discussed the case together in detail. Usually, they reached an agreement; if they did not, another physician was consulted for an independent opinion. This program dramatically decreased the number of low back patients, the number of days lost, and the number of patients sent to surgery.

Although knowledge of low back pain is limited, it is quite clear that enough is already known to adequately control the problem in industry. Instead of waiting for a major medical breakthrough to occur, emphasis should be placed on applying the knowledge that is already available. Low back pain control requires the combined efforts of workers, managers, unions, nurses, physicians, and others.

# Work-Related Disorders of the Neck and Upper Extremity

Lawrence J. Fine and Barbara A. Silverstein

A 31-year-old, right-handed man had been employed in a variety of automobile manufacturing jobs for 13 years. Two years ago he switched to a new plant and was assigned to a job that required him to move a spot welding machine beneath cars moving overhead. He had a minute to complete four welds on each car. The spot welder, which had metal handles, required substantial force for appropriate positioning, and it had to be repositioned four times for each car. The worker's wrists were in complete extension for a substantial portion of the job cycle.

When the worker started on this job, the weekday work shift was 9 hours long and Saturday work was required in most weeks. After 3 weeks on the job, he noted that he had pain in both wrists. He also noted numbness and tingling in the first four fingers of his left hand, first only at night, a few nights each week, after he had fallen asleep. When he awoke at night with the numbness, he would get up and walk around shaking his hands; in about 10 minutes he would be able to go back to sleep. Gradually, over the next several months, the numbness and pain worsened both in frequency and intensity. His left hand would feel numb by the end of the work shift, and any time he was driving, his hands would become numb. Since he liked his job and did not want to be placed on restriction, which would mean he could not work overtime, he decided to visit his private physician rather than the company physician. He also was not sure that the company physician would be very sympathetic to his complaints.

His physician found on physical examination that he had decreased sensitivity to light touch in the left index and middle fingers and a positive Phalen's test of the left

hand. She suspected carpal tunnel syndrome (CTS) and believed that the disorder might be work-related because the patient was young, male, and had no other risk factors, such as diabetes, past history of wrist fracture, or recent trauma to the wrist. The physician discussed job changes with the patient. She also prescribed wrist splints to be used only at night.

The splints relieved some of the nighttime numbness for a period. However, over the next 6 months, the patient's symptoms began to be present all of the time, and he thought that his left hand was becoming weaker. Similar symptoms also developed in his right hand.

The patient felt he could no longer do his job and returned to his physician. She noted that the Phalen's test was now positive bilaterally. She referred him to a hand surgeon and ordered nerve conduction tests because she was concerned that some surgeons do not always have these tests done before surgery. The nerve conduction test showed slowing of sensory nerve impulse conduction in the median nerve in the region of the carpal tunnel.

One year after the problem was first noted, he had surgery, first on the left hand and then on the right hand. Following surgery, the company placed him in a transitional work center for a 3-month period where he worked at his own pace and had no symptoms. He then returned to the assembly line with the restriction that he not use welding guns or air-powered hand tools. When he worked on the line, he occasionally had symptoms, but they were substantially less intense and less frequent than before.

He later transferred to a warehouse, because he felt that he would have a better chance of avoiding long layoffs there. He was placed on a job that required use of a stapling gun to seal packages. Three weeks after being placed in this job, his symptoms began to return with their former intensity. Through ordinary channels he immediately sought and was given a transfer to a position driving a fork lift truck. This change reduced, but did not eliminate, his symptoms. Currently he has numbness, tingling, and pain in the fingers of both hands about twice a month. Playing volleyball usually triggers a severe attack. With the use of nighttime splints, he can sleep through most nights without awakening. While he feels that his hands are weaker than before he developed his symptoms, he still is able to perform his job. He has decided that as long as his symptoms remain at this level, he will continue working.

This case illustrates the intermittent and progressive nature of most work-related disorders of the upper extremity, and particularly of CTS [39], the best known of the common work-related disorders of the upper extremity. Other examples of these disorders that may be related to work include de Quervain's disease [40], epicondylitis [41], rotator (or rotor) cuff tendinitis (mainly supraspinatus) [42], and tension neck syndrome [43]. This family of disorders may involve muscles (tension neck syndrome), tendons (supraspinatus tendinitis disease), joints (degenerative joint disease) [44], skin (calluses), nerves (CTS), or blood vessels (hand-arm vibration syndrome, or Raynaud's phenomenon of occupational origin) [45].

## Magnitude and Cost of the Problem

There is only limited information about the magnitude and the cost of this group of work-related musculoskeletal disorders. The U.S. Bureau of Labor Statistics' (BLS) Annual Survey of Occupational Injuries and Illnesses reported that the incidence of occupational illnesses and disorders associated with repeated trauma was 3 per 1,000 full-time workers in the private sector in 1991 [46]. There has been a steady increase from 1982, when the rate was 0.4 per 1,000. By contrast, in the same time period the rate for skin disorders has been more stable, from 0.67 in 1982 to 0.77 in 1991.

While no precise information is available on the location of these illnesses by body part, limited analysis of the BLS data suggests that the most common site of these disorders and illnesses is the upper extremity followed by the lower extremity (low back pain in the BLS system is usually recorded as an injury rather than a disorder or illness).

There is a little more information about the prevalence of CTS. One of the few population-based studies of occupational CTS using a medical record–based case definition is the workers' compensation record study in the state of Washington, which found that the rate of occupational CTS was 1.7 claims per 1,000 full-time workers during 1984 to 1988 [47]. About a quarter of these claims also indicated that CTS surgery had been performed. In Ontario, Canada, during 1988 the rate of occupational wrist tendinitis and CTS based on workers' compensation records was approximately 0.2 and 0.1 per 1,000 workers [48].

Self-reports of nonoccupational and occupational CTS and "prolonged" hand discomfort (20 days or more, or 7 or more consecutive days in the past 12 months) were collected in the 1988 Occupational Health Supplement to the annual National Health Interview Survey (NHIS). Approximately 8 percent of the active workers in the NHIS survey reported "prolonged" hand discomfort; about 1 percent reported that they had CTS [49]. Roughly 60 percent of the workers with CTS reported that their condition had been diagnosed by a medical person. Twenty percent of the workers with CTS and prolonged hand discomfort had missed work as a result of their condition compared to 6 percent of those with only prolonged hand discomfort.

Epidemiologic studies of workers in specific high-risk industries typically find that CTS cases consist of only a minority of all of the cases of hand and wrist disorders noted in the surveys [50]. Unfortunately, there are virtually no data on the prevalence of the other specific work-related disorders of the upper extremity such as trigger finger, epicondylitis, or rotator cuff tendinitis. While varying by specific occupation, these disorders are probably overall less common than CTS [41]. From a national perspective, while the precise prevalence of work-related musculoskeletal disorders of the upper extremity is unknown these disorders are likely the second most common occupational disorders after work-related low back disorders. Typical prevalence rates for CTS in workplaces with an average level of risk should be less than 1 percent.

## Pathophysiology

Clinical, laboratory, and epidemiologic studies all have contributed to the current understanding of the pathophysiology of work-related musculoskeletal disorders of the upper extremity and neck. Some investigators believe that work factors are rarely important.

While the current level of knowledge is incomplete, it nevertheless guides both treatment and preventive strategies. Five occupational factors are important in the etiology of these disorders: repetitive motions, forceful motions, mechanical stresses, static or awkward postures, and local vibration (Fig. 23-6).

### Repetition and Force

Repetitive motions of the hands, wrists, shoulders, and neck commonly occur in the workplace. A data-entry operator may perform 20,000 keystrokes per hour, a worker in a meat-processing plant may perform 12,000 knife-cuts per day, and a worker on an assembly line may elevate the right shoulder above the level of the acromion 7,500 times per day. These repetitive motions in an individual may eventually exceed the ability to recover from the stress, especially if forceful contrac-

Fig. 23-6. Schematic representation of pathophysiology of work-related disorders of the upper extremity and neck.

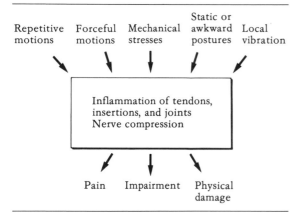

tions of muscles are involved in the repetitive motions.

The failure to recover usually implies the persistence of inflammation ("tissue reaction to injury"). In musculoskeletal work-related disorders, the sites of inflammation most commonly involve tendons, tendon sheaths, and tendon attachments to bones, bursae, and joints. This persistent inflammation can lead to nerve compression (CTS), chronic fibrous reaction in the tendon, tendon rupture (rotator cuff), calcium deposits, or fibrous nodule formations in a tendon, leading to a trigger finger [51].

Abrupt increases in the number of repetitive motions performed by the worker each day are clinically well recognized as a cause of tendinitis. Too many forceful contractions of muscles can cause corresponding tendons to stretch, compressing the microstructures of the tendons leading to ischemia, microscopic tears in tendons, progressive lengthening, and sliding of tendon fibers through the ground substance matrix. All these events can cause inflammation of tendons.

An important, but inadequately investigated, question is whether the repetitive stresses to the joints of upper limbs that occur in some occupations lead to the accelerated development of localized osteoarthrosis (LOA). Since LOA is not a specific disease but the final common pathway of biomechanical and pathologic changes in cartilage, subchondral bone, and bone surrounding joints, it is reasonable to assume that repetitive stresses can accelerate its development [44, 51].

### Posture, Stress, and Vibration

In addition to repetitive and forceful motions, three other exposure variables that influence the development of work-related musculoskeletal disorders are external mechanical stress, work performed in awkward or static postures, and segmental (localized) vibration.

Mechanical stress in tendons results from muscle contractions or when a tendon or other tissues are compressed because of contact between the body and another object. One of the major determinants of the level of the mechanical stress is the force of the muscle contractions. For example, a pinch that is very forceful will be more stressful than one that is not very forceful. Mechanical stress is often produced by handheld tools with hard sharp edges or the ends of short handles that press on soft tissues. The tool exerts just as much force on the hand as the hand does on the tool.

Mechanical stress to nerve or other soft tissues can occur when they come into contact with structures harder than themselves, particularly external hard or sharp objects. These stresses can lead to nerve compression. Examples include a digital neuritis associated with the edge of scissors handles or bowling ball holes coming into forceful contact with the sides of the fingers or thumb, and cubital tunnel syndrome in a microscopist who must position the elbow on a hard surface for long periods. Short-handled tools that dig into the base of the palm exert as much force on the hand, particularly the superficial branches of the median nerve, as the hand does on the tool.

Work performed in awkward or static postures is another important influence on the development of work-related musculoskeletal disorders. The level of mechanical stress produced by a muscle contraction varies with the posture of a joint. For example, it is believed that contraction of the finger flexors is more stressful if the wrist is flexed. Work with the arm elevated more than 60 degrees from the trunk is more stressful for the rotator cuff tendons than work performed with the arm at the trunk. Work performed in static postures that requires prolonged low-level muscle contractions of the upper limb or neck may also trigger chronic localized pain by an unknown mechanism.

Segmental vibration is transmitted to the upper extremity from impact tools, power tools, and bench-mounted buffers and grinders. The mechanism by which localized vibration from power tools contributes to the development of work-related Raynaud's phenomenon is not clear. Nevertheless, it has been associated with several types of power tools, such as chain saws, rock drillers, chipping hammers, and grinding tools (see box, Chap. 6).

Most of the effects thus described center on the tendon structures. The chronic effects of repetition and these other risk factors on muscles are not as well understood as the effects on tendons. Chronic or intermittent pain originating in muscles may be important in understanding several disorders including tension neck syndrome (costal-scapular syndrome) and overuse injuries in musicians [52]. Two types of muscle activity may be important in work-related disorders: low force with prolonged muscle contractions (moderate neck flexion while working on a video display terminal for several hours without rest breaks) and infrequent or frequent high-force muscle contractions (intermittent use of heavy tools in overhead work). Sustained static contractions can lead to increases in intramuscular pressure, which in turn may impair blood flow to cells within the muscle.

Motor nerve control of the working muscle may be important in sustained static contractions since even if the relative load on the muscle as a whole is low, the active part of the muscle can be working close to its maximal capacity. Thus, small areas of large muscles of the trapezius muscle may have disturbances in microcirculation that contribute to or cause the development of muscle damage (red ragged fibers), the reduction of strength, higher levels of fatigue, and sensitization of pain receptors in the muscle leading to pain at rest [53]. High levels of tension (strong contractions) can lead to muscle fiber Z-line rupture, muscle pain, and large delayed increases in serum creatine kinase. If not prolonged, these changes are reversible and completely repaired, often leading the muscle to be stronger.

It is hypothesized that if damage occurs daily due to work activity, the muscle may not be able to repair the damage as fast as it occurs, leading to chronic muscle damage or dysfunction. The mechanism of this damage at the cellular level is not understood. Work activities that lead to sustained relatively low-level muscle activity or higher-level muscular contractions may be a causal factor in some work-related musculoskeletal disorders.

### Nonoccupational Factors

In addition to occupational risk factors or exposures such as repetitive work, personal risk factors may influence the risk of developing these work-related disorders. For example, forceful repetitive activities such as wrist extension can occur in some recreational activities and contribute to the development of similar disorders. Personal risk factors, such as age, gender, and peak muscle strength, may contribute to the development of work-related disorders; however, those factors related to some specific disorders, such as rotator cuff tendinitis, have not been adequately studied to identify these.

The nonoccupational factors for CTS that have been most thoroughly studied include coexisting medical conditions, such as rheumatoid arthritis, diabetes mellitus, pregnancy, and acute trauma especially after Colles' fracture. Three additional possible nonoccupational risk factors are age, gender, and carpal tunnel size or shape. Carpal canal size, both small and large, has been proposed as a risk factor based on limited evidence [54].

For nonoccupational CTS, men have increasing risk with age, while in women the risk peaks at approximately age 50 [55]. In contrast, both men and women may experience occupationally related CTS at an earlier age [47]. While most clinic- or community-based studies report three times as many CTS cases among women as among men, studies from workplaces do not tend to see this gender difference. In a study of occupational CTS in Washington state, based on the workers' compensation system, the female-male ratio was 1.2 : 1 [47]. Few if any personal factors are useful and strong predictors of susceptibility to work-related disorders of the upper extremity.

### Psychosocial Factors

In addition to the physical factors described, psychosocial factors may be important in both the initial development of these disorders and the subsequent long-term disability that sometimes occurs. Few studies have rigorously investigated both psychosocial and physical factors, and their combined effects [56]. Psychosocial factors as they relate to musculoskeletal disorders may range from personality factors to the way in which work is organized. The effects of psychosocial factors may operate indirectly by altering muscle tension or other physiologic processes and through the latter may also influence the perception of pain [57]. Psychological factors may be particularly important in determining whether specific musculoskeletal disorders evolve into chronic pain syndromes. Overall, psychosocial factors appear to be more important in disorders of the neck/shoulder muscles than in tendon-related disorders of the forearm and the hand [58].

Studies that have addressed psychosocial factors have often used the demand-control-support model originally introduced by Karasek and Theorell [59]. In this model, high levels of psychological job demands may contribute to the development of work-related musculoskeletal disorders when they occur in an occupational setting where the worker has little ability to decide what to do and how to do a particular job task, and little opportunity to use or develop job skills. Further, these adverse effects are hypothesized to occur more frequently in a work environment where there is little social support from coworkers or supervisors. Nonoccupational psychosocial factors could also be important. Further studies are needed to better understand the complex interrelationships between physical occupational factors and occupational psychosocial factors.

A model has been developed to incorporate both physical and psychosocial factors in the development of work-related musculoskeletal disorders (Fig. 23-7). Exposures may be either to physical work factors or psychosocial factors. Dose

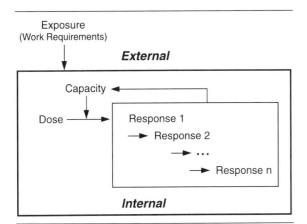

Exposure
(Work Requirements)

**External**

Capacity

Dose

Response 1

Response 2

...

Response n

**Internal**

Fig. 23-7. The proposed model contains sets of cascading exposure, dose, capacity, and response variables, such that the response at one level can act as a dose at the next level. In addition, the response to one or more doses can diminish (impairment) or increase (adaptation) the capacity for responding to successive doses.

also could be either physiologically or psychologically defined. Capacity could be either physiologically defined, such as strength of a specific tendon, or psychologically defined, such as the level of self-esteem. The internal processes resulting from a specific dose could occur in the spinal neural circuits or in the muscles of the forearm.

In summary, excessive repetitive or forceful motions, high levels of mechanical stress, work in static or awkward postures, and the use of vibrating power tools singularly or more frequently in combination can cause inflammation and chronic localized pain in the upper limb and neck. Precise dose-response relationships have not been developed for these risk factors and the precise role of the psychosocial factors needs to be further elucidated. At present it appears that when the exposure to several physical factors is high, then the risk of these disorders is substantially increased. When the level of exposure to physical factors is more moderate, then the overall level of risk may appear to be more dependent on the combination of personal attributes, physical factors, and psy-

chosocial factors. As with any occupational exposure, the risks will also depend somewhat on nonoccupational factors.

## Diagnosis

This broad group of work-related disorders of the neck and upper extremity has a diverse set of symptoms and physical findings. The evaluation of a patient for a suspected work-related disorder should have two major components: history of present illness and the work setting, and physical examination of the upper extremity and the neck [60].

The *history* of the present illness should fully characterize the symptoms by determining the location, radiation, duration, evolution, and exacerbating factors. An employee description of work activities is useful. The worker should describe the nature of his or her specific work tasks by risk factors (forceful exertions, repetitive activities, and other adverse exposures). For example, a worker who for 8 hours a day uses a vibrating hand tool during a repetitive task that is repeated every 30 seconds may be at high risk for wrist tendinitis. Similarly, a repetitive job that requires the arms to be elevated overhead during most of the work shift may increase the risk of a rotator cuff shoulder tendinitis. Because specific job tasks can vary within even a high-risk occupation, a careful history of specific job tasks is important.

When a worker who has been performing the same job for a considerable time period develops a disorder, the history should be directed not only at the chronic stable exposures but also at the acute factors. For example, if the worker uses a power screwdriver, perhaps the symptoms started when using screws from a "bad" batch that required more force for proper insertion. Other common acute risk factors are changes in work pace or length (i.e., longer or more frequent overtime either by lengthening the normal workday or by decreasing the number of days off), reducing the opportunity for recovery from fatigue and occult injury.

Despite the conscientious efforts of the employee and careful interviewing by the physician, description of work tasks may not be sufficient. In general, direct observation of the work process will provide the most accurate description of the risk factors associated with specific job tasks. In addition to visiting the workplace, the review of representative videotapes of job tasks, written description of job tasks based on industrial engineering data, and the results of ergonomic job analyses can all provide helpful information. While direct observation of the work is often required to determine with precision the level of risk factor exposure in specific job tasks, descriptions by workers will often identify many high-risk exposures with sufficient accuracy for a correct diagnosis.

Determining whether the patient has a predisposing medical condition such as a prior injury to the symptomatic area is also important. For example, in a study of all of the cases of CTS in Rochester, Minnesota, from 1961 through 1980 the following conditions were associated with CTS in more than 4 percent of the cases: Colles' fracture, other acute trauma, collagen vascular disease, arthritis of the wrist including rheumatoid arthritis, hormonal agents or oophorectomy, diabetes mellitus, and pregnancy [61]. Nonoccupational exposure to risk factors can be a potential confounding influence and should be elicited during the patient interview. For these nonoccupational exposures to be significant as causal factors they will need to be similar in intensity and frequency to the known occupational exposures.

Surveillance and epidemiologic studies have identified several industries and occupations associated with risks of CTS or other work-related musculoskeletal disorders. Being aware of these will alert physicians to the industries and occupations in which adverse exposures are more common. A few illustrative industries and occupations are listed in Table 23-4.

Finally, clinical experience, surveillance, and epidemiologic research suggest that many jobs with substantial exposure may adversely affect closely related muscles, tendons, or joints at the same time. As a result, workers in these high-risk jobs may present with one of several disorders such as carpal tunnel syndrome or de Quervain's disease.

The *physical examination* is an important part of the patient evaluation with work-related musculoskeletal disorders. An examination of the upper extremity typically involves inspection, palpation, assessment of the range of motion, evaluation of peripheral nerve function, and applicable provocative maneuvers of the upper extremity such as Phalen's test (Fig. 23-8).

One of the main objectives of the physical examination is to determine the precise structure(s) in the upper extremity that are the anatomic source of the symptoms. Numbness and paresthesias often result from peripheral nerve compression. Increased pain on resisted movements such as resisted wrist extension often result from inflammation of a tendon. While in a minority of cases it will not be possible to determine the precise source of the pain in the upper extremity, in the majority of cases it should be possible to determine the specific disorder that is present such as CTS or de Quervain's stenosing tenosynovitis. The severity of these disorders ranges from very mild with no significant impairment of the ability to work to very severe. The symptoms and physical signs of several of these disorders are described in the Chapter Appendix [62].

In addition to the disorders with specific findings on physical examination, workers in certain occupations (for example, keyboard operators, musicians, and newspaper reporters) often have an elevated rate of complaints of pain in the upper extremity or neck. These symptoms are similar to those of low back pain because a specific anatomic source of this pain often cannot readily be identified on clinical evaluation. As with low back pain, these pains are common, often intermittent in nature, and sometimes lead to substantial disability and impairment [52].

The diagnosis of a work-related musculoskeletal disorder is based on a three-step process. First is

**Table 23-4.** Illustrative examples of industries and occupations with high-risk job tasks

| Occupations and Industries | Disorders |
|---|---|
| OCCUPATIONS | |
| Seafood packers | Carpal tunnel syndrome [47] |
| Carpenters | Carpal tunnel syndrome [47] |
| Meat, poultry dealers | Carpal tunnel syndrome, other cumulative trauma disorders [47, 71] |
| Metal platers | Carpal tunnel syndrome [54] |
| Invasive cardiologists (removal of intra-aortic balloon) | Carpal tunnel syndrome [72] |
| Sausage makers | Epicondylitis [41] |
| Furniture packers | Carpal tunnel syndrome [73] |
| Dentists | Cervical spondylosis [74] |
| Rockblasters | Shoulder tendinitis [75] |
| Data-entry operators | Tension neck syndrome [74] |
| Instrumental musicians | Focal dystonias, overuse syndromes [75] |
| INDUSTRIES | |
| Pottery manufacturing | Various cumulative trauma disorders [71] |
| Mailing/addressing companies | |
| Hosiery manufacturing | |
| Meat and poultry slaughtering/ processing | Various cumulative trauma disorders [46] |
| Motor vehicle manufacturing | |
| Knit underwear mills | |
| Men's/boys' clothing manufacturing | |
| Motorcycles, bicycles, and parts manufacturing | |
| Luggage manufacturing | |
| Electrical engine equipment | |
| Household appliance manufacturing | |

the determination of whether the patient has a specific disorder such as flexor tendinitis of the forearm. This is usually based on the history and physical examination.

Second, there should be evidence from a detailed occupational history or, better yet, from direct observation of the workplace of substantial exposure to specific occupational risk factors. Analysis of health surveillance data such as Occupational Safety and Health Administration (OSHA) logs or workers' compensation records from the specific workplace may be particularly helpful in confirming that a specific job is associated with an ele-

vated risk of a work-related musculoskeletal disorder. Some employers, to facilitate return-to-work evaluations, will now provide physicians with a videotape of the job that the worker normally performs. This may be useful in determining the approximate level of exposure.

Third, nonoccupational causes should be considered as possible primary causal factors or as extenuating factors based on the history and physical examination. Review and analysis of the surveillance and epidemiologic studies of similar work may provide information on the relative contribution of occupational factors compared to non-

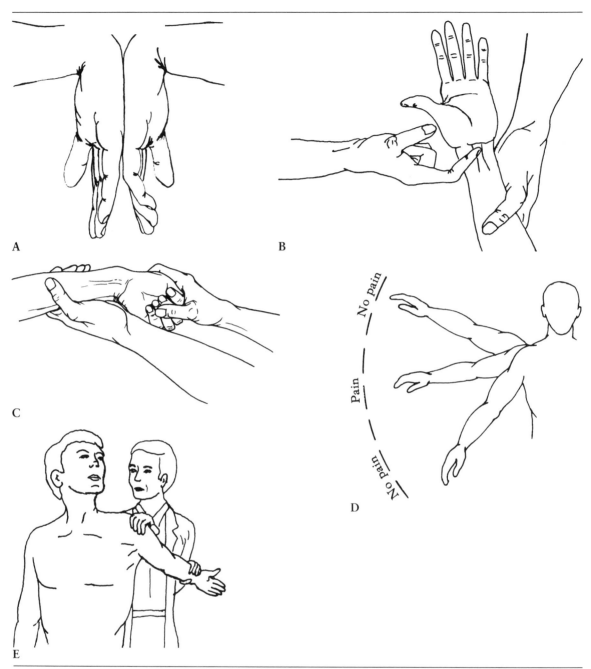

**Fig. 23-8.** A. Phalen's wrist flexion test for carpal tunnel syndrome. The results are positive if numbness and/or tingling occurs in the fingers within one minute. B. Tinel's sign for carpal tunnel syndrome. A light tapping elicits numbness and/or tingling in the fingers. C. Finkelstein's test for de Quervain's disease. Sharp pain around radial styloid and forearm, not just a pulling sensation. D. A painful arc is often seen with rotator tendinitis, particularly of the supraspinatus tendon. E. Adson's test for thoracic outlet syndrome. Obtain a radial pulse and have the patient cock the head and take a deep breath. A positive test is a diminished pulse and symptoms in the fingers. (Drawings by Mary Weed, Audiovisual Department, School of Public Health, University of Michigan, Ann Arbor, MI 48109-2029.)

occupational factors in the causation of a specific work-related musculoskeletal disorder in the patient's selected occupation and industry (Table 23-4). With the exception of the use of diagnostic tests for abnormalities in nerve conduction, elaborate diagnostic or laboratory studies are often not necessary unless the patient has a history of past trauma or symptoms suggestive of underlying systemic disease.

The most difficult part of the diagnosis of work-related musculoskeletal disorder is to determine the relative contribution of occupational factors to the etiology of the disorder. As with other diagnostic evaluation of work-relatedness, the critical question is whether the exposure has been of sufficient intensity, frequency, and duration. Because intense periods of high exposure as short as weeks in duration can cause carpal tunnel syndrome or other work-related musculoskeletal disorders, attention should be directed at estimating the intensity and frequency of exposure. It is not uncommon for exposure to occur to multiple risk factors at the same time, such as repetitive and forceful exertions of the hands or shoulder abduction and exposure to vibration from hand tools. Unfortunately, there are no simple rules of how to assess whether exposure has been of sufficient intensity and frequency to cause a disorder.

One study of CTS was based on cases referred for an independent medical examination for both diagnostic evaluation and determination of work-relatedness. The investigators used typical workers' compensation criteria and a standardized approach to assess exposure (frequently based on plant visits or review of videotape) and reported that approximately 60 percent of the confirmed CTS cases were work-related [63]. Fifteen percent of the patients were found not to have CTS but to have a different work-related disorder of the upper limb such as localized muscle "fatigue/myalgias," while an additional 21 percent had non-work-related disorders. This study emphasizes the need for thorough diagnostic evaluation to identify the specific disorder, and to assess exposure as carefully as is possible.

Conceptually, these work-related upper-limb disorders have some of the characteristics both of occupational and of work-related diseases as defined by the World Health Organization (WHO) (see box on p. 58). Because with high exposure the risk of disease can be quite high (i.e., a clear direct relationship between exposure and disease), even in these situations the physical signs and pathologic characteristics of the work-related and non-work-related cases will often be similar, in contrast to classic occupational diseases such as asbestosis or lead poisoning, which have clinically distinct features.

## Treatment and Prognosis

The goals of treatment are elimination or reduction in symptoms and impairment, and returning the employee to work under conditions that will protect his or her health. These goals can be most easily achieved by early and conservative treatment. Treatment of work-related musculoskeletal disorders early in the course has several advantages. The treatment is less difficult and costly. Surgical procedures can be avoided, periods of absence from work or stressful exposures will be shorter, and the effectiveness of treatment is greater [64, 65].

Since inflammation or nerve compression is the most common underlying cause of the symptoms of work-related musculoskeletal disorders, treatment is usually directed at two goals: to reduce inflammation or nerve compression, and to assist in the repair of any tissue damage. Symptomatic relief is provided by (1) the use of anti-inflammatory medications, (2) rest (sometimes facilitated by splints), and (3) application of heat or cold. Physical therapy techniques are used to assist in symptom relief, to ensure normal joint motion (stretching), and to recondition muscles after periods of rest or reduced use. If these more conservative measures fail to reduce symptoms and impairment for some conditions such as CTS, steroid injections or surgical treatments can be helpful [66]. Surgery, even in CTS, may be ineffective if the worker is returned to the old job without an effort to reduce the occupational exposures that were present. Since few scientifically valid studies have evaluated the long-term effectiveness of the treatment of the work-related musculoskeletal disorders of the limb and neck, an empirical approach is indicated.

Resting the symptomatic part of the upper extremity is the most important part of the treatment program. It can be achieved by reducing or eliminating worker exposure to the known risk factors. In addition to engineering changes, restricted duty, job rotation, or temporary transfer may be effective. In order for job transfer or rotation to be effective, the new job duties have to result in a net reduction in the level of exposure. Conducting an evaluation of the new duties to determine if a reduction in exposure will occur is often necessary. The magnitude of reduction in exposure required to facilitate recovery is often not known. In general, the more severe the disorder the greater the reduction in magnitude and duration will probably be required. Because of the adverse consequences of complete removal from the work environment, this should be used only in severe cases or when less drastic measures have failed.

Splints and other immobilization devices may provide rest to the symptomatic region. However, they may increase the level of exposure if the worker must resist the device in order to carry out regular job tasks. Such would occur on a job that required frequent wrist flexion while wearing neutral position wrist splints for CTS. Workers may also alter their work activities to adapt to wearing a splint in a way that leads to substantial stress on another region of the upper extremity such as the elbow or shoulder. Immobilization or prolonged rest may have direct adverse effects if either leads to muscle atrophy. As a result, careful monitoring of the worker who is on restricted duty, job transfer, or wearing an immobilization device is indicated. In addition, since it is difficult to predict the clinical course of these conditions and the empiri-

cal basis of many of the treatments for these disorders, frequent follow-up is desirable. Failure of the treatment plan to provide improvement over several weeks should lead to thorough re-evaluation of the treatment plan and its underlying assumptions. Many of these conditions will resolve within a few weeks with early treatment. The prognosis in general is good with early treatment and reduction in exposure.

Sometimes CTS and the other conditions of the upper extremity follow a course similar to that of chronic severe low back pain cases. With conservative treatment and appropriate adjustments in the work setting, the vast majority of cases should improve enough that the worker can successfully return to work, while a small minority of cases become chronic and very difficult to treat successfully with conventional approaches. In these severe cases of work-related disorders of the back and upper limb, the role of the physical capabilities of the worker, work demands, and psychosocial factors related both to the worker and the employer are all important in determining whether a worker successfully returns to work [67]. The ways in which these factors interact with each other are likely complex. The recognition that psychosocial factors such as job satisfaction or negative self-fulfilling beliefs by the patient, employer, or health care providers are important should not lead to ignoring the role of occupational physical exposures or "blaming of the victim" [68]. If the latter occurs, delayed recovery is often attributed to personal weakness, low job satisfaction, or desire for secondary gain [69]. Critical to the prevention of these severe chronic cases is early intervention, one reason that it is important to eliminate barriers to early reporting of symptoms.

It is increasingly recognized that comprehensive approaches that directly address all facets of the patient's situation may prove the most effective in returning the patient to work and reducing future impairment. As a consequence there has been a rapid development of comprehensive programs that ideally address the physical reconditioning of the worker, the psychosocial factors, and workplace factors such as ongoing exposure [67, 69].

The diagnosis and treatment of severe or chronic work-related musculoskeletal disorders is challenging. The identification of the level of exposure by patient history is difficult and usually direct observation of work is the preferred approach. There is substantial uncertainty about how to best measure exposure in some occupational settings especially in the office. There is a danger of both overdiagnosis and underdiagnosis, for example, assuming either that every case of CTS is work-related or that no case of CTS is work-related. Not only is the assessment of exposure difficult, but the scientific understanding of the exposure-disease relationship is still limited and imprecise. The danger exists of not recognizing when a case is becoming chronic and severe and when a multidisciplinary approach should be considered. Several observations are helpful when one is faced with challenges of diagnosing and treating these work-related conditions. A careful history and physical examination are important. An extensive objective assessment of the work environment may be required. In most cases, conservative treatment that preserves normal physical conditioning, that relies on a reduction of the level of occupational exposure while the patient remains at work, and that incorporates careful monitoring of the patient is a reasonable initial approach and is effective.

Prevention of these disorders requires the successful identification and remediation of adverse exposures.

## Preventive Strategy

Preventive strategy, largely experience-based, has not been comprehensively evaluated by scientific studies. The principles outlined below must be adapted to fit the specific characteristics of each working environment. They should be viewed as a guide rather than a blueprint, requiring ongoing scientific evaluation [70].

Three standard preventive strategies can be considered: (1) a reduction of the exposure to suspected occupational risk factors such as vibrating hand tools, (2) a conditioning process that increases the tolerance of workers to the suspected occupational risk factors, or (3) development of a replacement process that is highly predictive and reliable to identify those persons at unusually high risk of developing an upper-extremity disorder. The remainder of this chapter discusses the first strategy in detail. Before this discussion, however, brief comment is in order for the other two strategies.

Development of a replacement process is the least desirable of these strategies because there are no scientifically valid screening procedures to identify those persons at high risk of developing CTS, and this shifts the cost of reducing the incidence of symptoms onto the workers, who are denied employment or placement, and increases the cost of the hiring and replacement processes.

The second approach, a conditioning process that provides a period of time during which workers can gradually adapt their muscles and tendons to the new demands on them could be a useful approach for those persons in forceful- or repetitive-action jobs. Training of new workers in the most efficient and least stressful way of performing their jobs may also be useful, provided that the work tasks can be done in alternate ways, which are *both* less stressful and at least as fast. Similarly, workers with symptoms may, with training, be able to adapt an equally efficient, but less stressful, work method. Training activities have not been evaluated specifically. Several employers, perceiving long-term benefits in the "phasing-in period," have established transitional or training areas where employees may work at a reduced pace for a limited time.

Reduction in exposures, the standard preventive approach that directs attention to control of occupational factors, has the most promise. This approach often requires changes in the workstation, work process, or use of tools. Sometimes administrative changes, such as work restrictions, the use of personal protective equipment (for example, palm pads), or job rotation are useful alternatives. Job rotation of work requiring different types of motions of the upper extremity, however, may simply expose a larger number of workers to a considerable degree of risk.

To reduce exposure, the first step required for instituting changes in workstations or work processes is to analyze the specific characteristics of suspected high-risk jobs. While the job review can be conducted by an industrial engineer or occupational health professional with training in ergonomics, the involvement of those persons most knowledgeable about the job is important. Experience has shown that not only can operators and supervisors with limited technical training successfully identify many of the hazardous aspects of a specific job, but also specific solutions may not be effective or accepted without their involvement in the job review and the development of solutions.

## Reducing Exposure to Risk Factors

A job analysis performed on the patient with the spot welding job in the case at the start of this section would have identified several exposure factors. The job was repetitive and required forceful gripping of the handles of the welding gun. The wrists were extended through most of the job cycle.

After a job analysis has identified the potentially hazardous exposures associated with a specific job, specific solutions should be solicited from those knowledgeable about the job. With limited training in the control principles (discussed in the next section), engineers, production employees, and frontline supervisors often propose the most useful methods for eliminating hazardous risk factors. If several factors are present, it can be difficult to determine which is the most detrimental. Where possible, integrated solutions should be developed that reduce multiple risk factors at the same time.

Control of repetitiveness, forcefulness, awkward posture, mechanical stress, vibration, and cold are often possible, as illustrated below.

### Control of Repetitiveness
1. Use mechanical assists and other types of automation. For example, in packing operations, one can use a device, rather than the hands, to transfer parts.
2. Rotate workers between jobs that require different types of motions. Rotation must be viewed as a temporary administrative control, one used only until a more permanent solution can be found.
3. Implement horizontal work enlargement by adding different elements or steps to a job, particularly steps that do not require the same motions as the current work cycle.
4. Increase work allowances or decrease production standards. This control strategy is rarely looked on favorably by management.
5. Design a tool for use in either hand and also so that fingers are not used for triggering motions.

### Control of Forcefulness
1. Decrease the weight held in the hand by providing adjustable fixtures to hold parts being worked on. Many conventional balancers are available to neutralize tool weight. Articulating arms are being used in many plants to hold and manipulate heavy tools into awkward positions.
2. Control torque reaction force in power hand tools by using torque reaction bars, torque-absorbing overhead balancers, and mounted nut-holding devices. Control the time that a worker is exposed to torque reaction by using shut-off rather than stall power tools. Avoid jerky motions by handheld tools.
3. Design jobs so that a power grip rather than a pinch can be used whenever possible. (Maximum voluntary contraction in a power grip is approximately three times greater than in a pinch.)
4. Increase the coefficient of friction on hand tools to reduce slipperiness, for example, by plastic

sleeves that can be slipped over metal handles of tools.

5. Design jobs so that slides or hoists are used to move parts to reduce the amount of handling or carrying of parts by the worker.

### Control of Awkward Posture

The primary method for reducing awkward postures is to design adjustability of position into the job. Wrist, elbow, and shoulder postures required on a job are often determined by the height of the work surface with respect to the location of the worker. A tall worker may use less wrist flexion or ulnar deviation than a shorter worker. Additionally, awkward postures can be reduced by doing the following:

1. Altering the location or method of the work. For example, in automotive assembly operations, changing the line location where a part is installed may result in easier access.
2. Redesigning tools or changing the type of tool used. For example, when wrist flexion occurs with a piston-shaped tool that is used on a horizontal surface, correction may involve using an in-line type tool or lowering the workstation.
3. Altering the orientation of the work.
4. Avoiding job tasks that require shoulder abduction or forward flexion greater than 30 to 45 degrees, elbow flexion greater than 110 degrees, wrist flexion or extension greater than 30 to 45 degrees, and neck flexion greater than 20 degrees or frequent neck rotation.
5. Provide support for the forearm when precise finger motions are required to reduce static muscle loading in the arm and shoulder girdle.

### Control of Vibration

1. Do not use impact wrenches and piercing hammers.
2. Use balancers, isolators, and damping materials.
3. Use handle coatings that attenuate vibrations and increase the coefficient of friction to reduce strength requirements.

### Control of Mechanical Stress

1. Round or flare the edges of sharp objects, such as guards and container edges.
2. Use different types of palm button guards, which allow room for the operator to use the button without contact with the guard.
3. Use palm pads, which may provide some protection until tools can be developed to eliminate hand hammering.
4. Use compliant cushioning material on handles or increase the length of the handles to cause the force to dissipate over a greater surface of the hand.
5. Use different-sized tools for different-sized hands.
6. Avoid narrow tool handles that concentrate large forces onto small areas of the hand.

### Control of Cold and Use of Gloves

1. Properly maintain power tool air hoses to eliminate cold exhaust air leaks onto the workers' hands or arms.
2. Provide a variety of styles and sizes of gloves to ensure proper fit of gloves. While gloves may protect the hands from cold exposures, they often decrease grip strength (requiring more forceful exertion), decrease tactile sensitivity, decrease manipulative ability, increase space requirements, and increase the risk of becoming caught in moving parts.
3. Cover only that part of the hand that is necessary for protection. Examples include using safety tape for the finger tips with fingerless gloves and palm pads for the palm.

In summary, together work-related low back pain and disorders of the upper extremity are among the most common occupational health problems. Although scientific knowledge often limits our ability to determine precisely the role of occupational and nonoccupational factors in the diagnosis of these conditions, substantial progress can be made in reducing the severity of these disorders by applying the existing knowledge about the role of physical factors in these disorders, such as forceful repetitive hand work and frequent lifting of heavy objects. Work should be designed to reduce exposure to the known physical risk factors. Encouraging prompt and appropriately conservative medical evaluation of workers with these disorders can contribute to secondary prevention. Finally, for the minority of workers with these disorders who do not respond to conservative treatment including reduction in the level of exposure, it is likely that treatment programs that address all aspects of the problem—both the psychosocial and physical—have the greatest chance of preventing the permanent disability from these disorders.

# References

1. American Academy of Orthopaedic Surgeons. Musculoskeletal conditions in the United States. Park Ridge, IL: AAOS, 1992.
2. Andersson GBJ. Epidemiology of spinal disorders. In JW Frymoyer. ed. The adult spine. New York: Raven Press, 1991, pp. 241–74.
3. Pope MH, Andersson GBJ, Frymoyer JW, Chaffin DB. Occupational low back pain: Assessment, treatment and prevention. St. Louis: Mosby–Year Book, 1991, pp. 1–325.
4. Frymoyer J. The adult spine: Principles and practice. New York: Raven Press, 1991.
5. Spitzer WO, et al. Scientific approach to the assessment and management of activity-related spinal disorders: A monograph for clinicians. Report of the Quebec Task Force on Spinal Disorders. Spine 1987; 12:S1–S59.
6. Andersson GBJ. Epidemiologic aspects of low back pain in industry. Spine 1981; 6:53–60.
7. Klein BP, Jensen RC, Sanderson LM. Assessment of workers' compensation claims for back strains/sprains. J Occup Med 1984; 26:433–8.
8. Frymoyer JW, Pope MH. Epidemiologic insight into the relationship between usage and back disorder. In NH Hadler. ed. Current concepts in regional musculoskeletal illness. Orlando: Grune & Stratton, 1987, pp. 263–79.
9. Chaffin DB, Herrin GD, Keyserling WM. Preemployment strength testing: An updated position. J Occup Med 1978; 20:403–8.
10. Kelsey JL. An epidemiological study of acute herniated lumbar intervertebral discs. Rheumatol Rehab 1975; 14:144–59.
11. Kelsey JL, et al. Acute prolonged lumbar interver-

12. tebral disc. An epidemiologic study with special reference to driving automobiles and cigarette smoking. Spine 1984; 9:608–13.
12. Magora A. Investigation of the relation between low back pain and occupation. Ind Med Surg 1972; 41:5–9.
13. Keyserling WM, Punnett L, Fine LJ. Postural stress of the trunk and shoulders: Identification and control of occupational risk factors. In Ergonomic interventions to prevent musculoskeletal injuries in industry. Chelsea MI: Lewis, 1987, pp. 11–26.
14. Bigos SJ, Battie MC. Risk factors for industrial back problems. Semin Spine Surg 1992; 4:2–11.
15. Svensson H-O, Andersson GBJ. Low back pain in forty to forty-seven year old men: Work history and work environment factors. Spine 1983; 8:272.
16. Svensson H-O, Andersson GBJ. The relationship of low-back pain, work history, work environment, and stress: A retrospective cross-sectional study of 38 to 64 year old women. Spine 1989; 14:517–22.
17. Frymoyer JW, et al. Epidemiologic studies of low back pain. Spine 1980; 5:419–23.
18. Chaffin DB, Park KS. A longitudinal study of low-back pain as associated with occupational weight lifting factors. Ind Hyg Assoc J 1973; 34:513–25.
19. Snook SH, Campanelli RA, Hart JW. A study of three preventive approaches to low back injury. J Occup Med 1978; 20:478–81.
20. Snook SH. Low back pain in industry. In AA White, SL Gordon. eds. Symposium on idiopathic low back pain. St. Louis: Mosby, 1982, pp. 23–8.
21. Kelsey JL, et al. An epidemiologic study of lifting and twisting on the job and risk for acute prolapsed lumbar intervertebral disc. J Orthop Res 1984; 2:61–6.
22. Kelsey JL, Hardy RJ. Driving of motor vehicles as a risk factor for acute herniated lumbar intervertebral disc. Am J Epidemiol 1975; 102:63.
23. Heliovaara M. Occupation and risk of herniated lumbar intervertebral disc or sciatica leading to hospitalization. J Chron Dis 1987; 3:259–64.
24. Bigos SJ, et al. Back injuries in industry: A retrospective study. III. Employee-related factors. Spine 1986; 11:252–6.
25. Deyo RA, Diehl AK, Rosenthal M. How many days of bed rest for acute low back pain? A randomized clinical trial. N Engl J Med 1986; 315:1064–70.
26. Deyo RA. Conservative therapy for low back pain: Distinguishing useful from useless therapy. JAMA 1983; 25:1057.
27. Weber H. Lumbar disk herniation: A controlled, perspective study with ten years of observation. Spine 1983; 8:131–40.

28. Dillane JB, Fry J, Kalton G. Acute back syndrome: A study from general practice. Br Med J 1966; 2:82–4.
29. McGill CM. Industrial back problems: A control program. J Occup Med 1968; 10:174–8.
30. Battie MC. Minimizing the impact of back pain: Workplace strategies. Semin Spine Surg 1992; 4:20–8.
31. U.S. Department of Health and Human Services. Work practices guide for manual lifting. Washington, D.C.: Department of Health and Human Services, 1981. (NIOSH) publication no. 81–122.
32. Snook SH. The design of manual handling tasks. Ergonomics 1978; 21:963–85.
33. Himmelstein JS, Andersson GBJ. Low back pain: Risk evaluation and preplacement screening. Occup Med, State of the Art Rev 1988; 3:255–69.
34. Biering-Sorensen F. Physical measurements as risk indicators for low-back trouble over a one-year period. Spine 1984; 9:106–19.
35. Bergquist-Ullman M, Larsson U. Acute low back pain in industry. Acta Orthop Scand 1977; Suppl. no. 170.
36. Fitzler SL, Berger RA. Attitudinal change: The Chelsea back program. Occup Health Saf February 1982, pp. 24–6.
37. Fitzler SL, Berger RA. Chelsea back program: One year later. Occup Health Saf July 1983, pp. 52–4.
38. Wiesel SW, Feffer HL, Rothman RH. Industrial low back pain: A prospective evaluation of a standardized diagnostic and treatment protocol. Spine 1984; 9:199.
39. Phalen G. The carpal tunnel syndrome. Clinical evaluation of 598 hands. Clin Orthop 1972; 83:29.
40. Finkelstein H. Stenosing tendovaginitis at the radial styloid process. J Bone Joint Surg 1930; 12:509–40.
41. Kruppa K, et al. Incidence of tenosynovitis or peritendinitis and epicondylitis in a meat-processing factory. Scand J Work Environ Health 1991; 17:32–7.
42. Bland D, et al. The painful shoulder. Semin Arthritis Rheum 1977; 7:1,21–47.
43. Waris P, et al. Epidemiologic screening of occupational neck and upper limb disorders. Scand J Work Environ Health 1979; 5(Suppl. 3):25.
44. Halder N, et al. Hand structure and function in an industrial setting. Arthritis Rheum 1978; 21:210–20.
45. Cargile CH. Raynaud's disease in stonecutters using pneumatic tools. JAMA 1915; 64:582.
46. Bureau of Labor Statistics, U.S. Department of Labor, November 1992.
47. Franklin GM, Haug J, Heyer N, Checkoway H. Occupational carpal tunnel syndrome in Washington state, 1984–1988. Am J Public Health 1991; 81: 741–6.
48. Liss GM, Armstrong C, Kusiak RA, Gailitis MM. Use of provincial health insurance plan billing data to estimate carpal tunnel syndrome morbidity and surgery rates. Am J Ind Med 1992; 22:395–409.
49. Tanaka S, et al. Prevalence and work-relatedness of self-reported carpal tunnel syndrome in the United States—An analysis of 1988 National Health Interview Survey Data. Am J Public Health (in press).
50. Moore JS. Carpal tunnel syndrome. Occup Med 1992; 7:741–63.
51. Kelly WN, Harris ED, Ruddy S, Sledge CG. Textbook of rheumatology. Philadelphia: Saunders, 1981. Vol. 2.
52. Lockwood AH. Medical problems of musicians. N Engl J Med 1989; 320:221–7.
53. Armstrong TJ, et al. A conceptual model for work-related neck and upper-limb musculoskeletal disorders. Scand J Work Environ Health 1993; 19:73–84.
54. Hagberg M, Morgenstern H, Kelsh M. Impact of occupations and job tasks on the prevalence of carpal tunnel syndrome. Scand J Work Environ Health 1992; 18:337–45.
55. Stevens JC, et al. Carpal tunnel syndrome in Rochester, Minnesota. 1961 to 1980. Neurology 1988; 38:134–8.
56. Theorell T, Harms-Ringdahl K, Ahlberg-Hulten G, Westin B. Psychosocial job factors and symptoms from the locomotor system—a multi-causal analysis. Scand J Rehab Med 1991; 23:165–73.
57. Theorell T, Nordemar R, Michelsen H, Stockholm Music Study Group. Pain thresholds during standardized psychological stress in relation to perceived psychosocial work situation. J Psychosom Res 1993; 37:299–305.
58. Bongers PM, de Winter CR. Psychosocial factors and musculoskeletal disease. Mimeograph. Netherlands Institut Voor Praeventieve Gerzondheidszorg TNO, 1992.
59. Karasek RA, Theorell T. Healthy work. New York: Basic Books, 1990.
60. ANSI Z-365. Control of cumulative trauma disorders. Draft June 4, 1993.
61. Stevens JC, et al. Conditions associated with carpal tunnel syndrome. Mayo Clin Proc 1992; 67:541–8.
62. Silverstein BA, Fine LJ. Evaluation of upper extremity and low back cumulative trauma disorders: A screening manual. Ann Arbor: University of Michigan, 1984.
63. Moore JS. Clinical determination of work-related-

ness in carpal tunnel syndrome. J Occup Rehab 1991; 1:145–58.

64. Hales TR, Bertsche PK. Management of upper extremity cumulative trauma disorders. AAOHN 1992; 40:118–28.

65. Rempel DM, Harrison RJ, Barnhardt S. Work-related cumulative trauma disorders of the upper extremity. JAMA 1992; 267:838–42.

66. American Academy of Orthopaedic Surgeons. Clinical Policies—Carpal Tunnel Syndrome. July 11–13, 1991.

67. Feurstein M. A multi-disciplinary approach to the prevention, evaluation and management of work disability. J Occup Rehab 1991; 1:5–12.

68. Niemeyer LO. Social labeling, stereotyping, and observer bias in workers' compensation: The impact of provider-patient interaction on outcome. J Occup Rehab 1991; 1:251–67.

69. Parenmark G, Malmkvist AK. The effect of an outpatient rehabilitation program on occupational cervicobrachial disorders. J Occup Rehab 1992; 2:67–72.

70. Silverstein B, Fine LJ, Armstrong TJ. Carpal tunnel syndrome: Causes and a preventive strategy. Semin Occup Med 1986; 1:213–21.

71. Brogmus GF, Marko R. Cumulative trauma disorders of the upper extremities: The magnitude of the problem in U.S. industry. In W Karwowski, JW Yates. eds. Advances in industrial ergonomics and safety III. Philadelphia: Taylor and Francis, 1991, pp. 95–102.

72. Stevens K. The carpal tunnel syndrome in cardiologists (letter). Ann Intern Med 1990; 112:796.

73. Loslever P, Ranaivosoa A. Biomechanical and epidemiological investigation of carpal tunnel syndrome at workplaces with high risk factors. Ergonomics 1993; 36:537–54.

74. Hagberg M, Wegman DH. Prevalence rates and odds ratios of shoulder-neck diseases in different occupational groups. Br J Ind Med 1987; 44:602–10.

75. Stenlund B, Goldie I, Hagberg M, Hogstedt C. Shoulder tendinitis and its relation to heavy manual work and exposure to vibration. Scand J Work Environ Health 1993; 19:43–9.

## Bibliography

Armstrong TJ, Silverstein BA. Upper-extremity pain in the workplace, role of usage in causality. In MM Hadler. ed. Clinical concepts in regional musculoskeletal illness. New York: Grune & Stratton, 1987. Chap. 19.
*This chapter provides the clearest delineation of the association of upper-extremity disorders with work exposures.*

Cailliet R. Hand pain and impairment. 2nd ed. Philadelphia: Davis, 1981.
*A good introductory text with excellent illustrations.*

Deyo RA. Conservative therapy for low back pain: Distinguishing useful from useless therapy. JAMA 1983; 250:1057.
*Reviews the evidence supporting commonly used conservative therapies for low back pain. Methodologic criteria for validity and applicability were applied to 57 original articles describing trials of exercise, traction, use of corsets, bed rest, spinal manipulation, transcutaneous nerve stimulation, and drug therapy. The better studies are summarized with an indication of their design features and limitations.*

Nachemson A. Advances in low back pain. Clin Orthop 1985; 200:266.
*An objective and thorough review of current knowledge about low back pain. Topics include epidemiology, etiology, biomechanics, and treatment. Emphasis is placed on the benefits of patient education and motion, and the disadvantages of prolonged bed rest (inactivity) and repeat surgery.*

Quinet RJ, Hadler NM. Diagnosis and treatment of backache. Semin Arthritis Rheum 1979; 8:261.
*A very comprehensive, objective, and well-written review of the etiology, diagnosis, and treatment of low back pain. The authors discuss traction, drugs, diathermy, heat, cold, manipulation, corsets, braces, injection therapy, exercises, chemonucleolysis, and surgery.*

Rempel DM, Harrison RJ, Barnhardt S. Work-related cumulative trauma disorders of the upper extremity. JAMA 1992; 267:838–42.
*A very concise summary of the causes, diagnosis, and principles of treatment for common work-related disorders of the upper extremity.*

Rowe ML. Backache at work. Fairport, NY: Perinton, 1983.
*Describes the results of a 20-year clinical study of low back pain at a large company. Included in the study are 1,500 cases. The effectiveness of current selection techniques in preventing low back pain is discussed. Emphasis is also placed on preventing the disability.*

Wiesel SW, Feffer HL, Rothman RH. Industrial low-back pain: A prospective evaluation of a standardized diagnostic and treatment protocol. Spine 1984; 9:199. *Describes a standardized approach to the diagnosis and treatment of low back pain in employees at a large company. Two orthopedic surgeons monitored the course and treatment of employee low back pain and intervened when they believed it necessary. The program dramatically decreased the number of patients sent to surgery.*

APPENDIX

## Work-Related Disorders of the Upper Extremities

| Disorder | History | Physical examination |
|---|---|---|
| WRIST | | |
| Carpal tunnel syndrome | Pain, tingling, or numbness in medial sensory distribution of the hand. Nocturnal exacerbation. Problems with dropping things. | Positive Phalen's test (see Fig. 23–8). Positive Tinel's test (see Fig. 23–8). Thenar atrophy in severe cases. Rule out pronator teres syndrome, cervical root syndrome. |
| de Quervain's disease | Pain in anatomic snuffbox. May radiate up forearm. No history of radial or wrist fracture. | Positive Finkelstein's test (see Fig. 23–8) with sharp pain rather than just pulling sensation. Rule out radial nerve entrapment. |
| Trigger finger | Finger locks in extension or flexion. Requires assistance in unlocking. Nodule or tendon. | Nodule at base of digit palpable. Locking on flexion or extension of digits. |
| Ulnar nerve compression (Guyon canal syndrome) | Burning, tingling, or numbness in fourth and fifth digits. Clumsiness in fine movements. | Positive Tinel's sign at Guyon canal. Positive Phalen's test in ulnar distribution. Decreased pinch strength. Weakness on resisted abduction and adduction of digits. Rule out cervical root disorder, thoracic outlet syndrome, cubital tunnel syndrome. |
| Tendinitis, tenosynovitis | Localized pain and swelling over muscle-tendon structure. | Pain exacerbated by resisted motions. Fine crepitus on passive range of motion (ROM) possible. No pain on passive ROM. Pronounced asymmetrical grip strength. |
| ELBOW/FOREARM | | |
| Lateral epicondylitis (tennis elbow) | Pain at lateral epicondyle during rest or active motion of wrists and fingers. | Pain on resisted extension of wrist with fingers flexed. No pain or limitation on full passive ROM. Pain at epicondyle on palpation. Pain on resisted radial deviation. Rule out radial nerve entrapment. |
| Medial epicondylitis (golfer's elbow) | Pain at medial epicondyle during rest or active motion of wrist and fingers. | No pain on passive ROM. Pain on resisted wrist flexion and resisted forearm pronation. Pain at medial epicondyle on palpation. |
| Olecranon bursitis | Pain and swelling at olecranon. | No pain on passive or resisted ROM. Swelling around olecranon on palpation. Rule out rheumatoid arthritis. |
| Pronator teres syndrome | Burning pain in first three digits of hand and forearm. | Increased pain in forearm by resisted pronation with clenched fist and flexed wrist (Mill's test). Sensory impairment of thenar eminence. Rule out carpal tunnel syndrome. |

**SHOULDER**

| | | |
|---|---|---|
| Rotator cuff tendinitis (mainly supraspinatus) | Dull ache generally localized to deltoid area without neck or arm radiation. No symptoms of distal paresthesia. Nocturnal exacerbation. Subject may note "catch" on movement. | Diffuse tenderness over shoulder, especially over humeral head and lateral to acromion. If tenderness localized, it is most often over supraspinatus insertion. Weakness uncommon. *Supraspinatus:* Shrugs shoulder on abduction, painful arc at 70–90 degrees. Passive ROM normal. Pain on resisted abduction. *Infraspinatus:* Pain on resisted external rotation. Painful arc. Rule out rheumatoid arthritis. |
| Bicipital tenosynovitis | Pain localized to bicipital groove area; may radiate to anterior aspect of arm. No distal paresthesia. Nocturnal exacerbation. Subject able to use forearm when upper arm held against chest. Subject notes pain on abduction and rotation. | Positive Yergason's test (resisted supination), or positive Speed's test (resisted wrist flexion). Normal passive and active ROM. |
| Degenerative joint disease—acromioclavicular joint | Generalized aching shoulder pain exacerbated by motion. Least difficulty in morning but worse as day progresses. | Limitation is similar on active and passive ROM. Most discomfort is with mild abduction. Crepitus common. Tenderness on palpation directly over acromioclavicular articulation. Pain reproduced as arm abducted more than 90 degrees. Pain on shoulder shrug. |
| Degenerative joint disease—glenohumeral joint | Pain is very diffuse and nocturnal. | Tenderness to palpation along joint line. No deltoid or supraspinatus pain. Passive ROM full but painful. Active ROM retarded on flexion and extension. (Normal is 240 degrees in youth, 190 degrees at age 70. Normal abduction in youth is 166 degrees, 116 degrees at age 70.) |
| Thoracic outlet syndrome | Paresthesia usually in ulnar distribution of hand and arm. Pain and sensation of "weakness." Deep dull ache in arm and hand. Problem holding small objects. Nocturnal exacerbation common. | Positive Adson's test (see Fig. 23–8). Hyperabduction or costoclavicular test. Decreased grip strength. |

**NECK/SCAPULA**

| | | |
|---|---|---|
| Tension neck syndrome (costal-scapular syndrome) | Neck pain or stiffness. No history of herniated cervical disc, injury, or ankylosing spondylitis. | Muscle tightness, palpable hardening and tender spots. Pain on resisted neck lateral flexion and rotation. |
| Cervical root syndrome | Pain radiating from neck to one or both arms with numbness in hand(s). Exacerbated by cough. | Limited passive and active ROM. Radiating pain on passive motions. Positive foraminal test. Decreased pinprick in dermatome. Absence of joint findings. |

# 24
# Skin Disorders

Kenneth A. Arndt, Michael Bigby, and Serge A. Coopman

Any cutaneous abnormality or inflammation caused directly or indirectly by the work environment is an occupational skin disorder. Work-related cutaneous reactions and clinical syndromes are as varied as the environments in which people work. Skin disorders are the most frequently reported occupational diseases. A basic understanding of occupational skin disorders is therefore essential for everyone involved in occupational health.

An occupational skin injury is defined as an immediate adverse effect on the skin that results from instantaneous trauma or brief exposure to toxic agents involving a single incident in the work environment [1]. Occupational skin injuries account for 23 to 35 percent of all occupational injuries. Based on data collected in 1983 by the Bureau of Labor Statistics, it was estimated that the annual incidence of occupational skin injuries was 1.4 to 2.2 per 100 full-time workers. Lacerations and punctures are the most common skin injuries and in 1983 accounted for 82 percent of recorded occupational skin injuries. Thermal and chemical burns (14%), abrasions (3.4%), cold injuries (0.2%) and radiation injuries (0.04%) also occur [1].

Occupational skin diseases or illnesses also result from exposure to toxic agents or environmental factors at work. In contrast to occupational skin injuries, occupational skin diseases require prolonged exposures and involve longer intervals between exposure and occurrence of disease [1]. Skin diseases account for 30 to 35 percent of all reported occupational diseases in the United States

[1, 2]. However, in comparison with other occupational health problems, skin disorders are often more easily diagnosed and recognized as work-related.

The average annual reported incidence of occupational skin disease in the United States in 1982 was 0.7 cases per 1,000 workers. It is estimated that the actual incidence is 10 to 50 times higher than the reported incidence [3, 4]. In a joint European study of clinic patients with dermatitis, 30 percent of the men and 12 percent of the women had occupational dermatitis [5].

Occupational skin disease is also a leading cause of time lost from work. From 20 to 25 percent of all reported occupational skin disease cases lose an average of 11 workdays annually. However, at least one-third of skin disorders in workers may not be directly related to their jobs.

The annual cost of occupational skin disease in the United States is great: at least 200,000 lost workdays, an estimated direct economic cost (lost wages or productivity) of $9.6 million, and a total cost (adding the costs of replacement workers, indemnity, medical costs, and insurance) of $20 to $30 million. If this estimate is multiplied 10 to 50 times to compensate for underreporting, the actual annual cost may be $250 million to $1.25 billion [3, 4].

Occupational skin disorders are unevenly distributed among industries. A worker in agriculture, forestry, fishing, or manufacturing has three times the risk of developing a work-related skin disease of workers in other industries. The inci-

**Table 24-1.** Cases and incidence rate of occupational dermatologic conditions, in a segment of workers, by major industrial divisions—United States, 1984

| Industrial division | Number | Incidence rate* |
|---|---|---|
| Agriculture/forestry/ fishing | 2,233 | 28.5 |
| Manufacturing | 23,017 | 12.3 |
| Construction | 2,456 | 6.6 |
| Services | 7,973 | 5.0 |
| Transportation/utilities | 2,114 | 4.3 |
| Mining | 393 | 4.0 |
| Wholesale/retail trade | 3,770 | 2.1 |
| Finance/insurance/real estate | 563 | 1.1 |

*Per 10,000 full-time workers (2,000 employment hours/ full-time worker/year).
Source: Occupational injuries and illnesses in the United States by industry, 1984. U.S. Department of Labor Bureau of Labor Statistics. Bulletin 2259, 1986.

dence of occupational dermatologic conditions in the major industrial divisions in the United States is shown in Table 24-1. In other countries, particular occupational groups contribute the majority of cases: in England miners, in Germany steelworkers, and in Italy bricklayers [6].

## Skin: Structure and Function

To understand skin disorders, a basic review of skin structure and function is helpful. Skin is the boundary between humans and their environment and is therefore very often the first site exposed to environmental insults. Skin weighs 3 to 4 kg, constitutes 6 percent of body weight, and covers about 20 square feet (about 2 m²) of the average adult. It consists of three principal layers [7].

The *epidermis* is the most superficial layer (Fig. 24-1). Its outermost compartment, the anucleate stratum corneum or horny layer is very thin but supple and resilient. The stratum corneum acts as the principal barrier that retains water and interferes with the entrance of microorganisms and toxic substances. This barrier is quite impermeable to hydrophilic substances. Percutaneous absorp-

tion is greater with lipophilic compounds and through inflamed or abraded skin, and following occlusion by water-permeable materials (for example, waterproof clothes or rubber gloves) (see Chap. 13). Melanocytes of neural crest origin lie within the epidermis and synthesize the pigment melanin, which protects against ultraviolet radiation. Langerhans cells, which are dendritic antigen-presenting[1] cells important in the development of allergic contact dermatitis, also reside within the lower layers of the epidermis.

The *dermis* consists primarily of the fibrous protein collagen in a glycosaminoglycan[2] ground substance, both of which protect against trauma and envelop the body in a strong and flexible wrap. Also within the dermis are blood vessels, lymphatics, nerves, and the epidermal appendages: eccrine and apocrine sweat glands, sebaceous glands, and hair follicles. The epidermal appendages, especially the pilosebaceous unit (hair follicle and sebaceous gland), are important portals of entry for chemical irritants and allergens.

The third layer is the *subcutaneous tissue*. The thick, fatty subcutaneous tissue helps conserve the body heat and serves as an additional shock-absorbing buffer.

Certain aspects of normal or altered skin are particularly important for workers in an industrial environment. Induced or inherent alterations of barrier-layer function increase susceptibility to the effects of workplace exposures and open the skin to further damage. This phenomenon occurs in contact dermatitis, psoriasis, and atopic dermatitis. Workers with atopic dermatitis are estimated to have a thirteenfold higher prevalence of occupational irritant dermatitis [8]. Patients with psoriasis may develop psoriasis in areas exposed to trauma or irritation (Koebner's phenomenon). These two common skin diseases, if noted on pre-

[1]Dendritic cell that has the capacity to process (engulf, partially metabolize, and display on its surface) antigens and present antigens to lymphocytes.
[2]Polysaccharide (glycan) structure containing hexosamines (glycosamino) (hyaluronic acid, deymatin sulfate, and chondroitin sulfates).

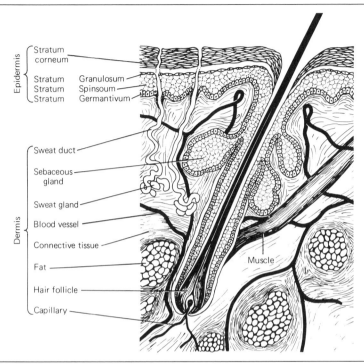

**Fig. 24-1.** Cross-section of human skin. The outermost stratum corneum is the principal barrier to chemical absorption. (From J Doull, CD Klaasen, MO Amdur. eds. *Casarett and Doull's Toxicology.* 2nd ed. New York: Macmillan, 1980:18. © 1980 by Macmillan Publishing Co.)

placement examination, may be sufficient reason to place a worker where exposure to irritating or sensitizing chemicals or to physical trauma does not occur.

Poorly pigmented skin is far more susceptible to ultraviolet light damage. Workers who tan poorly or not at all and who develop sunburns easily are more likely to develop basal cell and squamous cell skin cancers as a result of chronic exposure to sunlight. Such fair-skinned workers should protect their skin from ultraviolet damage by using sunscreens and wearing hats and long sleeves, especially if they work in outdoor occupations, such as agriculture, fishing, forestry, and construction.

Excessive eccrine (sweat) gland function results in hyperhidrosis (excessive perspiration), which may make it difficult to grasp objects. In the metal industry, malfunction of metal components occurs because of the problem of "rusters"—workers whose palmar sweat has a tendency to cause corrosion of metal objects. Another problem exacerbated by sweating results when otherwise harmless dusts, such as soda ash, may become hazardous by going into a solution after being deposited on wet (but otherwise normal) skin.

Disorders affecting the pilosebaceous follicles, such as acne, are worsened after exposure to heavy oils, greases, and hot and humid working conditions.

## Causes of Occupational Dermatoses

Those workplace agents that may induce skin disorders can be arbitrarily divided into categories as described in Table 24-2. Chemical agents produce

**Table 24-2.** Examples of workplace agents that induce skin disorders

| | |
|---|---|
| Chemical agents | Bacteria |
|   *Rhus* oleoresin (poison ivy and oak) |   Secondary superinfection |
|   Acids |   Impetigo |
|   Alkalis |   Furuncles |
|   Solvents |   Anthrax (infected hides) |
|   Oils |   Brucellosis (animals) |
|   Soaps and detergents |   Erysipeloid (fish and poultry) |
|   Plastics |   Mycobacteria infection (animals and fish tanks) |
|   Resins |   Tularemia (rodents) |
|   Paraphenylenediamine |   Cat-scratch disease (cats) |
|   Chromates |   Lyme disease (tick bites) |
|   Acrylates | Fungi |
|   Nickel compounds |   *Candida* infection (moist conditions) |
|   Rubber chemicals |   Dermatophytosis (animals, soil, and humans) |
|   Petroleum products not used as solvents |   Sporotrichosis (soil) |
|   Glass dust |   Blastomycosis (inhalation) |
| Plant and wood substances |   Coccidiodomycosis (inhalation) |
|   Pink rot celery | Ectoparasites |
|   Citrus fruit |   Cutaneous larva migrans |
| Physical agents |   Scabies |
|   Ionizing and nonionizing radiation |   Grain itch (mites) |
|   Wind |   Bites (ticks, fleas, mites, and spiders) |
|   Sunlight |   Swimmer's itch (schistosomes) |
|   Temperature extremes | Biting animals |
|   Humidity | Mechanical factors |
| Viruses |   Pressure |
|   Orf (sheep)* |   Friction |
|   Milker's nodule (cows) |   Vibration |
|   Herpes simplex (patients) | |
| Rickettsiae | |
|   Rocky Mountain spotted fever (ticks) | |
|   Murine typhus (fleas) | |
|   Tick typhus (ticks) | |
|   Rickettsialpox (mites) | |
|   Scrub typhus (mites) | |

*Agents of transmission or most common sources appear in parentheses.

the great majority of occupational dermatoses by inducing either irritant or allergic contact sensitivity reactions. Poison oak (*Rhus* oleoresin) was the most common cause of occupational skin disease in California in 1985, accounting for 28 percent of total cases and 21 percent of lost workday cases. The other most common offenders include acids, soaps, detergents, and solvents.

Plant and wood substances may induce contact dermatitis or a light-activated photocontact dermatitis, which occurs when contact with the photosensitizing substance is followed by exposure to sunlight. Dermatoses caused by vegetation are most commonly found among outdoor workers, especially farmers, construction laborers, lumber workers, and firefighters.

Among the physical agents, ultraviolet radiation can cause both acute and chronic skin disorders. Acute exposures to ultraviolet radiation can result in sunburn that may vary from erythema to severe blistering accompanied by fever, chills, and malaise. Shortwave ultraviolet radiation (UVB) damages epidermal cells. The subsequent release of inflammatory mediators causes vascular dilatation and influx of inflammatory cells in the dermis. Longer-wave ultraviolet light (UVA) can penetrate into the dermis and directly damage cells in the dermis. Acute ultraviolet exposure also causes increased production and dispersion of melanin, which causes darkening of the skin (tanning).

Chronic exposure to ultraviolet radiation causes solar elastosis, actinic keratoses, basal cell carcinomas, and squamous cell carcinomas. Solar elastosis is characterized by dryness and cracking of the stratum corneum, hyperpigmentation, decreased elasticity of the skin, and telangiectasia. Actinic keratoses are premalignant, erythematous, rough, scaly plaques that may develop into squamous cell carcinomas if left untreated. Solar ultraviolet radiation is responsible for the great majority of new skin cancers each year. All of the chronic effects of ultraviolet radiation occur most commonly and are most severe in lightly pigmented individuals who tan poorly and sunburn easily.

Ionizing radiation can also induce basal cell and squamous cell skin cancers. Chronic exposure to x-irradiation can cause a peculiar abnormality of the skin known as poikiloderma (areas of atrophy, telangiectasia, hyperpigmentation, and hypopigmentation) (see Chap. 15).

Exposure to cold temperatures may precipitate perniones (chilblains)[3] or Raynaud's phenomenon, or may cause frostbite. Working in hot and humid environments predisposes one to the development of intertrigo and miliaria (heat rash) (see Chap. 17). Low ambient humidity predisposes to dry skin and pruritus.

[3]Tender purple papules and nodules that develop on the hands and feet after exposure to cold weather.

Biologic agents are said to be the second most common cause of occupational skin diseases. Skin diseases caused by biologic agents are often difficult to diagnose. In contrast to most occupational skin disorders, it is often difficult to recognize that the skin disease is work-related. Making the correct diagnosis requires insight and thoroughness. Examples of occupational skin diseases caused by biologic agents include herpetic infections of the hands, as seen in dentists and respiratory therapists, and orf in sheep handlers (see Table 24-2).

Mechanical factors may cause callouses and fissures. Fibers that are too small to see with the naked eye, such as those of fibrous glass, may become embedded in the skin and cause pruritus and excoriation. The use of pneumatic devices, such as jackhammers and chain saws, is an often forgotten cause of occupational Raynaud's phenomenon.

## Reaction Patterns in Occupational Dermatology

Occupational skin diseases can be classified into several clinical patterns, including contact dermatitis, infections, pilosebaceous unit abnormalities, pigment disorders, and neoplasms. (Inflammation in the skin is called "dermatitis.") This system of classification can serve as a tool for remembering a wide variety of work-related clinical syndromes and can also serve as a reminder of etiologies of occupational skin diseases.

### Contact Dermatitis

The most common skin reaction seen in the industrial setting, contact dermatitis, accounts for approximately 90 percent of all occupational dermatoses. Contact dermatitis may be produced either by irritants or by allergic sensitizers. It occurs at the site of contact with the irritant or sensitizer, usually on exposed surfaces, especially the hands. Acute contact dermatitis is characterized by redness, swelling, blister formation, and exudation, leading to crusting and scaling. Thickening (lichenification), excoriations, and often hypo- or hyperpigmentation characterize chronic contact dermatitis.

*Primary irritant contact dermatitis* is a nonallergic reaction of the skin caused by exposure to irritating substances (Fig. 24-2). Any substance can act as an irritant, provided the concentration and duration of contact are sufficient. Most irritants are chemical substances, although physical and biologic agents may produce the same clinical picture. Approximately 80 percent of occupational contact reactions are of an irritant type.

Irritants can be classified as mild, relative, or marginal irritants that require repeated or pro-

**Fig. 24-2.** Chronic irritant hand dermatitis. Skin is thickened, scaling, and inelastic to touch, and shows a deep fissure.

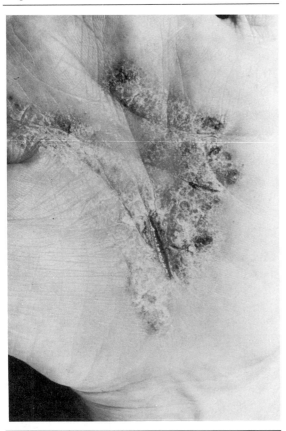

longed contact to produce inflammation (including soaps, detergents, and most solvents), and as strong or absolute irritants that will injure skin immediately on contact (including strong acids and alkalis). Exposure to strong acids and alkalis constitutes a medical emergency that should be treated by washing the area with copious amounts of cool water to limit tissue damage. Hydrofluoric (HF) acid is particularly damaging to the skin and may cause rapid, deep, and extensive tissue necrosis. Therapy for hydrofluoric acid burns may require injection of 5 percent calcium gluconate solution or application of a calcium gluconate gel or ointment after washing [9]. Follow-up care to prevent superinfection is essential for all chemical burns.

If exposure to mild irritants is constant, normal skin in some workers may become "hardened" or tolerant of this trauma, and contact can be continued without further evidence of inflammation.

*Allergic contact dermatitis* is a manifestation of delayed-type hypersensitivity and results from the exposure of sensitized individuals to contact allergens (Fig. 24-3). Most contact allergens produce sensitization in only a small percentage of those exposed. *Rhus* antigens, which induce sensitization in more than 70 percent of those exposed to poison ivy, oak, or sumac, are marked exceptions to this rule. The incubation period after initial sensitization to an antigen is 5 to 21 days, but the reaction time after subsequent reexposure is 6 to 72 hours. The normal reaction of a sensitized person after exposure to a moderate amount of poison oak or ivy is the appearance of a rash in 2 to 3 days and clearing within 1 to 2 weeks; with larger exposure, lesions appear more quickly (6–12 hours) and resolve more slowly (2–3 weeks). Contact sensitizers may less commonly lead to other cutaneous reaction patterns such as urticaria (hives). Health care workers have increased their use of rubber gloves to protect themselves from patients' body fluids since the emergence of the acquired immunodeficiency syndrome. This practice has led to an increase in the incidence of allergic contact dermatitis to rubber and latex [10].

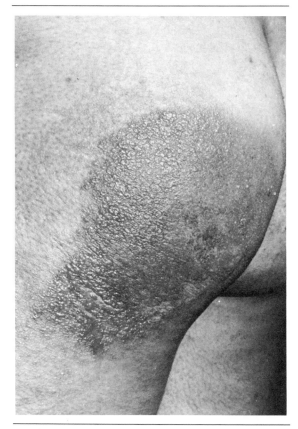

**Fig. 24-3.** Allergic contact dermatitis to MACE. This tear gas, methylchloroform chloracetophone, is a potent sensitizer. The patient was a security guard who sat down on a MACE spray can, the nozzle of which was pointed toward his buttocks.

Irritants and allergens cause itching as the primary symptom of contact dermatitis. Irritants also can cause an inelastic skin, discomfort due to dryness, and pain related to fissures, blisters, and ulcers (Fig. 24-4). Strong irritants can cause blistering and erosions; mild irritants or allergens may cause dermatitis with erythema, microvesicles, and oozing. Allergens most typically cause grouped or linear tense vesicles or blisters. Edema can occur and may be severe particularly on the face and the genital areas. Most often contact dermatitis can be

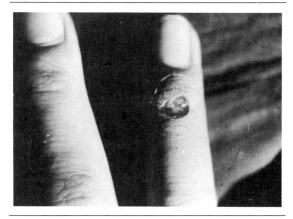

**Fig. 24-4.** Ulcer caused by contact with arsenic trioxide dust. This dust affected the whole community surrounding a gold smelting plant. (From DJ Birmingham, et al. An outbreak of arsenical dermatoses in a mining community. *Arch Dermatol* 1965; 91:457. Copyright 1965, American Medical Association.)

distinguished from other types of eczema/dermatitis not by the specific morphology of lesions but by their distribution and configuration—that is, the rash occurs in exposed or contact areas, often with a bizarre or artificial pattern of sharp margins, acute angles, and straight lines. "Airborne dermatitis" is caused by chemicals dispersed in the air in the form of vapors (for example, formaldehyde), droplets (for example, hairsprays, pesticides, and insecticides), or solid particles (industrial powders). The upper eyelid is frequently involved.

### Infections
Pyodermas induced by streptococci or staphylococci are the most common bacterial skin infections. These infections may occur as a result of trauma or as a complication of other occupational dermatoses. Barbers and cosmeticians who have contact in their work with customers suffering from contagious skin diseases are particularly at risk for bacterial and fungal infections. Lesions range from the superficial, such as impetigo, to the

deep, such as folliculitis, carbuncles, cellulitis, and secondary lymphangitis. Diagnosis is made by clinical appearance, Gram's stain, and culture. A less common infection is erysipeloid among meat and fish handlers and veterinarians; even rarer is anthrax among sheep handlers and animal hide and wool workers (see Chap. 18). A large outbreak of sporotrichosis in workers exposed to sphagnum moss was reported in 1988 [11].

Fungal infections with dermatophytes (ringworm) or the yeast-like fungus *Candida albicans* are often found in a local environment of moisture, warmth, and maceration; they therefore occur frequently in body folds and during warm seasons. The lesions of ringworm are annular, red, and scaling at the periphery with clearing in the center, whereas those of *Candida* are beefy red, weeping areas with satellite papules or pustules outside skinfold areas. Both organisms may involve the nail, but the paronychial area is most often affected by *Candida,* particularly in workers whose hands are often exposed to water such as dishwashers, hairdressers, and canning industry workers who handle fruit. In these individuals, the interdigital spaces of the hands are also predisposed. Demonstrating septate hyphae or budding yeasts and pseudohyphae on potassium hydroxide (KOH) examination will confirm the presence of fungal or yeast infection, and culture will delineate the type of organism.

*Herpes simplex* is the most frequently identified work-related viral skin infection in the United States. Health care workers, especially those who are exposed to oral secretions such as dental technicians, nurses, and anesthetists, may develop painful infections in their finger tips and around their nails (herpetic whitlow). These are often confused with felons or bacterial paronychial infections. Primary cutaneous infection by herpes simplex virus is also frequently observed in wrestlers and rugby players (herpes gladiatorum). Diagnosis is confirmed by finding viral giant cells on microscopic examination of scrapings from the vesicle floor (Tzanck preparation).

## Pilosebaceous Follicle Abnormalities

*Acne vulgaris,* a multifactorial disorder involving the pilosebaceous follicles, is usually first noted in teenage years and subsides by early adulthood. Heavy oils such as insoluble cutting oils and greases used by machine-tool operators (or machinists) may aggravate idiopathic acne or cause comedo-like follicular plugging and folliculitis (Fig. 24-5). Skin under saturated clothing is most at risk, but lesions are also found on the dorsal surfaces of the hands and on extensor surfaces of the forearms. "Oil boils" may develop as the result of entrapment of surface bacteria.

Some halogenated aromatic hydrocarbons will induce chloracne, an acneiform eruption consisting of comedones, hyperpigmentation, and the pathognomonic oil cysts on exposed skin sites. These disfiguring lesions can last for as many as 15 years. Though chloracne is not itself a disabling illness, it is important evidence of percutaneous absorption of chloracnegens. These chlorinated hydrocarbons have been associated with hepatic damage and malignancies in animals. Workers at risk include herbicide manufacturers and cable splicers and others exposed to polychlorinated bi-

Fig. 24-5. Oil folliculitis. These acne-like lesions were induced by insoluble cutting oils that had saturated work pants. (From American Academy of Dermatology set of teaching slides on occupational dermatitis.)

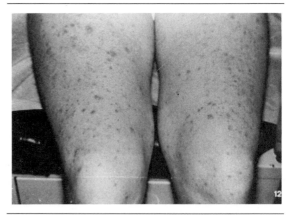

phenyls (PCBs) in dielectric applications (electrical insulation). Chloracne has been a side effect of recent massive environmental contamination by herbicides such as occurred in Seveso, Italy, in 1976, where an explosion in a nearby chemical plant sent a toxic cloud containing dioxin into the air. Dioxin, a trace contaminant of the chlorinated hydrocarbon 2,4,5-trichlorophenoxyacetic acid (2,4,5-T), is one of the most toxic substances known, second only to the neurotoxin botulin, and certain nerve gas and chemical warfare components. The dioxin-containing cloud settled on Seveso, a rural community of 5,000 people. There were 187 confirmed cases of chloracne, many in children; the long-term effects of this accident remain to be seen. Another exposure to dioxin occurred among inhabitants of and military personnel in Vietnam between 1962 and 1971, when Agent Orange, which contains 2,4,5-T, was used as a defoliant.

### Pigment Disorders

Occupational exposures can produce many pigments on the skin. Some are stains adhering to the stratum corneum, some are a result of systemic absorption or inoculation (tattoo) of heavy metals, but most are due to altered melanin pigmentation.

Postinflammatory hyper- and hypopigmentation are the most common pigment disorders (Fig. 24-6). Any dermatitis or other trauma to the skin, such as thermal or chemical burns, may lead to temporary increase or decrease in melanin pigmentation in that area. More heavily pigmented individuals show these findings most notably and with slower reversibility. If damage has been severe, melanocytes may have been destroyed and permanent depigmentation may occur, sometimes with scarring. Exposure to sun or other sources of ultraviolet light in the presence of photosensitizers such as tar, pitch, and psoralens will lead to enhanced erythema and, later, tanning.

An antioxidant used in rubber manufacturing, monobenzyl ether of hydroquinone, is the chemical most notorious for inducing permanent work-related loss of pigment (leukoderma). Metastatic

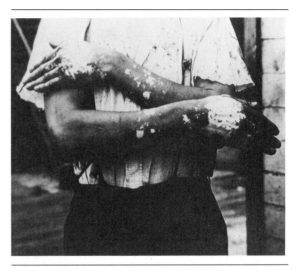

Fig. 24-6. Depigmentation caused by monobenzyl ether of hydroquinone. This chemical was used as an antioxidant in workers' gloves. (From EA Oliver, L Schwartz, LN Warren. Occupational leukoderma: Preliminary report. JAMA 1939; 113:927. Copyright 1939, American Medical Association.)

lesions of hypopigmentation not in sites of direct contact may also be found. In the recent past other phenolic compounds used as antioxidants or germicidal disinfectants have been found to produce pigment loss. This phenomenon results from a structural resemblance of these substances to tyrosine, an amino acid precursor of melanin synthesis.

### Neoplasms

Occupational neoplasms may be benign, premalignant, or cancerous (Fig. 24-7). Foreign-body granulomas or granulomatous inflammatory nodules due to beryllium or silica are important examples of benign lesions. (Interestingly, exposure to silica dust has also been implicated in the induction of scleroderma [12].) Foreign-body granulomas and fistulas also occur in the interdigital spaces of barbers when the skin is penetrated by small fragments of hair. Keratoses produced by exposure to

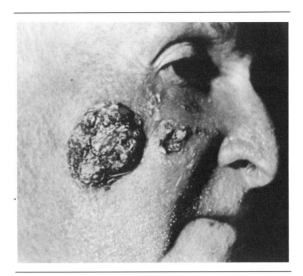

Fig. 24-7. Squamous cell carcinoma. This roofer had years of exposure to tars and sunlight. (From American Academy of Dermatology set of teaching slides on occupational dermatitis.)

shale oils or to ultraviolet light are examples of premalignant lesions. Examples of cancerous lesions include squamous cell carcinoma and basal cell carcinoma from chronic exposure to ultraviolet light; scrotal cancer from occupational exposure to hydrocarbons such as those in soot; and squamous cell carcinoma, often on the scrotum, historically among cotton spinners and currently among metal machinists exposed to carcinogens in lubricating oils. Oncogenic agents include: ionizing radiation; ultraviolet light; some insoluble oils and greases, especially shale oils; and degradation products of the incomplete combustion of woods, oils, and tar. A diagnostic skin biopsy is always necessary when a skin cancer is suspected.

### Disorders of Hair and Nails

Alopecia (hair loss) may be caused by exposure to thallium-containing rodenticides, chloroprene, boric acid, or high doses of ionizing radiation.

Nail abnormalities may follow mechanical or chemical injury to the nail matrix, or may result from infection with *Candida* or dermatophytes.

### Other Occupational Skin Disorders

The development of scleroderma-like lesions has been observed in those who work with polyvinyl chloride, particularly reactor cleaners who have been exposed to vinyl chloride, and in other individuals after exposure to perchlorethylene, a solvent used in dry-cleaning. In an Eastern European study of 61 patients with systemic sclerosis, 28 percent had undergone significant exposure to organic solvents [13]. An earlier Japanese study drew attention to an association between scleroderma-like skin changes and occupational exposure to epoxy resin [14]. The occurrence of scleroderma in South African coal miners with silicosis has been known for a considerable time.

A facial dermatosis characterized by erythema and rosacea-like lesions occurring in workers at video display terminals was originally described in Norway [15]. It is controversial whether "video display terminal dermatosis" is a true disease entity or the result of heightened awareness and recognition of preexisting skin conditions by workers who experience stress in the workplace. Most studies have found no association between video display terminals and skin disease.

## Diagnosis of Occupational Skin Disorders

Occupational skin disorders are diagnosed by an accurate, detailed, and discerning history; a careful physical examination; laboratory tests; and tests for allergic contact dermatitis.

The history is of utmost importance in making a diagnosis of occupational skin disorders. The history should include a detailed description of the patient's job and a complete list of chemical, physical, and biologic agents and mechanical factors to which the patient is exposed. The onset of the skin disorder in relation to starting or changing job duties is important. Occupational skin disorders often improve on weekends and during vacations. Up to one-third of skin disorders seen in workers are unrelated to their jobs, since exposure to irritants and allergens often occurs in the patient's home. Finally, all patients with contact dermatitis should be questioned about a past history of atopic dermatitis.

In the physical examination, emphasis should be placed on recognizing the patterns of occupational skin disorders. These disorders predominantly affect the hands, wrists, and forearms. The face, eyelids, and ears may also be involved. Examination of the entire cutaneous surface is recommended. Attention to spared areas as well as involved areas may provide clues to the etiology of the skin disorder. For example, phototoxic eruptions tend to spare areas covered by clothing, the upper eyelids, under the chin, and behind the ears. The appearance of acne lesions outside the typical acne distribution may be helpful in establishing the diagnosis.

Laboratory tests may include smears and cultures for viruses, bacteria, and fungi. A skin biopsy may be useful. A description of the laboratory tests used to help establish a diagnosis of skin disorders can be found in several references in the Bibliography.

Patch testing is used to document and validate a diagnosis of allergic contact sensitization and identify the causative agent (Fig. 24-8). It may also be of value as a screening procedure in patients with chronic or unexplained dermatitis to assess whether or not contact allergy is playing a causative role. The patch test is a unique means of in vivo reproduction of disease on a small scale since sensitization affects the whole body and may therefore be elicited at any cutaneous site; it is easier and safer than the "use" test because test items can be applied in low concentrations on small areas of skin for short periods of time. Patch testing is of no value in diagnosing irritant dermatitis except to exclude allergic contact dermatitis as a primary or contributing cause. Toxic chemicals or strong irritants should not be tested, although open patch tests are sometimes used for relative irritants such as shampoos or other detergents. Proper performance and interpretation of patch tests require considerable experience. Possible side effects in-

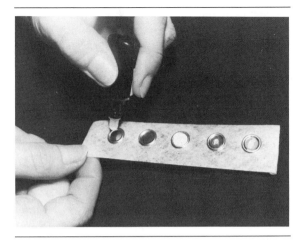

**Fig. 24-8.** Patch testing. Chemicals are applied to a Finn chamber made of aluminum, which is then taped to the patient's skin for 48 hours.

clude a severe local reaction, possible secondary autosensitization reaction, or actually sensitizing someone to the testing compound. Patch-test allergens are often available commercially; sometimes they must be prepared from the occupational agent suspected. These substances must be nonirritating and nontoxic. The selection of optimal patch-test preparations is the subject of much debate, and may vary from country to country according to their agricultural and industrial economies [16]. Patch-testing procedures and techniques of proper dilution of reagents can be found in several references in the Bibliography.

## Management of Skin Diseases

The treatment of occupational skin disease generally depends on accurate diagnosis of the clinical reaction pattern. While it may be possible to treat some disorders successfully without having an exact etiologic diagnosis, an exact diagnosis should always be made for purposes of workers' compensation and prevention of the disorder in other workers. There are no differences between the management of skin diseases caused by occupational and nonoccupational factors. The following is a brief summary of the more commonly used therapies; for detailed management strategies, texts on dermatologic therapy should be consulted.

### Contact Dermatitis

Acute exudative and vesicular contact dermatitis should be treated with compresses or dressings such as Burow's solution and topical anti-inflammatory agents. Topical corticosteroids are the anti-inflammatory agents of choice; they usually hasten resolution of the dermatitis and reduce itching. If the eruption is severe and accompanied by marked edema, a short course of oral corticosteroids may be necessary. Antihistamine drugs may reduce itching, and oral antibiotics are effective in eliminating secondary infection. Chronic contact dermatitis requires adequate lubrication and the skillful use of topical corticosteroids. Attempts to induce clinically relevant hyposensitization with purified allergens have not been successful.

### Infections

Systemic antibiotics are usually warranted for cutaneous pyodermas. For superficial infections, topical antibiotics may be effective (for example, mupirocin against staphylococcal and streptococcal infections, and silver sulfadiazine against many gram-negative organisms). The topical imidazole drugs miconazole and clotrimazole are almost always effective in eliminating ringworm (dermatophyte) or yeast (C. albicans) infection. Fungal infections of the scalp and the nail plate, however, should be treated with oral antifungal agents. Oral and intravenous acyclovir are available for the treatment of selected patients with herpes simplex infection. (Acyclovir is the only antiviral drug available to treat skin disorders.)

### Pilosebaceous Follicle Abnormalities

Acne and chloracne respond to topical and systemic treatment, but chloracne is far more recalcitrant and responds less completely. In most instances topical creams and gels containing tretinoin or benzoyl peroxide are the agents of choice. Some patients, however, may need treatment with oral antibiotics or isotretinoin. Lesions of chloracne often last months to years in spite of therapy.

### Pigment Disorders

Postinflammatory pigment changes slowly resolve with time. That part of postinflammatory hyperpigmentation reflective of increased epidermal melanocyte activity can be treated with hydroquinone-containing creams. Usually, however, "bleaching" creams are of limited value. The leukoderma caused by monobenzyl ether of hydroquinone or phenolic disinfectants is not amenable to treatment.

### Neoplasms

Premalignant keratoses can be treated with topical 5-fluorouracil (5-FU) or with liquid nitrogen cryosurgery, electrosurgery, or curettage. Cryosurgery, scalpel excision, and radiation therapy are appropriate for basal or squamous cell carcinomas. The best therapy in any instance depends on factors such as the size and site of the lesion and the patient's age and history of cutaneous carcinomas.

## Prognosis

The prognosis of occupational skin disorders depends on several variables including type of cutaneous reaction pattern, its exact cause (if determined), duration of eruption prior to diagnosis, type and effectiveness of treatment, patient compliance, and adequacy of preventive measures. Those workers with a specific allergic contact sensitivity may do well if they can avoid the allergen in work and home environments; in industrial settings it is almost always necessary to transfer such workers to another area of the plant. Workers with irritant contact reactions may be able to continue at work if the duration and intensity of exposure to contactants is decreased by environmental or protective measures. Those with atopy or a long history of dermatitis have a particularly dismal prognosis.

Persistence of what is presumed to be a work-related eruption even after the worker has been removed from the putative cause is not uncommon and may occur in the majority of cases [17, 18]. However, persistence of a work-related skin disorder should raise several potential questions: Was the correct diagnosis made and the best treatment prescribed? Has the patient conscientiously carried out the treatment plan? Has work exposure been eliminated, and are there other possible sources of contact in second jobs or at home? Are psychological factors playing a role, and is there any evidence of malingering? These questions are often difficult to answer definitely, just as it is often difficult to delineate the specific cause of an occupational dermatosis.

In 1970 the American Medical Association published guidelines on evaluating the degree of impairment and disability induced by occupational skin disorders; its criteria are shown in Table 24-3. As opposed to permanent skin impairment, functional loss is best evaluated by assessing the degree of itching, scarring, and disfigurement.

## Prevention

Occupational skin diseases are often preventable by a combination of environmental, personal, and medical measures.

### Environmental Measures

Environmental cleanliness is paramount in preventing occupational dermatoses. Maintaining a clean workplace involves the frequent cleaning of floors, walls, windows, and machinery; recognizing hazardous materials and either providing substitutes or altering or eliminating them from the workplace; ensuring proper ventilation, temperature, and humidity; and the use of exhaust hoods, splash guards, and other protective devices and systems.

**Table 24-3.** Criteria for evaluating permanent skin impairment

| Category | Impairment | Comments |
|---|---|---|
| Class 1 | 0–5% | With treatment there is no or minimal limitation in the performance of the activities of daily living, although certain physical and chemical agents might temporarily increase the extent of limitation. |
| Class 2 | 10–20% | Intermittent treatment is required, *and* there is limitation in the performance of some of the activities of daily living. |
| Class 3 | 25–50% | Continuous treatment is required, *and* there is limitation in the performance of many of the activities of daily living. |
| Class 4 | 55–80% | Continuous treatment is required, which may include periodic confinement at home or other domicile, *and* there is limitation in the performance of many of the activities of daily living. |
| Class 5 | 85–95% | Continuous treatment is required that necessitates confinement at home or other domicile, *and* there is severe limitation in the performance of the activities of daily living. |

Source: AMA Subcommittee on the Skin. Guides to evaluation of permanent impairment—the skin. JAMA 1970; 211:106. Copyright 1970, American Medical Association.

## Personal Measures

Personal cleanliness is a key element in preventing occupational skin disease. Washing facilities with hot and cold running water, towels, and proper cleansing agents must be easily accessible and strategically placed. The *mildest* soap that will clean the skin should always be used. Appropriate cleansing agents might include waterless hand cleaners for oils, greases, or adherent soils. Safety showers must be available if highly corrosive chemicals are being handled. If strong irritants are in the work environment, it is necessary for workers to shower at the end of each shift, or possibly more often. In some industries it is appropriate to supply clothing and laundering to ensure both the use of proper types of material as well as daily clothes changes. If water is not easily accessible for washing, waterless hand cleansers can be used. Solvents such as kerosene, gasoline, and turpentine should *never* be used for skin cleansing; they are quite damaging to the skin since they "dissolve" the cutaneous barrier and can either induce an irritant contact dermatitis or predispose to a cumulative insult contact dermatitis. A skin moisturizer should be used after handwashing, especially if frequent washing is necessary.

Protective clothing is often all that is needed to prevent a dermatitis by blocking contact of chemicals with the skin. The clothing should be chosen based on the skin site needing protection and the type of chemical involved (some solvents will dissolve certain fabrics or materials). Natural rubber gloves are impervious to most aqueous compounds but deteriorate after exposure to strong acids and bases. Very common allergens such as nickel salts penetrate rubber but not polyvinyl chloride glove material. Synthetic rubbers are more resistant to alkalis and solvents; however, some are altered by chlorinated hydrocarbon solvents. In Sweden, a database has been developed that contains test data on protective effects of gloves against chemicals [19]. It is always useful to wear absorbent, replaceable soft cotton liners inside protective gloves to make them more comfortable. Commercially available gear includes gloves of different lengths, sleeves, safety shoes and boots, aprons, and coveralls composed of materials such as plastic, rubber, glass fiber, metal, and combinations of these materials. Clothing that might become caught in machines must be avoided for safety reasons.

Protective creams, referred to as "barrier" creams, afford much less protection than does clothing. However, these creams can be valuable when gloves would interfere with the sense of touch required to perform the job or when use of a face shield might be awkward. Barrier creams should be applied to clean skin, removed when the skin becomes excessively soiled or at the end of each work period, and then reapplied. Proper use of a barrier cream not only provides some degree of protection but induces the worker to wash at least twice during the work shift.

There are four types of protective creams. *Vanishing creams* contain detergents, which remain on the skin and facilitate removal of soil when washing. *Water-repellent* creams leave a film of water-repellent substances such as lanolin, petrolatum, or silicone on the skin to help prevent direct contact with water-soluble irritants like acids and alkalis. *Solvent-repellent* creams repel oils and solvents and may leave either an ointment film or a dry, oil-repellent film on the skin surface. *Special creams* include sun shades; sunscreens absorbent of UVA, UVB, or both spectra of ultraviolet light; and insect repellents. Some common constituents of protective creams (for example, lanolin, propylene glycol, and sunscreens) can also induce contact dermatitis.

## Medical Measures

Careful screening of new workers in preplacement examinations will decrease the incidence of job-related dermatoses. Individuals with a history of atopic dermatitis should not work in occupations involving frequent exposure to harsh chemicals or water, such as certain machining, cooking, bottle-washing, and operating-room jobs. Those with psoriasis of the hands would do poorly in the same situation and furthermore may respond with a Koebner reaction in which psoriatic lesions develop in sites of heavy trauma. Such trauma includes scratches, abrasions, and cuts that disrupt the epidermis as well as rough handwork or continual kneeling.

Workers with dermatographism,[4] at high risk for annoying pruritic responses to trauma or to foreign bodies such as fibrous glass, should avoid these occupational exposures; workers with acne should not be employed in hot and humid workplaces or where they would be exposed to oil mists, heavy oils, or greases; and fair-skinned or sunlight-sensitive individuals should not work in intense ultraviolet light (see Chap. 17) or around potentially photosensitizing chemicals such as tar, pitch, and psoralens. Job applicants should be questioned concerning previous skin diseases, including childhood eczema and atopic diseases, contact dermatitis, psoriasis, fungal infections, and allergic reactions to drugs or other agents.

Preplacement patch testing is generally not advised; although it may occasionally identify a previously allergic person, the yield is very low and it has the greater risk of inducing contact sensitization. Chemical agents used in the workplace should undergo toxicologic testing to detect irritancy, allergenicity, acnegenicity, carcinogenicity, and other properties. When potentially hazardous substances are detected, they should be properly labeled, and workers should be educated about these hazards and how to avoid them.

Workers with severe, chronic, or unremitting allergic dermatoses should be transferred to other plant areas, if possible. By definition, allergy implies sensitivity to very low levels of an antigen, and it is usually not possible to continue working in the same site even though careful precautions are taken. Those with irritant dermatoses are often, but not always, able to continue working by

decreasing the duration and intensity of exposure to irritants. Relocation of workers is more easily accomplished within large industries; however, only one-third of the workforce is employed in such industries. Most cases of occupational dermatitis occur in small plants with poorly developed preventive services and less sophisticated or no supervisory and medical personnel.

## References

1. Centers for Disease Control. Leading work-related diseases and injuries. MMWR 1986; 35:561–3.
2. Division of Labor and Statistics. Occupational disease in California, 1985. San Francisco: California Department of Industrial Relations, 1987.
3. Mathias CGT. The cost of occupational skin disease. Arch Dermatol 1985; 121:332–4.
4. National Institute for Occupational Safety and Health. Pilot Study for Development of an Occupational Disease Surveillance Method. Cincinnati: NIOSH, 1975. (Publication no. 75–162.)
5. Malten KE, et al. Occupational dermatitis in five European dermatology departments. Berufsdermtososen 1963; 11:121–224.
6. Rycroft RJG. Occupational dermatosis. In RH Champion, JL Burton, FJG Eblingo. Textbook of Dermatology. 5th ed. Oxford: Blackwell, 1991.
7. Goldsmith LA. My organ is bigger than your organ. Arch Dermatol 1990; 126:301–2.
8. Shmunes E, Keil JE. Occupational dermatoses in South Carolina: A descriptive analysis of cost variables. J Am Acad Dermatol 1983; 9:861–6.
9. Trevino MA, Herrman GH, Sproue WL. Treatment of severe hydrofluoric acid exposures. J Occup Med 1983; 25:861–3.
10. Bubak ME, et al. Allergic reactions to latex among health-care workers. Mayo Clin Proc 1992; 67:1075–9.
11. Coles FB, et al. A multistate outbreak of sporotrichosis associated with sphagnum moss. Am J Epidemiol 1992; 22:444–8.
12. Haustein UF, et al. Silica-induced scleroderma. J Am Acad Dermatol 1990; 22:444–8.
13. Czirjak L, et al. Chemical findings in 61 patients with progressive systemic sclerosis. Acta Dermatol Venereol 1989; 69:533–6.
14. Yamakage A, et al. Occupational scleroderma-like disorders occurring in men engaged in the polymer-

[4]Urticaria due to physical factors, in which moderately firm stroking or scratching of the skin with a dull instrument produces a persistent, pale, raised wheal, with a red flare on each side.

ization of epoxy resins. Dermatologica 1980; 161: 33–44.

15. Berg M, Lidien S. Skin problems in video display terminal users. J Am Acad Dermatol 1987; 17: 682–4.

16. Móroni P, Peirini F. Patch testing and detective work in the workplace. Clin Dermatol 1992; 10:195–200.

17. Keczkes K, Bhate SM, Wyatt EH. The outcome of primary irritant hand dermatitis. Br J Dermatol 1983; 109:665–8.

18. Burrows D. Prognosis and factors influencing prognosis in industrial dermatitis. Br J Dermatol 1981; 21(Suppl. 105):65–70.

19. Mellstrom GA, Lindahl G, Nahlberg JE. Daisy. Reference database on protective gloves. Semin Dermatol 1989; 8:75–9.

## Bibliography

Adams RM. ed. Occupational medicine: State of the art reviews. Occupational skin disease. Philadelphia: Hanley & Belfus, 1986.

*A concise, well-written, and up-to-date treatise on this subject, which covers the basics of occupational skin diseases. The role of atopy in occupational skin disease, vibration syndromes, and AIDS in the workplace are among the interesting topics covered.*

Adams RM. Occupational skin disease. 2nd ed. Philadelphia: Saunders, 1990.

*A thorough and comprehensive general reference book. An essential book for the serious student of occupational skin disorders.*

AMA Subcommittee on the Skin. Guides to evaluation of permanent impairment—the skin. JAMA 1970; 211:106.

*This material was also published in the AMA volume Guides to the evaluation of permanent impairment. Chicago: American Medical Association, 143–8. Chap. 12.*

Arndt KA. Manual of dermatologic therapeutics: With essentials of diagnosis. 4th ed. Boston: Little, Brown, 1988.

*A practical manual. Discusses the pathophysiology, diagnosis, and treatment of common skin disorders seen in ambulatory patients. Patch testing is described.*

de Groot AC. Patch testing. Amsterdam: Elsevier, 1986.

*This book provides recommendations for test concentrations and vehicles for 2,800 allergens.*

Fisher AA. Contact dermatitis. 3rd ed. Philadelphia: Lea & Febiger, 1986.

*Essential, detailed reference on contact dermatitis. Contains a glossary that describes the proper patch-test concentrations of many common antigens.*

Maibach HI. Occupational and industrial dermatology. 2nd ed. Chicago: Year Book, 1986.

*A comprehensive, well-written book that includes the basics of occupational and industrial dermatology, dermatotoxicology, and specific industrial problems.*

Pigatto PD. guest ed. Industrial and occupational dermatitis. Clin Dermatol 1992; 10(2).

*A recent and extensive review from a European perspective. Most of the authors of the chapters are members of the Italian Group for the Study of Contact and Environmental Dermatitis (GIRDCA).*

# 25
# Eye Disorders

Paul F. Vinger and David H. Sliney

A 52-year-old metal worker was polishing a brass fixture on a buffing wheel. The fixture was torn from his grasp by the wheel and struck his left eye. In addition to a full-thickness laceration of the left upper eyelid, a severe laceration of the globe of the eye was apparent when he was evaluated at a hospital soon afterward. It was discovered then that the patient had a best-corrected vision in the uninjured right eye enabling him only to count fingers because of dense amblyopia ("lazy eye" secondary to unilateral uncorrected high myopia, or nearsightedness). Despite extensive surgical procedures, vision was lost in the injured left eye. Attempts to improve the vision in the uninjured right eye by optical means were not successful. He is now legally blind with no hope of recovery of useful vision. He can no longer drive or perform his usual work.

An 18-year-old arc-welding student stared at an electric welding arc while a piece of aluminum was being welded by another welder. He was outside a protective curtain and about 200 cm (about 6.5 ft) from the arc, yet was able to stare at the arc with his right eye for approximately 10 minutes. He sustained a retinal injury that initially resulted in marked visual loss. This loss slowly resolved over 16 months, leaving him with normal visual acuity and a residual, partially pigmented foveal lesion (*foveal* meaning in the central portion of the retina, which is required for normal reading and driving visual acuity and accurate color vision).

A scientist was working with a relatively weak neodymium-yag (neodymium-*y*ttrium-*a*luminum-*g*arnet) laser without safety goggles. He was not looking directly at the beam but heard a popping sound inside his eye accompanied by almost immediate obscuring of his vision. The laser burn, between the fovea and the optic nerve of his left eye, resulted in a large, permanent blind area in his visual field.

Every working day, there are over 2,000 preventable job-related eye injuries to workers in the United States. Occupational vision programs, including preplacement examinations and requirements for appropriate eye protectors in certain occupations, can prevent many of these injuries. Such programs could have prevented the loss of vision in the above situations.

## Causes of Occupational Eye Injuries

### Direct Trauma
Direct trauma is the most frequent cause of occupational eye injuries. Jobs in which there is the risk of high-speed flying particulate material as well as the tradition of working without eye protectors, such as automobile mechanics, present the highest risk (Table 25-1). Eye injuries from direct trauma are almost totally preventable with protective eyewear. Symptoms and signs of serious eye injury are shown in the box on p. 508.

### Chemicals
Many different types of chemicals are commonly involved in industrial eye injuries (see box on p. 509). These include alkalis, acids, esters, ketones, and other selected chemicals.

### Light, Laser, Heat, and Ionizing Radiation
Eye injuries can occur from essentially all portions of the electromagnetic spectrum; however, some sources of electromagnetic energy are far more

**Table 25-1.** Emergency room visits, Massachusetts Eye and Ear Infirmary, March 15 to September 15, 1985

3,185 eye trauma patients:
   48% at work—highest rate in auto repair
   5% of injuries deemed serious
   $2 million in hospital bills
   30 person-years of work lost
   9% involved in litigation

Source: OD Schein et al. The spectrum and burden of ocular injury. Ophthalmology 1988; 95:300–5.

hazardous to the eye because (1) the eye is more sensitive to the particular wavelengths, (2) the energy dose can be very high, or (3) the energy is delivered in a very brief interval (see Chap. 17).

Ionizing radiation is rarely a cause of industrial eye injury because standard precautions from exposure to ionizing radiation give adequate eye protection.

Exposure to excess heat can cause thermal burns to the lids and eye. Cataracts occur in unprotected glass blowers and furnace workers. Heat-absorbing or heat-reflecting protective eyewear is available. Other protective clothing or head or face shields may be indicated, depending on the severity of heat exposure.

Optical radiation is considered nonionizing radiation because photon energies for ultraviolet (UV) wavelengths greater than approximately 180 nm are insufficient to individually ionize atoms found in important biologic molecules (see Chap. 17). Unlike the nonthreshold biologic effects of ionizing radiation, such as x-rays, a threshold appears to exist for each biologic effect of optical radiation. In the UV and visible regions of the spectrum, photochemical damage mechanisms are demonstrable. Thermal injury mechanisms dominate for most pulsed laser exposures and infrared (IR) radiation exposures

The optical spectrum includes the UV, visible (light), and IR regions of the electromagnetic spectrum. Lasers, which can emit wavelengths in all parts of the spectrum, are unique sources of optical radiation, with extremely high brightness.

SYMPTOMS AND SIGNS OF SERIOUS EYE INJURY
Symptoms of serious eye injury indicating immediate referral are the following:

1. Blurred vision that does not clear with blinking
2. Loss of all or part of the visual field of an eye
3. Sharp stabbing or deep throbbing pain
4. Double vision

Signs of eye injury that require ophthalmologic evaluation are the following:

1. Black eye
2. Red eye
3. An object on the cornea
4. One eye that does not move as completely as the other
5. One eye protruding forward more than the other
6. One eye with an abnormal pupil size, shape, or reaction to light, as compared to the other eye
7. A layer of blood between the cornea and the iris (hyphema)
8. Laceration of the eyelid, especially if it involves the lid margin
9. Laceration or perforation of the eye

Although most workers are aware of the potential for lasers to cause eye injury, it must be stressed that more conventional light sources, especially with high output in the UV portion of the spectrum, such as welding arcs and sun lamps, can also be extremely hazardous. Figure 25-1 correlates the potential for retinal injury with the absorbed retinal irradiance of various light sources.

There are at least five separate types of hazards to the eye and skin from lasers and other more conventional optical sources:

1. UV photochemical injury to the skin (erythema and carcinogenic effects) and to the cornea

CHEMICALS COMMONLY INVOLVED
IN EYE INJURY

*Alkalis* are especially dangerous because of their ability to rapidly penetrate into the interior of the eye with severe consequences. (Ammonia penetrates into the interior of the eye within seconds and sodium hydroxide within minutes.) The severity of ocular injury is proportional to alkalinity and not to a specific cation. Many workers do not realize that wet plaster containing lime is sufficiently alkaline to result in blindness if not immediately and thoroughly removed from the eye.

*Acids* can burn the eye. Acid burns are usually less severe than alkali burns since acids do not penetrate into the eye as readily. However, since sulfuric acid is one of the most frequently used compounds in industry, permanent corneal scarring from acids is not rare.

*Carbon dioxide* poisoning may result in retinal degeneration, photophobia, abnormalities of eye movements, constriction of peripheral visual fields, enlargement of the blind spots, and deficient dark adaptation.

*Alkyl esters of sulfuric acid* are intensely irritating to the conjunctiva, cornea, and eyelid. Many esters are irritating to the conjunctiva.

*Hydrogen sulfide* causes a keratoconjunctivitis that is responsible for colored rings around lights and increased photophobia—a possible warning sign of early poisoning.

*Quinone vapor and hydroxyquinone dust* cause corneal and conjunctival pigmentation that can result in significant visual loss.

*Ketones* can be irritating to the eyes and mucous membranes.

*Methanol* can cause total blindness from optic atrophy.

Concentrated *nitric acid*, when splashed into the eye, produces immediate opacification of the cornea. Severe nitric acid burns cause blindness, symblepharon (adhesion of the eyelids to the globe of the eye), and phthisis (blind, soft eye).

Although *silver* results in argyrosis—the dramatic staining of the conjunctiva, cornea, and rarely the lens—significant associated visual loss has not been reported.

Organic *tin* compounds can cause intense chemical conjunctivitis associated with severe itching.

(photokeratitis) and lens (cataract) of the eye (180–400 nm).

2. Thermal injury to the retina of the eye (400–1,400 nm).
3. Blue-light photochemical injury to the retina of the eye (principally 400–550 nm).
4. Near-infrared thermal hazards to the lens (approximately 800–3,000 nm).
5. Thermal injury (burns) of the skin (approximately 340 nm–1 mm) and of the cornea of the eye (approximately 1,400 nm–1 mm).

### Company-Organized Sports and Exercise Programs

Many companies have physical fitness and sports programs that are important to the well-being, happiness, and ultimate on-the-job productivity of employees. However, many sports have an eye injury potential that can exceed the on-the-job eye injury risk. Hockey and the racket sports have very high eye-injury risk. Eye protection that meets American Society of Testing Materials (ASTM) standards should be mandated for these sports. Baseball, softball, basketball, and soccer have relatively high eye-injury risk. Safety glasses with polycarbonate lenses are indicated for these sports.

## Preplacement Examination and Safety Education

The purpose of preplacement examinations is to: (1) check for preexisting eye disorders, (2) identify

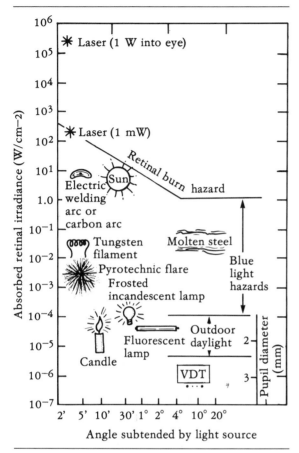

**Fig. 25-1.** Retinal irradiances (exposure dose rates) from representative light sources. Levels above $10^{-4}$ W/cm² may cause photochemical blue-light injury from fixating the source. Above 10 W/cm² (depending on image size), thermal burns may result from brief exposures. (From D Sliney, M Wolbarsht. Safety with lasers and other optical sources. New York: Plenum, 1980.)

individuals who are functionally one-eyed, (3) prescribe appropriate protective eyewear, and (4) ascertain that workers such as truck drivers meet standards for visual performance. The examination must be accompanied by education to teach the employee the potential for ocular injuries on the job, the importance of protection, and workplace rules regarding eye safety.

### Checking for Preexisting Disorders

In any work setting where there is eye injury risk, it is important that the employer document basic visual skills and rule out significant preexisting eye disease. In addition to guiding decisions about job placement and eye protection, this documentation protects both the employee and the company by providing baseline data that can be compared with results of subsequent screenings after any apparent eye injury and when the employee leaves the company.

For most occupations, satisfactory visual screening includes: central visual acuity (both for distant and near vision), muscle balance and eye coordination, depth and color discrimination, and horizontal peripheral fields. These screening tests can be measured by a nurse or a physician's assistant in 7 minutes or less on one of a variety of available binocular test instruments. These instruments are simple to operate, easy to transport, and relatively inexpensive, and they rarely require maintenance. For occupations that have a higher risk of eye injury, such as some work with high-powered lasers, screening by an ophthalmologist is preferable. Additional test procedures may be desirable, such as Amsler grid, fundus photos, peripheral visual fields, refraction, or a comprehensive eye examination; the value of particular test procedures can be discussed with the consulting ophthalmologist. Standardized reporting forms have been developed for these screening tests.

### Discovering the Functionally One-Eyed

A person is functionally one-eyed when loss of the better eye would result in a significant change in lifestyle due to poorer vision in the remaining eye. There is no question that a person with 20/200 or poorer best-corrected vision in one eye is functionally one-eyed since loss of the good eye would result in legal or total blindness and a burden both to the individual and society. On the other hand, most of us would function quite well with 20/40 or better vision in one eye. More difficult is advising employees with best-corrected vision in the poorer eye between 20/40 and 20/200. The loss of the ability to drive legally in most states would be a significant handicap to most persons and would significantly interfere with many present and potential future work and commuting situations. Therefore, we could safely conclude that an employee is effectively one-eyed if the best-correctable vision in the poorer eye is less than 20/40.

Every employee who tests less than 20/40 (with glasses, if worn) on the preplacement examination *must* be evaluated by an optometrist or an ophthalmologist to determine if the subnormal vision is simply due to a change in refraction. If the best-corrected vision in either eye is less than 20/40 after refraction, ophthalmologic evaluation to obtain a definitive diagnosis of the visual deficit and an accurate preplacement ocular evaluation are indicated.

If the employee is functionally one-eyed, the potential serious, long-term consequences of injury to the better eye should be discussed in detail prior to assigning work with intrinsic ocular risk. This discussion is essential even if the employee feels that life would not be changed if vision in the better eye were lost.

Effective eye protection is possible only when the employee understands the risks and is willing to cooperate with protective measures. Having the unconvinced employee wear an occluder over the better eye for several days will allow a better evaluation of the ability to function with the poorer eye. Usually, with an honest appraisal by the employee it is fairly easy to reach an agreement between the employer, the employee, and the ophthalmologist as to whether the employee is functionally one-eyed and the level of extra protection needed to decrease the risk of eye injury to the lowest possible level.

Most jobs that pose a high risk to unprotected eyes can be made quite safe with the use of appropriate protective devices. The employee deserves a careful explanation of the eye injury risk in the proposed job category, both with and without various types of eye protectors.

In addition to on-the-job protective eyewear, it is prudent for functionally one-eyed people to protect the good eye when they are not at work by wearing glasses made of polycarbonate lenses mounted in a sturdy frame. This is especially true of active people who are subject to eye injury in leisure activities. *The important role of glasses as a protective device cannot be overemphasized.*

### Prescribing Appropriate Protective Eyewear

Prescribing appropriate protective eyewear requires knowledge of the potential on-the-job risks and the best available means of protection. The nonexpert can get advice from an ophthalmologist, optometrist, or safety consultant who is experienced in eye hazards and protective eyewear.

All safety eyewear must meet the American National Standards Institute (ANSI) Z87.1 standard requirements. Again, polycarbonate plastic is best suited for use in a protective device unless special filtration or optical considerations make it impossible. Industrial safety lenses made of glass have only a fraction of the impact resistance of polycarbonate.

Since the total protection is decreased by up to 25 percent when side shields are removed (Fig. 25-2), dispensing safety eyewear without side shields cannot be justified for any work situation with a potential risk of flying particles or a significant risk of class 3 or class 4 laser exposure. Side shields are *always* indicated on safety eyewear (Fig. 25-3) unless the eyewear is to be used *only* in an office environment.

Goggles are indicated for (1) work where there is a higher potential for many fine flying particles, (2) use with certain lasers, (3) use over streetwear spectacles, (4) use with chemicals, and (5) welding that does not require a full-face shield (Figs. 25-4 and 25-5).

Face shields are required for arc welding (Fig. 25-6) or for use with tools that can project particles that pose an injury potential to the face, including the eyes. Protective eyeglasses or goggles

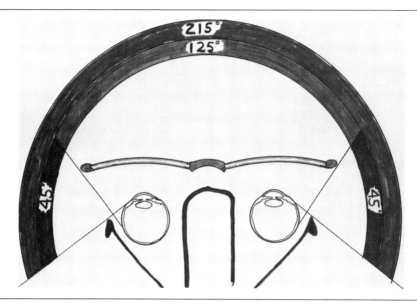

**Fig. 25-2.** View of the area of coverage of safety glasses without side shields. Note 90 degrees of unprotected eyes exposed to penetration by a fragment.

should *always* be worn under face shields, since workers frequently raise the shield to chip slag, examine a work piece, or breathe more easily—thus temporarily exposing the eyes to risk of injury.

*Laser eye protection* is designed to provide the greatest visual transmission along with an adequate optical density at the laser wavelengths. Most laser hazard controls are common sense procedures designed to limit personnel from the beam path and to limit the primary and reflected beams from occupied areas. The degree of control must be correlated with the injury potential of the laser in use (Table 25-2).

Selecting appropriate protective eyewear for laser use requires knowing (1) at least three output parameters of the laser—maximum exposure duration, wavelength, and output power (or energy); (2) applicable safe corneal radiant exposure; and (3) environmental factors, such as ambient lighting and the nature of the laser operation.

The laser wavelength(s) for which the type of eye shields were designed should be specified. Commercial protective eyewear is designed to greatly reduce or essentially prevent particular wavelength(s) from reaching the eye. Although most lasers emit only one wavelength, many lasers emit more, in which case each wavelength must be considered. It is seldom adequate to merely mark on the goggle that it will protect against radiation from a particular laser or it will protect against only the wavelength corresponding to the greatest output power. For example, a helium-neon laser may emit 100 mW at 632 nm and only 10 mW at 1,150 nm; however, safety goggles that absorb at the 632-nm wavelength may absorb little or nothing at the 1,150-nm wavelength. Hence, the wavelength range of use must be specified.

Eye protection filters for glass workers, steel and foundry workers, and welders are specified by *shades* (logarithmic representations of visual transmission). Typical shade values are the following:

| | |
|---|---|
| Acetylene flames | Shade 3 or 4 |
| Electric welding arcs | Shade 10 to 13 |
| Viewing the sun or plasma cutting/spraying | Shade 13 or higher |

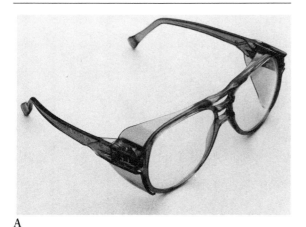

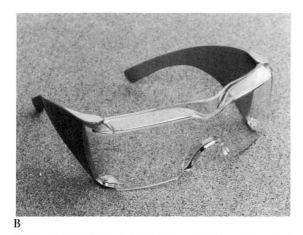

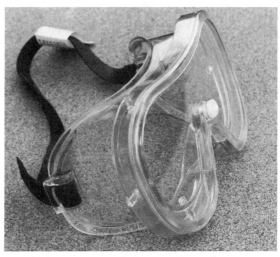

**Fig. 25-4.** Goggles, designed to protect eyes from chemical splash, suitable for use alone or over other spectacles.

**Fig. 25-3.** Safety wear with side shields, for use (A) by workers who require a prescription lens or (B) by workers who require eye protection, but do not need a spectacle lens for better vision.

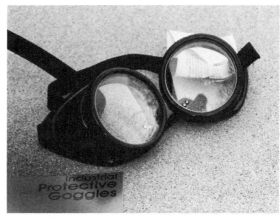

**Fig. 25-5.** Dust and impact goggles that could support protective lenses for impact, welding, or laser use.

These densities greatly exceed those necessary to prevent retinal burns but are required to reduce the luminance (brightness) to comfortable viewing levels. The user of the eye protection should therefore be permitted to choose the shade most personally desirable for the particular operation. Actinic UV radiation from welding arcs is effectively eliminated in all standard welding filters. Few people use welding goggles for arc welding because a welding helmet or shield is necessary to protect the face as well as the eyes from radiant energy.

Contact lenses give no eye protection and are contraindicated when the employee is exposed to chemicals, especially alkalis. The contact lens can be very difficult to remove when the employee has

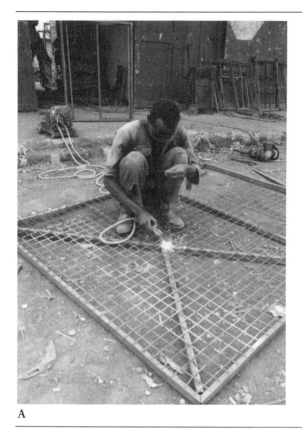

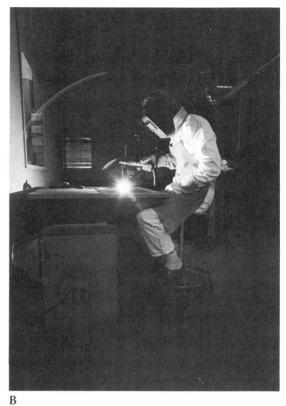

A                                                    B

**Fig. 25-6.** Use of proper eye protection in welding operations is necessary to protect against permanent eye damage. A. Inadequate protection. (Photograph by Barry Levy.) B. Adequate protection. (Photograph by Denny Lorentzen from *Newsletter*, National Swedish Board of Occupational Safety and Health, January 1981.)

**Table 25-2.** Laser hazard categories

Class 4: high power, can produce hazardous diffuse reflections and may also present a fire hazard or significant skin hazard.

Class 3: medium power, cannot produce hazardous diffuse reflections but does present a hazard when the beam is viewed directly.

Class 2: low power (<1 mW), are visible lasers safe for momentary (<0.25 sec) viewing; the eye's aversion response to bright light would normally preclude a person from staring into the light.

Class 1: nonhazardous, emit less than the recommended limits for intrabeam viewing for the maximal reasonable viewing duration.

a chemical corneal burn that involves extreme uncontrolled eyelid closure. The contact lens then will make irrigation far less effective since chemicals or caustic particles may be trapped beneath the lens, away from the flushing stream. Contact lenses are relatively contraindicated in areas where there is a large amount of dust, since particles trapped beneath the lens may increase the chance of corneal injury.

Contact lenses give no protection from UV keratitis (flash burn). Despite cases in the media reporting the "welding" of contact lenses to the cornea, a contact lens cannot be welded to the eye. All cases investigated have proven to be false reports. The pain that resulted was, in all investigated cases, due to UV keratitis because proper protection was not used over the contact lenses.

### Developing Occupational Group Standards for Visual Performance

Various job categories require different visual skills. A receptionist could be totally blind, whereas a precision machine worker might require better-than-average skills for near vision. However, some highly motivated but visually impaired employees may, with the help of low vision aids, function quite well in jobs that usually require good visual skills; they may do so as long as their placement on the job will not cause undue hazard to themselves or other employees. Thus, while visual guidelines are important, there may be exceptions.

Basic guidelines for visual skills associated with successful performance of various job tasks are noted in the Purdue Vision Standards.* However, these standards must be combined with information gathered at the workstation. This information includes observation of the employee's performance on the job so as not to discriminate against the visually handicapped but highly motivated employee who may be performing the job in a more satisfactory manner than a less-motivated, "hawk-eyed" coworker.

### Teaching Employees Company Rules on Eye Safety

Every company that has jobs with risk of eye injury *must* have written, enforced rules concerning eye safety. The employee must know both the rules and the consequences for not obeying them. A laissez-faire attitude on the part of the safety officer will result in noncompliance with the eye safety program, leading to eye injuries, disability, and litigation.

*Source: American Academy of Ophthalmology. Interprofessional Education Committee. The worker's eye. San Francisco: American Academy of Ophthalmology, 1981.

## First Aid and Referral Program for Occupational Eye Injuries

Chemicals must be copiously and thoroughly irrigated from the eye. All employees who might receive ocular chemical burns through their work must be taught the principle and methodology of prompt irrigation for any chemical that comes in contact with the eye. Emergency eyewash fountains must be located conveniently in chemical laboratories and in industrial chemical facilities. Eyewash fountains need to be tested regularly to make sure that they function properly.

Occupational health nursing personnel must be taught the symptoms and signs of serious eye injury (see box on p. 508), treatment of which consists of: (1) application of a dry, sterile eye pad to the injured eye; (2) the use of a protective shield if laceration of the globe of the eye is suspected; and (3) prompt referral to an ophthalmologist. The nurses must have constant access to immediate ophthalmologic consultation by a prearranged agreement with a hospital emergency department that has ophthalmologic coverage *or* an independent ophthalmologist (or group of ophthalmologists) who agrees to give full-time coverage for serious eye injuries.

## Management of Eye Injuries

1. *Immediate emergency action followed by a referral to an ophthalmologist* is indicated for all chemical injuries. Any chemical splashed into the eye(s) must be considered a vision-threatening emergency. Forcibly keep the patient's eyelids open while irrigating with water from any source for at least 5 minutes; *then* refer the patient to an ophthalmologist. Inform the ophthalmologist of the nature of the chemical contaminant.

2. *Injuries that require prompt referral* include all injuries with signs or symptoms of serious eye injury (see box on p. 508). Patch the injured eye lightly with a dry, sterile eye pad. If laceration of the eye is suspected, add a protective shield over the sterile eye pad. Instruct the patient not to

tightly squeeze the eye shut because it greatly elevates the intraocular pressure. Calmly transport the patient to the ophthalmologist.

3. *Injuries that are treatable at the site* include conjunctival foreign body, dislodged contact lens, and spontaneous nontraumatic asymptomatic subconjunctival hemorrhage. Conjunctivitis, with normal vision and a clear cornea, can be treated with an antibiotic eye ointment for several days. If there is no improvement, referral to the ophthalmologist is indicated.

*Never* put eye ointment in an eye about to be seen by the ophthalmologist. The ointment makes clear visualization of the retina very difficult.

*Never* give a patient a topical anesthetic to relieve pain, such as from a flash burn. The prolonged use of topical anesthetics can result in blindness from corneal breakdown.

*Never* treat a patient with a topical steroid unless directed by the ophthalmologist. Topical steroids can make several conditions much worse, such as herpes simplex keratitis, fungal infections, and some bacterial infections.

If in doubt as to how severe an ocular symptom or sign is, *always err on the side of caution* and refer the employee to the ophthalmologist for diagnosis and treatment.

# Other Requirements for Eye Safety Programs

Site evaluation and effective preventive eye care in the workplace need a great deal of improvement. Full-site evaluation and determination of visual and safety needs require input from an occupational health team including occupational and primary care physicians, ophthalmologists, nurses, optometrists, opticians, industrial hygienists, laser safety officers, and other safety personnel.

The occupational health team evaluates and preserves vision and ocular health by assessing:

The visual requirements needed to adequately and safely perform the job

The worker's visual skills

The safety of various job tasks

The illumination and visual/ergonomic conditions of the worksite

The intrinsic safety of the worksite

The availability and suitability of protective eyewear

Medical access and a system for first aid and definitive care in the event of injury

Obviously stated safety rules easily seen by all workers at the site

A definite statement concerning enforced company penalties for violations of safety rules

# Safety at the Workplace

## Direct Trauma

Prevention of eye injury from direct trauma requires a combination of: making equipment safer with proper shields; positioning workers so that flying particles from one worker's area do not enter the space of a nearby worker; prescribing, dispensing, and maintaining protective eyewear; and ensuring that safety eyewear is worn at all times.

## Light and Laser Hazards

Three factors enter into any analysis of light and laser hazards: (1) the type of laser or light source and the potential hazards of associated equipment, (2) the environment, and (3) potentially exposed individuals. Since many combinations are possible, numerous, rigid laser safety regulations should be avoided.

Since bright, continuous visible sources elicit a normal aversion or pain response that can protect the eye from injury, visual comfort can often be used as an approximate hazard index for the design of goggles and other hazard controls. Almost all conceivable accident situations require a hazardous exposure to be delivered within the period of the blink reflex. Few arc sources are sufficiently large and bright enough to be a retinal burn hazard under normal viewing conditions, but if the arc or tungsten filament is greatly magnified by an optical projection system, it is possible for hazardous irradiances to be imaged on a sufficiently large area of the retina to cause a burn. If an arc were initiated at a close viewing range (a few meters for all but the most powerful xenon searchlights, or a few inches from a welding arc, most movie projection equipment, or movie lamps) a retinal burn could result. Several hazard-reduction options are available to prevent individuals from viewing the source at close range.

The probability of hazardous *laser* retinal exposure is almost always remote. The pencil beam from most lasers is so small that direct entry into the 2- to 7-mm pupil of the eye is unlikely unless deliberate exposure occurs or unless an extremely careless atmosphere exists in the laser work area. However, the perception of a low likelihood of injury is probably the greatest single problem that exists with laser safety programs. When workers who do not follow precautions or who do not wear eye protectors are not injured, overconfidence, a lack of trust in the health and safety professionals, and a continued disregard for safety programs result. The only solution is a sound program of education, coupled with strict enforcement of company safety regulations. If workers understand that the laser hazard is somewhat similar to Russian roulette, they are more likely to take precautions. Better-educated workers may also be less likely to attribute all eye irritation or vision changes they experience to work with the lasers.

## Safety Enforcement Policies

It is not possible to overstate the importance of eye injury prevention in terms of worker pain and suffering, the medical costs to society, and the direct and indirect costs to industry. Safety is as much a concern of management as it is of the occupational health team. Management must ensure that safety rules are followed, that overall planning includes safety, and that safety activities are promoted—through newsletters or membership in the Wise Owl Club, which is sponsored by the National Society to Prevent Blindness.

## Bibliography

American Academy of Ophthalmology, Interprofessional Education Committee. The worker's eye. San Francisco: American Academy of Ophthalmology, 1981.
*Text and slides on workers' eye safety programs.*
American National Standards Institute (New York). Standards:
ANSI Z87.1—1989 practice for occupational and educational eye and face protection.
ANSI Z136.1—1986 safe use of lasers.
ANSI Z49.1—welding and cutting.
Duke-Elder S, MacFaul PA. System of ophthalmology injuries. St. Louis: Mosby, 1972. Vol. 14
*A complete description of injuries with an excellent bibliography.*
Sliney D, Wolbarsht M. Safety with lasers and other optical sources. New York: Plenum, 1980.
*A detailed text with multiple references.*
Vinger PF. The eye and sports medicine. In TD Duane. ed. Clinical ophthalmology. Philadelphia: Harper & Row, 1985. Vol. 5, Chap. 45.
*Charts on polycarbonate included. Safety in sports programs featured.*

# 26

# Disorders of the Nervous System

Edward L. Baker, Jr., and Richard Schottenfeld

The nervous system, comprised of the brain, spinal cord, and peripheral nerves, is a complex system responsible for both voluntary and involuntary control of most body functions. These are accomplished through a process of receiving and interpreting stimuli as well as transmitting information to the effector organs. The adverse impact of stressors from the work environment (physical, chemical, and psychological) are experienced in a variety of ways. Of the many means by which these effects can be categorized, we have chosen the somewhat arbitrary distinctions between neurologic and behavioral effects on the one hand, and psychiatric effects on the other, to organize this information for the reader—Eds.

## Neurologic and Behavioral Disorders

### Edward L. Baker, Jr.

A 29-year-old man was seen following 8 years of employment in a chlor-alkali plant where he was primarily employed in maintenance and operation of the electrolytic cells. Four years after beginning work in the plant he began to notice increased nervousness and irritability. His nervousness continued for 2 years; he then began to experience episodes of severe depression. At that time he also experienced a tremor of the hands, bleeding gums, easy fatiguability, increased salivation, and loss of appetite. He sustained an injury to his left Achilles tendon and was away from work for 7 months, during which time most of his symptoms improved. Tremu-

lousness, nervousness, and depression, however, remained.

This man and his wife reported that prior to his employment at the plant he was outgoing, calm, and patient. He had been a military policeman in the Marines and did not experience emotional upsets during his tour of duty despite significant stress.

Urine mercury monitoring, which had been performed by his employer during his entire period of employment, had demonstrated numerous values over 500 μg per liter, the highest of which was 736 μg per liter in his fifth year of employment (normal range in general population 5–30 μg per liter).

Physical examination performed at the end of his 7-month removal from work showed no evidence of tremor, a mild loss of pinprick sensation on the dorsal aspect of his arms, and an otherwise normal neurologic exam. Lines of increased pigmentation were observed at the gingival margins of several teeth.

Neuropsychological testing showed normal levels of intellectual functioning. He showed mild defects in his ability to perform mental calculations and in his immediate verbal and visual memory. Written spelling was particularly impaired with an inability to copy simple sentences. He could not concentrate on various tasks and, as a result, his performance was erratic with incorrect answers to simple questions and correct answers to more difficult ones. He was emotionally labile in the test situation, appearing anxious and depressed. He displayed average performance on tests of manual dexterity.

This patient's illness was manifest primarily by emotional disturbances that had secondary effects on standardized tasks of psychological performance. He showed no particular deficits in memory, psychomotor performance, learning ability, or recall of current events.

His most striking deficit was one of impaired concentration, which resulted in erratic performance on various tests. These effects were still detected months after he was removed from mercury exposure.

During recent years increasing concern has developed over the occurrence of neurobehavioral disorders among workers in various occupations. In many instances, as in this case study, specific chemical substances have been identified that are responsible for characteristic pathologic processes within the nervous system. In other cases groups of substances such as solvents have been associated epidemiologically with manifestations of nervous system disease. Although exposure to industrial toxins has been known for hundreds of years to affect behavior, recent studies have applied quantitative methods to the study of behavioral aberrations following toxin exposure and have demonstrated a wide range of clinical and subclinical effects for numerous substances. It has been shown that many neurotoxic agents produce a dose-related spectrum of impairment, ranging from mild slowing of nerve conduction velocity or prolongation in reaction time to neuropathy and frank encephalopathy.

Disorders with predominantly psychiatric manifestations have been described in some workers, ranging from acute psychosis and "mass psychogenic illness" to chronic neurasthenia (a condition characterized by mildly impaired responses to behavioral tests and symptoms of persistent fatigue). Although specific chemical substances have been identified that may be associated with certain of these psychiatric syndromes, etiologic mechanisms are unclear.

In view of the increasing diversity of industrial hazards, neurologic disorders are likely to follow the introduction of some new substances into the workplace. This happened in the 1970s when an industrial catalyst, dimethylaminopropionitrile (DMAPN), was found to be associated with bladder neuropathy in workers producing polyurethane foam; it also recently occurred when peripheral neuropathy in employees in a coated-fabrics plant was traced to the introduction of a neurotoxic solvent, methyl *n*-butyl ketone (MBK).

## Neurologic Disorders

### Pathophysiology

**Peripheral Nervous System Effects.** Two basic forms of damage to peripheral nerves have been identified as responsible for the peripheral neuropathies associated with occupational exposure to neurotoxins. *Segmental demyelination* results from primary destruction of the neuronal myelin sheath, with relative sparing of the axons. This process begins at the nodes of Ranvier and results in slowing of nerve conduction. There is characteristically no evidence of muscle denervation, although disuse atrophy may occur if paralysis is prolonged. As remyelination begins during the recovery phase, recovery is rapid and usually complete in mild to moderate neuropathies.

*Axonal degeneration* is associated with metabolic derangement of the entire neuron and is manifest by degeneration of the distal portion of the nerve fiber. Myelin sheath degeneration may occur secondarily. Nerve conduction rates are usually normal until the condition is relatively far advanced. Distal muscles show changes of denervation. Recovery may occur by axonal regeneration but is very slow and incomplete.

In many instances, axonal degeneration and segmental demyelination may coexist, presumably due to secondary effects derived from damage to each system. Therefore, although the above descriptions of classic manifestations of these syndromes hold in experimental models, the clinical manifestations of neuropathy in exposed individuals may represent a combination of both pathologic processes.

**Central Nervous System Effects.** Recent studies, including investigations of lead, chlordecone (Kepone), and carbon monoxide, have shown significant disruption of neurotransmitter metabolism, affecting dopamine, norepinephrine, gamma-aminobutyric acid (GABA), and serotonin, which correlates with behavioral aberrations in experimental animals. Furthermore, many industrial solvents cause acute depression of central nervous system (CNS) synaptic transmission resulting in drowsiness and weakness. Such mechanisms are undoubtedly responsible for the poorly understood manifestations of CNS toxicity induced by workplace substances.

### Combined Peripheral and Central Nervous System Effects.

Certain industrial neurotoxins cause distal degeneration of axons in both the central and peripheral nervous systems. This form of axonal degeneration was originally described as "dying back" neuropathy. In view of the association of central and peripheral nervous system degeneration, it has been recently suggested that this process be referred to as central-peripheral distal axonopathy. Substances associated with this effect include acrylamide, n-hexane, MBK, carbon disulfide, and organophosphorus compounds, the most notable of which is tri-ortho-cresyl phosphate (TOCP).

Characteristically, distal degeneration occurs within the long nerve fiber tracts of both the peripheral and central nervous systems. Once degeneration begins peripherally, it becomes more severe in the initially affected nerve segments while progressing centrally to involve more proximal segments of nerve fibers. Within the spinal cord the long ascending and descending tracts (the spinocerebellar and corticospinal tracts) appear to be the most severely affected. Involved fiber tracts demonstrate axonal swellings, which are often focal and are associated with neurofilament accumulation within the axon. Although the length of the axon is a key determinant of fiber susceptibility, fiber diameter may also be important: Large-diameter, myelinated fibers are more frequently affected.

The precise locus of the metabolic derangement that is responsible for these manifestations of axonal damage is unknown. Chemical substances may bind to the inactivate intra-axonal enzyme systems required for maintenance of normal axonal transport mechanisms.

### Manifestations

### Peripheral Nervous System.

Virtually all of the industrial toxins that affect the peripheral nervous system cause a mixed sensorimotor peripheral neuropathy. The initial manifestations of this disorder consist of intermittent numbness and tingling in the hands and feet; motor weakness in the feet or hands may develop somewhat later and progress to the development of an ataxic gait or an inability to grasp heavy objects. Although the distal portion of the extremities is involved initially and to a greater degree, severe cases may also manifest proximal muscle weakness and muscle atrophy. Nerve biopsies in affected individuals have shown axonal swellings and paranodal myelin retraction. Extensor muscle groups usually manifest weakness before flexors.

Although the manifestations are fairly consistent from one toxin to another, certain specific characteristics are unique to individual agents (Table 26-1). Painful limbs and increased sensitivity of the feet to touch are particularly characteristic of arsenical neuropathy. Sensory involvement predominates in the relatively rare neuropathy seen with alkyl mercury poisoning. Both motor and sensory disorders are observed in the neuropathies associated with exposure to n-hexane, MBK, and acrylamide.

The peripheral neuropathy associated with lead exposure is unusual because only the motor system is involved. The most characteristic early manifestation of lead neuropathy is wrist extensor weakness. Reports of involvement of the lower extremities resulting in ankle drop were made during the 1930s, when cabaret dancers consumed lead-contaminated illicit whiskey and developed lead neuropathy in the muscles that they used most actively. Overt wrist drop, which was a characteristic manifestation of lead neuropathy in reports of many years ago, is quite rare today.

The development of these syndromes is usually

**Table 26-1.** Peripheral nervous system effects of occupational toxins*

| Effect | Toxin | Comments |
| --- | --- | --- |
| Motor neuropathy | Lead | Primarily wrist extensors |
| | | Wrist drop and ankle drop rare |
| Mixed sensorimotor neuropathy | Acrylamide | Ataxia common |
| | | Desquamation of hands and soles |
| | | Sweating of palms |
| | Arsenic | Distal paresthesias earliest symptom |
| | | Painful limbs, especially in calves |
| | | Hyperpathia of feet |
| | | Weakness prominent in legs |
| | Carbon disulfide | Peripheral neuropathy rather mild |
| | | CNS effects more important |
| | Carbon monoxide | Seen only after severe intoxication |
| | DDT | Only seen with ingestions |
| | n-hexane and methyl n-butyl ketone (MBK) | Distal paresthesias and motor weakness |
| | | Weight loss, fatigue, and muscle cramps common |
| | Mercury | Predominantly distal sensory involvement |
| | | More common with alkyl mercury exposure |
| | Organophosphate insecticides (selected agents) | Delayed onset following single exposure (usually nonoccupational) |

*This table and subsequent tables include most but not all of the neurotoxic substances associated with listed conditions.

insidious. Very slow development of numbness and tingling of the fingers and toes occurs over several weeks and may then be followed by motor weakness. Of particular interest is the case of several toxins, including acrylamide, n-hexane, and MBK, in which the neuropathy may progress even after workers are removed from exposure. This deterioration persists for 3 to 4 weeks after removal from exposure; at that point recovery may begin. The duration of the recovery process is proportional to the degree of severity of neuropathy: Less severely affected cases may totally resolve over a 3- to 6-month period, whereas individuals with advanced disease may show persistent signs and symptoms 1 to 2 years later.

Physical examination of affected individuals shows a characteristic distribution of sensory loss, particularly to pain and temperature discrimination (Fig. 26-1). Frequently vibration sensation is impaired and touch perception, particularly with acrylamide poisoning, is lost. Tremor of the hands is particularly common in several types of chemical intoxication. In most instances the tremor is a resting tremor that is not increased with movement. The tremor seen with chlordecone (Kepone) poisoning is a frequent manifestation of the disease and has characteristic features: irregular, nonpurposive, and most severe when the limb is static but unsupported against gravity. In contrast the tremor seen with mercury poisoning is fine and affects the eyelids, tongue, and outstretched hands. Motor weakness in toxic neuropathies is characteristically found in distal muscles of the arms and legs (Fig. 26-1). Intrinsic muscles of the hands and feet are particularly affected in neuropathies caused by n-hexane, MBK, and acrylamide. Exten-

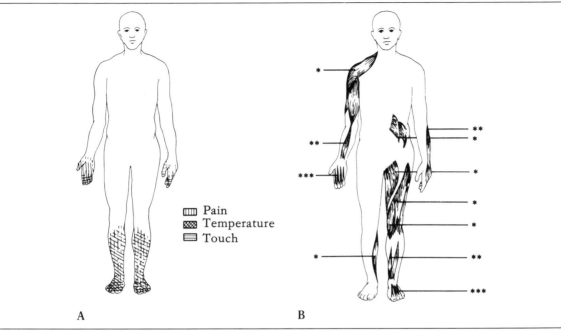

**Fig. 26-1.** A. Pattern of sensory loss in a severe case of MBK neuropathy. B. Distribution of muscle weakness in MBK neuropathy with degree of weakness proportional to number of asterisks. (From N Allen. Solvents and other industrial organic compounds. In PJ Vinken, GW Bruyn eds. Intoxications of the nervous system. Part I [vol. 36] in Handbook of clinical neurology. Amsterdam: Elsevier/North-Holland Biomedical Press, 1979.)

sor weakness of the forearms is characteristic of lead neuropathy. Impaired coordination is often seen in individuals with motor weakness in the extremities; cerebellar pathology need not be present for these manifestations to occur. In summary, distal sensory and motor impairment characterized by numbness and weakness of the hands and feet is followed by more proximal involvement as the toxic neuropathy develops.

*Other Neurologic Manifestations.* A wide variety of additional manifestations may be seen that are specific to individual toxins (Table 26-2). Movement disorders that resemble Parkinson's disease have been reported in individuals exposed to carbon disulfide, carbon monoxide, and manganese; hypotonia, dystonia, and other disorders of locomotion occur in individuals with excessive expo-

sure to these substances. In the case of manganese toxicity, significant improvement following drug therapy was seen in the characteristic mask-like facies of a patient with occupational exposure to this toxin (Fig. 26-2).

A characteristic abnormality of eye movements called opsoclonus can be caused by chlordecone (Kepone) exposure. It consists of irregular bursts of involuntary, abrupt, rapid jerks of both eyes simultaneously, usually horizontal, but multidirectional in severely affected individuals.

Seizures are often seen in individuals with acute excessive exposure to industrial toxins. Organochlorine insecticides such as DDT and chlordane have been associated with seizures following acute ingestion of large doses. Seizures are a rare manifestation of lead encephalopathy in adults.

Cranial nerve involvement is uncommon with

**Table 26-2.** Other neurologic manifestations of occupational toxins

| Manifestation | Agent |
|---|---|
| Ataxic gait | Acrylamide |
|  | Chlordane |
|  | Chlordecone (Kepone) |
|  | DDT |
|  | *n*-hexane |
|  | Manganese |
|  | Mercury (especially methyl mercury) |
|  | Methyl *n*-butyl ketone (MBK) |
|  | Methyl chloride |
|  | Toluene |
| Bladder neuropathy | Dimethylaminopropionitrile (DMAPN) |
| Constricted visual fields | Mercury |
| Cranial neuropathy | Carbon disulfide |
|  | Trichloroethylene |
| Headache | Lead |
|  | Nickel |
| Impaired visual acuity | *n*-hexane |
|  | Mercury |
|  | Methanol |
| Increased intracranial pressure | Lead |
|  | Organotin compounds |
| Myoclonus | Benzene hexachloride |
|  | Mercury |
| Nystagmus | Mercury |
| Opsoclonus | Chlordecone (Kepone) |
| Paraplegia | Organotin compounds |
| Parkinsonism | Carbon disulfide |
|  | Carbon monoxide |
|  | Manganese |
| Seizures | Lead |
|  | Organic mercurials |
|  | Organochlorine insecticides |
|  | Organotin compounds |
| Tremor | Carbon disulfide |
|  | Chlordecone (Kepone) |
|  | DDT |
|  | Manganese |
|  | Mercury |

the peripheral neurotoxins mentioned above. However, trichloroethylene has a predilection for the trigeminal facial nerves and has been associated with facial numbness and weakness. Carbon disulfide exposure is also associated with cranial neuropathies.

Excesses of CNS tumors have been reported among workers in the petrochemical industry; studies are currently being performed to determine if these are work-related.

An unusual manifestation of neurotoxicity was seen several years ago in a group of workers exposed to an industrial catalyst, dimethylaminopropionitrile (DMAPN). This substance caused a neuropathy in the bladder, resulting in urinary retention, urinary hesitancy, and sexual dysfunction. Although the symptoms improved after removal of the affected individuals from exposure to this substance, symptoms and signs persisted in some individuals for at least 2 years.

### Diagnosis

Electrophysiologic tests that assess peripheral nerve function, including electromyograms (EMGs) and nerve conduction measurements, are important tools in assessing the extent and severity of neurologic disorders in workers exposed to industrial toxins. These techniques are often useful in the evaluation of individual patients. Recently, noninvasive techniques that measure sensory thresholds for vibration and temperature have been developed to monitor diabetic patients for the occurrence of sensory neuropathy. These techniques are also efficient tools for reliable screening of workers with significant exposure to neurotoxic agents or with early sensory symptoms. In addition to detection of toxic neuropathy, these instruments may also be useful in detection of compression neuropathies, such as carpal tunnel syndrome.

Electroencephalograms (EEGs) have also been used in the evaluation of workers exposed to neurotoxins. However, these have not usually been as useful as nerve conduction tests. EEGs may be of value as an adjunct to the assessment of altered

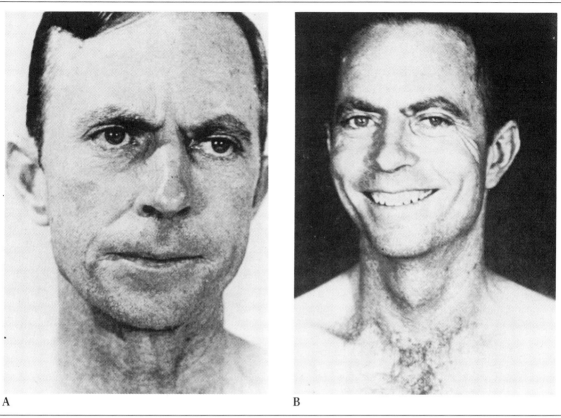

A                                    B

**Fig. 26-2.** A. Mask-like facies of patient with manganese toxicity prior to therapeutic trial with L-dopa. B. Full facial expression of same patient being maintained on L-dopa. (From HA Rosenstock, DG Simons, JS Meyer. Chronic manganism: Neurologic and laboratory studies during treatment with levodopa. JAMA 1971; 217:1355. Copyright 1971, American Medical Association.)

states of consciousness of unknown etiology. A more promising extension of EEG use is the measurement of cortical-evoked potentials following auditory or visual stimuli; for example, prolonged latency of visually evoked responses has been reported in individuals chronically exposed to *n*-hexane.

## Behavioral Disorders

### Manifestations

Excessive exposure to industrial toxins may result in behavioral effects, ranging from mild symptoms of fatigue to persistent impairment of nervous system function. In view of the vagueness of many behavioral manifestations of neurotoxin exposure, standardized psychometric testing has greatly facilitated the evaluation of these disorders. In general, neurotoxins particularly affect psychomotor performance by causing slowness in response time, impaired eye-hand coordination, and diminished concentration ability. Emotional effects are also seen and consist of irritability and, at times, emotional lability. Recent memory may be disrupted, manifest in testing situations as an inability to learn new material. Aspects of cognitive functioning that are usually not affected by toxins include remote memory and fund of general information. Two categories of chronic behavioral effect have been described: chronic symptoms alone (or organic affective syndrome) or symptoms plus abnormalities of performance or standard neurobehavioral tests (chronic toxic encephalopathy).

Although few toxins have unique behavioral effects, several substances deserve particular attention (Table 26-3). Carbon disulfide affects all levels of the CNS and may result in bizarre clinical syndromes including acute psychosis. Heavy overexposure has been associated with suicide in at least one worker. Although neurotoxins may cause both behavioral effects and peripheral neuropathy in the same individual, one effect usually predominates.

Most chlorinated hydrocarbon solvents in current use in industry cause a relatively brief "high" following exposure to significantly elevated concentrations in air. Intentional abuse of industrial solvents by individuals desiring these intoxicating effects has been reported to cause permanent damage to the peripheral and central nervous systems. Such use should obviously be proscribed in view of the potentially severe consequences.

### Diagnosis

Standardized psychometric testing using measures of memory, intelligence, attention, dexterity, reaction time, personality, and general psychomotor function is very useful in evaluating exposed individuals as well as groups of workers. These neurobehavioral tests have been adapted for computer administration to facilitate reproducibility in testing groups and to improve data-handling efficiency. Computerized testing has been used in epidemiologic and clinical research to evaluate health effects of nervous system toxins. Interpretation of test results must take into account confounding factors such as age, education, alcohol consumption, and preexisting neurologic disease in order to evaluate correctly the etiologic role of toxin exposure. The most important feature of the diagnostic process is a carefully obtained occupational history that identifies specific neurotoxins and assesses the magnitude and duration of exposure to each. The work history is particularly important in evaluating behavioral disorders since these conditions are often attributed to factors unrelated to work.

**Table 26-3.** Behavioral effects of occupational toxins

| Manifestation | Agent |
| --- | --- |
| Acute psychosis or marked emotional instability | Carbon disulfide |
| | Manganese |
| | Toluene (rare) |
| Acute intoxication | Solvents |
| | Carbon monoxide |
| Chronic behavioral symptoms | Acrylamide |
| | Arsenic |
| | Lead |
| | Manganese |
| | Mercury |
| | Methyl n-butyl ketone (MBK) |
| | Organotin compounds |
| | Organic solvents |
| | Styrene |
| Chronic toxic encephalopathy | Organic solvents |
| | Lead |
| | Carbon disulfide |
| | Styrene |

## Management and Control

Management of occupationally induced neurologic problems consists primarily of identification of the offending agent and removal of the worker from continued exposure. In some episodes—for example, that of DMAPN exposure—removal of the offending agent from the workplace may result in cessation of the development of new cases. Some workers with known exposure may develop mild, early symptoms of neurotoxicity; objective demonstration of functional impairment using standardized tests is essential in the management of individual cases. Workers with evidence of toxin-related symptoms or functional impairment should be removed from exposure until these deficits resolve and exposure in the workplace is terminated.

Prevention of occupationally induced neurologic disorders can be accomplished through workplace medical and environmental control programs. The goal of environmental control is to reduce concentrations of neurotoxic substances in the worker's environment by various manipulations. Medical strategies designed to reduce neurologic morbidity include preplacement evaluation and periodic medical monitoring. The goal of preplacement evaluation as it relates to neurologic disorders is to avoid placement of individuals with preexisting disease (such as peripheral neuropathies) in jobs with exposures that might exacerbate these conditions. Furthermore, conditions that might impair workers' ability to perform their jobs, such as uncontrolled epilepsy in persons operating hazardous machinery, would be grounds for medical exclusion of such individuals from these jobs.

Periodic medical monitoring programs are becoming more common in industries where neurotoxins are used. An important element of such monitoring programs is the measurement of the neurotoxic agent in biologic fluids. The most common such application occurs in industries where lead and mercury are used.

Periodic monitoring of lead-exposed workers should include a work and medical history; physical examination, with special attention to the nervous system; blood and urine studies to evaluate hematologic and renal effects of lead exposure; and, most importantly, determination of blood concentration of lead and zinc protoporphyrin (ZPP). The content of such exams is mandated by the federal Occupational Safety and Health Administration (OSHA) standard on occupational exposure to lead, in which specific guidelines are given for job transfer of workers with excessive concentrations of lead in their blood. The OSHA standard for inorganic lead requires that employers make routine blood-lead monitoring available to all employees exposed to lead above the action level of 30 μg per cubic meter, regardless of whether respirators are worn. The standard requires that testing be repeated every 6 months when the most recent blood-lead level is less than 40 μg per dL. If the employee's blood-lead level is greater than 50 μg per dL and this level is confirmed by a second blood-lead level (which must be obtained within 2 weeks of the employer's receipt of the first level), the employee is to be removed from any job in which exposure is above the action level of 30 μg per cubic meter. Such workers must be retested monthly and not returned to an exposed job until their blood lead is below 40 μg per dL on two analyses. If a worker's blood lead is greater than or equal to 40 μg per dL but less than or equal to 60 μg per dL the worker must be retested every 2 months. If the average of the last three blood-lead measurements taken within the last 6 months is greater than 50 μg per dL, a worker must also be removed from exposure and retested monthly until the blood lead is less than 40 μg per dL. Any worker removed from a job because of elevated blood lead is protected by the medical removal protection (MRP) provision of the OSHA lead standard. This provision requires an employer to "maintain the worker's earnings, seniority, and other employment rights and benefits (as though the worker had not been removed) for a period of up to 18 months."

The evaluation of mercury-exposed workers is similar with three exceptions. Urine mercury determinations are used rather than blood measurements; there is no enzymatic test such as the ZPP test that measures the metabolic toxicity of mercury exposure; and finally, there is no comprehensive OSHA standard for occupational mercury exposure that prescribes the content of periodic medical evaluations and medical action levels for job transfer. Workers exposed to cadmium and arsenic should be monitored periodically with urinary determinations of these two metals in addition to standard medical evaluations.

Workers chronically exposed to solvents should have periodic medical histories and physical examinations with attention to the nervous system. Standardized behavioral tests show promise as periodic monitoring tools, and measurement of urinary metabolites of solvents is sometimes helpful as an adjunct to other medical monitoring techniques.

Pesticide-exposed workers, particularly those using organophosphate insecticides, should be periodically evaluated with red blood cell cholinesterase levels to assess their degree of pesticide exposure. Although some recommendations have been made that periodic nerve conduction testing should be performed in addition to standard medical history and physical examination, this test is not suitable for routine monitoring of asymptomatic workers.

Treatment of occupational neurologic disease beyond removal of the worker from continued toxic exposure may consist of the administration of drugs designed to remove the offending agent or counteract its effects. Chelating drugs, such as ethylene diamine tetraacetic acid (EDTA), dimethylsuccinic acid (DMSA), and penicillamine, are given as treatment for symptomatic poisoning by lead and other heavy metals. These drugs should only be given as treatment for symptomatic disease and not prophylactically to lower blood levels of the metal; they have known toxicity, which may add to the toxic effects of the metals and may also increase gastrointestinal absorption of the metal. Workers should be removed from exposure to the offending agent prior to initiation of drug therapy.

Treatment of organophosphate insecticide poisoning is accomplished primarily by giving atropine, a pharmacologic antagonist of the pesticide. If patients are seen very soon after exposure, other drugs (oximes) can be given to regenerate inhibited cholinesterase enzyme.

Ultimately, prevention of occupational diseases of the nervous system rests on adequate testing of chemicals prior to their introduction into the workplace and in environmental measures designed to reduce exposure. The Toxic Substances Control Act (TSCA) addresses the issue of premarket testing, and the Environmental Protection Agency (EPA) has specified criteria for neurologic evaluation of chemical substances. Biologic assays of organophosphate compounds have successfully predicted those substances that will be neurotoxic to humans. Substances such as n-hexane and MBK, which produce an axonal neuropathy in exposed humans, have been shown to produce similar effects in animals, and the neurologic disorder associated with Kepone toxicity was seen in experimental animals several years before it was reported in exposed humans. Therefore, testing of industrial substances by administration of toxins to experimental animals is essential in the identification of substances with neurotoxic potential.

In rare instances structural similarity alone has proved useful in predicting toxicity. N-hexane and MBK are metabolized to 2,5-hexanedione, which is thought to be responsible for the neurotoxic manifestations of these two industrial chemicals. Thus, investigation of structure-activity relationships may be of value in identifying substances with potential neurotoxicity. In those instances where neurotoxicity is suspected because of the chemical structure of the compound, animal tests are still required.

As standardized tests of neurologic function become increasingly available, field studies of industrial toxins using these techniques will be used to determine the appropriate levels of industrial exposure. These levels, referred to as threshold limit values (TLVs) or permissible exposure limits (PELs), have in the past been based on informed opinion of experts. In the future, as epidemiologic studies become more precise in assessing the neurotoxic hazard of these substances, control measures and specific exposure standards will be based on much more objective information.

## Effects of Selected Neurotoxins

### Lead

The most commonly encountered workplace substance with clearly recognized neurotoxic effects is lead (see also Chaps. 13, 27, 29, and 31). The National Institute for Occupational Safety and Health (NIOSH) has estimated that over 1 million U.S. workers are daily exposed to lead (Fig. 26-3). The manifestations of lead neurotoxicity as currently encountered differ significantly from those seen in reports from the earlier part of this century when more overt disorders were observed. The most common neurologic finding in workers exposed to lead is impaired CNS function manifested by symptoms of fatigue, irritability, difficulty in concentrating, and inability to perform tasks requiring sustained concentration. These symptoms are associated with abnormalities on standardized neuropsychological testing showing impairment of verbal intelligence, memory, and perceptual speed. Symptoms of arm weakness characteristically affecting extensor muscle groups are also seen in the early phases of lead toxicity. Often, weakness occurs before abnormalities are seen on nerve conduction testing. Such abnormalities tend to de-

**Fig. 26-3.** Current work practice rules require significant personal and environmental protection in lead exposures. A. Lead battery worker is protected mainly by local exhaust ventilation. B. Automobile lead grinder is protected by air-supplied hood and floor exhaust ventilation. (Photographs by Earl Dotter.)

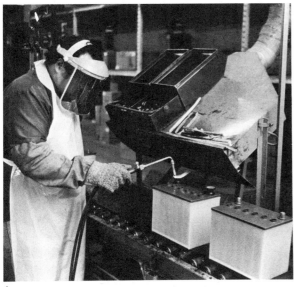

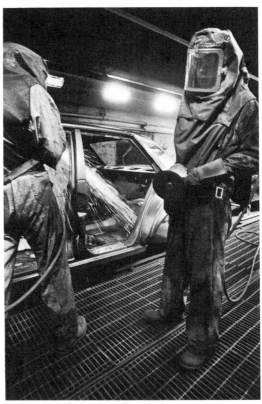

A                                                                          B velop in individuals with blood-lead levels in the range of 60 μg per deciliter and become more apparent as the blood-lead level rises. After removal from exposure, these symptoms and abnormalities resolve slowly over weeks to months, the duration depending on their initial intensity and other factors.

Neurologic abnormalities following lead exposure usually occur after hematologic toxicity as manifested by elevated ZPP level and reduction in blood hemoglobin concentration. Permanent renal damage occurs much later than neurologic dysfunction and characteristically develops only after at least 5 years of lead exposure. In contrast, neurologic abnormalities may develop within 2 to 3 months of the onset of work in a lead environment, particularly in those places where exposure is relatively poorly controlled. Abnormalities of nerve conduction tend not to occur before at least 6 to 8 months of chronic exposure to lead.

## Mercury

Although disease as striking as that experienced by Lewis Carroll's Mad Hatter no longer occurs in plants in the United States, behavioral effects of exposure to elemental mercury are seen. Erethism, a set of behavioral symptoms classically associated with mercury toxicity, is characterized by unusual shyness, anxiety, inability to concentrate, and irritability. Standardized memory tests have been shown to be affected in individuals with urine mercury concentrations of 200 μg per liter or above. A fine tremor of the hands is associated with mercury poisoning, and computer-assisted analysis of EMGs has shown a shift in the frequency of normal forearm tremor as an early manifestation of mercury toxicity. Peripheral neuropathy is not a recognized feature of elemental mercury poisoning. Measurement of mercury in urine and blood is a useful tool in the assessment of workplace exposure. Urine mercury levels above 300 μg per liter are considered excessive.

Organic mercurials, particularly alkyl mercury compounds such as methyl mercury, have a strong affinity for the CNS, and severe neurologic effects have been associated with excessive exposure (see also Chap. 27). The best-described episode of organic mercury poisoning occurred in Minamata, Japan, where early symptoms of poisoning consisted of distal paresthesias, cerebellar disorders, visual impairment, deafness, and mental disturbances. Sensory deficits were seen with loss of position sense, impaired two-point discrimination, astereognosis, and mild hypalgesia. Visual impairment characteristically consisted of constriction of visual fields. Mental disturbances were characterized by agitation alternating with periods of stupor and mutism. The more severe cases exhibited dystonic flexion postures. Peripheral neuropathies were not seen in this group of individuals.

The devastating and usually irreversible effects on the nervous system of organic mercury poisoning should be prevented through restriction of the use of these substances. To that end, the practice of treating seed grain with organic mercurial fungicides has been curtailed by the EPA following outbreaks of neurologic disease in the United States and Iraq among persons ingesting food inadvertently contaminated with these substances.

## Organophosphate Insecticides

Acute organophosphate insecticide poisoning is characterized by the inhibition of acetylcholinesterase with resulting overactivity of cholinergic components of the autonomic nervous system, inhibition of conduction across myoneural junctions in skeletal muscle, and interference of CNS synaptic transmission. Manifestations of acute toxicity include meiosis, blurring of vision, chest tightness, increased bronchial secretion, and wheezing. Gastrointestinal effects are also seen, including abdominal cramps, nausea, and vomiting. Increased sweating, salivation, and lacrimation are also characteristic features.

Atropine is the drug of choice for treating the acute manifestations of organophosphate insecticide poisoning. Repeated doses are given to the point of atropinization, and subsequent doses of the drug may be required since the duration of action of atropine is less than that of organophosphate insecticides. Since organophosphate compounds bind irreversibly to cholinesterase, reactivation of the enzyme system occurs only through synthesis of additional cholinesterase molecules. Therefore, recovery of normal cholinesterase concentrations in red blood cells is slow, and repeated exposure may result in cumulative depression of cholinesterase stores. Recovery following an acute episode of poisoning is usually complete within 7 days unless anoxia has occurred during the acute phase of the episode. Measurement of red blood cell cholinesterase concentrations is valuable during the acute intoxication episode and is also used for surveillance of occupationally exposed workers. Plasma cholinesterase concentrations are of less value in occupational settings since many factors may alter them.

A syndrome of delayed neurotoxicity has been reported with certain organophosphate compounds (although not with organophosphate pesticides currently used in the United States). This syndrome develops 8 to 35 days after exposure to the organophosphorus compounds. Progressive weakness begins in the distal lower extremities, and toe and foot drop often develop; finger weakness and wrist drop follow lower-extremity manifestations. Sensory loss is minimal. Deep tendon reflexes are frequently depressed. The disease may progress for 1 to 3 months following onset, and recovery is very slow.

Recent studies of workers occupationally exposed to organophosphates have revealed some evidence of psychomotor impairment and abnormal EEG. Further studies are required to assess the extent and nature of these disorders. Evaluation of patients exposed to organophosphate insecticides should include, in addition to work history, a neurologic exam with attention to manifestations of autonomic nervous system dysfunction. Measurement of red blood cell cholinesterase concentration is valuable; cholinesterase levels correlate reasonably well with manifestations of clinical toxicity. Migrant workers are at risk for the acute and chronic effects of exposure to organophosphate insecticides used in agriculture. Unfortunately, this population has not been adequately studied and often migrant workers do not receive adequate protection from pesticide exposure (see Chap. 35).

### Organic Solvents

Exposure to organic solvents occurs daily for over one million U.S. workers. The most frequently used include toluene, xylene, trichloroethylene, ethanol, methylene chloride, and methyl chloroform. Although chemically heterogeneous, these compounds are often discussed as a group because of toxicologically similar effects and the high frequency of exposure to various combinations of these substances (Fig. 26-4).

Acute narcosis follows exposure to high concentrations of solvent vapors, and lower levels may produce a transient intoxication syndrome similar to that seen with ethanol consumption.

To facilitate the characterization of persistent health effects of solvent exposure, a nomenclature has been developed by a World Health Organization (WHO) working group and by a workshop of invited experts held in the United States. The mildest form of effect, organic affective syndrome (or type 1 solvent health effect), is characterized by symptoms of irritability, fatiguability, difficulty in concentrating, and loss of interest in daily events. This type of effect is typically reversible. The second, a more severe form of effect, mild chronic toxic encephalopathy, is characterized by objective abnormalities on neurobehavioral testing and by symptoms that are similar to those of organic affective syndrome (type 1 effect) but are more pronounced. Sustained personality or mood change (type 2a effect) or impairment in intellectual function (type 2b) may be seen at this level of effect, singly or in combination. Severe chronic toxic encephalopathy (type 3 effect) is characterized clinically as a type of dementia with global deterioration of memory and other cognitive functions;

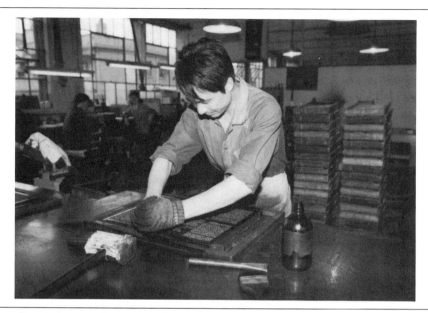

**Fig. 26-4.** Printer cleaning type with organic solvent is exposed via skin through permeable cloth gloves and air via evaporation from work surface and open bottle. (Photograph by Barry Levy.)

reversibility is unlikely. Workers exposed to solvents may exhibit any of these three syndromes depending on the intensity and duration of their exposure. Epidemiologic studies have frequently shown a decrease in reaction time, dexterity, speed, and memory among workers with prolonged solvent exposure. Relatively few abnormalities have been demonstrated in peripheral nervous system function; nerve conduction abnormalities have been reported in one study of mixed solvent exposure. Measurement of urinary metabolites such as hippuric acid in toluene exposure may be of value in monitoring exposed populations. Further research is needed to develop a more complete approach to prevention of solvent-induced disease.

## Mass Psychogenic Illness

*Mass psychogenic illness* (MPI) can be defined as the collective occurrence of physical symptoms and beliefs about the origin of these symptoms among a group of persons in the absence of a plausible biologic explanation. Reports of MPI have described workers employed at repetitive, boring tasks in workplaces having physical as well as emotional stressors. Symptoms are vague (often headache, dizziness, nausea, and weakness) and not consistent among outbreaks. The onset of an MPI outbreak has been described as precipitous, with many cases occurring over a few hours; it has been reported to follow a "trigger stimulus," which is often a noxious odor. Recurrence of similar symptoms in those initially affected are also common. Studies using psychometric testing have purported to identify "susceptible individuals" who are at risk for MPI. The poorly described nature of this entity increases the likelihood that attention will be focused on the worker when no obvious environmental agent is readily found. For this reason investigation of suspected outbreaks of MPI should focus intently on excluding environmental toxins as etiologic agents.

## Diagnosis and Management

In practice the determination that an outbreak of acute illness is due to psychogenic factors is often impossible. Exclusion of toxic agents as etiologically responsible is often very difficult in view of the paucity of understanding of the effects of workplace toxins and the complexity of exposures in the work environment. Since efforts to identify susceptible workers shift the focus away from improving the work environment, this approach is not in keeping with accepted public health practice. Many descriptions of MPI have stressed that women are more frequently affected than men; this difference in attack rates may well relate to traditional hiring practices in which women are assigned to more repetitive, boring jobs than men. Chronic stress-related complaints have often been described in plants in which MPI has occurred, suggesting that workplace factors may play an important role in the genesis of MPI. Primary attention should be directed to alleviation of chronic sources of stress in the workplace (see Chap. 19). Investigations that merely identify so-called susceptible individuals as a means of controlling this problem will fail to achieve satisfactory results and will often infringe on workers' rights.

## Psychiatric Disorders

Richard Schottenfeld

Mr. A, who is 39 years old and married, had an excellent work record as a machinist until 1 year ago, when he was involved in an unsuccessful effort to organize his workplace. Since then, he reports that his supervisor has continuously criticized his performance, assigned him jobs that he was not trained to do, and threatened to terminate his employment. Mr. A has become increasingly anxious, depressed, and preoccupied about losing his job. He believes that he will never be able to work again and blames himself for his predicament. He has become somewhat reclusive, feels too embarrassed to leave his home, and reports problems in sleeping, appetite and weight loss, and a loss of interest in his hobbies or family life. He experienced similar symptoms at age 23, following the breakup of a romantic relationship, but managed to work throughout that episode and recovered, after several months, without treatment.

It is well accepted that psychological functioning and emotional status can be profoundly influenced by the work environment. As illustrated by the case example, problems associated with the work setting and work relationships as well as perceptions about these may lead to psychological and emotional distress, ranging from mild to quite severe. Psychiatric disorders may also affect one's ability to work effectively in response to normal demands. Psychiatric evaluation is necessary after occupational disruptions, not only when hallucinations, delusions, or other severe psychiatric symptoms occur, but also following traumatic or distressing occupational exposures, during or after occupational injuries or illnesses, during prolonged periods of disability, and when unusually severe functional impairment occurs with an injury or illness.

Organic and nonorganic causes of psychiatric disorders both need to be considered. Exposures to lead, mercury, manganese, organic solvents, or other neurotoxins are common causes of work-related psychiatric disturbances [1, 2]. Nonorganic occupational causes of psychological distress include stress resulting from the physical environment at work, work tasks and related responsibilities, organizational structure and morale, interpersonal relationships at work, shiftwork (see Chap. 20), and traumatic events, including occupational illnesses or injuries [3, 4]. Occupationally related nonorganic psychiatric disorders include post-traumatic stress and adjustment, somatoform, substance abuse, anxiety, and depressive disorders.

Nonorganic psychological disorders are considered a category of leading occupational health problems by NIOSH, with an estimated one-third of all workers reporting moderate to high stress levels at work and experiencing adverse psychological effects as a result (see also Chap. 19) [3, 5].

## Mechanisms

In order to understand the psychiatric consequences of traumatic occupational exposures it is useful to rely on a biopsychosocial model. Such a model is constructed to account for the roles of toxic exposure and physical trauma as well as psychological and biological vulnerability and social factors in influencing the onset and course of post-traumatic psychiatric disorders [6].

Biologic vulnerability refers to individual differences both in sensitivity and in response to the same exposure and in susceptibility to development of psychiatric symptoms and disorders. Psychological factors affecting development of symptoms include the individual's cognitive assessment of the severity of danger, personal meaning attached to trauma, and effectiveness of coping skills and ability to modulate intense emotions that frequently follow exposure [7–10]. These emotions include anxiety, anger, helplessness, guilt, and shame. Social factors also influence symptoms and severity of psychiatric distress [11, 12]. A supportive social environment can help an individual cope with distressing emotions, while a climate of social unrest, such as during times of economic hardship, labor-management disputes, or intensified racial conflict, or community-wide misunderstanding about the actual risks of exposure can compound adverse effects.

## Toxic Effects of Occupational Exposure

Many types of heavy metals, solvents, pesticides, and other chemicals can adversely affect the central nervous system and cause toxic or organic psychiatric syndromes. Focal neurologic signs may or may not be present, depending on the duration, severity, and specific toxicity of exposure. Some exposures may lead mainly or entirely to psychiatric symptoms without other neurologic manifestations.

Following are descriptions of some of the more spectacular and primarily psychiatric manifesta-tions of toxic exposures as well as neuropsychiatric disorders associated with acute and chronic exposure to organic solvent mixtures.

### Lead, Mercury, Manganese, and Other Metals

Severe intoxications with many metals, including inorganic lead, mercury, manganese, and tin, often occur with signs and symptoms of encephalopathy, such as delirium, headache, and seizures, or with other physical signs that suggest the diagnosis of a toxic neuropsychiatric disorder [13–16]. Prodromal symptoms of intoxication, however, as well as symptoms of chronic or lower-level exposures to some of these metals may occur without obvious signs of encephalopathy or intoxication [1]. Sometimes, profound psychological and emotional changes due to toxic exposures may lead unsuspecting health care providers to overlook signs of toxic exposure (see Chap. 13).

### Organic Solvent Syndromes

By the mid-1980s six solvents and solvent mixtures were considered to meet scientific criteria for proven human neurotoxicity while evidence for human neurotoxicity has continued to be inconclusive regarding other solvents [17, 18]. Of those solvents generally accepted as neurotoxic, carbon disulfide, toluene, trichloroethylene, and perchlorethylene cause neuropsychiatric disturbances, while n-hexane and methyl butyl ketone (MBK) result in peripheral neuropathies without CNS involvement. High doses of toluene are sometimes self-administered to create a euphoric state, but chronic use causes central nervous system dysfunction, including memory loss, emotional lability, anxiety, and irritability, and signs of corticobulbar and cerebellar dysfunction (nystagmus, slurred speech, and ataxia) [19, 20]. Trichloroethylene and perchlorethylene cause sensory and motor cranial neuropathies, and chronic exposure has inconsistently been linked to emotional disturbances and cognitive deficits.

While acute solvent exposures at high concentrations clearly cause intoxication and acute psychiatric disturbances, chronic exposure to solvent mixtures and episodic acute solvent intoxications have been inconsistently linked, in epidemiologic studies, to increased rates of neuropsychiatric disorders and disability [20–25]. Among clinical studies of solvent-exposed workers seeking treatment, cognitive impairment (deficits in short-term memory, visuomotor performance, and reaction time) and emotional disturbances (depression, irritability, and anxiety) are commonly reported [26, 27]. However, there is some evidence that no association exists in individual workers between the presence of cognitive dysfunction and psychiatric symptoms. Most studies report no progression of such disorders following removal from exposure, and many report improved psychological and cognitive functioning over time after removal from exposure [28]. A history of episodic peak exposure with acute symptoms of solvent intoxication is associated with an increased probability of demonstrable cognitive deficits and persistence of deficits of dysfunction.

Acute solvent intoxication, with symptoms resembling alcohol intoxication and often accompanied by headache, confusion, flushing, tinnitus, and ataxia, is common in situations involving short-term exposure at excessively high levels [29]. The relationship between chronic solvent exposure at levels that ordinarily do not exceed the accepted exposure limits and chronic or persistent psychiatric syndromes is more controversial, however, and results of epidemiologic studies are often conflicting. Several studies suggest that about 25 percent of solvent-exposed workers who report at least occasional episodes of acute intoxication at work experience chronic symptoms of fatigue, memory and concentration difficulties, and depressed or irritable mood, compared to reports at less than half this rate among nonexposed control subjects. Inconsistent results and confusion about the impact of chronic, low-level solvent exposure have resulted from problems in documenting exposure histories and differences among studies in the instruments used to assess psychiatric symptoms and cognitive functioning, in the definitions used to diagnose psychiatric disorders, and in the choice of controls.

## Indirect Effects: Psychological and Emotional Reactions to Work Loss, Work Stress, and Traumatic Exposures

Because the work environment can profoundly affect psychological functioning and emotional status, it is critically important to recognize the severe impact on psychiatric function that may result from work loss (including disability), job stress, and psychological reactions to exposure or trauma, even without any direct or toxic neurologic insult.

### Psychiatric Impact of Unemployment and Disability

Besides its central function of providing an income or source of livelihood, work is a primary source of social status and self-esteem and provides structure for the day, an outlet for physical and mental activity, and an opportunity for creativity and social interactions [30, 31]. Not surprisingly, then, unemployment, layoff, disability, and retirement can adversely affect psychiatric functioning. Increased rates of suicide, psychiatric hospitalization, and crime are found to follow periods of increased unemployment. Unemployed workers and those threatened with unemployment report lowered self-esteem and heightened feelings of anger, anxiety, humiliation, depression, and somatic distress [32]. Even financially secure retirees report high levels of psychological distress, demonstrating the importance of noneconomic factors associated with the stress of not working. These psychiatric symptoms may also be associated with mild cognitive deficits, including impaired memory, concentration, and problem-solving, which further interfere with regaining employment or rehabilitation.

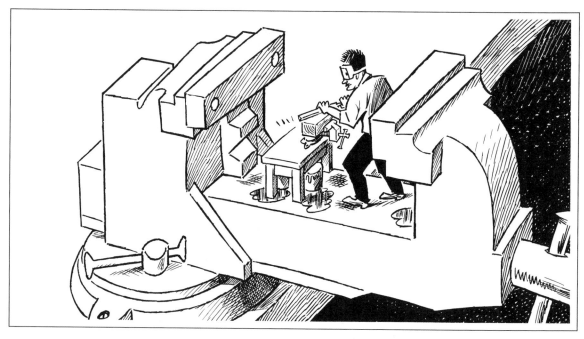

(Drawing by Nick Thorkelson)

### Occupational Stress

Occupational stress, broadly defined, refers to features of the workplace that adversely affect psychological and emotional health and well-being (see Chap. 19). Stress may result from the physical work environment, work tasks and responsibilities, interpersonal relationships, and organizational structure [4, 5]. Psychological and emotional symptoms associated with occupational stress include, most prominently, anxiety, depression, irritability, malaise, fatigue, and disturbed sleep and appetite. European and Canadian studies indicate that about one-third of workers report experiencing moderate to high levels of stress at work and adverse psychological effects, while data from the U.S. suggest that over 10 percent of the workforce experience high levels of job stress, making job stress the second most prevalent occupational hazard, following exposure to loud noise. Psychological disorders also are the fastest growing area of workers' compensation claims in many states [5].

### Psychiatric Reactions to Traumatic Exposure

Psychological and emotional functioning can be profoundly disrupted by traumatic events. Traumatic experiences include life-threatening or extremely frightening occupational injury, illness, or chemical exposure, or witnessing the severe injury or death of a fellow worker. These traumatic events are outside the range of usual human experience, will probably be experienced by almost anyone as severely distressing, and are usually accompanied acutely by feelings of intense fear, terror, or helplessness [33]. Psychiatric sequelae of traumatic events may be severe and protracted. These sequelae include anxiety, depression, adjustment, substance use, conversion, and classic posttraumatic stress disorders [10, 34, 35].

While the most extreme traumatic experiences are associated with the greatest incidence of severe psychiatric disorders, less extreme trauma can also lead to adjustment disorders, associated with anxious, depressed, or mixed emotional features or physical complaints [36, 37]. Less extreme occupational trauma or stressors include relatively minor exposures, injuries, or illnesses as well as intensified levels of work stress.

Rates of post-traumatic stress disorders associated with occupational exposure will depend on severity and duration of exposure, sensitivity of instruments used to assess symptoms, and criteria used to diagnose a disorder. Almost all studies document an exposure gradient for the development of post-traumatic stress disorders, with the highest incidence of psychiatric disorders occurring among persons most severely or directly affected. Following the Mt. St. Helens eruption in Washington state in 1980, 11 percent of men and 21 percent of women who suffered personal injury, loss of a close relative, or extreme property damage experienced at least one disaster-related psychiatric disorder (compared to rates of 1 percent in men and 2 percent in women who were not directly affected) [37]. Similarly, most studies document a two- to fivefold increased risk for post-traumatic stress disorder among Vietnam veterans who experienced high levels of combat stress compared to those with no combat or low to medium levels of combat stress.

*Substance abuse and dependence* constitute the most prevalent adult psychiatric disorders [38]. Dependence is characterized by loss of control over alcohol or drug use; persistent use despite adverse medical, social, and occupational consequences; and tolerance and physical dependence. Alcohol- and drug-dependent patients typically deny their problematic substance use. They also experience increased rates of other psychiatric disorders, including anxiety and depression. In the absence of an accurate history of substance use, these comorbid psychiatric disorders may be incorrectly attributed to environmental or occupational causes (toxic exposure or stress).

*Mass psychogenic illness* is the collective occurrence of a set of physical symptoms and related beliefs among a set of individuals without an identifiable pathogen [39, 40]. A number of related characteristics of a circumstance should be present before the explanation of MPI should be invoked. Generally MPI episodes are associated with either or both stressful environmental conditions (such as noxious odors or excessive heat) and psychosocial stress (disputes or interpersonal strife concerning work relationships or job demands). Often there is a clear precipitating event, such as exposure to new odors, fumes, or chemicals. Cases tend to spread along a visual or verbal chain of transmission and most often are found among women or children. Finally, the illness is characterized predominantly by subjective, nonspecific, or transitory symptoms or symptoms related to anxiety (nausea, dizziness, lightheadedness, sleepiness, weakness, headache).

## Psychiatric Assessment

Psychiatric assessments in occupational medicine practice are directed at elucidating the etiology of psychiatric symptoms and disproportionate disability—that is, functional disability exceeding that expected on the basis of known medical impairments—and facilitating treatment and rehabilitation.

In situations that suggest acute changes in mental status, such as intoxication or delirium, one should obtain sufficient information to exclude nonoccupational causes of these disorders. A complete evaluation of acute mental status changes requires a thorough neurologic examination, detailed mental status evaluation, laboratory evaluation, and specialized diagnostic tests. Laboratory evaluation needs to include assessment of plasma electrolytes; serum calcium, magnesium, and creatinine; blood urea nitrogen (BUN); liver function tests; blood alcohol concentration; thyroid function; and appropriate evaluations for suspected toxins, such as lead. Also needed are a complete blood count, urinalysis, and testing of blood or urine for drugs of abuse. Blood gases may be needed to detect hypoxia.

A *complete psychiatric evaluation* is indicated in the following circumstances: (1) when the general evaluation reveals evidence of psychiatric distress; (2) following any severe traumatic experience, including occupational exposure, injury, or illness; (3) when there is prolonged disability; or (4) when symptoms or disability exceed those expected.

## Prevention

Because work-related psychological disorders have been identified as a leading occupational health problem, NIOSH has proposed a national strategy to protect and promote the psychological health of workers. The strategy focuses mainly on reducing job stress and providing employee mental health services [5] (see Chap. 19).

Efforts to prevent stress-related disorders focus on ameliorating major areas of job stress; providing job security and career opportunity, a supportive social environment, and meaningful, creative, rewarding work; and making every effort to ensure worker participation in decision making and control of the work environment.

Although reducing job stress is a laudable goal, major changes in the structure of work are unlikely at present, given economic pressures, including demands for increased productivity and competitiveness. In fact, the evidence is compelling that projected changes in the economy, workplace technology, and workforce will lead to *increased* stress in the coming years. Projected changes include job displacement, movement into lower-skill, lower-paying jobs with little opportunity for advancement, and conflicting role demands for working parents with child care responsibilities [5]. Against this background, work stress may be inevitable. Cultural norms supporting the idea that work should be comfortable or enjoyable may be creating stress since they can be incompatible with the demands of competition and productivity.

While eliminating job stress entirely is an unrealistic goal, reduction of many environmental and psychosocial stressors can improve productivity, decrease stress-related disorders, and improve rehabilitation efforts. Stress-management programs targeted at employees may provide some benefits, especially if accompanied by organizational and workplace changes, when they are indicated. These programs typically teach relaxation techniques, boundary- and goal-setting, and time management skills and also encourage recreation and regular exercise.

Specific strategies are useful in preventing stress disorders associated with shiftwork. Physiologic adaptation to shiftwork, with consequent improved sleep and lessened fatigue, may be facilitated by carefully timed exposure to bright lights and darkness and by modifications in work-schedule design (see Chap. 20).

NIOSH recommendations also include enriching psychological health services for workers. The growth of employee assistance programs (EAPs), which provide evaluation and referral for impaired workers or workers with psychological or emotional problems, has led to increased access to services in some settings. Most workers, however, do not have access to EAP, and recent moves to reduce or eliminate health coverage for psychiatric disorders and chemical dependency will lead to even greater difficulties.

Drug and alcohol testing in the workplace has also been promoted as a way to prevent substance abuse. Workplace drug and alcohol testing, however, may create substantial problems if implemented unfairly or improperly conducted, and stringent guidelines need to be followed to ensure their success. In order to be effective, drug and alcohol testing in the workplace should be conducted as part of a broader program of prevention and treatment services [41].

## References

1. Schottenfeld RS, Cullen MR. Organic affective illness associated with lead intoxication. Am J Psychiatry 1984; 141:1423–6.
2. Hogstedt C, Lundberg I. Epidemiology of occupational neurobehavioral hazards: Methodological ex-

periences from organic solvent research. Rev Epid Sante Publique 1992; 40 (Suppl.):S7–S16.

3. Keita GP, Jones JM. Reducing adverse reaction to stress in the workplace: Psychology's expanding role. Am Psychol 1990; 45:1137–41.

4. Cooper CL. Identifying stresses at work: Recent research developments. J Psychosom Res 1983; 27:369–76.

5. Sauter SL, Murphy LR, Hurrell JJ. Prevention of work-related psychological disorders. Am Psychol 1990; 45:1146–58.

6. Engel GL. The clinical application of the biopsychological model. Am J Psychiatry 1980; 137:535–44.

7. MacFarlane AC. The aetiology of post-traumatic morbidity: Predisposing, precipitating and perpetuating factors. Br J Psychiatry 1980; 154:221–8.

8. Mendelson G. The concept of posttraumatic stress disorder: A review. Inter J Law Psychiatry 1987; 10:45–62.

9. Modlin HC. The postaccident anxiety syndrome: Psychosocial aspects. Am J Psychiatry 1966; 123:1008–12.

10. Schottenfeld RS, Cullen MR. Occupation-induced posttraumatic stress disorders. Am J Psychiatry 1985; 142:198–202.

11. Mechanic D. Social structure and personal adaptation: Some neglected dimensions. In GV Coelbo, et al., Coping and Adaptation. New York: Basic Books, 1974, pp. 32–44.

12. Cassel J. The contribution of the social environment to host resistance. Am J Epidemiol 1976; 104:107–23.

13. Schottenfeld RS. Psychologic sequelae of chemical and hazardous materials exposures. In JB Sullivan, GR Kreiger. eds. Hazardous materials toxicology: Clinical principles of environmental health. Baltimore: Williams & Wilkins, 1992.

14. Smith PJ, Langold GD, Goldberg J. Effects of occupational exposure to elemental mercury on short term memory. Br J Ind Med 1983; 40:413–9.

15. Vroom FQ, Greer M. Mercury vapor intoxication. Brain 1972; 95:305–18.

16. Baker EL, et al. Occupational lead neurotoxicity: Improvement in behavioural effects after reduction of exposure. Br J Ind Med 1985; 43:507–16.

17. Spencer PS, Schaumburg HH. Organic solvent neurotoxicity. Scand J Work Environ Health 1985; 11:53–60.

18. Baker EL. Organic solvent neurotoxicity. Ann Rev Public Health 1988; 9:223–32.

19. Benignus VA. Neurobehavioural effects of toluene: A review. Neurobehav Toxicol Teratol 1981; 3:407–15.

20. Cherry N, et al. Neurobehavioural effects of repeated occupational exposure to toluene and paint solvents. Br J Ind Med 1985; 43:291–300.

21. Flodin U, Edling C, Axelsson O. Clinical studies of psychorganic syndromes among workers with exposure to solvents. Am J Ind Med 1984; 5:287–95.

22. Gregersen P, et al. Neurotoxic effects of organic solvents in exposed workers: An occupational, neuropsychological, and neurological investigation. Am J Ind Med 1984; 5:201–25.

23. Edling C, Ekberg K, Ahlborg G. Long-term follow-up of workers exposed to solvents. Br J Ind Med 1990; 47:75–82.

24. Maizlish NA, et al. Behavioural evaluation of workers exposed to mixtures of organic solvents. Br J Ind Med 1985; 42:579–90.

25. Moen BE, et al. Reduced performance in tests of memory and visual abstraction in seamen exposed to industrial solvents. Acta Psychiatr Scand 1990; 81:114–9.

26. Morrow LA, et al. Alterations in cognitive and psychological functioning after organic solvent exposure. J Occup Med 1990; 32:444–50.

27. Morrow LA, et al. Risk factors associated with persistence of neuropsychological deficits in persons with organic solvent exposure. J Nerv Ment Dis 1991; 179:540–5.

28. Spurgeon A, et al. Neurobehavioral effects of long-term occupational exposure to organic solvents: Two comparable studies. Am J Ind Med 1992; 22:325–35.

29. Bruhn P, et al. Prognosis in chronic toxic encephalopathy. Acta Neurol Scand 1981; 64:259–72.

30. Jenkins R, et al. Minor psychiatric morbidity and the threat of redundancy in a professional group. Psychol Med 1982; 12:799–807.

31. Warr P. Psychological aspects of employment and unemployment (editorial). Psychol Med 1982; 12:7–11.

32. Linn MW, Sandifer R, Stein S. Effects of unemployment on mental and physical health. Am J Public Health 1985; 75:502–6.

33. American Psychiatric Association. Diagnostic and statistical manual of mental disorders (DSM-III-R). Washington, D.C., 1987.

34. Feinstein A. Posttraumatic stress disorder: A descriptive study supporting DSM-III-R criteria. Am J Psychol 1989; 23:22–6.

35. Malt U. The long-term psychiatric consequences of accidental injury: A longitudinal study of 107 adults. Br J Psych 1988; 153:810–8.

36. Green BL, Lindy JD, Grace MC. Buffalo Creek sur-

vivors in the second decade: Stability of stress symptoms. Am J Orthopsychiatry 1990; 60:43–5.

37. Shore JH, Wollmer WM, Tatum EL. Community patterns of posttraumatic stress disorders. J Nerv Ment Dis 1989; 177:681–5.
38. Robins LB, et al. Lifetime prevalence of specific psychiatric disorders in three sites. Arch Gen Psychiatry 1984; 41:949–58.
39. Colligan MJ. Mass psychogenic illness: Some clarification and perspectives. J Occup Med 1981; 23:635–8.
40. Colligan MJ, Pennebaker JW, Murphy LR. Mass psychogenic illness: A social psychological analysis. New Jersey: Lawrence Erlbaum Associates, 1982.
41. Schottenfeld RS. Drug and alcohol testing in the workplace—objectives, pitfalls and guidelines. Am J Drug Alcohol Abuse 1989; 15:413–27.

# Bibliography

## Neurologic and Behavioral Disorders

Baker EL, Feldman RG, French JG. Environmentally related disorders of the nervous system. Med Clin North Am 1990; 74:325–45.
*A review of neurologic disorders caused by chemical and physical factors encountered in the workplace or the general environment.*

Chang YC. An electrophysiological followup of patients with n-hexane polyneuropathy. Br J Ind Med 1991; 48:12–7.
*Electroneurographic and evoked potential study of 11 Taiwanese printers showed persistent abnormalities of peripheral nerve and CNS electrophysiology even though most workers regained motor and sensory functions.*

Cherry N, Gautrin D. Neurotoxic effects of styrene: Further evidence. Br J Ind Med 1990; 47:29–37.
*A report of a study of 70 Canadian factory workers showing neurobehavioral and neurologic effects of chronic styrene exposure.*

Cranmer JM, Goldberg L. eds. Proceedings of the Workshop on Neurobehavioral Effects of Solvents. Neurotoxicology 1987; 7:1–95.
*A comprehensive review of solvent-related health effects developed by a workshop of international experts.*

He FS, et al. Neurological and electroneuromyographic assessment of the adverse effects of acrylamide on occupationally exposed workers. Scand J Work Environ Health 1989; 15:125–9.
*A study of 71 Chinese acrylamide workers showing peripheral nervous system and cerebellar dysfunction.*

Heyman A, et al. Peripheral neuropathy caused by arsenical intoxication. N Engl J Med 1956; 254:401.
*Largest series of cases of arsenical neuropathy. Careful discussion of prognosis and treatment.*

Kurland LT, et al. Minamata disease. World Neurol 1960; 1:370.
*Extensive discussion of historic outbreak of methyl mercury poisoning.*

Landrigan PJ. Current issues in the epidemiology and toxicology of occupational exposure to lead. Toxicol Ind Health 1991; 7:9–14.
*A recent authoritative update on health effects of occupational lead exposure.*

Linz DH, Barrett ET, Pflaumer JE, Keith RE. Neuropsychological and postural sway improvement after Ca EDTA chelation in mild lead intoxication. J Occup Med 1992; 34:638–49.
*An interesting case report illustrating the use of recent neurodiagnostic techniques in evaluating occupational lead intoxication.*

Namba T, et al. Poisoning due to organophosphate insecticides—acute and chronic manifestations. Am J Med 1971; 50:475.
*A clinical review with excellent discussion of treatment.*

Reels HA, et al. Assessment of the permissible exposure level to manganese in workers exposed to manganese dioxide dust. Br J Ind Med 1992; 49:25–34.
*A report of a comprehensive epidemiologic study of 92 exposed workers combined with an assessment of the PEL for manganese.*

Sharp DS, et al. Delayed health hazards of pesticide exposure. Ann Rev Public Health 1986; 7:441–71.
*A review of the delayed health effects of organophosphate insecticides and related compounds.*

Snoeij NJ, et al. Biological activity of organotin compounds—an overview. Environ Res 1987; 44:335–53.
*A review of organotin neurotoxicity.*

Spencer PS, Schaumberg HH. eds. Experimental and clinical neurotoxicology, Baltimore: Williams & Wilkins, 1980.
*In-depth discussion of the pathophysiology of neurotoxin-induced disease.*

Taylor JR, et al. Chlordecone intoxication in man. Neurology 1978; 28:626.
*A complete description of a severe outbreak of occupational neurologic disease.*

Vinken PJ, Bruyn GW. eds. Handbook of clinical neurology. Intoxications of the nervous system, parts I and II. Amsterdam: Elsevier, 1979. Vols. 36 and 37.

*A collection of comprehensive monographs on various neurotoxins. An excellent reference work.*

White RF, Proctor SP. Research and clinical criteria for development of neurobehavioral test batteries. J Occup Med 1992; 34:140–8.

*A comprehensive discussion of the issues related to the use of neurobehavioral testing in the evaluation of workers at risk for toxic encephalopathy.*

World Health Organization, Nordic Council of Ministers. Chronic effects of organic solvents on the central nervous system and diagnostic criteria. Copenhagen: WHO Regional Office for Europe, 1985.

*An important summary of a consensus WHO workshop on the nature of organic solvent neurotoxicity.*

### Psychiatric Disorders

Colligan MJ. Mass psychogenic illness: Some clarification and perspectives. J Occup Med 1981; 23:635–8.

*This article examines mass psychogenic illness from a variety of perspectives.*

Sauter SL, Murphy LR, Hurrell JJ. Prevention of work-related psychological disorders. Am Psychol 1990; 45:1146–58.

*This article reviews the scientific literature regarding work stress and its impact on psychological and emotional well-being.*

Schottenfeld RS. Psychologic sequelae of chemical and hazardous materials exposures. In JB Sullivan, GR Kreiger. eds. Hazardous materials toxicology: Clinical principles of environmental health. Baltimore: Williams & Wilkins, 1992.

*This chapter provides an overview of the psychiatric issues that arise as a consequence of exposure to toxic substances.*

# 27
# Reproductive Disorders

Maureen Paul

The prevention of reproductive system disorders is an important public health priority. These problems include abnormalities that affect the reproductive function of both men and women as well as a wide range of untoward pregnancy outcomes. In the United States, approximately one in seven married couples is involuntarily infertile. Between 10 and 20 percent of pregnancies end in clinically recognized spontaneous abortion, while rates of very early peri-implantation loss are even higher. Among newborns in the United States, approximately 7 percent are of low birthweight (<2,500 gm), and 3 percent have major congenital malformations.

While the causes of many reproductive system disorders remain unknown, scientific interest in an etiologic role for occupational exposures has increased dramatically. A number of economic, social, and scientific changes eventually converged to bring attention to this issue. Foremost among these changes was the unprecedented entry of women into the labor force after World War II. In the United States, the proportion of women in the civilian workforce increased from 23 percent in 1950 to nearly 60 percent today. Two-thirds of these women are of reproductive age, and each year over one million infants are born to women who are employed during gestation.

The years during and after World War II also heralded revolutionary changes in industry, resulting in the birth of agribusiness and the petrochemical industry. Concern about the chemicals being introduced into commerce ultimately led to new laws and to new research to improve understanding of environmental risks of these chemical agents. In addition, a number of events highlighted the issue of reproductive hazards specifically. The drug thalidomide, prescribed as an anti-emetic and sedative to pregnant women, was linked to limb malformations and other defects in newborns. In utero exposure to diethylstilbestrol (DES) resulted in anomalies of the reproductive tract and later development of vaginal cancer in daughters of the treated women. In Japan, contamination of fish with methyl mercury and contamination of cooking oil with polyhalogenated biphenyls led to serious developmental toxicity in children exposed prenatally. These tragedies served to break the prevailing belief that the placenta acted as a protective barrier for the fetus. Moreover, in 1977 a situation occurred that brought new dimensions to the problem. At a pesticide formulation plant in northern California, male workers with long-term exposure to dibromochloropropane (DBCP) were found to have decreased sperm counts and impaired fertility. Although DBCP was banned from production in the United States, many workers who were azoospermic on initial examination remained so several years after cessation of exposure (see box).

These events led reproductive toxicologists and epidemiologists to examine a multitude of workplace and environmental exposures for potential adverse reproductive and developmental effects in both sexes. By the mid-1980s the National Institute for Occupational Safety and Health (NIOSH)

DBCP: A POTENT REPRODUCTIVE TOXIN

In 1977 a small group of men in a northern California chemical plant noticed that few of them had recently fathered children. Investigation of the full cohort of production workers subsequently found a strong association between decreased sperm count and exposure to DBCP, a brominated organochlorine used as a nematocide since the mid-1950s. The spermatotoxic effects in some of the exposed men were sufficient to render them sterile. Testicular biopsies showed the seminiferous tubules to be the site of action and spermatogonia to be the target cell. The relationship between reduced sperm count and exposure to DBCP, both in its manufacture and use, has been confirmed in studies of other plants in the United States and abroad. Follow-up of workers after cessation of exposure shows that spermatogenic function is eventually recovered in those less severely affected. However, many of the azoospermic men have remained azoospermic.

included reproductive disorders among the 10 leading work-related illnesses and injuries in the United States, and the World Health Organization (WHO) called for international multidisciplinary collaboration to identify agents that impair reproductive function and the populations at risk of exposure.

Today, occupational health physicians and nurses, as well as obstetrician-gynecologists and other primary care clinicians, encounter patient concerns about fertility and pregnancy risks that might result from workplace exposures. Addressing these issues can be difficult due to their emotional character and to the enormous gaps that still exist in the scientific understanding and regulation of reproductive and developmental toxicants.

# Reproductive and Developmental Toxicology

Reproductive processes in the male and female are complex and incompletely understood. The major components of the reproductive system are the hypothalamic-pituitary axis and the gonads. In a precisely regulated hormonal milieu, normal human reproduction proceeds from formation and transport of the germ cells through fertilization, implantation, and prenatal and postnatal development. Toxic agents can act at one or many sites to disrupt this chain of events, resulting in reproductive dysfunction or aberrant pregnancy outcomes.

## Spermatogenesis

Spermatogenesis in humans is an ongoing process of cell division that requires approximately 74 days to complete. Proceeding from basement membrane to lumen of the seminiferous tubule, stem cell spermatogonia undergo successive mitotic and meiotic divisions to form spermatocytes and then spermatids containing 23 chromosomes. The spermatids undergo morphologic transformation to spermatozoa before entering the lumen of the seminiferous tubule. These sperm cells mature further and acquire motility and fertilizing capacity during passage through the epididymis, where they are primarily stored before ejaculation. This process is under the influence of the anterior pituitary gland's luteinizing and follicle-stimulating hormones (LH and FSH, respectively). In the testis LH stimulates testosterone production, which, together with FSH, acts to initiate and regulate sperm production.

**Specific Agents.** Occupational agents can disrupt sperm production either directly, by injuring testicular cells, or indirectly, by interfering with the hormonal regulation of spermatogenesis. In addition, toxic agents may also impair sexual function by reducing libido or by inhibiting erection and ejaculation. The stage(s) of spermatogenesis affected by a toxicant determines both the time required for clinical expression of the injury and the prospects for recovery. As long as the stem cell precursors are spared, spermatogenic damage is reversible over time. Fortunately, this appears to be the case with most substances studied so far. Table 27-1 lists some occupational agents that are known or suspected to affect male reproductive function adversely [1]. A number of physical and chemical agents have been found to disrupt spermatogenesis. Perhaps the best known spermatotoxin is DBCP, the first substance discovered to cause infertility in American workers. Men exposed for at least 3 years to this nematocide were found to be azoospermic or severely oligospermic, with elevated levels of serum FSH, while the sperm counts and gonadotropin levels of workers with short-term exposure were normal. Testicular biopsies from men with chronic exposure revealed a near absence of spermatogonia and spermatocytes. In fact, DBCP is one of the few occupational agents found to target primitive spermatogonia, explaining the long-term sterility seen in some workers. While the manufacture of DBCP has been banned in the United States, it remains a low-level groundwater contaminant in some states. Another pesticide, ethylene dibromide, has been associated with post-testicular effects including decreased sperm velocity, motility, and viability.

Among the heavy metals, lead is the best-studied spermatotoxin [2]. In investigations of workers exposed to lead in battery manufacture, blood-lead levels above 40 µg/dL have been associated with decreased sperm counts and aberrant sperm motility and morphology. Total urinary gonadotropin levels were unaffected in these workers, suggesting a direct toxic effect of lead on the gonads. Recent evidence suggests, however, that lead may also act at the level of the hypothalamus and pituitary to impair endocrine function.

The ethylene glycol ethers, 2-methoxyethanol and 2-ethoxyethanol, as well as their acetates, are organic solvents used in industry as jet-fuel deicers; as components of inks, cleaners, and finishers; in coating and dyeing operations; and in the manufacture of printed circuit boards. These agents cause testicular atrophy and disruption of the sem-

**Table 27-1.** Selected occupational agents with suspected effects on male reproductive function

| Adverse effects | Examples |
| --- | --- |
| Decreased libido | Heavy metal poisoning (for example, lead, manganese) |
| Hormonal alterations | Manufacture of oral contraceptives |
| | Estrogen agonists (for example, polychlorinated biphenyls, organohalide pesticides) |
| | Lead |
| Spermatotoxicity | Heat |
| | Ionizing radiation ($\geq 15$ rad) |
| | Lead |
| | Inorganic mercury |
| | Dibromochloropropane (DBCP) |
| | Ethylene dibromide |
| | Carbaryl |
| | Chloroprene |
| | Carbon disulfide |
| | Ethylene glycol ethers |

Source: Adapted from B Baranski. Effects of the workplace on fertility and related reproductive outcomes. Environ Health Perspect 1993; 101 (Suppl. 2):86.

iniferous tubules in several laboratory animal species, and they have been associated with decreased sperm counts in exposed workers [3]. The ethylene glycol ethers target meiotic spermatocytes; at high doses, effects on spermatogonia and late spermatids have also been reported. The ethylene glycol ethers are metabolized in the body to alkoxyacetic acids, which are responsible for their reproductive toxicity. Since the propylene glycol ethers are not biotransformed to these toxic derivatives, they are being used as safer substitutes in some industries.

Two physical agents that are known to affect semen parameters are ionizing radiation and heat. Oligospermia can occur after x-ray doses of 15 rad, and temporary azoospermia after 30 rad. While usual occupational radiation exposures are well below these levels, higher exposures do occasionally occur, as during certain nuclear reactor incidents. Even a 1 to 2°C rise in scrotal temperature can temporarily affect sperm production. Semen analyses in men working outdoors in hot weather reveal reductions in sperm concentration and motility, although the clinical significance of these findings has not been studied.

Little is known about the effects of occupational agents on sexual function or on hormonal regulation of reproduction in men. Gynecomastia and decreased libido have been reported in men involved in the manufacture of oral contraceptives. In addition, agents that affect the central nervous system (CNS) or that cause severe debilitation may affect sexual function. For example, decreased libido has been associated with severe lead and manganese poisonings. Although not directly studied in humans, some chemicals, such as the polyhalogenated biphenyls and organohalide pesticides, are structurally similar to the reproductive sex steroid hormones, raising the possibility that they could disrupt male reproduction by binding to endogenous hormone receptors.

### Oogenesis

Unlike the male who has a renewing pool of spermatogonia that proliferate throughout life, the female receives a fixed endowment of germ cells before birth. The number of germ cells in the female reaches a maximum of approximately 7 million by the twentieth week of gestation. Through a natural process of atresia, this falls to approximately 400,000 by puberty, only about 400 of which will become dominant follicles capable of ovulation and fertilization during the normal reproductive life span. When the germ cell pool is nearly depleted, menopause ensues.

In the female fetus, oogonia actively proliferate, and variable numbers enter the first meiotic division to become primary oocytes. These cells remain dormant until shortly before ovulation, when the first meiotic division is completed. Meiosis II occurs at time of fertilization.

During each menstrual cycle, a number of follicles (oocytes surrounded by supporting granulosa cells) begins to develop. The initial stages of follicle development are gonadotropin-independent, but further growth and selection of a dominant follicle depend on pituitary FSH. As the follicle grows, circulating estradiol levels increase, enhancing oocyte development and stimulating proliferation of endometrial tissue. A critical blood level of estrogen triggers a midcycle surge of LH, which is required for ovulation of the dominant follicle to occur. After release of the oocyte from the ovary, LH induces luteinization of the remaining granulosa cells to form the corpus luteum. Continued production of estrogen and progesterone by the corpus luteum prompts vascularization and biochemical changes within the endometrium necessary to support a conceptus, should fertilization occur. In the absence of fertilization, the corpus luteum degenerates, resulting in a dramatic drop in circulating sex steroid hormones and sloughing of the endometrium with menstruation.

The length of the menstrual cycle varies among women, with a normal range of 22 to 35 days. Durations of flow up to 7 days are acceptable. Disturbances in ovulation manifests clinically as infertility or menstrual dysfunction and can result from direct ovarian toxicity or from disruption of hormonal interrelationships along the hypothalamic-pituitary-gonadal axis.

*Specific Agents.* Little is currently known about ovarian toxicity in humans, in part because of the relative inaccessibility of the female germ cell. In women undergoing therapeutic irradiation, ovarian doses required to induce temporary or permanent amenorrhea decrease with advancing age as a result of the natural depletion of the germ cell pool over time. Exposures in the range of 250 to 500 rad cause permanent sterility in most women over age 40, while most younger women experience only temporary menstrual disturbances. Doses below 60 rad are without effect in most age groups.

Women who smoke cigarettes experience menopause somewhat earlier than nonsmokers. Laboratory animal studies suggest that this effect may be due to accelerated atresia of oocytes induced by the polycylic aromatic hydrocarbons in cigarette smoke [4].

Menstrual disorders have been reported among workers in numerous occupations [1, 4], including women working in formulating oral contraceptives and dental workers exposed to metallic mercury vapor. While early reports suggested menstrual irregularities in women occupationally exposed to aromatic hydrocarbons, more recent studies of workers exposed to styrene or toluene have not confirmed these findings. High levels of physical stress can disturb hypothalamic function, accounting for the amenorrhea experienced by some athletes, dancers, and other women who exercise strenuously.

In a recent investigation, reduced fertility was reported in dental assistants exposed to high levels of nitrous oxide. The probability of conception in each menstrual cycle was nearly 60 percent lower among women exposed to unscavenged nitrous oxide for 5 or more hours per week than among unexposed women [5].

### Genotoxicity

Damage to genetic material takes two major forms: (1) point mutations, involving the addition, deletion, or substitution of one or a small number of nucleotides in the DNA sequence, and (2) chromosomal abnormalities, expressed as changes in chromosome number or structure. Genetic alterations induced in germ cells, if compatible with germ cell survival and division, may be transmitted to future generations. Deleterious mutations can also arise in somatic cells of the developing embryo and result in teratogenesis or other adverse outcomes.

Most numerical chromosomal abnormalities are incompatible with germ cell survival or cause early death of the zygote. Surviving infants often suffer physical, behavioral, and intellectual impairments. Some structural chromosomal changes have no adverse effects, while others are associated with mental retardation, anomalies, reduced fertility, and malignancy. Point mutations are more often transmitted without cell death. The effects of autosomal dominant and X-linked mutations are discernible in first-generation progeny, while recessive mutations may not be expressed for many generations.

Using bacterial assays, increased mutagenic activity has been detected in the urine of workers exposed to anesthetic gases, chemotherapeutic agents, or epichlorohydrin. Chromosomal aberrations have been measured by metaphase spread analysis of the lymphocytes of workers exposed to clastogenic (chromosome-breaking) agents. Induction of chromosomal aberrations in these somatic cells implies a potential germ cell hazard as well, although this relationship has yet to be validated. Increased frequencies of chromosomal aberrations have been reported in radiation workers and in workers exposed to chemicals such as benzene, styrene, ethylene oxide, epichlorohydrin, arsenic, chromium, and cadmium. While these assays are useful as biologic markers of exposure to genotoxicants, they do not predict specific reproductive health effects in individuals.

Epidemiologic study of toxicant-induced genetic effects in human populations is exceedingly difficult due in part to the background incidence of spontaneous mutations, to the multifactorial etiology of many adverse outcomes, and to the infeasibility of measuring the effects of recessive mutations that occur at low frequency in remote generations. Despite the widespread use of muta-

genic agents in industry, none have been specifically linked to adverse genetic effects in humans.
This is true even for ionizing radiation, which is
mutagenic in every tested species. The large studies
of children born to atomic-bomb survivors have
not yet documented significant increases in any of
six genetic indicators, including untoward pregnancy outcomes, childhood mortality, sex chromosome aneuploidy, balanced chromosomal exchanges, protein mutations, or childhood cancer
[6].

Since chromosomal anomalies frequently result
in pregnancy loss, some investigators have studied
the association between environmental factors and
karyotypic abnormalities in spontaneous abortion
specimens. In these studies, parental occupation
was not associated with chromosomally abnormal
abortion; however, a few "environmental" factors,
such as maternal cigarette smoking and fever during pregnancy, increased the risk of loss of chromosomally normal fetuses.

The risk of adverse pregnancy outcomes after
preconception exposure of men to toxic agents is
an area of active research [7]. A number of mechanisms have been postulated for these male-me-
diated effects, including germ cell mutagenesis.
While findings have yet to be replicated and precise mechanisms clarified, increased rates of pregnancy loss have been reported in the wives of men
exposed to lead, inorganic mercury, anesthetic
gases, organic solvents, and other agents. Limited
studies also suggest that certain paternal occupations may pose an increased risk for development
of childhood cancers. For example, some studies
have found elevated rates of nervous system cancers in the children of men employed in electrical
occupations or in the petrochemical industry.

### Pregnancy

Fertilization usually occurs within 12 hours of
ovulation in the distal portion of the fallopian
tube. The early zygote undergoes a series of cell
divisions to form the blastocyst, which implants in
the uterus 5 to 6 days after conception. The pre-
implantation phase of development is often re-

ferred to as the "all-or-none" period. This terminology derives from ionizing radiation studies
showing that irradiation at high enough doses may
cause death of the conceptus, but that sublethal
doses are unlikely to result in teratogenic effects
because of effective cellular repair processes at this
stage of development.

The embryonic period extends from the 17th to
the 56th day postconception and is characterized
by a precisely timed sequence of organogenesis.
The embryo at this stage is acutely sensitive to teratogenic insult. The remaining fetal period is
marked by significant growth of the conceptus and
by the continued differentiation and maturation of
some organ systems, such as the endocrine, immune, and central nervous systems. Therefore, exposure to toxic agents in the second and third
trimesters of pregnancy may reduce fetal growth
or result in functional or neurobehavioral abnormalities in offspring.

Clinical manifestations of developmental toxicity depend on the properties of the agent, the timing and dose of exposure, genetic susceptibility,
and other factors. In addition, many developmental endpoints are interrelated, as illustrated by
the high rates of pregnancy loss observed among
malformed fetuses. Some agents, such as thalidomide and DES, affect the embryo at doses far below those that induce maternal toxicity; others,
such as methyl mercury and cyclophosphamide,
are harmful to conceptuses only at maternally
toxic doses.

Numerous physiologic alterations occur during
pregnancy that modify the absorption, distribution, metabolism, and excretion of occupational
chemicals (Table 27-2). Transfer of chemicals
across the placenta occurs primarily by passive diffusion. Chemicals that are lipophilic and of low
molecular weight would be expected to cross the
placenta quite readily.

Physiologic alterations of pregnancy may also
modify physical work capacity. For example, with
advancing gestation, increased protuberance of the
abdomen coupled with exaggerated lordosis of the
lumbar spine shift the center of gravity posteriorly.

**Table 27-2.** Some physiologic changes of pregnancy that may affect toxicokinetics

| Physiologic parameter | Effect |
| --- | --- |
| Delayed gastric emptying<br>Reduced intestinal motility | Increases absorption of ingested agents |
| Increased tidal volume<br>Increased minute ventilation | Increases absorption and elimination of inhaled agents |
| Increased plasma volume<br>Increased total body water | Decreases blood concentrations of chemicals |
| Decreased plasma proteins, especially albumin | Increases bioavailability of agents |
| Increased body fat | Decreases blood concentration<br>Increases fat storage of lipid-soluble agents |
| Increased renal blood flow<br>Increased glomerular filtration rate | Increases renal elimination of polar metabolites |

In addition, the mobility of the pelvic joints increases as a result of ligamentous relaxation. These changes result in postural instability and may cause low back discomfort. Therefore, work modifications may be indicated during the second half of pregnancy for women whose jobs involve prolonged sedentary postures or tasks that require delicate balance, such as heavy lifting or climbing.

Pregnant workers subjected to prolonged standing or strenuous exertion may also be intolerant of work in hot, humid environments. Reduction of cardiac output created by decreased venous return, coupled with peripheral vasodilation to dissipate the heat generated by both the fetus and the employee's own increased metabolic rate, may lead to dizziness or syncope in these settings.

*Specific Agents.* Only a few of the thousands of occupational agents in widespread use have been adequately evaluated for developmental toxicity in humans (Fig. 27-1). Table 27-3 lists common physical, chemical, and biologic agents for which there is epidemiologic evidence of adverse effects on pregnancy.

With rare exception, contemporary studies from industrialized nations reveal better pregnancy outcomes among women in the workforce compared to unemployed women, a finding that may be related in part to the economic and health care ben-

efits derived from the work experience. At the same time, a quite consistent body of evidence suggests that women who perform strenuous work may be at increased risk of preterm delivery [8]. While definitions of strenuous work differ in these studies, findings are most consistent for women whose jobs involve at least two of many selected stressors, such as prolonged standing, physically stressful postures, heavy lifting or carrying, and long work weeks. One study found that the risk was greatest among women who had predisposing medical or obstetric risk factors for early delivery, such as an incompetent cervix or a history of preterm birth.

In less developed nations, women both inside and outside of the traditional workforce commonly engage in home-based economic activities, such as agricultural work and tending livestock. In addition, their household duties range from cleaning, cooking, and child care to hauling of wood and water. The effects of these activities on pregnancy outcome deserve further attention, since they typically involve long hours, physically stressful postures, and strenuous tasks. To date, limited data on women in less developed nations suggest that home-based work, particularly work that involves prolonged standing, may reduce birthweight of newborns.

Depending on the gestational timing of expo-

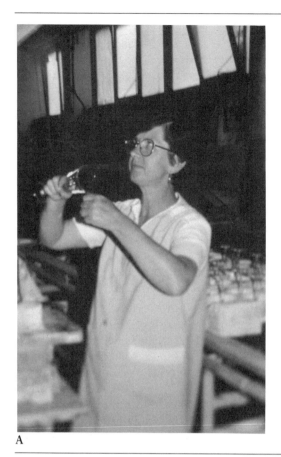

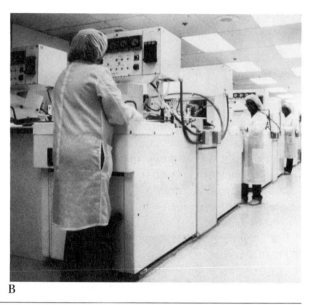

A    B

**Fig. 27-1.** Pregnant workers in seemingly clean work environments may be exposed to reproductive hazards.
A. Pregnant quality control worker in Hungarian leaded glass factory licks fingers between inspecting glasses that
may have lead dust on them. (Photograph by Barry Levy.) B. Semiconductor "clean rooms" have extremely low
dust levels but can contain high air levels of organic solvents such as glycol ethers. (Photograph from Rom WN
[ed.] *Environmental and Occupational Medicine*, 2nd ed. Boston: Little, Brown, 1992, p. 1053.)

sure, high-dose ionizing radiation can cause death
of the embryo, growth retardation, or birth defects, including microcephaly, eye malformations,
and mental retardation. However, usual occupational exposures are far below those expected to
produce these effects. Prenatal x-ray exposures in
the range of 2 rad have been associated in many
studies with a modest increased risk for childhood
leukemia. The Nuclear Regulatory Commission
(NRC) stipulates that the total dose to the embryo-

fetus due to occupational exposure of a declared
pregnant woman not exceed 0.5 rem, with avoidance of substantial variations in dose rate [9].

Ongoing longitudinal studies suggest that low-
level exposure to lead in utero can cause subtle
neurobehavioral deficits during the early years of
life. While the Occupational Safety and Health
Administration (OSHA) lead standard recommends that blood-lead levels of prospective parents and the fetus/newborn not exceed 30 μg/dL,

cognitive deficits have been noted with prenatal exposures as low as 10 to 20 μg/dL. Limited follow-up studies to date suggest that these developmental delays do not persist in school-aged children unless postnatal blood-lead levels remain elevated. Associations with preterm delivery, fetal growth deficits, and minor malformations have been reported with less consistency. Although lead can induce spontaneous abortions at high doses, a recent study of women residing near a lead smelter in Yugoslavia found no increased risk of spontaneous abortion with blood-lead levels ranging from 5 to 40 μg/dL [10].

A number of studies suggest a modest increased risk of major malformations, including oral clefts, gut atresia, and CNS anomalies, among children born to women who work in occupations with mixed organic solvent exposure, such as laboratory workers. However, these studies lack quantitative exposure data and fail to identify specific offending agents. Recreational abuse of toluene has been reported to cause an embryopathy similar to the fetal alcohol syndrome, although the effects of toluene at lower exposures typical of workplace settings have not been adequately investigated [11]. In a recent large study of semiconductor workers, an elevated risk of spontaneous abortion was found among female fabrication workers exposed to photoresist/developer solutions containing glycol ethers, xylene, or n-butyl acetate (Fig. 27-1B). This finding is particularly intriguing given the extensive animal evidence of developmental toxicity from exposure to the ethylene glycol ethers. Other chemicals reported to increase the risk of pregnancy loss after occupational exposure include waste anesthetic gases, ethylene oxide, and antineoplastic agents [1].

Despite worldwide concern about the toxicity of pesticides, information on their human developmental effects is sparse. Many pesticides are mutagenic or teratogenic in laboratory animals, and limited epidemiologic investigations have reported increased risks for spontaneous abortion, stillbirths, or birth defects among farmworkers and residents living in communities with high pesticide usage. In the United States alone, there are approximately 21,000 registered pesticide products containing over 700 active and 1,200 "inert" ingredients. While many of the highly toxic chlorinated hydrocarbon pesticides have been banned from production or use in the United States, these chemicals persist as environmental contaminants and are still in widespread use in developing nations.

Biologic agents present a hazard to a wide range of workers, including health care workers, veterinarians, public safety personnel, hazardous waste workers, day care workers, and schoolteachers. Rubella virus, cytomegalovirus (CMV), and toxoplasmosis pose a teratogenic risk, while human immunodeficiency virus (HIV), hepatitis B virus (HBV), and perinatal varicella infection may result in significant infant morbidity and mortality. In addition, infection during pregnancy with human parvovirus B19, the etiologic agent of fifth disease, has been associated with nonimmune fetal hydrops and pregnancy loss. In general, universal precautions provide adequate protection against viruses that are transmitted through close contact with infected body fluids (CMV, HIV, and HBV), but not against airborne viruses (rubella and parvovirus B19). At-risk workers should be offered available vaccinations, preferably before employment. Rubella vaccine, a live virus vaccine, should be given at least three months before pregnancy; hepatitis B vaccine is not contraindicated during pregnancy. Susceptible pregnant workers should avoid contact with individuals infected with rubella or human parvovirus B19. While temporary job transfer may decrease the risk of infection in these workers, it does not completely eliminate it, since these viruses are usually also ubiquitous in the community.

## Clinical Evaluation and Management

### Steps in the Clinical Work-up

The most common clinical situations that require knowledge of occupational reproductive hazards include preconception counseling, evaluation of

**Table 27-3.** Selected occupational agents with suspected effects on pregnancy

| Agent | Reported effects | Recommendations |
|---|---|---|
| PHYSICAL AGENTS | | |
| Strenuous work | Preterm delivery. Women with medical or obstetric conditions predisposing to preterm delivery may be at particular risk. | Lifting aids. Rest breaks. Light duty options. Preterm delivery prevention programs. |
| Ionizing radiation | Growth deficits, CNS malformations, mental retardation at high doses. Possible low risk of genetic defects, childhood cancer at doses < 5 rad. | Exposure monitoring. Shielding. Minimize time of exposure. Increase distance from source. Occupational limit < 0.5 rem total dose during pregnancy. |
| CHEMICAL AGENTS | | |
| Lead | Neurobehavioral deficits in infants associated with prenatal blood-lead levels as low as 10–15 µg/dL. | Standard hierarchy of controls. Air and blood-lead monitoring. Medical removal protection. |
| Waste anesthetic gases | Spontaneous abortion | Standard hierarchy of controls. Air monitoring. NIOSH recommends that exposures to $N_2O$ not exceed 25 ppm. Follow OSHA *Work Practice Guidelines for Personnel Dealing with Cytotoxic Drugs* [15]. |
| Antineoplastic agents | Spontaneous abortion | |
| Organic solvents | Modestly increased risk of birth defects for mixed solvent exposure (some studies—doses lacking). Fetal loss rates increased in semiconductor workers exposed to EGEE/ EGME. Toluene abuse → "fetal solvent syndrome." | Standard hierarchy of controls. OSHA proposed exposure limits: 0.5 ppm for EGEE, EGEEA 0.1 ppm for EGME, EGMEA |
| Ethylene oxide | Spontaneous abortion | Standard hierarchy of controls. Exposure monitoring. NIOSH recommended limit < 0.1 ppm. |
| Polychlorinated biphenyls (PCBs) | Congenital PCB syndrome at high doses; excreted efficiently into breast milk. Low-level dietary exposure related to mild neonatal growth and neurobehavioral deficits in some studies. | USFDA tolerance limit: 1.5 ppm in cow's milk and dairy products. No longer produced in U.S. Exposure risk for workers who repair PCB machinery. Measure serum levels when excessive exposure suspected. |

**Table 27-3. (continued).**

| Agent | Reported effects | Recommendations |
|---|---|---|
| BIOLOGIC AGENTS | | |
| Hepatitis B virus (HBV) | Neonatal chronic carrier state. Chronic liver disease and mortality. | Universal screening of pregnant women. Vaccine not contraindicated during pregnancy. Postexposure HBIG for susceptible workers. |
| Human immuno-deficiency virus (HIV) | Morbidity and mortality for adults and infected neonates. | Universal precautions. Postexposure prophylaxis. |
| Cytomegalovirus (CMV) | Neonatal death, malformations, developmental deficits. Seroconversion rates in health care workers using adequate precautions not increased compared to community controls. | Universal precautions. Serology. |
| Rubella virus | Spontaneous abortion, stillbirth, congenital defects with infection during first 16 weeks of pregnancy. | Isolation precautions. Document immunity by serology preplacement. Vaccine (>3 months before pregnancy). Susceptible workers should not care for patients with rubella infection. |
| Varicella-zoster virus | Maternal pneumonia serious. Malformation risk ~5% for infection in first ½ of pregnancy. Neonatal morbidity/mortality if maternal infection < 5 days before or < 2 days after delivery. | Isolation precautions. Limit patient contact based on history of immunity—not pregnancy per se. Postexposure VZIG prophylaxis for susceptible workers. |
| Human parvovirus B19 | Nonimmune fetal hydrops. Fetal death. | Serology. Serial maternal serum α-fetoprotein and ultrasounds in B19 IgM-positive women. Community viral reservoir so removal of susceptibles may lessen but not eliminate risk of infection. Workers may return to job 21 days after last reported case. |

Key: NIOSH = National Institute for Occupational Safety and Health; OSHA = Occupational Safety and Health Administration; USFDA = United States Food and Drug Administration; ppm = parts per million; EGEE/EGEEA = ethylene glycol monoethyl ether and its acetate; EGME/EGMEA = ethylene glycol monomethyl ether and its acetate; HBIG = hepatitis B immune globulin; VZIG = varicella-zoster immune globulin; IgM = immuno-globulin M.

the infertile couple, and assessment of workers who are pregnant or who have experienced an untoward pregnancy outcome. In all of the situations, it is essential to answer the following three questions:

1. *To what agent(s) is the patient potentially exposed, and is there evidence to suggest that this agent(s) causes adverse reproductive or developmental effects?*

Since reproductive disorders have multiple etiologies, the history of work and general environmental exposures should be taken on both the male and the female partner. Physical as well as chemical exposures need to be noted. As mentioned earlier, for example, strenuous work may particularly exacerbate the risk of preterm delivery in women who have delivered early in the past. No physical findings are pathognomonic for work-related reproductive disorders; however, the physical examination may contribute signs of exposure (such as dermatitis in a solvent-exposed worker) or organic pathology contributing to the problem (such as uterine fibroids in a woman with menstrual irregularity).

Even after taking a comprehensive history, questions frequently remain about the precise identity of chemicals handled on the job. Material safety data sheets (MSDSs) contain essential information about hazardous product ingredients and should be carefully reviewed. However, reproductive and developmental toxicity data on MSDSs may be sparse or missing entirely. In a recent review of nearly 700 MSDSs for lead and the ethylene glycol ethers, 62 percent failed to mention reproductive system effects; those that did were 18 times more likely to mention developmental toxicity than adverse male reproductive effects [12].

Additional data on reproductive and developmental toxicity of occupational agents are available from many sources, including computerized databases, toxicology "hotlines," reference books, and government agencies. A selected list of these resources is provided in Appendix B.

2. *Is the patient actually exposed to the agent(s) and, if so, what is the timing and dose of exposure?*

Through the occupational history, the clinician can determine whether exposures are episodic or chronic in nature and gather information about protective measures that can reduce exposure. Since teratogens exert their effects during specific critical periods of organogenesis, every effort should be made to establish gestational age at the time of exposure precisely. Abnormal semen parameters should prompt a search for gametotoxic exposures in the several months before the onset of the problem. Occasionally, exposures in the more distant past are important. For example, 90 percent of absorbed lead is stored in bone; conditions that increase bone turnover, such as menopause and perhaps pregnancy, may increase blood-lead levels.

Worksite walkthroughs, the assistance of industrial hygienists, and the use of biologic markers, when available, greatly enhance understanding of actual exposures. Note, however, that in only a few instances in the U.S. are occupational standards established with reproductive risks in mind (lead, ethylene oxide, DBCP, and ionizing radiation). Hence, exposure data should not be considered simply in terms of whether regulatory limits are exceeded [13]. NIOSH's recommended exposure limits (RELs) do consider available reproductive and developmental effects data, but are not updated often.

3. *Given the information collected, does the patient's exposure to the agent(s) pose a reproductive or developmental risk?*

The final step in the work-up involves assimilating exposure and health effects data to estimate the degree of risk to the patient. In addition to the properties of the agent and the characteristics of exposure, the health professional must consider biologic factors that modify risk, such as age, nutritional status, or preexisting medical or reproductive problems. For example, the risk of fetal chromosomal abnormalities increases in women

35 years of age and older, and cigarette smoking is associated with subfertility, earlier age at menopause, spontaneous abortion, and fetal growth deficits. Deficiencies of iron, zinc, and calcium increase gastrointestinal absorption of lead.

Intervention is clearly warranted when exposure to any chemical or physical agent exceeds regulatory exposure limits. Because few legally mandated limits are designed to protect against reproductive system effects, even lesser exposures to known or suspected reproductive hazards may deserve attention. When the reproductive risk is uncertain due to inadequate toxicity data, the clinician can take reasonable measures to decrease exposures; however, the success of these efforts may vary, depending on the resources and cooperation of individual employers. Some workers may be unwilling to accept even small risks and will have the financial security to leave their jobs; others may feel that the socioeconomic and health consequences of job loss far outweigh uncertain risks from workplace exposures. In these circumstances, practitioners should carefully explore the options available to patients and assure that their decisions are as well informed as possible.

### Risk Prevention and Management

There are two primary ways by which occupational health specialists can prevent or reduce work-related health risks. The first is through patient education and counseling. The second is by intervening in the workplace to reduce or eliminate deleterious exposures.

*Counseling.* Reproductive problems are intensely personal; patients who believe that their workplace exposures may be contributing to the problem typically feel anxious and vulnerable. Counseling these patients requires time and space free from distractions, attentive listening, and a compassionate attitude. Information should be conveyed in an understandable and nonjudgmental fashion. Since patients may not retain all information conveyed in the counseling session, it is helpful to summarize key points in a follow-up letter.

Uncertainties or limitations in the data must be clearly conveyed. Frequently, patients' perceptions of risks will be distorted, and counseling can help to place the risk in proper perspective. For example, a pregnant woman with a blood-lead level of 20 $\mu$g/dL may fear that her child will be "mentally retarded"; the clinician should explain that, while close follow-up of the infant is advisable, the developmental delays associated with low-level prenatal lead exposure are subtle and often do not persist. In addition, the concept of relative risk should be put in perspective. For example, a two-fold increased risk for fetal loss may elevate the miscarriage rate from 15 to 30 percent, while doubling the risk of a malformation that occurs with a baseline frequency of 1 per 1,000 live births would result in 1 additional affected infant in 1,000.

In all cases, the clinician should provide information on background rates of adverse reproductive outcomes, as well as their multifactorial etiologies. Frequently, the potential risks from a workplace exposure will be small compared to spontaneous risks or those attributable to nonoccupational causes. Through this type of comprehensive counseling, patients are better able to make informed choices and to accept clinicians as educators and advocates, while understanding that a perfect outcome can never be guaranteed.

*Controlling Exposure.* When exposures are of concern, clinicians should make every effort to eliminate potential hazards through consultation with employers and regulatory agencies. The traditional industrial hygiene hierarchy (see Chap. 6) that emphasizes engineering controls is especially important for chemical exposures. Bulky protective clothing and respirators are particularly uncomfortable during the latter part of pregnancy due to weight gain, increased metabolic heat load, and physiologic changes in respiratory parameters. Sometimes, however, short-term use of personal protective equipment, while more effective controls are being developed, may provide a satisfactory alternative to removing workers from their jobs. If these measures cannot be implemented in a timely fashion or do not control exposures adequately, the employer may be willing to transfer the worker to a less hazardous job.

In addition to control of chemical exposures, attention also needs to be directed to the control of ergonomic risk factors that particularly affect the pregnant woman (see box). Administrative controls can be used on a short-term basis to increase tolerance of and decrease risk associated with strenuous work, hot environments, or prolonged static postures. For example, more frequent rest breaks and rotation between seated and standing jobs may reduce fatigue and improve circulation, including circulation to the uterus and placenta.

Failing these alternatives, temporary work leaves can be considered. In nations such as France and Finland, liberal maternity and paternity leaves allow for broad latitude in addressing these problems. In the U.S., however, leave options are more limited. The OSHA lead and cadmium standards are the only occupational regulations that specifically allow for compensated job removal of workers with medical conditions that may be exacerbated by exposure. Pregnancy is not considered a disabling condition under the Americans with Disabilities Act. Some states and many private employers have short-term disability insurance programs for workers with physical or medical conditions that interfere with their ability to perform their jobs. However, disability benefits are frequently denied to workers with reproductive concerns on the basis that speculative fetal risk or conditions such as infertility are not strictly work disabling. While such interpretations are arguable from a legal standpoint, many workers lack the resources to challenge denial of benefits. Workers' compensation is also an inadequate remedy, since it also applied to job-disabling conditions and requires proof of the work-relatedness of illnesses and injuries, a criterion difficult to fulfill given the scientific uncertainties and multifactorial etiologies of most reproductive system disorders. As a

---

## THE IMPACT OF ERGONOMIC RISK FACTORS ON REPRODUCTION
Laura Punnett

There is reason to expect poor tolerance of the pregnant worker's uterus and the fetus to ergonomic stressors such as heavy physical work, prolonged standing, and static non-neutral trunk postures. There is a physiologically plausible common mechanism for the effect of these exposures on pregnancy. A wide variety of stressors, including fatigue and psychosocial strain, affect the sympathetic nervous system and cause the release of hormones such as catecholamines and prostaglandins into the maternal circulation. Catecholamines, such as norepinephrine, tend to stimulate uterine contractility; uterine irritability causes cervical changes; the two together initiate the onset of labor. Furthermore, epinephrine levels are elevated in the presence of anxiety or stress. Norepinephrine and epinephrine increase blood pressure and decrease uteroplacental blood flow (UPBF) and placental function. The resulting decreased progesterone production leads to an increase in prostaglandin and to cervical changes.

During exercise, catecholamine and prostaglandin levels have also been shown to increase, with similar effects on uterine contractility. In addition, the circulatory response to exercise involves an increase in sympathetic nervous system activity, which decreases circulation to the uterus in order to increase it to the skeletal muscle.

Thus, exercise is associated with visceral vasoconstriction. Animal studies suggest that the uterus is not protected during this reaction and that UPBF is decreased as a result. Because fetal nutrition is dependent on placental blood flow, it is likely that prolonged strenuous exercise will result in fetal deprivation. It appears that this effect is largely independent of maternal nutritional status; it is not known how it can be modified by general physical fitness. It is biologically plausible that ergonomic strain is relevant even very early in pregnancy, because hypoxia in the first trimester could affect fetal enzymes. A placenta compromised by hypoxia from the beginning of pregnancy might support fetal growth only to a limited stage of development.

It is also important to distinguish static from dynamic exercise in terms of the cardiovascular requirements of each. Local exercise does not have the same effect as whole-body work on redistribution of the circulation, but local static exertion has been shown to produce marked strain on the cardiovascular system. Thus, there may be more reason to expect an effect on UPBF from whole-body exercise, but the importance of prolonged static exertion of local muscle groups needs further investigation. The relative importance of static and dynamic exercise remains confusing. For example, regular physical exercise also increases plasma volume. Moderate aerobic exercise has been positively associated with fetal growth among well-nourished, low-risk physically fit women, but rest during the last 6 weeks of pregnancy also increases fetal weight. However, there is no increase in preterm delivery in women who participate regularly in sports.

Prolonged standing, which affects venous return, decreases plasma volume, and activates the sympathetic nervous system, would be expected to have the same effect on placental perfusion. In addition, growth of the uterus is associated with a loss of the normal lumbar spine curve. As the spine is projected forward, the major blood vessels are compressed, resulting in decreased UPBF. Prolonged standing, especially in forward flexed postures, could further aggravate the decrease in UPBF. The effects of such non-neutral trunk postures might be more likely to occur later in pregnancy when there is decreased room for the pregnant uterus.

The epidemiologic findings for studies of ergonomic risk factors and pregnancy outcome are mixed, complicated in part by the need to include the many other known risk factors for low birthweight and prematurity, as well as by the selection of higher-risk women out of the workforce. Heavy physical work has been shown, in some studies, to be associated with preterm delivery and low birthweight for gestational age. In particular, frequent heavy lifting (such as loads greater than 25 lb lifted over 50 times per week) is associated with uterine contractions, spontaneous abortions, prematurity, and low birthweight. Long hours at work (more than 45 hours per week), especially in physically strenuous jobs, have been linked to decreased gestational age. Finally, although not a uniform finding, some studies have shown increased risk of low birthweight in women who stand for most of the workday.

Variable shiftwork, in addition to operating as a psychosocial stressor, may affect circadian rhythms (body temperature, hormone secretion) and thus reproductive hormones. Anovulation and menstrual disorders are postulated to result, in addition to spontaneous abortion. Shiftwork has been associated with an increase in first-trimester miscarriages, preterm deliveries, and decreased birthweight for gestational age.

An additional impact of ergonomic issues might be through interaction with chemical exposures. Physical exertion results in increased ventilation rates (as does pregnancy itself). A higher tissue dose might, therefore, result from the same environmental concentration.

last resort, employees who leave their jobs because of hazardous conditions may be eligible for unemployment benefits [14].

Workplace interventions should be initiated only with the full knowledge and consent of the worker. While those with cooperative employers are likely to welcome these measures, others may fear employer retaliation or job loss. Obviously, the clinician must be ready and willing to advocate for the at-risk worker. However, given the complexities of these problems, the uncertainty of risk in many cases, and the limited options available to some workers, decisions ultimately belong to the well-informed patient.

## Specific Clinical Encounters

### Evaluation of the Infertile Couple

Occupational health specialists may be asked to determine whether or not exposures in the workplace are contributing to a couple's fertility problems. Because of the multifactorial etiology of infertility, consideration of workplace reproductive hazards is only one part of a more comprehensive evaluation of the male and female.

The occupational work-up of the infertile couple involves identification of agents that affect libido, hormonal regulation, or gonadal function as well as characterization of the timing and dose of exposure. The physical examination may reveal important abnormalities, such as gynecomastia, decreased testicular size, or organic pathology relevant to the problem.

Treatment of infertility includes addressing all potential contributing factors, including reduction of workplace exposures that may impair reproductive function. Often, the only way to determine if an occupational agent is responsible for the problem is to see if abnormalities, such as low sperm count, improve after cessation of exposure. Exposure abatement at the workplace is the best solution; obtaining disability leave in these circumstances is problematic, since causation is often uncertain, and infertility does not interfere with job performance per se.

*Case 1.* A 27-year-old male complains of inability to conceive with his spouse for 13 months. He is employed at an automobile radiator repair shop. His job involves cleaning radiators with a caustic soda solution, disassembling them with an oxygen-acetylene torch, and repairing and then resoldering the units with lead-tin solder. His workroom, which is shared with three other workers, has two windows that are left open on warm days. He wears overalls that are laundered at home, gloves when handling the cleaning solutions, and appropriate shields when using the torch. A one-pack-a-day smoker, he, like his coworkers, often smokes and eats in his work area. His wife, a 25-year-old female who has never been pregnant, is employed as a waitress. An infertility work-up by her gynecologist reveals no abnormalities. The histories are otherwise unremarkable, and his physical examination is normal.

A semen analysis reveals a sperm count of 18 million sperm/ml with mildly abnormal motility and morphology. His other laboratory test results include a blood-lead level of 63 μg/dL and a zinc protoporphyrin (ZPP) of 178 μg/dL, with a normal complete blood count (CBC) and renal function tests. His wife has a blood-lead concentration of 22 μg/dL, a ZPP of 65 μg/dL, and blood indices consistent with a mild iron deficiency anemia.

This case involves lead poisoning due to inhalation of lead fumes during soldering and to contamination of the workspace with lead dust. In addition, the worker's habit of eating and smoking in contaminated areas may increase lead exposure through ingestion and volatilization of lead residues on cigarettes. As illustrated, lead poisoning may present as reproductive system impairment with few, if any, other systemic symptoms.

Excessive lead absorption is common among radiator repair workers. For example, in one study, the blood-lead levels of 80 percent of radiator repair mechanics surveyed exceeded 30 μg/dL. Home laundering of workclothes laden with lead dust can result in exposure to family members, and most likely accounts for the modestly elevated blood-lead level in this worker's spouse. Elevation of ZPP reflects heme enzyme inhibition, which, in her case, probably results from both lead absorption and iron deficiency.

This patient is eligible for medical removal protection under the OSHA lead standard, which requires temporary removal of workers with blood-lead levels of 60 μg/dL or higher, without loss of wages or benefits. This rule also applies to workers with medical conditions that might be exacerbated by exposure to lead, and thus may be instrumental in protecting pregnant or reproductively impaired workers who have lower blood-lead levels.

The OSHA lead standard also calls for institution of control measures to decrease exposure, which in this case might involve improved ventilation systems, provision of respirators, better housekeeping, prohibition of eating and smoking in work areas, and employer laundering services. Before returning to work, this radiator mechanic should be counseled about the hazards of lead and ways to minimize exposures through safe work practices and personal hygiene measures, including smoking cessation. Reporting this case of lead poisoning to OSHA would trigger a workplace inspection and better assure that effective control measures are put into place to protect all workers.

Blood-lead levels should be normalized in both the male and female before conception; therefore, contraceptive counseling is important. As in this case, a finding of blood-lead levels over 10 μg/dL before or during pregnancy should prompt action to identify and remove sources of exposure. Correction of iron deficiency helps to lessen lead absorption. Treatment for the mechanic could include chelation therapy and follow-up would include serial semen analyses to monitor recovery of sperm parameters.

### Evaluation of the Pregnant Worker

One of the most challenging situations confronting clinicians is evaluation and counseling of the pregnant worker. Many women do not seek prenatal care early in pregnancy, and deleterious exposures may have already occurred. While the preconception setting allows ample time for evaluation and preventive intervention, pregnancy creates a need for expeditious assessment and action. In most cases, occupational health specialists will work jointly with obstetricians or family practitioners in caring for patients.

Comprehensive histories should be taken on both members of the couple to gather information on occupational, environmental, medical, obstetric, genetic, and demographic factors that can influence pregnancy outcome adversely. Every effort should be made to identify potential developmental hazards and to establish both the dose and gestational timing of exposure precisely. In addition, the occupational health specialist should carefully explore the employment and benefit options available to at-risk patients.

*Case 2.* A 33-year-old female pregnant with her second child seeks advice at 8 weeks' gestation. She is a nurse employed on the pediatric ward of an urban hospital caring for children with a variety of illnesses, including some patients undergoing chemotherapy for childhood cancers. Although she practices universal precautions* routinely, she is concerned about a recent outbreak of fifth disease among children on her ward. She works 12-hour rotating shifts three to four times per week. Her obstetric history includes a normal delivery at 34 weeks' gestation 6 years ago. Her husband works as a radiology technician at the same hospital, and radiation badge monitoring reveals negligible exposure. Laboratory tests show that she is immune to rubella and has no serologic evidence of prior hepatitis B or human parvovirus B19 infection.

Health care workers may be exposed to a number of occupational reproductive hazards. Exposures that must be considered in this case include antineoplastic drugs, strenuous working conditions, and biologic agents such as HBV and human

*Universal precautions is an approach to infection control in which all human blood and certain body fluids are treated as if known to be infectious.

parvovirus B19. In addition, infection with CMV is common among preschool-aged children and immunosuppressed patients.

Epidemiologic studies suggest that the risk of spontaneous abortion is increased among nurses occupationally exposed to chemotherapeutic agents during pregnancy; one study also found an association with major malformations in offspring. However, exposures in these studies may have been substantial, since the nurses worked in areas with high usage of antineoplastic agents and often prepared the drugs before administering them to patients. Preparation of chemotherapeutic drugs outside of biologic safety cabinets can result in significant exposures. While there are no occupational limits for exposure to antineoplastic agents, OSHA has published guidelines for the safe handling of such drugs that should be followed strictly [15].

The nurse in this case has serologic studies that indicate she is immune to rubella but susceptible to infection with HBV. As an at-risk health care worker, she should be offered HBV vaccination, which is not contraindicated during pregnancy. Primary infection with CMV during pregnancy may cause congenital defects and developmental impairment in offspring. However, several studies have shown that, when adequate precautions are taken, the risk of CMV infection for pediatric nurses does not differ from that of community controls. Although not performed in this case, serologic testing is available to determine the CMV status of workers.

Her serologic studies also reveal that she is susceptible to infection with human parvovirus B19 (immunoglobulin G negative); while her negative immunoglobulin M (IgM) suggests that recent infection has not occurred, only 80 percent of women with recent infection have detectable IgM antibody levels. Human parvovirus B19 infection during pregnancy has been associated with non-immune fetal hydrops and fetal loss, which often occurs between the tenth and twentieth weeks of gestation. The Centers for Disease Control estimate that the maximum risk of B19-associated fe-

tal death is in the range of 1.5 to 2.5 percent in cases in which the antibody status of the pregnant woman is unknown, and is less than 10 percent after documented maternal infection [16].

This situation requires careful counseling and management; in addition, consultation with perinatologists or infectious disease specialists, or both, is advisable. Since human parvovirus B19 is transmitted through aerosol droplet spread, as well as through contact with infected blood products, universal precautions are not completely protective. Therefore, it is reasonable to consider transfer options for this nurse until the outbreak of fifth disease has subsided. However, she must understand that this measure will not protect against community-acquired infection, a point particularly pertinent since she has a young child in her household. Given the 20 percent rate of false-negative IgM in patients with recent infection, prudent follow-up might include serial ultrasound tests to monitor for fetal hydrops.

In addition to the psychological and emotional challenges inherent in caring for ill patients, health care workers are often exposed to ergonomic stressors. As illustrated in this case, nursing jobs may involve long hours and rotating shifts, as well as heavy lifting when moving patients. With a history of early delivery, this nurse has a predisposition to preterm delivery, which may be exacerbated by strenuous working conditions. Therefore, job modifications, such as reduced hours, increased rest breaks, and avoidance of heavy lifting, should be considered during the third trimester of pregnancy. In addition, she should be counseled about the signs and symptoms of preterm labor and have more frequent cervical examinations during the third trimester to monitor for cervical dilatation.

*Case 3.* A 26-year-old female, at 7 weeks' gestation with her first pregnancy, has been employed at a small, nonunionized furniture manufacturing plant for 4 years. Her job involves applying an adhesive to the backs of furniture cushions with a medium-sized brush and setting them into couch and chair frames. Other workers in her immediate area finish the wooden furniture frames with solvent-based cleaners and lacquers. The only ventilation in the room consists of a ceiling fan, and no personal protective equipment except gloves is available. Review of MSDSs reveals that the adhesive is toluene-based and that the other chemicals used by nearby workers include acetone, xylene, and methylene chloride. During a recent OSHA inspection, the woman's 8-hour time-weighted average exposure to toluene was 80 ppm (OSHA's permissible exposure limit [PEL] is 100 ppm). Airborne concentrations of the other solvents ranged from one-third to one-half of the PELs. The worker is concerned about the effects of these chemicals on her pregnancy. However, she is reluctant to voice her concerns due to fear of employer harassment or job loss. Although her husband works at a dry-cleaning plant, the couple depend on her job for adequate income and health benefits. No disability insurance plan is available through the state or her employer.

This case is among the most difficult that occupational health specialists will encounter, since it involves both scientific uncertainty as well as limited employment and benefit options for the worker. While some studies suggest that mixed organic solvent exposure during pregnancy may increase the risk for spontaneous abortion or congenital defects, little information is available on specific agents or the doses required to induce adverse developmental effects in humans. Accumulated case series suggest that recreational abuse of toluene at doses high enough to cause narcosis (~500 ppm) may be teratogenic, but effects at lower exposures, typical of occupational settings, have not been adequately investigated. In addition, both toluene and xylene at high doses are fetotoxic in laboratory animals, and methylene chloride is metabolized to carbon monoxide in vivo.

From a public health perspective, even the uncertain and limited data on these organic solvents would seem to warrant minimization of exposures during pregnancy. However, the degree to which this goal is achievable may vary according to the resources and goodwill of the employer, as well as the financial status of the worker. In stable, large industries, employers are often willing to temporarily transfer exposed workers while implementing more effective controls to reduce exposures. In small firms, like the one in this case, transfer options are limited and employers may be unable to bear the cost of new engineering controls. Since this employer is not violating OSHA standards, it is unlikely that OSHA will compel the employer to decrease exposures further. At the same time, OSHA limits for these organic solvents do not necessarily protect against adverse developmental outcomes, so that a potential, albeit uncertain, risk to the pregnancy remains.

In these situations, workers who are employed in low-wage, nonunionized jobs with few protections or benefits face difficult choices. This worker may ultimately decide that attempts at intervention in the workplace are worth the potential risks of employer retaliation; she may choose to leave work and pursue unemployment benefits or she may decide to stay on the job, preferring uncertain occupational risks over the adverse health and financial consequences of unemployment. Whatever she chooses, the health care provider should assure that her decisions are well-informed. If she remains at work, counseling regarding safe work practices and simple control measures, such as respirator use, is crucial. In addition, referral to legal professionals may be warranted to assure that her rights are fully protected.

As is so poignantly exemplified here, there is a tremendous need in the U.S. for policy reform in the area of reproductive health hazards. Recently, workers have won important legal cases involving gender discrimination in the workplace and denial of disability or unemployment benefits to pregnant women exposed to potential hazards. However, these cases are extremely costly and beyond the resources of most workers. Like many public health issues, addressing the problem of occupational reproductive hazards will require not only scientific advances, but also more stringent regulation of reproductive hazards and fundamental changes in the policies that govern the protections and accommodations available to affected workers [14].

In conclusion, reproduction is an exceedingly complex process vulnerable to insult at many stages, and targets of reproductive injury include the male and female worker as well as the conceptus. Concerted scientific inquiry into the reproductive and developmental effects of occupational toxicants is relatively new, leaving considerable gaps in our knowledge of specific agents, their mechanisms of action, and their adverse effects.

At the same time, workers are turning increasingly to health care providers with concerns about potential reproductive hazards. Evaluation of patients includes identifying possible harmful exposures, defining the characteristics of exposure, and making estimates of risk based on the best available data. Clinicians can play vital roles in encouraging employers to decrease hazards and in providing supportive advocacy and counseling to workers. In addition, there is a great need for more involvement of health care providers in the critique and reformulation of policies that affect workers with occupational reproductive concerns.

# References

1. Baranski B. Effects of the workplace on fertility and related reproductive outcomes. Environ Health Perspect 1993; 101 (Suppl. 2):81–90.
2. Winder C. Reproductive and chromosomal effects of occupational exposure to lead in the male. Reprod Toxicol 1989; 3:221–33.
3. Occupational Safety and Health Administration. 29 CFR Part 1910. Occupational exposure to 2-methoxyethanol, 2-ethoxyethanol and their acetates (glycol ethers); proposed rule. Fed Register 1993; 58:15526–632.
4. Mattison DR. Clinical manifestations of ovarian toxicity. In RL Dixon. ed. Reproductive toxicology. New York: Raven Press, 1985, pp. 109–30.
5. Rowland AS, et al. Reduced fertility among women employed as dental assistants exposed to high levels of nitrous oxide. N Engl J Med 1992; 327:993–7.
6. Neel JV, et al. The children of parents exposed to atomic bombs: Estimates of the genetic doubling dose of radiation for humans. Am J Hum Genet 1990; 46:1053–72.
7. Colie CF. Male mediated teratogenesis. Reprod Toxicol 1993; 7:3–9.
8. Marbury MC. Relationship of ergonomic stressors to birthweight and gestational age. Scand J Work Environ Health 1992; 18:73–83.
9. Paul ME. Physical agents in the workplace. Semin Perinatol 1993; 17:5–17.
10. Miller RK, Bellinger D. Metals. In M Paul. ed. Occupational and environmental reproductive hazards: A guide for clinicians. Baltimore: Williams & Wilkins, 1993, pp. 233–52.
11. Donald JM, Hooper K, Hopenhayn-Rich C. Reproductive and developmental toxicity of toluene: A review. Environ Health Perspect 1991; 94:237–44.
12. Paul M, Kurtz S. Analysis of reproductive health hazard information on material safety data sheets for lead and the ethylene glycol ethers. Am J Ind Med 1994; 25:403–415.
13. United States Congress, General Accounting Office. Reproductive and developmental toxicants: Regulatory actions provide uncertain protection. Washington, D.C.: General Accounting Office, 1991.
14. Clauss CA, Berzon M, Bertin J. Litigating reproductive and developmental health in the aftermath of UAW v. Johnson Controls. Environ Health Perspect 1993; 101 (Suppl. 2):205–20.
15. Yodaiken RE. OSHA work practice guidelines for personnel dealing with cytotoxic drugs. Am J Hosp Pharm 1986; 43:1193–204.
16. Centers for Disease Control. Risks associated with human parvovirus B19 infection. MMWR 1989; 38:81–97.

# Bibliography

El Batawi MA, et al. Effects of occupational health hazards on reproductive functions: Report by a WHO meeting. Geneva: World Health Organization, 1987.

Koren GM. ed. Maternal-fetal toxicology: A clinicians' guide. New York: Marcel Dekker, 1990.

Paul M. ed. Occupational and environmental reproductive hazards: A guide for clinicians. Baltimore: Williams & Wilkins, 1993.

Schardein JE. Chemically induced birth defects. New York: Marcel Dekker, 1985.

Scialli AR. A clinical guide to reproductive and developmental toxicology. Boca Raton, FL: CRC Press, 1991.

United States Congress, Office of Technology Assessment. Reproductive hazards in the workplace. Washington, D.C.: U.S. Government Printing Office, OTA-BA-266, 1985.

# 28

# Cardiovascular Disorders

Gilles P. Thériault

"Two young men employed in the mineral assay industry developed noninflammatory cardiomyopathy. By review of clinical findings, elicitation of occupational and environmental histories, worksite evaluations, and ascertainment of tissue cobalt levels, Nevada Public Health authorities confirmed these cases to be due to occupational cobalt exposure. Hair and heart cobalt levels were elevated for the cases, but control samples had no detectable cobalt" [1].

A 37-year-old man, whose work consisted of moving cars containing 180-kg rolls of wire from one side of a plant to the other, developed an acute myocardial infarction. One morning, at the end of his night shift, while trying to free his loaded cart that had become stuck in a hole in the floor, he felt an acute pain in his chest. On arrival at the hospital, an extensive myocardial infarction was diagnosed. Even though this man smoked a pack of cigarettes daily and had a father who had died from heart disease, the workers' compensation board awarded him a settlement for "an injury resulting from an accident at work."

A 55-year-old man with a past history of mild angina pectoris had been hired as a parking attendant in an underground parking garage. On a particularly cold winter day, when business had been heavier than usual, severe chest pain and shortness of breath developed. When he arrived at the hospital, his carboxyhemoglobin (COHb) level was found to be 10 percent. He died during the night of myocardial infarction. Measurements of the garage air taken the following day showed levels of carbon monoxide (CO) of up to 100 ppm.

One of the great achievements of medicine in developed countries over the last three decades has been the decline in cardiovascular disease (CVD) and, in particular, coronary heart disease (CHD) among people aged 45 to 64. This is the result of many measures, some preventive, such as changes in dietary habits, smoking, and exercise, and some curative, such as improvement in the management of heart disease victims. Nevertheless, CVD remains, even today, the leading cause of death worldwide [2] and a great deal of effort has to be maintained in the fight against this problem.

Because CVD causes so much mortality, preventing even a small increase in risk due to occupational exposure can involve large numbers of people and represent an important public health measure.

Personal risk factors that contribute to the development of CHD have been well studied, but the contribution of working conditions to this disease has been explored very little. In 1981 the American Heart Association recognized this gap in knowledge and recommended that occupational epidemiologic studies be performed [3].

## Risk Factors for Coronary Heart Disease

Risk factors associated with CHD can be divided into three categories: personal, hereditary, and environmental. As shown in Table 28-1, personal risk factors include sex, age, race, high serum cholesterol, high blood pressure, and cigarette smoking. There are strong interactions between these factors that act synergistically, such that a smoker

Table 28-1. Personal risk factors associated with CHD

| Risk factor | Feature |
| --- | --- |
| Sex | Mortality for women lags behind that of men by about 10 years |
| Age | Risk increases with age |
| Race | Before age 60, white men have lower death rates than nonwhite men; the inverse is true after 60 |
| High serum cholesterol | Risk estimated at 1.7–3.5 |
| High blood pressure | Risk estimated at 1.5–2.1 |
| Cigarette smoking | Risk estimated at 1.5–2.9 |

with high blood pressure and high serum cholesterol is eight times more at risk of developing CHD than a nonsmoker who has normal serum cholesterol and blood pressure [4].

There are other personal risk factors, such as obesity and diabetes, but their roles in causing CHD are minor compared with those cited above. In certain families, the risk of CHD is high and is correlated with the number of blood relatives who have developed the disease and the early age at which they developed it [5].

## Occupation as a Risk Factor for Coronary Heart Disease

While the association between personal risk factors and CHD is well documented, our knowledge of the role of occupational risk factors is still limited. Several chemical and physical agents have been suspected of causing CHD in workers chronically exposed to them. However, scientific evidence indicates a direct causal relationship for very few of them. For most of these agents, the evidence is based on isolated case reports or on a few unconfirmed studies. Table 28-2 lists some occupational hazards associated with cardiovascular disorders.

## Carbon Monoxide

The potential for exposure to carbon monoxide in industry is high. This odorless and colorless gas is produced in most processes where there is fire, combustion, or oxidation. High exposures may occur in many workplaces such as steel and iron foundries, petroleum refineries, pulp and paper mills, and plants where formaldehyde and coke are produced. One of the most common and insidious sources is the internal combustion engine; workers in garages and enclosed parking spaces may be chronically exposed to fairly high levels of CO. Firefighters, apart from the usual hazards of their work, may be exposed to excessively high levels of CO in smoke.

Carbon monoxide causes a variety of signs and symptoms, dependent on concentration of exposure (Table 28-3). Exposure to high concentrations of CO ($> 1,500$ ppm) can cause sudden death by anoxia. Exposure to low concentrations decreases myocardial oxygen consumption, concomitantly increases coronary flow and heart rate, and lowers exercise tolerance of healthy persons. When a person already suffers from a certain degree of coronary insufficiency, such consequences may manifest by an increase of the S-T segment depression on electrocardiogram (ECG), the onset of angina pectoris [8], and occasionally by acute myocardial infarction.

However, the association between chronic exposure to low levels of CO and the development of coronary atherosclerosis leading to CHD has yet to be shown. Recent literature indicates that low exposure to CO accelerates the development of atherosclerosis in laboratory animals when combined with a diet rich in saturated fats, especially when exposure consists of intermittent peaks [9]. The few studies conducted so far among working groups have been unable to show a distinct relationship between chronic exposure to CO and the development of CHD. The known association of CHD with cigarette smoking, combined with recent observations that workers intermittently exposed to peaks of CO have higher risk of

**Table 28-2.** Some occupational hazards associated with cardiovascular disorders

| Hazard | Effect | Strength of evidence |
|---|---|---|
| Carbon monoxide | Atherosclerosis | Weak |
| Carbon disulfide | Atherosclerosis | Strong |
| Certain aliphatic nitrates | Coronary spasm | Strong |
| | Atherosclerosis | Satisfactory |
| Lead | Hypertension (renal) | Weak |
| Cadmium | Hypertension (renal) | Insufficient |
| Arsenic | Coronary heart disease | Insufficient |
| Physical inactivity | Coronary heart disease | Strong |
| Noise | Transient high blood pressure | Strong |
| | Long-term high blood pressure | Insufficient |
| Shiftwork | Coronary heart disease | Weak |
| Halogenated solvents | Arrhythmia | Satisfactory |
| Chronic hand-arm vibration | Vibration white finger | Strong |

**Table 28-3.** Progressive effects of exposure to carbon monoxide[a]

| 8-hour average concentration (ppm) | Carboxyhemoglobin[b] concentration (%) after equilibrium | Main signs and symptoms |
|---|---|---|
| 0 | 0.1–1.0 | No signs or symptoms. Normal endogenous level. |
| 25–50 | 2.5–5 | No symptoms. Compensatory increase in bloodflow to certain vital organs. Patients with severe cardiovascular disease may lack compensatory reserve. |
| 50–100 | 5–10 | Visual light threshold slightly increased. |
| 100–250 | 10–20 | Tightness across the forehead. Slight headache. Visual evoked response abnormal. Possibly slight breathlessness on exertion. May be lethal to fetus. May be lethal for patients with severe heart disease. |
| 250–450 | 20–30 | Slight or moderate headache and throbbing in the temples. Flushing. Nausea. Fine manual dexterity abnormal. |
| 450–650 | 30–40 | Severe headache, vertigo, nausea and vomiting. Weakness. Irritability and impaired judgment. Syncope on exertion. |
| 650–1,000 | 40–50 | Same as above, but more severe with greater possibility of collapse and syncope. |
| 1,000–1,500 | 50–60 | Possibly coma with intermittent convulsions and Cheyne-Stokes respiration. |
| 1,500–2,500 | 60–70 | Coma with intermittent convulsions. Depressed respiration and heart action. Possibly death. |
| 2,500–4,000 | 70–80 | Weak pulse and slow respiration. Depression of respiratory center leading to death. |

[a]Carboxyhemoglobin and carbon monoxide equivalents obtained from the formula developed by Gobbato and Mangiavacchi [6]. Main signs and symptoms extracted from Kurppa and Rantanen [7].
[b]Varies with pulmonary ventilation rate, endogenous carboxyhemoglobin production, blood volume, barometric pressure, and relative diffusion capability of the lungs.

heart disease, keeps this question open to further research.

### Carbon Disulfide

Of all the chemicals for which an association with heart disease has been studied, carbon disulfide ($CS_2$) shows the most convincing evidence. Although this chemical is used mostly as a solvent and in the production of organic chemicals, paints, fuels, and explosives, its use in the viscose rayon–producing industry revealed this association (Fig. 28-1). Mortality studies of viscose rayon workers who were exposed to $CS_2$ have shown that they are two to five times at greater risk of dying from heart disease than unexposed workers. Reduction of exposures reduces the risk to workers [10]. In one study, the excess mortality declined from a relative risk of 4.7 to 1.0 over a 15-year period after implementation of exposure reduction measures [11].

The mechanism by which $CS_2$ causes heart disease is not known, although it is hypothesized that it may be through changes in cholesterol metabolism with promotion of atherosclerosis of the coronary arteries.

### Nitroglycerin and Other Aliphatic Nitrates

Some aliphatic nitrates are potent vasodilators of coronary vessels; this property has long been used for the treatment of angina pectoris. However, it has been reported that some workers exposed continuously to nitroglycerin, and in particular to ethylene glycol dinitrate, during the manufacturing of explosives have suffered from angina pectoris on withdrawal from exposure (Fig. 28-2). This phenomenon, which occurs on weekends or on vacations, disappears on return to work. The mechanism involved is thought to be a coronary spasm that develops after the chemically induced vasodilation has ceased. The reversal of this spasm by

**Fig. 28-1.** Worker tending machines that spool rayon thread from carbon disulfide. Worker exposure to carbon disulfide was high until this process was enclosed, which reduced worker exposure and, by recycling the carbon disulfide, saved the company a substantial amount of money [10]. (Photograph by Barry Levy.)

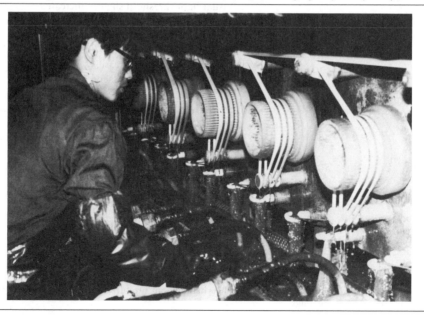

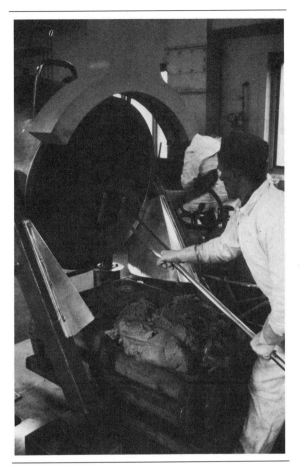

**Fig. 28-2.** Dynamite kneading involves exposure to nitrates, which, on days off, can result in rebound vasospasm of coronary arteries. Note local exhaust and protective clothing. (Photograph courtesy of C. Hogstedt.)

the administration of nitroglycerin has actually been observed under angiography during the withdrawal period.

Studies have reported elevated risk for CHD after some 20 years of exposure, which seems to indicate that nitro compounds are not only responsible for acute vasospastic reactions but also increase the risk of CHD after long exposure. The mechanism by which nitro compounds generate atherosclerosis remains unknown.

## Metals

There has been much speculation on the potential for lead, cadmium, and arsenic to cause CHD among workers with long chronic exposure to these chemicals. Kristensen [12] has made an extensive review of the epidemiologic literature on the subject.

Much research has been conducted on the relationship between lead exposure and high blood pressure. A pattern has emerged to the effect that workers exposed to lead have shown high mortality due to cerebrovascular diseases, very likely mediated by hypertensive diseases. No clear association with CHD has been reported. Most studies have shown an increased mortality due to chronic renal diseases among lead-exposed workers (see Chap. 31).

For several years in the 1960s and early 1970s cadmium was believed to cause high blood pressure among exposed workers. This was supported by laboratory studies on animals. Most recent studies have not confirmed this hypothesis and today we can state with a good deal of certainty that cadmium exposure does not entail an increased risk of CHD among workers exposed.

In his review of the epidemiologic literature, Kristensen [12] found only three studies that addressed the issue of arsenic exposure and CVD. In all three, the exposure was arsenic trioxide. Excess mortality from CHD was reported in copper smelter workers. It was difficult, however, to attribute the excess mortality to arsenic. Reasonable evidence of an association between arsenic exposure and CHD is still lacking.

## Noise

High levels of noise, exceeding 85 dBA (decibels on the "A" scale), are common in the workplace. There are few factories, smelters, or mines where hazardous noise is not a problem. The association between chronic exposure to high noise levels and hearing loss is well-documented (see Chap. 16).

Some researchers have proposed that noise can also damage the cardiovascular system indirectly by causing high blood pressure and, over a long period, atherosclerosis of the heart and blood vessels. Intermittent and impact noise would seem to be more harmful than continual noise in this respect. However, reports have been rather inconsistent on this issue and observations are frequently confounded by methodologic inadequacies.

Acute exposure to high levels of noise initiates cardiovascular responses that mimic the effects of acute stress: These include increases of blood pressure and heart rate; blood levels of catecholamines and lipids, such as low-density lipoproteins and fatty acids; and vascular tone of peripheral vessels. These changes are transitory, however, and disappear a short time after exposure ends [13]. Long-term effects of exposure to noise, such as chronic high blood pressure, coronary atherosclerosis, or ischemic heart problems, have yet to be demonstrated, if indeed they do exist.

### Physical Inactivity

Of all the occupational factors that have been associated with work, inactivity is the one that seems to carry the closest association with CHD. From his review, Kristensen [14] concluded that clear evidence emerged to the effect that physical inactivity is causally related to an excess risk of both CVD and CHD. The relative risk for CVD can be estimated to be at least 2.0 when inactive people are compared to active ones.

### Psychological Stress and the Psychosocial Work Environment

Among less well-defined risks of CHD are a wide array of psychological stress factors. The most widely studied of these is the type A behavior pattern in "an individual who chronically struggles to obtain an unlimited number of goals in the shortest possible time, often in competition with other people or opposing forces in the environment" (see Chap. 19) [15].

An extensive review of the evidence on the association between CHD and type A behavior [16] concluded that population studies demonstrate type A behavior to be a risk factor for coronary heart disease among healthy working men, but not for recurrent events or for mortality in men who have had a first heart attack or who are suffering from angina. Subsequent studies pointed out that anger and hostility seem to play an important role in this association between type A behavior and coronary heart disease.

Contrary to previous beliefs, white-collar workers who are exposed to the more stressful psychological environment of the decision-making process have shown lower mortality and incidence rates of CHD than blue-collar workers. This effect can be explained by the high socioeconomic status of white-collar workers; it could also indicate a risk associated with the physical stresses and exposures to pollutants of the blue-collar working environment.

In the early 1980s Karasek and associates [17] proposed a model, referred to as a job strain model, by which a work situation can be classified bidirectionally according to the degree of monotony of a job and to the level of control one can exercise over his or her work. Jobs characterized by high monotony, understimulation, high predictability, and lack of control would entail the highest risk of CHD (see Chap. 19).

Attempts to test the Karasek model in real-life situations seem to have been rather successful. Most such studies have been conducted among urban bus drivers. They have reported that the risk of CHD for workers exposed to strainful work situations can be estimated to be between 1.3 and 4.0, depending on various studies. It is proposed that the mechanism behind this phenomenon is an increase in circulating hormones such as plasma testosterone and noradrenaline, and an increase in blood pressure. Under the same intervention, cortisol in plasma increased more among passive than among active workers. This job strain model could explain the different CHD risks of the white- and blue-collar workers.

Shiftwork and excessive overtime have recently been suspected of being associated with CHD [18]. More evidence is needed for such associations to be confirmed (see Chap. 20).

## Occupation as a Risk Factor for Cardiovascular Disorders

Some cardiovascular disorders other than CHD have also been associated with exposure to chemical and physical agents at work. Among the most noteworthy are myocarditis, congestive heart failure, cardiac arrhythmias, Raynaud's phenomenon, and skin telangiectasia.

In the mid 1960s an epidemic of fatal cardiomyopathies was reported among heavy beer drinkers after several breweries added a foam-stabilizing, cobalt-containing substance to the beer. It has been suggested that the synergistic effects of alcohol, cobalt, and a protein-poor diet were at the root of the cobalt-induced cardiomyopathy, symptoms of which resemble thiamine deficiency [19]. Until then, no such cardiopathy had been reported as resulting from exposure at work despite awareness that in the hard metal and other cobalt-using industries, such exposure existed. Since then, four cases of cobalt cardiomyopathy have been reported among exposed workers; the last two were identified in the mineral assay industry [1]. This may reflect that such a disease has long existed among cobalt-exposed workers but has been misdiagnosed or overlooked until now.

In their advanced stages, silicosis, asbestosis, severe asthma following exposure to toluene diisocyanate (TDI), and other pulmonary diseases may develop into right-sided heart failure. This condition, called chronic cor pulmonale, can be regarded as the terminal stage of a long chronic evolution of the disease.

Acute exposures to some halogenated and non-halogenated industrial solvents, such as toluene, xylene, chloroform, and trichloroethylene, and to fluorocarbon aerosol propellants have been associated with sudden death. The mechanism underlying this effect is presumably a fatal cardiac arrhythmia or ventricular fibrillation due to sensitization of the heart muscular fibers to epinephrine. Case reports indicate that these sudden deaths are usually preceded by high levels of exposure to the solvents and concurrent stress, resulting in activation of the sympathetic nervous system. Epidemiologic studies have not revealed increases of CVD mortality among painters or other groups of workers exposed to organic solvents.

Chronic exposure of the hands to vibration from vibrating tools, such as pneumatic drills, hammers, chisels, riveting tools, metal grinders, and chain saws, has been associated with a vascular syndrome affecting the fingers. This syndrome, called Raynaud's phenomenon, vibration white finger (VWF), or hand-arm vibration syndrome, manifests by an episodic whitening of the fingers accompanied by numbness or complete loss of sensation. The toes can be similarly affected. On recovery, there is reddening and tingling of the affected areas accompanied by pain. In forestry, the prevalence of this phenomenon has been estimated to be over 30 percent [20]. After several years of exposure, the syndrome becomes so disabling that the affected worker is forced to leave the job. Recovery takes place slowly once exposure has ceased (see Chap. 17).

Another vascular phenomenon that has been associated with a specific occupation is skin telangiectasis in aluminum workers. Primary aluminum reduction workers have developed numerous red spots on their chest, back, and upper limbs. These maculae are clusters of telangiectasias. Apart from their unesthetic appearance, they do not seem to carry any other health significance. Neither the mechanism involved nor the causal chemical is known at this point, although it is proposed that a fluoride element bound to a hydrocarbon molecule excreted by the sweat may account for the phenomenon [21].

## Cardiovascular Disorders and Cigarette Smoking

Although antitobacco campaigns have succeeded in decreasing the number of smokers, many workers still smoke cigarettes. It is therefore appropriate to stress the relationship between smoking and CHD.

Most studies have estimated the risk of CHD among smokers to be in the order of 2.5 as compared with nonsmokers. It seems that this risk is associated more closely with the number of cigarettes smoked per day than with the number of years of smoking. Recent investigation demonstrates that this risk is reversible after a person stops smoking: The risk decreases to the level of a nonsmoker after 10 years of abstention [22].

## Screening for Coronary Artery Disease in Asymptomatic Workers

The use of exercise stress testing has been proposed as a means of screening out from strenuous jobs those persons who are at high risk of developing ischemic heart disease. This concept stemmed from the results of several studies showing that symptomatic persons undergoing exercise stress testing who present a lowering of the S-T segment on ECG develop three to five times more CHD after 5 years than those without this ECG change [23].

This type of screening may seem attractive, particularly in situations in which persons are working under conditions that may represent a higher risk of CHD, such as regular exposure to low levels of CO or working in strenuous jobs. However, many sound arguments militate against this approach: (1) the low reliability of exercise stress testing in predicting the development of CHD, (2) discrimination in hiring of workers on unproven grounds, (3) the unavailability of preventive measures for those identified as being at higher risk, (4) the association of risk with numerous other factors, and (5) the existence of risk associated with the testing itself.

After weighing all considerations, the benefits that can be gained from exercise stress testing to screen out persons potentially at risk of coronary artery disease appear to be substantially outweighed by the drawbacks. The procedure cannot be recommended for asymptomatic persons.

## Return to Work After Myocardial Infarction

There is a 5 to 10 percent mortality during the first year after a myocardial infarction. After a 1-year survival, mortality goes down to approximately 3 percent annually. Factors associated with a poor prognosis are the extent of the damage caused to the myocardium (expressed by a poor left ventricular ejection fraction), a ventricular irritability with persistent ventricular ectopic activity, persistent angina, or the presence of associated diseases such as diabetes mellitus and high blood pressure.

After an uncomplicated attack of myocardial infarction or an uncomplicated surgical bypass, a worker can resume normal activities within 6 to 8 weeks. Return to normal working could be gradual and extended over a period of up to 3 months, although this is not always necessary.

One of the challenges of modern medicine is to adequately match the heart attack victim left with a handicap to a work activity commensurable with his or her residual capacities. There are no magic formulas to that effect and much is left to the discretion of the attending physician. There exists a system that is very useful for that purpose; it is called the metabolic equivalence system (METS). It consists of assessment through treadmill or cycle ergometry testing of the amount of oxygen consumption expressed in METS (1 MET = an oxygen consumption of 3.5 ml/kg body weight/min) that the infarct victim can consume before showing signs of cardiac stress.

Once the infarct victim's METS is known, the physician can refer to an occupational equivalence table that classifies working activities according to their energy requirements. In so doing, the physician can match the residual physical capacity of the patient to the energy demand of a set of occupations. The same METS system is used by transportation departments in deciding on limitations to the driving of public vehicles, emergency vehicles, and heavy trucks.

In the past, much caution has been used in recommending an individual's return to work after a heart attack to a job in which the safety of fellow workers or of the general public was directly concerned, such as driving public transportation vehicles, piloting aircraft, and erecting scaffolding. Recent successes in the management of heart victims and the observation that the risk of a recurrent attack is low have brought important changes in those perceptions so that today it is common policy to allow resumption of these occupations after a period (often of 1 year) of absence of symptoms.

## Coronary Heart Disease and Workers' Compensation

Although CHD is essentially a personal rather than an occupational disease, it is sometimes brought to the courts of law under the allegations that it resulted from the stress or strain of a specific work activity. The assumption is that work has contributed in an appreciable degree to the precipitation of the disease or aggravated a preexisting condition. In certain circumstances, such cases can be recognized as legally work-related.

In most North American workers' compensation programs, CHD is considered to be an injury caused by accident rather than an occupational disease. The presence of an accident originally meant that some "unusual exertion" was a neces-sary precondition, but its definition has varied much with time and place [24].

It is reasonable to assume that most courts of law will accept cases when four conditions are met: (1) the asserted heart pathology is well demonstrated; (2) the CHD has followed an exertive activity, not encountered normally in the execution of the work (often this is in relation to an emergency situation); (3) the heart attack took place immediately or in a reasonable period of time after the effort; and (4) a physician states that the exertion, more probably than not, triggered the attack.

There seems to be general agreement that firefighters and police officers are at high risk for CHD and, accordingly, several states have favorably considered compensation cases for these workers. The impetus for such an attitude has been a concern over the physical and emotional stresses of both occupations, and, in addition, the chemical hazards encountered in fighting fires.

## Impact of Work on the Frequency of CVD

Some authors have attempted to quantify the impact of work on cardiovascular diseases. To do so, they have estimated what is called etiologic fractions. These estimates are based on the assumed relative risk resulting from one exposure and the prevalence of such an exposure in a working population. "The etiologic fraction is that proportion of the disease that would not have occurred had the risk factor not occurred in the population" [25].

Such a risk assessment for Danish workers was published by Olsen and Kristensen in 1991 [25]. It is reproduced in Table 28-4. According to these estimates, 51 percent of premature cardiovascular deaths among men and 55 percent among women would not have occurred if none of the occupational risks factors had existed (the figures are 16 and 22 percent when sedentary work is not included among risk factors). These estimates are re-

**Table 28-4.** Etiologic fractions of work environment risk factors for premature cardiovascular diseases in Denmark

| Risk factor | Prevalence of exposures (%) | | Relative risks | Etiologic fractions (%) | |
|---|---|---|---|---|---|
| | Men | Women | | Men | Women |
| Monotonous, high-paced work | 6 | 16 | 2.0 | 6 | 14 |
| Shiftwork | 20 | 20 | 1.4 | 7 | 7 |
| Noise | 7 | 4 | 1.2 | 1 | 1 |
| Chemical exposures | Low | Low | >1.0 | 0–1 | 0 |
| Passive smoking | 12 | 13 | 1.3 | 2 | 2 |
| "Sedentary" work | 90* | 90* | 2.0 | 42 | 42 |
| All occupational risk factors | | | | 51 | 55 |
| All occupational risk factors except "sedentary" work | | | | 16 | 22 |

*Only those 72 percent who are also physically inactive during leisure time will gain any benefit from physical activity at work.
Source: Olsen O, Kristensen TS. Impact of work environment on cardiovascular diseases in Denmark. J Epidemiol Commun Health 1991; 45:4–10.

markably high, although the premises on which they are based look reasonable.

# References

1. Jarvis JQ, Hammond E, Meier R, Robinson C. Cobalt cardiomyopathy. A report of two cases from mineral assay laboratories and a review of the literature. J Occup Med 1992; 34:620–6.
2. Trends and determinants of coronary heart disease mortality: International comparison. Int J Epidemiol 1989; 18 (Suppl. 1).
3. Harlan WR, et al. Impact of environment on cardiovascular disease. Report of the American Heart Association Task Force on Environment and the Cardiovascular System. Circulation 1981; 63:242A–71A.
4. Feinleib M. Risk assessment, environmental factors and coronary heart disease. J Am Coll Toxicol 1983; 2:91–104.
5. Barrett-Connor E, Khaw KT. Family history of heart attack as an independent predictor of death due to cardiovascular disease. Circulation 1986; 69:1065–9.
6. Gobbato F, Mangiavacchi D. Previsione del rischio di ossicarbonismo acuto. Nomogramma per il calcolo della carbossiemoglobina nel sangue in fun-
zione della concentrazione del CO in aria, del tempo di esposizione e della ventilazione polmonare. (Prevention of the hazard of acute carbon monoxide poisoning. A nomogram for calculating blood COHb on the basis of the carbon monoxide concentration in air, the length of exposure and lung ventilation.) Lavoro Umano 1977; 29:129–40.
7. Kurppa K, Rantanen J. In L Parmeggiani. ed. Encyclopedia of occupational health and safety. 3rd ed. Geneva: ILO, 1983. Pp. 395–9. Vol. 1.
8. Anderson EW, et al. Effect of low-level carbon monoxide exposure on onset and duration of angina pectoris. Ann Intern Med 1973; 79:46–50.
9. Weir FW, Fabiano VL. Re-evaluation of the role of carbon monoxide in production or aggravation of cardiovascular disease processes. J Occup Med 1982; 24:519–25.
10. Liang YX, Qu DZ. Cost benefit analysis of the recovery of carbon disulfide in the manufacturing of viscose rayon. Scand J Work Environ Health 1985; 11 (Suppl. 4):60–3.
11. Nurminen M, Hernberg S. Effects of intervention on the cardiovascular mortality of workers exposed to carbon disulphide: A 15 year follow-up. Br J Ind Med 1985; 42:32–5.
12. Kristensen TS. Cardiovascular diseases and the work environment. A critical review of the epidemiologic literature on chemical factors. Scand J Work Environ Health 1989; 15:245–64.

13. Delin CO. Noisy work and hypertension. Lancet 1984; 2:931.
14. Kristensen TS. Cardiovascular diseases and the work environment. A critical review of the epidemiologic literature on nonchemical factors. Scand J Work Environ Health 1989; 15:165–79.
15. Dorian B, Taylor CB. Stress factors in the development of coronary artery disease. J Occup Med 1984; 26:747–56.
16. Matthews KA, Haynes SG. Type A behavior pattern and coronary disease risk. Update and critical evaluation. Am J Epidemiol 1986; 123:923–60.
17. Kasarek R, et al. Job decision latitude, job demands and cardiovascular disease: A prospective study of Swedish men. Am J Public Health 1981; 71:694–705.
18. Knutsson A, Akerstedt T, Jonsson BG, Orth-Gomer K. Increased risk of ischaemic heart disease in shift workers. Lancet 1986; July 12:89–91.
19. Morin Y, Daniel P. Québec beer drinkers cardiomyopathy: Etiological considerations. Can Med Assoc J 1967; 97:925–8.
20. Thériault GP, De Guire L, Gingras S. Raynaud's phenomenon in forestry workers of the Province of Québec. Can Med Assoc J 1982; 126:1404–8.
21. Thériault GP, Harvey R, Cordier S. Skin telangiectases in workers at an aluminum plant. N Engl J Med 1980; 303:1278–81.
22. Rosenberg L, Kaufman DW, Helmrich SP, Shapiro S. The risk of myocardial infarction after quitting smoking in men under 55 years of age. N Eng J Med 1985; 313:1511–14.
23. Hltaky MA. Exercise stress testing to screen for coronary artery disease in asymptomatic persons. J Occup Med 1986; 28:1020–5.
24. Barth PS, Hunt MA. Occupational disease in the law. In Workers' compensation and work-related illnesses and diseases. Cambridge, MA: MIT Press, 1980. Pp. 92–116.
25. Olsen O, Kristensen TS. Impact of work environment on cardiovascular diseases in Denmark. J Epidemiol Commun Health 1991; 45:4–10.

## Bibliography

Benowitz NL. Cardiovascular toxicology. In J Ladou. ed. Occupational medicine. San Mateo, CA: Appleton & Lange, 1990. Pp. 237–46.

*A review of the toxicity of cardiotoxic chemicals, their mode of action with a description of the clinical symptoms of poisoning, and their treatment and prevention. A good overview of cardiovascular environmental toxicology.*

Epstein FP. The epidemiology of coronary heart disease. J Chronic Dis 1965; 18:735–74.

*A thorough review of the epidemiology of CHD, including mortality, incidence and prevalence, and the importance and reduction of known risk factors. Old reference, but its findings are still applicable today.*

Kristensen TS. Cardiovascular diseases and the work environment. A critical review of the epidemiologic literature on (1) non-chemical and (2) chemical factors. Scand J Work Environ Health 1989; 15:165–79 and 245–64.

*A comprehensive review (over 2,000 references) of all identifiable epidemiologic literature on cardiovascular diseases and work. A remarkable achievement.*

Scott A. Employment of workers with cardiac disease. J Soc Occup Med 1985; 35:99–102.

*Despite all the advances in management of the cardiac victims, it is still a sad fact that many patients do not return to gainful employment. The author discusses this issue in the socioeconomic context of modern workplaces.*

Stamler J, Wentworth D, Neaton JD. Is relationship between serum cholesterol and risk of premature death from coronary heart disease continuous and graded? JAMA 1986; 256:2823–8.

*A very large study that illustrates remarkably well the risks associated with personal risk factors, age, serum cholesterol, high blood pressure, and smoking.*

Trends and determinants of coronary heart disease mortality: International comparison. Int J Epidemiol 1989; 18 (Suppl. 1).

*The papers in this supplement provide information presented at a workshop on "Trends and Determinants of Coronary Heart Disease Mortality. International Comparison." It is a broad, comprehensive look at CHD mortality from the view of international comparisons of mortality, morbidity, risk factors, and medical care.*

Turino GM. Effect of carbon monoxide toxicity: Physiology and biochemistry. Circulation 1981; 63:253A–9A.

*A critical review of the evidence of CO toxicity on the cardiorespiratory system.*

# 29
# Hematologic Disorders

Bernard D. Goldstein and Howard M. Kipen

The hematologic system is a primary endpoint of effect for a variety of occupational health problems. It is also a conduit of unwanted material to other organ systems and often an early indicator of important effects in other tissues. In addition, a number of the most important problems in the workplace are due to chemical agents that may produce more than one hematologic effect [1, 2].

## Agents That Interfere with Bone Marrow Function

### Benzene: Aplastic Anemia and Acute Myelogenous Leukemia

The potent hematotoxicity of benzene was first described in workers in the nineteenth century. Life-threatening aplastic anemia appears to be an inevitable consequence of exposure to high levels of benzene. Acute myelogenous leukemia in association with benzene exposure was originally reported in 1927, and the causal relationship has since been established through epidemiologic research [3].

The control of benzene exposure in the workplace (Fig. 29-1) and in the general environment has been a subject of much interest and controversy during the past decade. A major reason for the controversy surrounding the regulatory control of benzene is that, among the organic chemicals that are known to be human carcinogens, it is produced in the highest volume (9.7 million tons in the United States in 1985) and has the greatest potential of exposure for workers and the general public. The National Institute for Occupational Safety and Health (NIOSH) estimates that up to 2 million American workers may be exposed. Benzene is an integral component of petrochemical feed stocks and is present in gasoline in the United States in the range of 1.0 to 1.5 percent. It is a useful intermediate in organic synthesis and is frequently used in research and commercial laboratories. Benzene is also formed during coke oven operations. Although an excellent solvent, it can and should be largely replaced in this role by much less toxic solvents, such as toluene. Benzene, however, is likely to remain a ubiquitous component of our society for the near future.

In 1991 three doctors from Brazil described an occupational health disaster that had developed among workers in the steel industry outside of São Paulo. They reported in 1984 that 680 workers were removed from work because of hematologic abnormalities, and that this had progressed beyond 1,000 workers as of 1991. Data were presented on 95 workers with repeated neutrophil counts below 2,000/mm³ who also had bone marrow biopsies or aspirates.

The average white blood cell (WBC) count was 3,770 while the average hemoglobin was 14.5 gm/dL, hematocrit was 44.6 percent, and mean corpuscular volume (MCV) was 93 fl. Bone marrow examinations showed total hypocellularity in 78 percent, granulocytopenia in 83 percent, megakaryocytopenia in 65 percent, and erythropenia in 51 percent. Thus, the dominant effects in this group appeared to be on leukocytes, although the sample was selected based on WBC counts. The authors were aware of three acute leukemias, two aplastic anemias, and three cases of myelodysplastic syndrome.

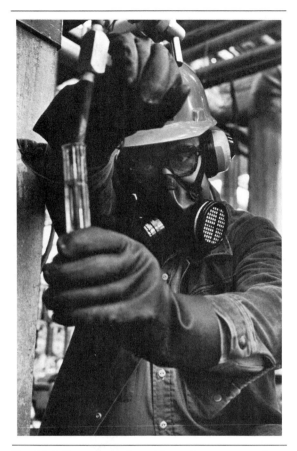

**Fig. 29-1.** Benzene worker with respiratory protection and impermeable gloves. (Photograph by Earl Dotter.)

Given that no formal cohort was constructed and followed, it is not clear whether this represented complete case ascertainment.

Benzene exposures in this working group occurred in a coke by-products production plant. Limited sampling information described the benzene exposures as being at least 10 ppm on a chronic basis. This may be an underestimate in light of the widespread bone marrow depression in those affected. Surveillance of populations in the U.S. since the 1950s has not yielded similar examples of such widespread hematologic effects of benzene [4].

The current U.S. occupational standard for benzene is 1 ppm TWA (time weighted average). In 1977, following discovery by NIOSH of a group

of rubber workers with a fivefold increased risk of acute myelogenous leukemia, the Occupational Safety and Health Administration (OSHA) attempted to lower the workplace standard for benzene to 1 ppm, first by an emergency temporary standard and then through a formal rule-making process. Both approaches were overturned by the courts, the latter in a 5-to-4 U.S. Supreme Court decision, which in part called on OSHA to calculate the benefits of its action. In 1987, using updated information on the rubber worker cohort, OSHA established the 1 ppm standard [5].

The mechanism by which benzene produces hematotoxicity has not been determined. Benzene does not produce bone marrow damage; one or more metabolites do. Approximately 50 percent of inhaled benzene is excreted by exhalation; the remainder is metabolized to a variety of products, particularly phenol. Measurement of urinary phenol has been used as a marker of benzene exposure. Although this is a useful technique to confirm relatively high-level exposure such as may occur in spills or accidents, the variation in background levels of urinary phenol, which are presumably from dietary sources, appears to preclude use of this assay as a technique to determine benzene exposure at levels present in a modern, well-regulated workplace. Benzene can also be measured in blood or in exhaled breath, both assays being in equilibrium with total body benzene. While useful for determining instantaneous benzene body burden, the relatively steep slope of the disappearance curve of benzene following exposure makes such assays inappropriate as indicators of quantitative exposure. Studies in humans have determined that the half-life of benzene is relatively short, benzene being no longer detectable in the body approximately 1 week following exposure. Other potentially useful urinary markers of benzene exposure, such as muconic acid, are currently undergoing evaluation.

In laboratory animals, the metabolism of benzene has been reported to be inhibited by simultaneous exposure to toluene, resulting in protection against benzene-induced hematotoxicity.

However, this protection does not occur at relatively low exposure levels in animals; in addition, toluene does not appear to inhibit benzene metabolism in humans exposed to usual workplace concentrations. In animal studies, benzene hematotoxicity has been shown to be potentiated by ethanol and by lead; however, the relevance of these findings to humans is yet to be determined. A potential interaction of note is the report that Japanese atom bomb survivors who developed leukemia were more likely to have also had an occupational exposure to benzene [6].

Studies of the toxicology of benzene in laboratory animals have clearly demonstrated benzene-induced aplastic anemia in a variety of species. However, only recently has it been possible to demonstrate tumorigenicity in laboratory animals, predominantly carcinomas and lymphatic tumors, in addition to a weak leukemic effect. While various lymphatic tumors have been associated with benzene exposure in humans, causality does not yet appear to be fully proven [7] (Table 29-1). At present, the evidence that benzene is causally related to human nonhematologic neoplasms is minimal.

Table 29-1. Relationship of benzene exposure to hematologic disorders

Causality proven
  Pancytopenia: aplastic anemia
  Acute myelogenous leukemia and variants (including acute myelomonocytic leukemia, acute promyelocytic leukemia, and erythroleukemia)
Causality reasonably likely
  Chronic lymphocytic leukemia
  Paroxysmal nocturnal hemoglobinuria (PNH)
  Acute lymphoblastic leukemia
  Multiple myeloma
  Lymphoma: lymphocytic and histiocytic
  Myelofibrosis and myeloid metaplasia
Causality suggested but unproven
  Hodgkin's disease
  Chronic myelogenous leukemia
  Thrombocythemia

Benzene not only destroys the pluripotential stem cell responsible for red blood cells, platelets, and granulocytic white blood cells, but it also causes a rapid loss in circulating lymphocytes in laboratory animals and humans. Based on studies in animals and the lymphocytopenic effects in humans, the potential for benzene effect on the immune system in workers has been suggested but not demonstrated. There is evidence that benzene results not only in a decrease in number but also in structural and functional abnormalities in circulating blood cells. An increase in red cell MCV and a decrease in lymphocyte count may be useful parameters for surveillance of potentially exposed workers. Cytogenetic abnormalities are common in significant benzene hematotoxicity and, with advances in techniques, may become useful in surveillance.

Aplastic anemia is frequently a fatal disorder, with death usually occurring due to infection related to leukopenia or hemorrhage due to thrombocytopenia. Studies of groups of workers with overt evidence of benzene hematotoxicity have often been initiated following the observation of a single individual with severe aplastic anemia. For the most part, those individuals who did not succumb relatively quickly to aplastic anemia demonstrated recovery following removal from benzene exposure. A follow-up study of a group of workers who previously had significant benzene-induced pancytopenia revealed minor residual hematologic abnormalities 10 years later [8]. An occasional individual in these groups with initially relatively severe pancytopenia was observed to proceed from aplastic anemia through a preleukemic phase to the eventual development of acute myelogenous leukemia. This development is not unexpected since individuals with aplastic anemia from any cause appear to have a higher-than-expected likelihood of developing acute myelogenous leukemia. Accordingly, it has been suggested that acute myelogenous leukemia is not a direct consequence of a benzene effect on the genome, but rather occurs indirectly through the production of aplastic anemia, or at least significant pancytopenia. If true, this would imply that workplace control of benzene that prevents pancytopenia would be sufficient to also preclude a risk of myelogenous leukemia. However, based on currently available evidence, there is no reason to alter the present prudent public health approach of assuming that there is no threshold for the carcinogenic effect of benzene. In other words, we assume that every molecule of benzene to which an individual is exposed has some finite risk, albeit small, of producing a somatic mutation that may result in acute myelogenous leukemia.

Review of leukemia cases that have been reported to be associated with exposure to benzene reveals not only acute myelogenous leukemia but also a number of variants of this disorder, including acute myelomonocytic leukemia, promyelocytic leukemia, and erythroleukemia, the last of which is a relatively rare variant that has been disproportionately reported. Even in cases not specifically designated as erythroleukemia, evidence of erythroid dysplasia is relatively commonly noted in the bone marrow. Perhaps related is the observation of an increased MCV of erythrocytes as a fairly common and early manifestation of benzene hematotoxicity.

A typical case report of acute myelogenous leukemia in an individual heavily exposed to benzene is described below:

A 29-year-old white man went to his physician with complaints of nonspecific malaise and bleeding gums. On physical examination, he was noted to be febrile and to have exquisite sternal tenderness. Laboratory findings included hematocrit, 32 percent; white blood count, 28,000/mm³; undifferentiated blast forms, 40 percent; and platelet count, 28,000/mm³. The bone marrow findings were diagnostic of acute myelogenous leukemia. Cytogenetic studies were not performed until after the patient had undergone chemotherapy. Although abnormalities were observed, the findings could not clearly be related to the etiology of the acute leukemia.

The patient had been working in the chemical industry since age 20, when he received an associate degree in laboratory technology. Since that time, he had taken

courses at two universities to earn a bachelor's degree in chemistry. Control of chemical exposure in the student laboratories of all three academic institutions was negligible to modest. Benzene was present in each. In only one laboratory course was there any specific instruction concerning the control of chemical hazards in the laboratory. His initial job was in the control room of a petrochemical plant, where he primarily checked dials. He rarely was outdoors or in the chemical area but did participate in the clean-up of occasional spills.

From 23 to 27 years of age, he worked as a technician in the quality control laboratory of a chemical company that produced chlorinated hydrocarbon pesticides. On about two-thirds of workdays, his job was to test the extent of chlorination of the product. The procedure included a solvent extraction in which 50 ml of benzene was added to each of 30 samples on a laboratory bench, and the samples were then placed into a hood containing a heating device. After a specified time, the 30 beakers were removed from the hood and, while still hot and bubbling, were placed on a laboratory bench. After titration and analysis, the residual material was dumped into a sink and the viscous residue was washed vigorously with hot water. He reported that the smell of benzene was particularly notable during the washing procedure, and on occasion he would become lightheaded. This feeling would clear in a few minutes if he left the room or stood by an open window.

During this period, his supervisor, who did most of the same procedures and had also been exposed to lindane (gamma benzene hexachloride), developed fatal aplastic anemia. Benzene was used in the laboratory as a general solvent and kept in bottles out of the hood.

Two years before the development of acute myelogenous leukemia, he began work in another chemical plant as a laboratory technician. In this laboratory he also performed chloride analysis, but acetone was used as the extractant and benzene was kept in the hood. In addition, the latter laboratory regularly received visits from industrial hygienists with monitoring equipment, and they presented lectures about laboratory safety.

### Other Hematologic Disorders
### Due to Benzene
Benzene has also been associated with other myeloproliferative disorders, including chronic myelogenous leukemia and myelofibrosis and myeloid

metaplasia; however, evidence is less convincing for a causal relationship with benzene exposure than it is for acute myelogenous leukemia. It is not surprising that cases of the relatively rare disorder paroxysmal nocturnal hemoglobinuria (PNH)have been reported in benzene-exposed workers. This paraneoplastic disorder is related both to aplastic anemia and to acute myelogenous leukemia. Lymphoproliferative disorders, including Hodgkin's and non-Hodgkin's lymphoma, acute and chronic lymphatic leukemia, and multiple myeloma, have also been reported in association with benzene exposure [9]. Again the evidence of a causal relationship to benzene is suggestive but not conclusive.

### Other Causes of Aplastic Anemia and Hematologic Neoplasia

Other agents in the workplace have been associated with aplastic anemia, the most notable being radiation. The effects of radiation on bone marrow stem cells have been employed in the therapy of leukemia. Similarly, a variety of chemotherapeutic alkylating agents produce aplasia and pose a risk to workers responsible for producing or administering these compounds. Radiation, benzene, and alkylating agents all appear to have a threshold concentration below which aplastic anemia will not occur. Protection of the production worker becomes more problematic when the agent has an idiosyncratic mode of action in which minuscule amounts may produce aplasia; chloramphenicol is an example of such an agent. A variety of other chemicals have been reported to be associated with aplastic anemia, but it is often difficult to determine causality. An example is the pesticide lindane. Case reports have appeared, generally following relatively high levels of exposure, in which lindane is associated with aplasia. This finding is far from being universal in humans, and there are no reports of lindane-induced bone marrow toxicity in laboratory animals treated with large doses of this agent. Bone marrow hypoplasia has also been associated with exposure to ethylene glycol

ethers, trinitrotoluene (TNT), pentachlorophene, and arsenic.

Hematologic neoplasms have been reported to occur in other occupational situations. There is some evidence that (1) farmers have a higher risk of lymphoma; (2) production workers exposed to ethylene oxide, used primarily as a sterilant, have an increased incidence of acute myelogenous leukemia (although this increase was not found in one large cohort of sterilization workers); and (3) much more controversially, workers exposed to electromagnetic fields may possibly be at greater risk of leukemia [10–12]. Multiple myeloma has been associated with radiation and with solvent exposure. The reported association of toluene with aplastic anemia and leukemia almost certainly is incorrect, because this represents contamination of toluene with benzene.

## Agents That Affect Red Blood Cells

### Agents That Interfere with Hemoglobin Oxygen Delivery

Certain toxins produce adverse effects by interfering with the orderly delivery of oxygen from red cell hemoglobin to tissues (see Chaps. 13 and 28).

*Carbon Monoxide.* Carbon monoxide (CO) binds relatively firmly with the oxygen-combining site of hemoglobin, thereby preventing the uptake of oxygen from the lungs. This effect is magnified because once one or more of the four oxygen-combining sites on a hemoglobin molecule is occupied by CO, it becomes more difficult for the oxygen on the molecule to be released at the tissue level. This "shift to the left" of the oxygen dissociation curve accounts for the potential lethality of carboxyhemoglobin (COHb) concentrations as low as 25 to 35 percent of total hemoglobin. The affinity of hemoglobin for CO is more than 200 times greater than it is for oxygen; that is, a gas mixture of 1,000 ppm CO and 20 percent oxygen (200,000 ppm) would result in about one-half oxyhemoglobin and one-half COHb at equilibrium. At the normal rate of respiration, equilibration occurs slowly, requiring approximately 8 to 12 hours. The rate of COHb level change depends on the rate of respiration, thereby putting active workers at greater risk.

There is a natural background level of approximately 0.5 percent COHb because of the formation of CO during metabolism. A pack-a-day cigarette smoker will achieve COHb levels of about 5 percent. The U.S. workplace standard for carbon monoxide is 50 ppm TWA, which will result in approximately 8 to 9 percent COHb at the end of an 8-hour workday. There is also a 400-ppm short-term exposure limit (STEL)—a 15-minute time-weighted average not to be exceeded at any time during a workday. There is roughly an additive effect of COHb levels from cigarette smoke and from ambient exposures.

In a workplace, CO poisoning is usually caused by incomplete combustion coupled with improper ventilation. Carbon monoxide is also formed through the metabolism of certain exogenous agents, most notably methylene chloride.

There is some evidence that COHb levels in the range of 5 percent are associated with a minimal decrement in psychomotor function, suggesting that at these or higher levels there may be an increased risk of performing tasks wrong, leading to industrial accidents [13]. Individuals with preexisting cardiovascular disease have been reported to have a decrease in exercise tolerance and earlier development of acute angina or intermittent claudication, with effects occurring at levels ranging down to perhaps 2.5 percent COHb.

Detection of CO poisoning depends primarily on clinical suspicion. Complaints include headache, weakness, lassitude, and mental obtundation. In severe cases, the blood has a characteristic cherry red color. Treatment includes removal from the contaminated air and ventilation with oxygen.

*Methemoglobin-Producing Compounds.* Methemoglobin is another form of hemoglobin that is incapable of delivering oxygen to the tissues.

Hemoglobin iron must be in the reduced ferrous state in order to participate in the transport of oxygen. Under normal conditions, oxidation to methemoglobin, with iron in the ferric state, goes on continuously, resulting in approximately 0.5 percent of total hemoglobin in the form of methemoglobin in the steady state. Reduction to ferrous hemoglobin occurs through the activity of an NADH-dependent methemoglobin reductase.

Clinically significant methemoglobinemia has been a not uncommon event in industries using aniline dyes. Other chemicals that frequently cause methemoglobinemia in the workplace have been nitrobenzenes, other organic and inorganic nitrites and nitrates, hydrazines, and a variety of quinones [14] (Table 29-2).

Cyanosis, confusion, and other signs of hypoxia are the usual symptoms. In chronically exposed individuals, blueness of the lips may be observed at levels of methemoglobinemia (approximately 10 percent or greater) that are without other overt consequences. The blood has a characteristic chocolate brown color. Treatment consists of avoiding further exposure. With significant symptoms, usually at methemoglobin levels greater than 40 percent, therapy with methylene blue or ascorbic acid can accelerate reduction of the methemoglobin level.

There are inherited disorders that lead to persistent methemoglobinemia, either due to heterozygosity for an abnormal hemoglobin or homozy-

Table 29-2. Selected agents implicated in environmentally and occupationally acquired methemoglobinemia

Nitrate-contaminated well water
Nitrous gases (in welding and silos)
Aniline dyes
Food high in nitrates or nitrites
Moth balls (containing naphthalene)
Potassium chlorate
Nitrobenzenes
Phenylenediamine
Toluenediamine

gosity for deficiency of red cell NADH-dependent methemoglobin reductase. Individuals who are heterozygous for this enzyme deficiency will not be able to decrease elevated methemoglobin levels caused by chemical exposures as rapidly as will individuals with normal enzyme levels.

In addition to oxidizing the iron component of hemoglobin, many of the chemicals that cause methemoglobinemia, or their metabolites, are also relatively nonspecific oxidizing agents, which at high levels can cause a Heinz body hemolytic anemia. This process is characterized by oxidative denaturation of hemoglobin, leading to the formation of punctate membrane-bound red cell inclusions known as Heinz bodies, which can be identified with special stains. Oxidative damage to the red cell membrane also occurs. While this may lead to significant hemolysis, the compounds listed in Table 28-2 primarily produce their adverse effects through the formation of methemoglobin, which may be life threatening, rather than through hemolysis, which is usually a limited process. In essence, two different red cell defense pathways are involved: (1) the NADH-dependent methemoglobin reductase required to reduce methemoglobin to normal hemoglobin and (2) the NADPH-dependent process through the hexose monophosphate (HMP) shunt, leading to the

maintenance of reduced glutathione as a means to defend against oxidizing species capable of producing Heinz body hemolytic anemia (Fig. 29-2). Heinz body hemolysis can be exacerbated by the treatment of methemoglobinemia patients with methylene blue because it requires NADPH for its methemoglobin-reducing effects. Hemolysis will also be a more prominent part of the clinical picture in individuals with deficiencies in one of the enzymes of the NADPH oxidant defense pathway or an inherited unstable hemoglobin. Except for glucose 6-phosphate dehydrogenase (G6PD) deficiency, described later in this chapter, these are relatively rare disorders.

Another form of hemoglobin alteration produced by oxidizing agents is a denatured species known as sulfhemoglobin. This irreversible product often can be detected in the blood of individuals with significant methemoglobinemia produced by oxidant chemicals. Sulfhemoglobin is the name also given, and more appropriately, to a specific product formed during hydrogen sulfide poisoning (see Chap. 13).

### Hemolytic Agents: Arsine

The normal red blood cell survives in the circulation for 120 days. Shortening of this survival can lead to anemia if not compensated by an increase

Fig. 29-2. Red blood cell enzymes of oxidant defense and related reactions.

$$GSH + GSH + (0) \xrightarrow{\text{Glutathione Peroxidase}} GSSG + H_2O$$

$$GSSG + 2NADPH \xrightarrow{\text{Glutathione Reductase}} 2GSH + 2NADP$$

$$\text{Glucose-6-Phosphate} + NADP \xrightarrow{\text{G6PD}} \text{6-Phosphogluconate} + NADPH$$

$$Fe^{+++} \text{ Hemoglobin (Methemoglobin)} + NADH \xrightarrow{\text{Methemoglobin Reductase}} Fe^{++} \text{ Hemoglobin}$$

in red cell production within the bone marrow. There are essentially two types of hemolysis: (1) intravascular hemolysis, in which there is an immediate release of hemoglobin within the circulation, and (2) extravascular hemolysis, in which red cells are destroyed within the spleen or the liver.

One of the most potent intravascular hemolysins is arsine gas ($AsH_3$). Inhalation of a relatively small amount of this agent leads to swelling and eventual bursting of red blood cells within the circulation. It may be difficult to detect the causal relation of workplace arsine exposure to an acute hemolytic episode. This is partly because the delay between exposure and onset of symptoms but primarily because the source of exposure is often not evident. Arsine gas is made and used commercially, often now in the electronics industry. However, most of the published reports of acute hemolytic episodes have been through the unexpected liberation of arsine gas as an unwanted by-product of an industrial process, for example, if acid is added to a container made of arsenic-contaminated metal. (A characteristic untoward exposure is described below.) Any process that reduces arsenic, such as acidification, can lead to the liberation of arsine gas. As arsenic can be a contaminant of many metals and organic materials, such as coal, arsine exposure can often be unexpected. Stilbene, the hydride of antimony, appears to produce a hemolytic effect similar to that of arsine.

NIOSH has recommended an immediate danger to life and health (IDLH) level of 6 to 30 ppm for 30 minutes, and the National Academy of Sciences Committee on Toxicology has recommended an emergency exposure limit of 1 ppm for 1 hour. Death can occur directly due to complete loss of red blood cells. (A hematocrit of zero has been reported.) However, a major concern at arsine levels less than those that produce complete hemolysis is acute renal failure due to the massive release of hemoglobin within the circulation (see Chap. 31). At much higher levels, arsine may produce acute pulmonary edema and possibly direct renal effects. Hypotension may accompany the acute episode. There is usually a delay of at least a few hours be-

tween inhalation of arsine and the onset of symptoms. In addition to red urine due to hemoglobinuria, the patient will frequently complain of abdominal pain and nausea, symptoms that occur concomitantly with acute intravascular hemolysis from a number of causes [15].

Treatment is aimed at maintenance of renal perfusion and transfusion of normal blood. As the circulating red cells affected by arsine apear to some extent to be doomed to intravascular hemolysis, an exchange transfusion in which arsine-exposed red cells are replaced by unexposed cells would appear to be optimal therapy. As in severe life-threatening hemorrhage, it is important that replacement red cells have adequate 2,3-diphosphoglyceric acid (DPG) levels so as to be able to deliver oxygen to the tissue.

Two maintenance workers were assigned to clean up a clogged drain with a mixture of sodium hydroxide, sodium nitrate, and aluminum chips, which together act to form hydrogen gas. Arsine was formed from the combination of hydrogen with arsenic, which was residual in the drain from a use 5 years before. Both men noted the development of a sewer-like odor during the 2 to 3 hours during which they worked on the drain. One man noted a headache, followed by numbness of tongue and cheeks, weakness, and nausea while at work. After being home for a few hours, he sought medical attention. The second patient first noted abdominal discomfort at the end of the workday and while at home experienced nausea, vomiting, and hematuria. He was treated at an emergency department that evening with "stomach medicine" and after being anuric all night was admitted the next morning to a local hospital. Both patients were treated for acute renal failure with partial recovery in one and a need for maintenance dialysis in the other patient [16].

A variety of other hemolytic agents are found in the workplace. As discussed before, for many the toxicity of concern is methemoglobinemia. Other hemolytic agents include naphthalene and its derivatives. In addition, certain metals, such as copper, and organometals, such as tributyl tin, will shorten red cell survival, at least in animal models.

Mild hemolysis can also occur during traumatic physical exertion (march hemoglobinuria); a more modern observation is elevated white blood counts with prolonged exertion (jogger's leukocytosis). The most important metal that affects red cell formation and survival in workers is lead.

### Hematologic Aspects of Lead Poisoning

Occupational exposure to dusts and fumes that contain lead compounds is a frequent concern of medical personnel who evaluate workers in a variety of occupational and environmental settings. In addition to occupations with well-recognized risks, such as battery makers, secondary lead smelter workers, and foundry workers, the list of potentially lead-exposed occupations includes more commonly encountered groups, such as firing range personnel, jewelry and pottery workers, bridge workers and other iron workers (Fig. 29-3), welders, and painters. The last three groups are at risk when sanding or burning through lead pigment containing paints, particularly in a marine

setting. Exposure usually is from inhalation of dust or lead oxide fumes. Skin absorption occurs readily only with organic lead compounds, such as tetraethyl lead (a gasoline antiknock additive no longer used in the United States); poor work habits and hygiene can predispose to ingestion and inhalation of lead on cigarettes. The finer the lead particle generated at work (as in lead fume from burning), the greater proportion of lead absorbed from the respiratory tract. An understanding of hematologic aspects of lead poisoning is important, in part, because the erythrocytic cells of the bone marrow and peripheral blood represent a major target for lead toxicity as well as an easily sampled window into its systemic effects (see also Chaps. 13, 26, 27, and 31).

### Pathophysiology of Lead Hematotoxicity

Although lead is known to inhibit most of the enzymes in the heme biosynthetic pathway, its most pronounced effect is inhibition of the final enzy-

Fig. 29-3. Overexposures to lead occur in iron workers. Man at left is exposed to lead as he cuts apart a ship. Man at right is obtaining air sample for lead level determination. Protection against lead exposures is essential for all its uses. (Photograph courtesy of NIOSH.)

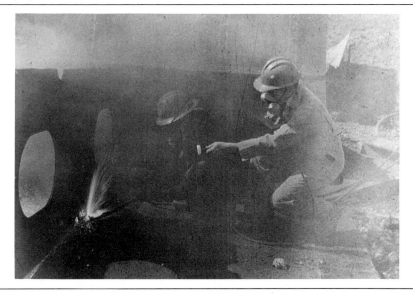

matic reaction in heme formation, in which heme synthetase (ferrochelatase) catalyzes incorporation of ferrous iron into the heme ring (Fig. 29-4). The resultant decrease in intra-erythroid levels of iron-containing heme releases earlier reactions in the biosynthetic pathway from feedback inhibition by the end product, particularly for the irreversible first reaction, the synthesis of Δ-amino-levulinic acid from succinyl-CoA and glycine, catalyzed by Δ-ALA synthetase. Increased production of Δ-ALA, and decreased incorporation of iron into protoporphyrin IX causes accumulation of abnormally high levels of all constituents of the pathway, particularly of the penultimate protoporphyrin IX. These high intracellular levels of erythrocyte protoporphyrin provide the biochemical basis for one group of valuable diagnostic tests in the evaluation of lead toxicity.

Interference with heme formation leads to a series of predictable abnormalities in red cell maturation. Bone marrow examination of the lead-intoxicated patient, while rarely clinically indicated, will reveal erythroid hyperplasia and sideroblastic changes in which the more mature cells display iron-staining granules in a perinuclear arc. Of greater clinical relevance are the peripheral red cell abnormalities. Due to a combination of decreased red blood cell production and reduced survival time (from membrane abnormalities), normochromic microcytic or normochromic normocytic anemia is the classic finding, although anemia is only expected with the combination of high blood levels and chronic exposures. Examination of the peripheral smear may demonstrate increased punctate basophilic stippling of red blood cells (stippled cells) and reticulocytosis. Decreased osmotic fragility may also be demonstrated in the laboratory.

It is of utmost importance that neither absence of the above hematologic changes nor absence of other signs and symptoms of clinical lead poisoning (such as neurologic dysfunction) be used to rule out the presence of significantly high lead burdens in either individuals or populations. Development of overt hematologic disease from lead

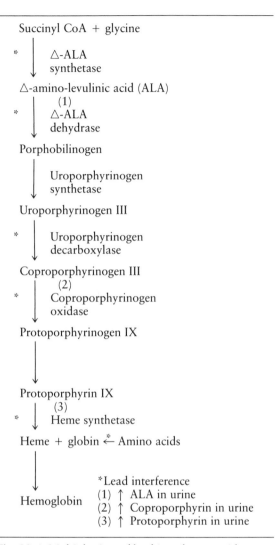

Fig. 29-4. Multiple sites of lead interference with hemoglobin synthesis. (From WN Rom. Environmental and occupational medicine. Boston: Little, Brown, 1982.)

may be expected to result only after serious breaches of safety procedures and of recommended exposure limits, such as those of the 1978 OSHA lead standard. Air concentrations are limited to a TWA of 50 $\mu g/m^3$, personal hygiene standards are set, and mandatory biologic monitoring of blood-lead levels is now the law for those with significant exposures to lead [17]. In the United States, OSHA has now issued an interim rule revising its regulations to include the previously exempted construction workers. Ideally, elevation of biologic indices, such as blood lead and zinc protoporphyrin (ZPP), the latter of which is not specified in the 1978 OSHA standard, will be recognized before overt hematologic disease supervenes.

In chronic lead intoxication, the marrow produces erythrocytes with a modestly decreased survival due to membrane abnormalities, and thus there is some hemolytic component to a resulting anemia. The unusual occurrence of acute lead intoxication due to massive inhalation of dust, as has occurred in some painters when sanding leaded paint from older homes, may result in acute hemolysis similar to that encountered following arsine exposure. The diagnosis is usually evident from the occupational history.

### Hematologic Tests for Diagnosis of Lead Poisoning

The most commonly used test is direct measurement of the blood-lead (PbB) concentration, routinely performed in clinical laboratories by atomic absorption. Only a few milliliters of whole venous blood are required; however, significant unreliability of laboratory values has been demonstrated. Since lead is a ubiquitous contaminant of industrialized societies, background levels in adults approximate 5 to 15 μg/dL, although neurologic dysfunction has been suggested, especially in children, at the upper end of this "normal" range. Values greater than 35 μg/dL commonly indicate significant exposures. The OSHA lead standard is designed to control airborne exposures so that most workers' PbB will be less than 40 μg/dL, although it does not specify worker removal from exposure until blood lead reaches 50 μg/dL.

Blood-lead levels best reflect recent exposure, that is, exposure within 2 to 3 weeks. Large amounts of lead are readily incorporated into bone and maintained in equilibrium with blood and soft tissue levels. Thus chronic or intermittent expo-

sure may lead to relatively moderate elevations of PbB (30–60 μg/dL) in the face of a substantial total body burden. In situations in which individuals have the opportunity for chronic or intermittent exposures, PbB may be an incomplete index of both body burden and toxicity, and the following two alternatives are indicated to supplement this evaluation.

As implied above, lead inhibition of heme synthetase results in large accumulations of various heme precursors within developing erythrocytes, the most prevalent of which is protoporphyrin IX. Increases in erythrocyte protoporphyrins (EPs) can be measured by extraction of the porphyrins from whole blood, followed by spectrophotometry or fluorometry. Additionally, they can be measured in urine, a common approach in the work-up of other abnormalities of porphyrin metabolism. A more recent and highly useful test is the fluorometric assay for intraerythrocytic ZPP, which has been shown to correlate almost perfectly with free erythrocyte protoporphyrin (FEP) determinations [18]. Zinc is the most abundant intracellular heavy metal, apart from iron, and readily complexes with excess EP, forming a specific fluorescent product. During extraction, zinc is usually removed—hence the term *free erythrocyte protoporphyrin*. The direct assay of ZPP with a hematofluorometer can be performed in the field using only microcapillary amounts of whole blood. Rather than assaying a level of lead, it represents a sensitive indicator of biochemical dysfunction. Elevated protoporphyrin measurements are not specific for lead inhibition of heme synthesis; this parameter is commonly elevated in iron deficiency anemia. Thus, all abnormal values must be interpreted in the context of PbB and serum iron determinations.

It is important to recognize differences in the interpretation of PbB results, compared with those of ZPP [19]. Zinc protoporphyrin measures intraerythrocytic abnormalities developed during bone marrow maturation; since the red cells of even a lead-intoxicated individual circulate for over 100 days, ZPP reflects the cumulative average inhibition of heme synthesis over the preceding 3 to 4 months. It remains elevated for the life of an individual cell. However, PbB reflects more recent lead exposure. Thus, in an intermittently exposed worker, ZPP may be elevated from exposures of 1 to 2 months previously, whereas the blood lead could be normal after initially rising and subsequently falling as lead is redistributed to bone and excreted slowly by the kidney. Although no clear guideline has been established, in many laboratories a ZPP greater than 100 µg/dL is said to be beyond the usual range. Even lower levels may be of concern in protecting against lead-induced neurologic dysfunction, especially in children.

Finally, occult lead intoxication, especially if exposures have taken place more than 3 months before, may be demonstrated by a diagnostic challenge with calcium ethylenediaminetetraacetic acid (EDTA). This metal chelator will bind lead cations in bone and soft tissue. Excretion of greater than 600 µg of lead in a 24-hour urine specimen suggests previous significant exposure. In the presence of renal insufficiency, 72-hour urine collections may be required [20].

## Other Hematologic Disorders

### White Blood Cells

There are a variety of drugs, such as propylthiourea (PTU), that are known to affect the production or survival of circulating polymorphonuclear leukocytes relatively selectively. In contrast, nonspecific bone marrow toxins affect the precursors of red cells and platelets as well. Workers engaged in the preparation or administration of such drugs should be considered at risk. There is one report of complete granulocytopenia in a worker poisoned with dinitrophenol. Alteration in lymphocyte number and function, and particularly of subtype distribution, is receiving more attention as a possible subtle mechanism of effects due to a variety of chemicals in the workplace or general environment, particularly chlorinated hydrocarbons, dioxins, and related compounds. Validation of the health implications of such changes is not complete.

### Coagulation

Similar to leukopenia, there are many drugs that selectively decrease the production or survival of circulating platelets, which could be a problem in workers involved in the preparation or administration of such agents. Otherwise, there are only scattered reports of thrombocytopenia in workers. One study implicates toluene diisocyanate (TDI) as a cause of thrombocytopenia purpura. Abnormalities in the various blood factors involved in coagulation are not generally noted as a consequence of work. Individuals with preexising coagulation abnormalities, such as hemophilia, often have difficulty entering the workforce. However, although a carefully considered exclusion from a few selected jobs is reasonable, such individuals are usually capable of normal functioning at work.

## Hematologic Screening and Surveillance in the Workplace

### Markers of Susceptibility

Due in part to the ease in obtaining samples, more is known about inherited variations in human blood components than about those of any other organ. Extensive studies sparked by recognition of familial anemias have led to fundamental knowledge concerning the structural and functional implications of genetic alterations. Of pertinence to occupational health are those inherited variations that might lead to an increased susceptibility to workplace hazards. A number of such testable variations have been considered or actually used for the screening of workers. The rapid increase in knowledge concerning human genetics makes it a certainty that in the future we will have a better understanding of the inherited basis of variation in human response, and we will be more capable of predicting the extent of individual susceptibility through laboratory tests (see Chaps. 3 and 33).

Before discussing the potential value of currently available susceptibility markers, the major ethical considerations in the use of such tests in workers should be emphasized. It has been questioned whether such tests favor exclusion of workers from a site rather than maintain a focus on improving the worksite for the benefit of the workers. Some distinction has been made between the use of susceptibility markers as a screening device at a preplacement examination and such use as part of an ongoing evaluation of employed workers. At the very least, before embarking on the use of a susceptibility marker at a workplace, the goals of the testing and consequences of the findings must be clear to all parties.

The two markers of hematologic susceptibility for which screening has taken place most frequently are sickle cell trait and G6PD deficiency. The former is at most of marginal value in rare situations, and the latter is of no value whatsoever in most of the situations for which it has been advocated.

Sickle cell disease is a fairly common disorder in which the individual is homozygous for hemoglobin S (HbS). It is a relatively severe disease that often, but not always, precludes entering the workforce. The HbS gene may be inherited with other genes, such as HbC, which may reduce the severity of its effects. The basic defect in individuals with sickle cell disease is the polymerization of HbS, leading to microinfarction. Microinfarction can occur in episodes, known as sickle cell crises, and can be precipitated by external factors, particularly those leading to hypoxia and, to a lesser extent, dehydration. With a reasonably wide variation in the clinical course and well-being of those with sickle cell disease, employment evaluation should focus on the individual case history. Jobs that have the possibility of hypoxic exposures, such as those requiring frequent air travel, or those with a likelihood of significant dehydration, are not appropriate.

Much more common than sickle cell disease is sickle cell trait, the heterozygous condition in which there is inheritance of a gene for HbS and one gene for HbA. Individuals with this genetic pattern have been reported to undergo sickle cell crises under extreme conditions of hypoxia. Some consideration has been given to excluding individuals with sickle cell trait from jobs where hypoxia is a common risk, probably limited to the jobs on military aircraft or submarines, and perhaps on commercial aircraft. However, it must be emphasized that individuals with sickle cell trait do very well in almost every other situation. For example, athletes with sickle cell trait had no adverse effects from competing at the altitude of Mexico City (2,200 m, or 7,200 ft) during the 1968 Summer Olympics. Accordingly, with the possible few exceptions described above, there is no reason to consider exclusion or modification of work schedules for those with sickle cell trait.

Another common genetic variant of a red blood cell component is the A form of G6PD deficiency. It is inherited on the X chromosome as a sex-linked recessive gene and is present in approximately one in seven black males and one in 50 black females in the United States. As with sickle cell trait, G6PD deficiency provides a protective advantage against malaria. Under usual circumstances, individuals with this form of G6PD deficiency have red blood counts and indices within the normal range. However, due to the inability to regenerate reduced glutathione, their red blood cells are susceptible to hemolysis following ingestion of oxidant drugs and in certain disease states. This susceptibility to oxidizing agents has led to workplace screening on the erroneous assumption that individuals with the common A variant of G6PD deficiency will be at risk from the inhalation of oxidant gases. In fact, it would require exposure to many times higher than the levels at which such gases would cause fatal pulmonary edema before the red cells of G6PD-deficient individuals would receive oxidant stress sufficient to be of concern [21]. G6PD deficiency will increase the likelihood of overt Heinz body hemolysis in individuals exposed to aniline dyes and other methemoglobin-provoking agents (Table 29-2), but in these cases, the primary clinical problem remains the life-threatening methemoglobinemia. While knowledge of G6PD status might be useful in such cases primarily to guide therapy, this knowledge should not be used to exclude workers from the workplace.

There are many other forms of familial G6PD deficiency, all far less common than the A variant. Certain of these variants, particularly in individuals from the Mediterranean basin and Central Asia, have much lower levels of G6PD activity in their red blood cells. Consequently the affected individual can be severely compromised by ongoing hemolytic anemia. Deficiencies in other enzymes active in defense against oxidants have also been reported, as have unstable hemoglobins that render the red cell more susceptible to oxidant stress in the same manner as in G6PD deficiency.

### Surveillance

One of the most difficult tasks in occupational medicine is to distinguish between statistical abnormality and clinical abnormality in the interpretation of laboratory tests obtained as part of surveillance. Surveillance differs substantially from clinical testing in both the evaluation of ill patients and the regular screening of presumably healthy individuals. In ill patients, a laboratory value just beyond normal limits is unlikely to explain the cause of the illness. Similarly, physicians evaluating apparently healthy individuals will tend to discount an unsupported finding of one laboratory test just beyond normal limits. In contrast the laboratory tests chosen for a surveillance program are in general those for which any abnormality is a matter of concern due to the nature of the job. These tests are not intended for diagnostic purposes, although they may be useful to supplement normal diagnostic testing. In an appropriately designed surveillance program, the aim is to prevent overt disease by picking up subtle early changes through the use of laboratory testing. Therefore, a highly abnormal finding should automatically trigger a response—or at least a thorough review—by physicians.

To respond appropriately, the statistical basis of the "normal" laboratory value must be understood. For blood counts, it has been traditional to describe the "normal" range as including 95 percent of the distribution of blood counts in healthy people. This range implies that 1 of 20 clinically normal individuals will be statistically abnormal in any one blood count, 1 in 40 being higher than normal and 1 in 40 being lower than normal. This situation presents a problem when reviewing blood counts in that clinical information can be obtained by findings beyond either end of the normal range. For most hematotoxins, such as benzene, one is primarily concerned with the lower end of the range. The problem of making a distinction between statistical abnormality and clinical abnormality is further compounded by the number of tests in use and the relatively large number of workers who may be under surveillance. Consider that in a normal individual, blood counts for platelets, white cells, and red cells might each have a 1 in 40 chance of a count below the normal range. In a study of 100 healthy individuals with no known exposure to hematotoxins, it would not be surprising if perhaps 6 were found to have a statistically abnormal low count for one of these parameters. This finding would be the baseline of false-positives if a physician were evaluating 100 workers potentially exposed to benzene.

In the initial review of hematologic surveillance data in a workforce potentially exposed to a hematotoxin such as benzene, there are two major approaches that are particularly helpful in distinguishing false-positives. The first is the degree of the difference from normal. As the count gets further removed from the normal range, there is a rapid drop-off in the likelihood that it represents just a statistical anomaly. Second, one should take advantage of the totality of data for that individual, including normal values, keeping in mind the wide range of effects produced by benzene. For example, there is a much greater probability of a benzene effect if a slightly low platelet count is accompanied by a low-normal white blood cell count, a low-normal red cell count, and a high-normal MCV. Conversely, the relevance of this same platelet count to benzene hematotoxicity can be relatively discounted if the other blood counts are at the opposite end of the normal spectrum. These same two considerations can be used in judging whether the individual should be removed from the workforce while awaiting further testing and whether the additional testing should consist only of a repeat complete blood count (CBC).

If there is any doubt as to the cause of the low count, the entire CBC should be repeated. If the low count is due to laboratory variability or some short-term biologic variability within the individual, it is less likely that the blood count will again be low. Comparison with preplacement or other available blood counts should help distinguish those individuals who have an inherent tendency to be on the lower end of the distribution. Detection of an individual worker with an effect due to a hematologic toxin should be considered a sentinel health event, prompting careful investigation of working conditions and of coworkers (see "Surveillance" in Chap. 3).

The wide range in normal laboratory values for blood counts can present an even greater challenge since there can be a substantial effect while counts are still within the normal range. For example, it is possible that a worker exposed to benzene or ionizing radiation may have a fall in hematocrit from 50 to 40 percent, a fall in the white blood cell count from 10,000 to 5,000/mm$^3$, and a fall in the platelet count from 350,000 to 150,000/mm$^3$—that is, more than a 50 percent decrease in platelets; yet all these values are within the "normal" range of blood counts. Accordingly, a surveillance program that looks solely at "abnormal" blood counts may miss significant effects. Therefore, blood counts that decrease over time while staying in the normal range need particular attention.

Another challenging problem in workplace surveillance is the detection of a slight decrease in the mean blood count of an entire exposed population—for example, a decrease in mean white blood cell count from 7,500 to 7,000/mm$^3$ because of a widespread exposure to benzene or ionizing radiation. Detection and appropriate evaluation of any such observation require meticulous attention to standardization of laboratory test procedures, the availability of an appropriate control group, and careful statistical analysis. For instance, cigarette smoking increases WBC counts by about 25 percent and thus smoking habits should be accounted for in making intergroup comparisons.

## References

1. Wintrobe MM, et al. Clinic hematology. Philadelphia: Lea & Febiger, 1993.
2. Williams WJ, et al. Hematology. New York: McGraw-Hill, 1990.
3. Laskin S, Goldstein BD. eds. Benzene toxicity, a clinical evaluation. J Toxicol Environ Health Suppl. 2, 1977.
4. Ruiz MA, Vassallo J, De Souza C. A morphological study of the bone marrow of neutropenic patients exposed to benzene of the metallurgical industry of Cubatao, São Paolo, Brazil (letter). J Occup Med 1991; 33:83.
5. Rinsky RA, et al. Benzene and leukemia. An epidemiologic risk assessment. N Engl J Med 1987; 316:1044–50.
6. Ishimaru T, et al. Occupational factors in the epidemiology of leukemia in Hiroshima and Nagasaki. Am J Epidemiol 1971; 93:157–65.
7. Goldstein BD. Clinical hematotoxicity of benzene. In Carcinogenicity and toxicity of benzene. Princeton, NJ: Princeton Scientific, 1983, pp. 51–61. Vol. 4.
8. Hernberg S, et al. Prognostic aspects of benzene poisoning. Br J Ind Med 1966; 23:204.
9. Goldstein BD. Is exposure to benzene a cause of human multiple myeloma? Trends in cancer mortality in industrial countries. Ann NY Acad Sci 1990; 609:225–34.
10. Steenland K, et al. Mortality among workers exposed to ethylene oxide. N Engl J Med, 1991; 324:1402–7.
11. Hogstedt C, Aringer L, Gustavsson A. Epidemiologic support for ethylene oxide as a cancer-causing agent. JAMA 1986; 255:1575–8.

12. Savitz DA, Pearce NE. Occupational leukemias and lymphomas. Semin Occup Med 1987; 2:283–9.

13. National Academy of Sciences, Committee on Medical and Biologic Effects of Environmental Pollutants. Carbon monoxide effects on man and animals. Washington, D.C.: NAS, 1977, pp. 68–167 Chap. 5.

14. Smith RP. Toxic responses of the blood. In Casarett and Doull's toxicology: The basic science of poisons. 3rd ed. New York: MacMillan, 1986.

15. Fowler BA, Wiessberg JB. Arsine poisoning. N Engl J Med 1974; 291:1171–4.

16. Parish GG, Glass R, Kimbrough R. Acute arsenic poisoning in two workers cleaning a clogged drain. Arch Environ Health 1979; 34:224–7.

17. U.S. Department of Labor, Occupational Safety and Health Administration: Occupational exposure to lead: Final standard. Fed Register 43:52952–53014 and 43:54353–616, 1978; and U.S. Department of Labor, Occupational Safety and Health Administration. Lead exposure in construction: Interim final rule. Fed Register 58:26590–649, 1993.

18. Lamola AA, Joselow M, Yamane T. Zinc protoporphyrin (ZPP): A simple, sensitive, fluorometric screening test for lead poisoning. Clin Chem 1975; 21:93–7.

19. Fischbein A, et al. Zinc protoporphyrin, blood lead and clinical symptoms in two occupational groups with low-level exposure to lead. Am J Ind Med 1980; 1:391–9.

20. Lilis R, Fischbein A. Chelation therapy in workers exposed to lead. JAMA 1976; 235:2823–4.

21. Amoruso MA, et al. Estimation of risk of glucose 6-phosphate dehydrogenase–deficient red cells to ozone and nitrogen dioxide. J Occup Med 1986; 28:473–9.

## Bibliography

Cullen MR, Robins JM, Eskenazi B. Adult inorganic lead intoxication: Presentation of 31 new cases and a review of recent advances in the literature. Medicine 1983; 62:221–47.
*A clinically oriented review with a good perspective on what is relevant.*

Lilis R, et al. Prevalence of lead disease among secondary lead smelter workers and biological indicators of lead exposure. Environ Res 1977; 14:255–85.
*A complete clinical and laboratory evaluation of a cohort of highly exposed workers that clearly describes the relationship between ZPP, blood lead, and clinical findings.*

Linet MS. The leukemias: Epidemiological aspects. New York: Oxford University Press, 1985.
*An excellent in-depth review of the epidemiology of leukemia. Contains valuable summary tables. The approach to the existing literature is both informative and critical.*

Nielsen B. Arsine poisoning in a metal refining plant: Fourteen simultaneous cases. Acta Med Scand Suppl. 496, 1969.
*Contains five papers describing various aspects of an episode of arsine poisoning at a metal refining plant, including industrial hygiene studies, the clinical picture, and examination of the renal circulation in affected individuals.*

# 30
# Hepatic Disorders

Glenn S. Pransky

More than 100 chemicals are known to be toxic to the human liver, and many of these are frequently encountered in the workplace. Usually, hepatotoxicity of a particular substance has not been recognized until acute liver disease followed occupational exposure. Similar hepatotoxic effects can often be easily reproduced in laboratory animals. These investigations provide a method for predicting whether a new chemical is likely to cause acute hepatitis (but not chronic liver disease). As a result of substitution with less hepatotoxic alternatives and improved exposure control, the incidence of acute occupational hepatitis has decreased considerably.

In contrast to acute liver disease, causes of chronic liver diseases are much more difficult to determine. Animal models that allow prediction of effects after many years of low-level exposure do not exist. Although most cases are due to nonoccupational causes, such as alcohol, viral hepatitis, or autoimmune disease, epidemiologic studies have shown higher rates of hepatic carcinoma and cirrhosis in certain occupational groups, including rubber manufacturers and smelter workers. The specific etiologic chemical in these situations is often unknown.

Reports of industrial and experimental effects implicate haloalkanes (such as carbon tetrachloride), haloaromatics (such as polychlorinated biphenyls [PCBs]), azo dyes, nitrosamines, and nitroaromatics (such as dinitrobenzene) as types of organic compounds that are frequently hepatotoxic. Variation in toxicity exists within each class;

for example, haloalkane toxicity increases as the number of atoms per molecule decreases, the number of halogen atoms increases, and the atomic weight of the halogen increases. Realization of these relationships has led to replacement, where possible, of the industrial solvents carbon tetrachloride ($CCl_4$) and tetrachloroethane ($C_2H_2Cl_4$) with methylene dichloride ($CH_2Cl_2$) and trichloroethylene ($C_2HCl_3$), which has substantially reduced the incidence of haloalkane-induced hepatotoxicity. Inorganic toxins include antimony, arsine, chromium, iodine, phosphorus, thallium, and thorium.

## High-Risk Occupations

Occupations with exposure to hepatotoxins are found in many different industries including munitions, rubber, cosmetics, perfume, food processing, refrigeration, paint, insecticide and herbicide, pharmaceutical, plastics, and synthetic chemicals. Usually these workers are exposed by inhalation of fumes. Most hepatotoxins have pungent odors that warn of their presence, preventing accidental oral ingestion of large amounts; however, ingestion of imperceptible amounts of hepatotoxins over long periods of time may cause injury. Skin absorption has been a significant cause of disease only with trinitrotoluene (TNT) exposure in munitions workers and with methylenedianiline exposure in epoxy resin workers.

Table 30-1 indicates the effects and typical work

**Table 30-1.** Some causes of occupational liver disease

| Disease produced | Type of agent | Example | Types of workers exposed |
|---|---|---|---|
| ACUTE HEPATITIS | | | |
| Acute toxic hepatitis | Chlorinated hydrocarbons | Carbon tetrachloride Chloroform | Solvent workers, degreasers, cleaners, refrigeration workers |
| | Nitroaromatics | Dinitrophenol (DNP) Dinitrobenzene | Chemical indicator workers Dye workers, explosives workers |
| | Ether | Dioxin | Herbicide and insecticide workers |
| | Halogenated aromatics | Polychlorinated biphenyls (PCBs) | Electrical component assemblers |
| | | DDT Chlordecone (Kepone) } | Insecticide workers, fumigators, disinfectant workers |
| | | Chlorobenzenes | Solvent workers, dye workers |
| | | Halothane | Anesthesiologists |
| Acute cholestatic hepatitis | Epoxy resin | Methylenedianiline | Rubber workers, epoxy workers, synthetic fabric workers |
| | Inorganic element | Yellow phosphorus | Pyrotechnics workers |
| Acute viral hepatitis, type B | Virus | Hepatitis B | Health care workers (see Chap. 18) |
| Subacute hepatic necrosis | Nitroaromatic | TNT | Munitions workers |
| CHRONIC LIVER DISEASE | | | |
| Fibrosis/cirrhosis | Alcohol | Ethyl alcohol | Imbibing bartenders, wine producers, whiskey producers |
| | Virus | Hepatitis B and C | Day care workers, health care workers (see Chap. 18) |
| | Inorganic element | Arsenic | Vintners, smelter workers |
| | Haloalkene | Vinyl chloride | Vinyl chloride workers |
| Angiosarcoma | Haloalkene | Vinyl chloride | Vinyl chloride workers |
| Biliary tree carcinoma | Unknown agents | — | Rubber workers |

exposures of several toxic chemicals; Table 30-2 lists some occupations with exposures to hepatotoxic chemicals.

## Pathophysiology

Most agents cause liver disease only after activation by hepatic enzymes. The liver performs two types of reactions on foreign compounds to enhance their removal from the body: *conjugations* (additions of side chains to increase water solubility) and *biotransformations* (oxidation, reduction, and hydration) (see Chap. 13). Degradation reactions may activate hepatotoxins into unstable intermediates capable of damaging hepatocytes; these reactions are chiefly responsible for toxic injury to the liver. In the metabolism of vinyl chloride (Fig. 30-1), for example, it is the unstable epoxide that is presumed to be responsible for the carcinogenicity of the chemical; another intermediate, the aldehyde, may cause acute hepatotoxic-

Table 30-2. Examples of occupations with exposure to hepatotoxic chemicals

| | |
|---|---|
| Airplane hangar employees | Leather workers |
| Airplane pilots (insecticides) | Linoleum makers |
| Boat builders (styrene) | Nurses (chemotherapeutic drugs) |
| Cement (rubber, plastic) workers | Painters, paint makers |
| Chemical industry workers | Paint remover makers and users |
| Chemists | Paraffin workers |
| Cobblers | Perfume makers |
| Degreasers | Petroleum refiners |
| Dry cleaners | Pharmaceutical workers |
| Dye workers | Photographic material workers |
| Electrical transformer and condenser makers | Polish (metal) makers and users |
| Electroplaters | Printers |
| Enamel makers and enamelers | Pyroxylen-plastics workers |
| Extractors, oils and fats | Rayon makers |
| Fire extinguisher makers | Refrigerator workers |
| Galvanizers | Resin (synthetic) makers |
| Garage workers | Rubber workers |
| Gardeners (insecticides) | Scourers (metal) |
| Gas (illuminating) workers | Shoe factory workers |
| Glass (safety) makers | Soap makers |
| Glue workers | Straw hat makers |
| Ink makers | Thermometer makers |
| Insecticide makers | Varnish workers |
| Insulators (wire) | Waterproofers |
| Lacquer makers and lacquerers | |

Source: HJ Zimmerman. Hepatotoxicity: The adverse effects of drugs and other chemicals on the liver. New York: Appleton-Century-Crofts, 1978, p. 307.

ity. Some agents, such as halothane, affect only a small percentage of those exposed. These chemicals are probably metabolized to intermediates that may cause autoimmune hepatotoxicity in sensitized individuals.

Inducing agents are factors that increase levels of degrading enzymes and thus enhance production of toxins. In small doses, most hepatotoxins are themselves inducing agents; other factors that induce enzymes are DDT and phenobarbital, high-protein diets, and fasting. Variations in thyroid and adrenal hormones may increase enzyme levels. Similar enzyme alterations from alcohol ingestion make heavy drinkers more susceptible than others to chlorinated hydrocarbon exposure. Also, hepatotoxin exposure may significantly alter drug and hormone metabolism.

## Classes of Occupational Liver Disease

Practically any type of liver disease can be caused by an occupational exposure. To the physician, these illnesses appear as either (1) acute hepatitis occurring soon after exposure, or (2) chronic liver disease becoming clinically evident after years of exposure.

Workplace exposures can cause liver disease in a variety of ways. Although true incidence is difficult to determine, the most common occupational liver disease in the United States is believed to be *viral hepatitis, type B*, due to parenteral exposure to hepatitis B virus (see Chap. 18). Chemicals at work may contribute to liver disease by intensifying the effects of nonoccupational agents, such as viruses and alcohol. Several drugs, notably isoniazid (INH), phenobarbital, phenytoin, cytotoxic agents, androgens, and estrogens, may enhance the effects of workplace hepatotoxins by enzyme induction or by subclinical liver damage. Exposure to low levels of several different hepatotoxic agents in the workplace may cause much more toxicity than equivalent levels of a single agent. As clinical, laboratory, and pathologic features rarely implicate a specific chemical etiology, the relative importance of specific occupational and nonoccupational factors in an individual case can be difficult to determine.

### Acute Hepatitis
The incidence of acute toxic hepatitis has declined as many compounds found to be responsible have

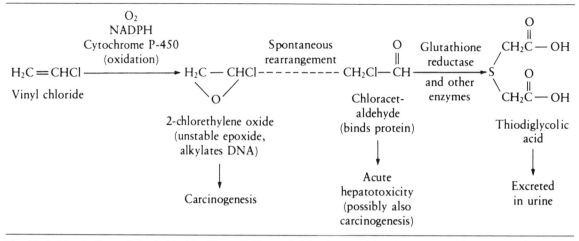

**Fig. 30-1.** Metabolism of vinyl chloride. (From T Green, DE Hathaway. The chemistry and biogenesis of S-containing metabolites of vinyl chloride interactions. Chem Biol Interact 1977; 17:137.)

been replaced with less hepatotoxic substitutes. The few cases still reported are usually caused by accidental inhalation of chemical fumes known to be hepatotoxic. The symptoms are similar to some of those of acute viral hepatitis (headache, dizziness, drowsiness, nausea, and vomiting), but they begin 12 to 48 hours after exposure, and patients remain afebrile. A history of exposure and appropriate liver function tests are sufficient to diagnose acute toxic hepatitis. Examination of liver tissue reveals zonal, massive, or submassive necrosis, often with fatty infiltration; jaundice and hepatomegaly are evident on physical exam. Patients usually recover within 4 to 6 weeks. Complications and death occur infrequently and are most often associated with extrahepatic diseases such as renal failure, which can result from the liver dysfunction or from direct toxicity of the substance to other organs.

The following case is typical of acute toxic hepatitis:

A 39-year-old man was exposed to high levels of carbon tetrachloride fumes when the ventilating system malfunctioned at the degreasing plant where he worked. Immediately after the exposure, he felt lightheaded and weak but was better several hours later. He noticed that his appetite was decreased the next day and presented to a physician complaining of increasing malaise.

Physical exam was normal, except for a tender liver edge palpable four fingerbreadths below the costal margin and minimal abdominal distension. Laboratory tests revealed a total serum bilirubin of 2.2 mg/dL, SGOT 1100, LDH 980, and a normal alkaline phosphatase.

The patient was unable to eat for the next 3 days at home and noticed dark urine for 5 days after this visit. He was able to slowly return to a normal diet over the next week but still felt generally weak 1 month later; follow-up exam then revealed a normal-sized liver and normal liver function tests.

Dinitrophenol and methylenedianiline cause acute cholestatic hepatitis, which begins with fever, chills, and pruritus, in addition to the usual symptoms of acute toxic hepatitis. If the initial injury to the liver is severe, it can be rapidly fatal. However, the liver damage associated with this disease is usually less extensive than that seen in acute toxic hepatitis, and most patients will recover within several days.

A variant of acute toxic hepatitis known as subacute hepatic necrosis is seen after months of exposure to TNT, PCBs, and tetrachloroethane. After weeks of skin, gastrointestinal, and neurologic complaints, symptoms of acute toxic hepatitis appear. Unlike acute toxic hepatitis, however, this variant may cause cirrhosis in survivors.

### Chronic Liver Disease

Prolonged, often asymptomatic, exposure to toxic agents can lead to chronic liver disease, which is usually manifest as cirrhosis or cancer. Because of the prolonged latency period (onset of symptoms 10–30 years after first exposure), the etiologic link to a specific agent is difficult to establish, and workers can be exposed for years before a compound is recognized to be toxic. For example, before the association between vinyl chloride exposure and liver angiosarcoma was recognized, an estimated 1 million workers were occupationally exposed to this chemical. Arsenic and thorium dioxide, as well as vinyl chloride, have been associated with hepatic angiosarcoma.

The following is a case history of angiosarcoma in a vinyl chloride worker. Three cases of this rare tumor occurred within 3 years at a plant that manufactured polyvinyl chloride (PVC). The physician and director of environmental health at the plant noticed this cluster of cases and discovered that they were associated with vinyl chloride exposure.

A 36-year-old white man was admitted to the hospital because of tarry stools. He had worked for 15 years as a chemical helper and autoclave cleaner in the manufacture of polyvinyl chloride (Fig. 30-2) from vinyl chloride monomer. Past history was unremarkable. Physical examination was notable for pallor and black stools. Liver and spleen were not palpable. Although an upper GI series was interpreted as normal, a tentative diagnosis was made of a bleeding duodenal ulcer. Four months later, he was readmitted for persistently tarry stools. At this time his liver and spleen were palpable. Liver function tests were only slightly abnormal. A barium swallow test suggested esophageal varices. A liver scan was interpreted as being compatible with a large lesion of the left lobe, extending into the right lobe.

An exploratory laparotomy revealed marked enlargement of the liver and spleen, with the liver adherent to

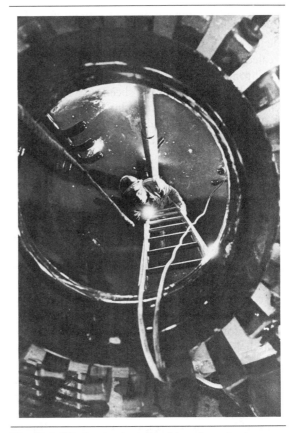

Fig. 30-2. Worker in vinyl chloride polymerization chamber is at risk of hepatic injury from exposure to vinyl chloride. This work illustrates a more common hazard, the potential for oxygen deprivation from work in confined spaces. (From HF Mark, the Editors of Life. LIFE SCIENCE LIBRARY/Giant Molecules. Photograph by Gordon Tenney. Time-Life Books Inc. Publisher. © 1966 Time Inc.)

the anterior surface of the stomach. A biopsy of the liver revealed angiosarcoma.

The patient was treated with radiotherapy and chemotherapy. He was able to return to work for a short time. Twenty months after his first hospitalization he died [1].

This report, with several associated cases, was published in 1974 and immediately generated a multinational epidemiologic investigation of cancer mortality in vinyl chloride plants. A high incidence of cancer, including angiosarcoma, was revealed.

Chronic exposures to most agents that cause acute hepatitis have not been associated with chronic liver disease, partly due to the lack of clinical features that would distinguish occupational from nonoccupational chronic liver disease and to the high incidence of chronic liver disease in the nonexposed population. Therefore, a causal relationship in any individual between work exposure and later development of cirrhosis or cancer is difficult to prove. Only by study of groups of exposed workers can it be proven that a substance causes chronic liver disease.

An abnormally high incidence of chronic liver disease has also been reported in refrigeration engineers, chemists, dry cleaners, rubber manufacturers, and workers exposed to tetrachloroethane and plutonium. Hepatocellular carcinoma (malignant hepatoma) in humans has not yet been clearly associated with occupational exposures.

Chronic liver disease is often first recognized when portal hypertension appears. Liver biopsy may show cirrhosis, but in the case of arsenic and vinyl chloride exposures, subcapsular or diffuse fibrosis and angiosarcoma may be found. In advanced cases severe hepatic dysfunction is typical. Prognosis is poor, with 75 percent mortality within 5 years. Even then the value of such medical monitoring is not proved.

## Tools for Diagnosis

Certain tests, developed for use in the diagnosis of patients with liver disease, have been used to screen workers with potentially hepatotoxic exposures. Most detect subtle liver damage by measuring serum liver enzymes or hepatic clearance of metabolites from blood and are good for confirming acute symptomatic liver disease. Unfortunately, these tests are not very sensitive for detection of early abnormalities in liver function (before

symptoms appear) and are rarely specific for chemically induced liver disease (see Chap. 3). Typically, the occupational physician is faced with an asymptomatic worker who is exposed to a variety of potential hepatotoxins at work, drinks alcohol, and has abnormal liver enzymes on routine blood testing. A careful exposure history, review of alcohol intake, observations in coworkers, and follow-up after removal from exposure are necessary to distinguish between occupational and nonoccupational disease.

In subclinical chronic liver disease, abnormal values usually appear only after permanent damage has taken place. As the latency period of chronic liver disease may be several decades, periodic liver tests must be performed for many years after exposure has ceased to enable early detection of disease progression. Research has focused on the development of tests to enable detection of changes before they become irreversible. Unfortunately, no single test can sensitively detect change in the four major functional areas of the liver: detoxification/metabolic, reticuloendothelial/phagocytic, biliary excretion, and vascular.

A few tests are available that can help quantify the amount of previous exposure to a hepatotoxin. These include tests that can detect arsenic, vinyl chloride, and carbon tetrachloride metabolites in urine and can determine exposure levels to solvents in workplace air. Some tests are inexpensive, give reasonably quantitative results, and help assure that hepatotoxin exposure is within acceptable limits. However, the distinction between etiologies of liver disease is rarely clear, and it may become necessary to insist on removing the affected worker from all potentially hepatotoxic medications and exposures and to follow the individual with periodic tests of liver function.

## Management and Prevention

The management of occupational liver disease is identical to that of nonoccupational liver disease. A multifaceted approach, with emphasis on recognition of hazards and use of environmental controls, is needed to prevent occupational liver disease. Work situations should be designed to minimize direct employee contact with hepatotoxins. Preplacement screening should focus on the identification of factors such as alcohol or barbiturate abuse or chronic liver disease that could make the worker particularly susceptible to the effects of hepatotoxic exposure. Though many who work with potentially hepatotoxic substances are routinely screened by periodic liver function tests, false-positive and false-negative results are common and may be difficult to evaluate. The appearance of confirmed abnormalities should initiate a careful investigation of the workplace, removing the affected worker from further exposure until the cause is identified and controlled. A worker with occupationally related liver disease should not return to the original job unless the substance is removed or adequate environmental control of it is established. Epidemiologic and laboratory studies to identify hepatotoxins should be given high priority. Substances capable of producing chronic hepatic disease can be identified by long-term epidemiologic studies only if exposures are well-characterized, and if age, alcohol intake, lifestyle, diet, and nonoccupational liver disease are carefully controlled.

# Reference

1. Creech JL, Johnson MN. Angiosarcoma of the liver in the manufacture of vinyl chloride. J Occup Med 1974; 16:150.

# Bibliography

Zimmerman HJ. Hepatotoxicity. New York: Appleton, 1978, p. 597.

Schiff L. Diseases of the liver. 6th ed. Philadelphia: Lippincott, 1987.

Tamburro CH. Chemical hepatitis. Med Clin North Am 1979; 63:545.
*Excellent general references. Zimmerman's book is listed first because it is a comprehensive source on hepatotoxicity due to chemicals and drugs (it includes chapters on occupational and environmental liver toxicity). Schiff's book is an exhaustive reference on liver disease, with detailed information on management, toxic hepatitis, and cirrhosis. Tamburro's article, an overview of hepatotoxic chemicals, contains examples of liver biopsies of each type of toxic liver injury, as well as a detailed description of the indocyanine green clearance test.*

Dossing M, Skinhoj P. Occupational liver injury: Present state of knowledge and future perspective. Int Arch Occup Environ Health 1985; 56:1.
*An excellent review of the state-of-the-art and controversies in identification of occupational hepatotoxins.*

Herip DS. Recommendations for the investigation of abnormal hepatic function in asymptomatic workers. Am J Ind Med, 1992; 21:331–9.
*This article provides a logical approach to evaluation of workers exposed to potential hepatotoxins who have asymptomatic elevations of liver function tests.*

Hodgson MJ, Goodman-Klein BM, Van Thiel DH. Evaluating the liver in hazardous waste workers. In M Gochfeld, EA Favata. eds. Hazardous waste workers. Occup Med State of the Art Rev, 1990; 5:67–78.
*An excellent review of theoretical and practical issues involved in screening workers for occult liver disease.*

Popper H, et al. Environmental hepatic injury in man. In H Popper, F Schaffner. eds. Progress in liver disease. New York: Grune & Stratton, 1979, pp. 605–38.
*A current and thorough overview of occupational and other environmental liver disease, with attention to mechanisms and experimental data. Good review of vinyl chloride problem.*

Selikoff IJ, Hammond EC. eds. Toxicity of vinyl chloride–polyvinyl chloride. Ann NY Acad Sci 1975; 246.
*Several hundred pages by various authors on experimental, clinical, and epidemiologic data on vinyl chloride carcinogenesis.*

Tamburro CH, Liss GM. Tests for hepatotoxicity: Usefulness in screening workers. J Occup Med 1986; 28:1034.
*A thorough review of various tests for screening exposed workers for early signs of hepatotoxicity.*

# 31
# Renal and Urinary Tract Disorders

Ruth Lilis and Philip J. Landrigan

Acute and chronic kidney failure are major causes of illness and death in the United States. Approximately 75,000 Americans suffer from end-stage renal disease (ESRD), and each year approximately 4,000 new cases are reported, for an annual incidence in the United States of about 50 cases per million [1].

The proportion of ESRD that may be caused by occupational exposures is not known. However, a large number of known and suspected nephrotoxins are used in American industry (Table 31-1).

For most cases of ESRD, no etiologic information is available. Several factors account for this absence of information. Exposures to nephrotoxins frequently go unnoticed. Few renal toxins produce easily recognizable acute syndromes; instead they produce chronic disease after many years of exposure and long latency [2]. Because the kidneys have great reserve capacity and can function adequately despite progressive loss of nephrons, work-related kidney disease is typically not diagnosed until considerable dysfunction has occurred. By that time, the specific signatures of certain toxins, such as the intranuclear inclusion bodies of lead intoxication, have disappeared. Biopsies or postmortem examinations of tissue specimens from most patients with ESRD look very much alike; regardless of etiology, they are characterized by nonspecific glomerulosclerosis, tubular dilation, and chronic interstitial inflammatory and fibrotic changes. Thus, histopathologic diagnosis of occupationally induced ESRD is seldom possible.

*The kidney is a target organ for a number of toxic chemical compounds.*

Renal excretion is the major route of elimination for many toxic compounds. The relatively high renal blood flow, about one-fourth of total cardiac output, exposes the renal structures to a relatively high toxic burden. Concentration of toxins in the glomerular ultrafiltrate through active reabsorption contributes further to the intensity of toxic exposures. The considerable endothelial surface represented by the extensive capillary network in the kidney, the presence in renal tubular cells of numerous important enzyme systems, the local synthesis of active peptides (for example, renin and prostaglandin), and the generally high metabolic rate of the organ are additional factors increasing the vulnerability of the kidneys to chemical toxins. These agents can adversely affect the delicate balance between bloodflow, glomerular filtration, tubular reabsorption, and filtrate concentration.

## Acute and Chronic Renal Effects of Occupational and Environmental Agents

Acute nephropathies are the result of severe, usually short-term overexposures to toxic chemicals. These compounds can injure the kidney either directly, due to their intrinsic nephrotoxic effects, or indirectly as the result of systemic, prerenal toxic effects. Simultaneous toxicity to other organs,

**Table 31-1.** Estimated numbers of workers in the United States with potential occupational exposures to proven or suspected nephrotoxins as of 1990

| Agent | Total number of workers potentially exposed |
| --- | --- |
| Lead and compounds | 1,674,927 |
| Cadmium and compounds | 93,630 |
| Mercury and compounds | 617,743 |
| Uranium and compounds | 8,544 |
| Solvents | 2,505,136 |
| Arsenic and compounds (including arsine) | 61,102 |
| Pesticides | 1,838,611 |
| Beryllium and compounds | 44,468 |

Unpublished provisional data as of 7/1/90, NIOSH National Occupational Exposure Survey (1981–1983). U.S. Dept. of Health and Human Services.

such as the liver, brain, and lungs, can occur, complicating clinical presentation and therapeutic management.

Pathogenic mechanisms in acute nephropathies are complex. Impaired glomerular filtration is frequently the prime abnormality and aberrant tubular reabsorption can be a secondary event. Tubular necrosis is often found and usually results in nonselective and almost complete reabsorption of glomerular filtrate. Increased renin production in the juxtaglomerular apparatus and disturbances in renal prostaglandin synthesis have also been documented. Reduction of renal cortical blood flow and development of arterial and arteriolar vasoconstriction are thought to be major mechanisms in acute nephropathies of toxic etiology [3].

Sudden marked renal ischemia is an additional important causal mechanism resulting in acute nephropathies. It can occur as a result of systemic hypotension (due to dehydration, diarrhea, and shock) or massive hemolysis. Less frequently, physical agents, such as extreme heat (especially with concomitant extreme physical exercise), crush injuries, or high-voltage electrical injuries (resulting in muscle necrosis—rhabdomyolysis), can lead to acute post-traumatic renal failure.

Chronic nephrotoxicity due to occupational or environmental exposure has typically been associated with long-term absorption. The mechanisms by which certain chemical compounds leading to chronic nephropathies have not been completely elucidated even for etiologic agents that have long been known to result in renal function impairment, such as lead. Functional tubular cell damage can remain subclinical for years; glomerular function impairment can occur simultaneously with the slight and slowly progressing tubular injury. The result of this sequence of events is slow reduction in the number of functional nephrons, most often with concomitant development of interstitial fibrotic changes. This process can remain subclinical for years, until it reaches the critical level of nonfunctional nephrons, with resulting renal insufficiency, as expressed in significant reduction of glomerular filtration rate (GFR; creatinine clearance) and increase in blood urea nitrogen (BUN) and creatinine.

More recently immunologic mechanisms have been found to be involved in the development of solvent-related glomerulopathies. Antibodies to solvent-altered basement membranes have been demonstrated and autoimmune glomerulonephritis has been found to occur more often in persons exposed to solvents. This area is being actively investigated.

## Nephrotoxicity of Metals

*Mercury.* Mercury nephrotoxicity may follow accidental or intentional ingestion of mercuric salts. Acute tubular injury and even tubular necrosis can result. Such severe nephrotoxicity is extremely unusual in occupational or environmental mercury poisoning.

Under present day circumstances of occupational or environmental exposure, the nephrotoxicity of mercury is usually limited to a moderate proximal tubular dysfunction; the clinical correlate is low-grade proteinuria. More sensitive tests have recently been introduced, such as measurements of urinary enzymes, including N-acetyl-β-D-glucosaminidase (NAG), to assess early renal tubular dysfunction in mercury-exposed workers [4]. Another sensitive indicator of impaired renal function in mercury-exposed persons is urinary excretion of beta-galactosidase.

Urinary mercury excretion higher than 50 μg per liter (a level less than that in most previous studies) was recently shown to be associated with a significantly increased NAG excretion; a previous study had found an increase of urinary beta-galactosidase when U-Hg (mercury in urine) exceeded 50 μg/gm creatinine. Although the clinical predictive value of tubular enzymuria is not yet completely evaluated, it seems appropriate to protect workers against any renal effect. Some authorities have recommended a limit for U-Hg of 50 μg/per liter or lower, corresponding to an air level of about 25 μg/m$^3$.

Glomerular injury, due to toxic effects mediated by an autoimmune reaction, with formation of autoantibodies against glomerular structures has been reported in animal experiments [4]. Glomerular injury seldom has been described in humans. A few cases of nephrotic syndrome in mercury workers have been reported; recently case reports have documented glomerular lesions mediated by immunologic mechanisms.

Recently, an industrial episode of acute elemental mercury overexposure was reported from a chloralkali plant in the United States [5]. Fifty-three employees performing maintenance work were exposed, and 11 were followed closely because of higher U-Hg excretion (range, 59–193 μg/liter). Proteinuria was present in one person; BUN and serum creatinine were normal. Excretion of enzymes was not assessed, but a renal tubular defect in bicarbonate handling was suggested by hyperchloremia and a positive urinary anion gap; serum chloride was found to decrease with time, closely following the decrease in urinary and blood mercury levels. This episode illustrates the continuing risk of mercury overexposure and the need to appropriately protect workers. Sensitive methods for the assessment of renal tubular function, such as measurement of urinary NAG and beta-galactosidase, might prove to be useful additions for monitoring employees with potential mercury exposure.

*Lead.* The acute toxic effects of lead on the kidney are characterized by proximal tubular dysfunction and formation of intranuclear inclusion bodies composed of a lead-protein complex [6]. Mitochondrial abnormalities, related to impairment of cellular respiration and phosphorylation, are present in the proximal tubular cells. Aminoaciduria, glucosuria, and hyperphosphaturia (Fanconi's syndrome) are characteristic clinical features of acute lead nephropathy; renal tubular dysfunction is frequently present in acute episodes of childhood lead poisoning (mostly due to ingestion of lead-based paint). Acute lead poisoning in adults, due to occupational lead exposure, is exceedingly rare today in industrialized countries. The incidence in developing countries is not known.

Chronic lead nephropathy was well documented in the early decades of this century when heavy occupational lead exposure was widespread and severe lead poisoning was frequent. Progressive renal damage eventually resulting in renal failure (Bright's disease) was common in lead-exposed workers [7].

With relatively less heavy lead exposure, there is a slow deterioration of renal function, with progressive reduction in renal blood flow and glomerular filtration rate. Increases in serum creatinine, BUN, and, in some cases, uric acid can occur [8, 9]. This chronic deterioration in function is more marked with higher lead exposure. Thus, a dose-response effect has been shown to exist [10].

A 61-year-old black man was examined during a clinical field survey of secondary lead smelter workers. He appeared to be chronically ill and complained of marked fatigue, weakness, muscle pain, loss of appetite, weight loss, frequent headache, and some deterioration of his memory. He had been employed at the same facility for 34 years. He had been repeatedly tested for blood-lead levels; over the last several years of his employment, a blood-lead test had been mandatory every 2 months. The patient's statement was that his blood-lead level had been "always high." Also noteworthy was the fact that he had been treated with more than five courses of chelation therapy over the years. This fact confirmed that the blood-lead levels had been significantly elevated. On repeated occasions, he had been removed from his work because of high blood-lead levels. The last such episode was in 1970. The past medical history was negative for other diseases.

In February 1973 the patient had been examined by his physician, whose help he sought because of tiredness, muscle pain, abdominal pain, constipation, and weight loss. Because of the intensity and persistence of these symptoms, he had to be admitted to a hospital. The blood-lead level was found to be elevated, at 83 μg/dL. Slight anemia (hemoglobin, 13.1 gm/dL), a finding not unusual for lead poisoning, was also present. Kidney impairment was indicated by an elevated BUN (25 mg/dL), coarse granular casts in the urine, and an elevated serum uric acid (8.3 mg/dL and 8.9 mg/dL). Chelation therapy with penicillamine, 500 mg 4 times a day, was started and relieved most of the symptoms. Ten months after this episode an elevated serum creatinine level (2.1 and 2.2 mg/dL) and uric acid (8.9 mg/dL) were again found. The creatinine clearance was markedly reduced to 43 ml per 1.73 m² (normal is 80–140 ml). This marked reduction in the glomerular filtration rate indi-

cated renal insufficiency. A repeated creatinine clearance test again showed a much depressed value of 35 ml. The blood-lead level was 60 μg/dL, although the patient had discontinued his lead exposure for months.

In adults, lead nephropathy develops as an insidious, progressive, chronic interstitial nephritis, characterized by the absence of proteinuria (including low molecular weight proteins, such as $\beta_2$-microglobulin) or albuminuria. The urinary excretion of the lysosomal enzyme NAG seems to be an early marker of lead nephrotoxicity [4]. In children, lead nephropathy often manifests itself as proximal tubular dysfunction [11].

Nonenzymatic markers of tubular injury, brush-border antigens in urine, have recently been found to be particularly useful for early detection of nephrotoxicity [12]. Mutti and associates [12], have developed monoclonal antibodies to several proximal tubular brush-border proteins.

A high-affinity lead-binding protein in the rat kidney has recently been identified [13]; it was shown to be a specific cleavage product of $\alpha_2$-microglobulin, which is a member of the retinol-binding protein superfamily. Increase in the urinary excretion of this protein has been noted in rats exposed to lead in drinking water after 2 weeks of exposure.

The renal pathology in chronic lead nephropathy can affect all structures of the nephron. Diffuse damage to proximal tubules and tubular atrophy have been observed. With progressive renal insufficiency, interstitial fibrosis and loss of glomeruli, periglomerular fibrosis, and glomerular obsolescence are the most marked abnormalities, together with arteriolar endothelial proliferation [9].

Heavy environmental exposure of children to lead in Queensland, Australia, earlier in this century resulted in endemic childhood lead poisoning. Subsequently, endemic nephropathy with clinically overt renal failure was detected in numerous young and middle-aged adults in Queensland. A high lead body burden, demonstrated by positive calcium disodium ethylene diaminetetraacetic acid (EDTA) chelation (urinary lead excretion exceeding 600 μg/24 hr after administration of 1 gm EDTA), confirmed lead as the etiologic agent.

Children with asymptomatic lead poisoning due to lead paint in old buildings in Paris were found to have increased urinary excretion of β$_2$-microglobulin in 8 of 27 cases; urinary NAG was found to be increased in a similar proportion of cases. The use of these sensitive methods allows early detection of nephrotoxicity [14] in childhood lead poisoning.

Other environmental lead exposure that has resulted in renal functional impairment has been chronic ingestion of drinking water with high lead content (in excess of 100 μg/liter). Chronic consumption of lead-contaminated "moonshine" whiskey has also been reported to produce severe lead poisoning including "saturnine gout."

Increased susceptibility to lead toxicity, including nephrotoxicity, has been shown to be associated with iron deficiency. Iron deficiency is common in women in developing countries, particularly during pregnancy.

Mortality studies of lead-exposed workers indicate excess death rates from chronic nephritis and from "other renal sclerosis," as well as "other hypertensive disease" (other than essential hypertension) [15]. While this pattern of mortality reflects previous high lead exposure in certain industrial plants, the effects of recent lower-level occupational and environmental exposures are still not completely assessed. A no-effect level for lead with regard to renal function has not been established.

Experimental studies on rats conducted to explore the reversibility of lead nephropathy after cessation of lead exposure and administration of the chelating agent dimercaptosuccinic acid (DMSA) have not shown a favorable long-term effect on the progression of lead nephropathy [16].

Analysis of bone biopsies from patients with end-stage renal disease who were undergoing dialysis in three European countries showed that about 5 percent had elevated bone lead comparable to levels found in occupationally exposed populations [17]. Thus, the contribution of lead nephropathy to the number of cases with end-stage renal disease may be substantial. The use of x-ray fluorescence analysis to measure lead in bone represents a major methodologic advance in the evaluation of cumulative lead body burden; it is especially valuable in assessing dose-response relationships for long-term effects of lead exposure, including renal disease [18].

*Cadmium.* Acute high-dose overexposure to cadmium compounds, especially cadmium oxide fumes, has been reported to result from welding, soldering, and cutting cadmium metal and cadmium-containing alloys. The major target organ under such circumstances is the lung, and severe, sometimes fatal chemical pneumonitis is the major clinical manifestation. In some of these cases, renal lesions, mainly affecting the tubular epithelium, have been observed. Marked proteinuria occurs. Bilateral renal cortical necrosis has been reported.

Chronic renal toxicity due to long-term exposure is the best-documented adverse health effect due to cadmium. It has been confirmed in numerous studies, in both humans and in experimental animals. It has been found under circumstances of both occupational and environmental exposure.

Increased urinary excretion of low molecular weight proteins is the most outstanding feature of chronic cadmium nephropathy. Cadmium oxide fume or dust, cadmium sulfide, and cadmium stearate have all been found to be nephrotoxic and to produce proteinuria under conditions of long-term exposure. The low molecular weight proteinuria is characterized by increased excretion of β$_2$-microglobulin (on which a sensitive test for biologic monitoring is based), muramidase, ribonuclease, orosomucoid, transferrin, and retinol-binding protein (RBP). Recently, retinol-binding protein has also been used for biologic monitoring; a sensitive and accurate radioimmunoassay has been developed.

Other features of proximal tubular dysfunction such as aminoaciduria and glycosuria have been found in some cases of cadmium nephropathy. Increased urinary levels of NAG, a lysosomal enzyme abundant in renal tubular cells and released into the urine during tubular cell damage, have been reported.

Glomerular dysfunction, with significantly increased urinary albumin loss, decreased GFR, and increased serum creatinine levels have been documented in persons with long-standing cadmium nephrotoxicity [19]. Cadmium nephropathy, nevertheless, rarely results in chronic renal failure in humans.

New markers of nephrotoxicity have recently been proposed for detection of nephrotoxic effects in cadmium-exposed workers: urinary protein 1, a sex-linked, $\alpha_2$-microprotein, and transferrin, a high molecular weight protein, assayed by means of sensitive immunoassays [20].

Urinary protein 1, as well correlated with urinary cadmium as are $\beta_2$-microglobulin ($\beta_2$-M), RBP, or NAG, has the advantage of excellent stability in urine and could therefore be of particular value for screening purposes. Transferrin, measured by the new immunoassay, is generally a more sensitive marker of glomerular dysfunction than albuminuria.

High molecular weight proteinuria is now being reported in cadmium-exposed workers with lower urinary cadmium levels, in the range of 2 µg/gm creatinine to 10 µg/gm creatinine, without increased excretion of low molecular weight proteins ($\beta_2$-M, RBP). Previously, cases with initial glomerular dysfunction might not always have been detected. In such cases, renal insufficiency may be more likely to develop.

Urinary excretion of the enzymes NAG and alanino-amino-peptidase (AAP) was found to be significantly higher in a cadmium-exposed group than in control subjects [21]. The urinary enzyme levels were correlated with urinary cadmium.

The mechanism of cadmium nephrotoxicity is attributed to slow accumulation of cadmium in the kidney cortex. Cadmium in plasma is transported bound to the protein metallothionein. The cadmium-metallothionein complex is readily filtered through the glomerulus and then almost completely reabsorbed by the proximal tubular epithelium. Renal excretion of cadmium is slow and the half-life in the renal cortex is estimated to be several decades. When the concentration of cadmium in the renal cortex exceeds a certain "critical level," estimated to be in the range of 170 to 300 mg/kg, proteinuria can be detected, indicating disruption of proximal tubule reabsorption. The kidney cadmium concentration does not generally increase further after proteinuria has ensued; some of the proximal tubular cells with highest cadmium concentration are disrupted; their cadmium is lost in the urine. The critical urinary cadmium level at which proteinuria is expected has been 10 µg/gm creatinine; as indicated above, this "critical" urinary cadmium level must now be reconsidered. When screening of cadmium-exposed workers reveals urinary excretion in excess of 5 µg/gm creatinine, exposure must be discontinued to prevent overt clinical nephropathy.

Most studies in humans indicate that chronic cadmium nephropathy is not reversible and that proteinuria and slight decrements in glomerular function can persist and even progress for years after cessation of exposure.

A recent follow-up study of cadmium workers removed from exposure in a nonferrous smelter revealed that, while cadmium concentrations in blood and urine decreased significantly over the 5 years after cessation of exposure, serum creatinine increased significantly; none of the urinary low and high molecular weight proteins that were initially elevated returned to normal. These results confirm that cadmium nephropathy is not reversible. In addition, the increase of serum creatinine and serum $\beta_2$-microglobulin indicated a progressive reduction of GFR, about five times greater than expected [22].

In a multifaceted study of cadmium alloy workers in Great Britain, increased excretion of both high molecular and low molecular weight proteins; increased enzymuria; significant decreases in the renal reabsorption of calcium, phosphate, and urate; and reduced GFR were found. A cumulative cadmium exposure index and the liver cadmium concentration were significantly correlated with almost all the variables that showed a significant difference between the exposed and matched controls. Most abnormalities detected were noted in those with a cumulative exposure equivalent to about 20 years' exposure at 50 $\mu g/m^3$, the current occupational exposure limit used in many countries. Elevated NAG excretion was found at even lower cumulative exposure indices [23]. Authors of a study of workers in a cadmium recovery facility in the U.S. came to very similar conclusions [24], including the cumulative cadmium exposure at which nephrotoxicity occurs and the recommendation for a lower permissible occupational exposure limit for airborne cadmium.

Environmental cadmium contamination has occurred in Japan and has produced Itai-Itai (Ouch-Ouch) disease in populations that ingest cadmium-contaminated rice and other foodstuffs. Patterns of renal dysfunction similar to those described above have been found. In addition, osteomalacia, with pain in back and legs, especially in postmenopausal women, is characteristic of this syndrome and thought to be due to the synergistic effects of dietary deficiencies and cadmium-induced disturbances in tubular reabsorption of calcium and phosphorus.

Recently, cadmium-induced nephrotoxicity was examined in Chinese, Malay, and Indian female workers in a factory that manufactured nickel-cadmium batteries in Singapore [25]. Urinary NAG was the marker that detected the largest proportion of abnormalities in the exposed group; a statistically significant increase in NAG excretion was seen with urinary cadmium levels of from 3 $\mu g$ per liter upward. Similar results were reported in a group of women occupationally exposed to cadmium in a nickel-cadmium battery plant in the United States [26]. The only abnormalities detected were increased excretion of the enzymes NAG and AAP, although the urinary excretion exceeded 10 $\mu g/gm$ creatinine in one-third of the group. The mean age of women in this study was less than 45 years. It was thought that cadmium

nephrotoxicity in women is more marked after menopause, as the experience with Itai-Itai disease in Japan indicates.

The concern for adverse effects of cadmium exposure has increased considerably over the past decades. The growing production of cadmium (doubling every 10 years), its documented accumulation in the environment, its long biologic half-life, and better understanding of its nephrotoxicity are important factors for this growing concern.

It is now recognized that the criteria for acceptable cadmium absorption established in active industrial workers, a urinary concentration of 10 $\mu g/gm$ creatinine, corresponding to 200 mg cadmium per kilogram in renal cortex (wet weight), might underestimate the risk for other groups in the general population, particularly the elderly (with declining renal function) and postmenopausal women. This is suggested by a large collaborative study on effects of environmental cadmium contamination on the exposed general population in Belgium [27]. This study has been prompted, in part, by higher mortality from renal diseases in both males and females in areas with high environmental cadmium contamination.

*Uranium.* Soluble uranium compounds are markedly nephrotoxic. Overt clinical nephropathy with proteinuria and increased BUN and serum creatinine has occurred after accidental occupational exposure to uranium hexafluoride and oxyfluoride. Restoration of function has generally occurred in such cases. Uranyl nitrate is a potent nephrotoxic agent that has been extensively used in experimental models for the study of renal tubular dysfunction [4].

Acute uranium nephrotoxicity, well-studied in animals but less so in humans, has been shown to produce morphologic changes of renal proximal tubular cells, glycosuria, aminoaciduria, increased excretion of small molecular weight proteins, and, at higher levels of exposure, albuminuria and acute renal failure.

While no concerted effort has been made to up-date the basic concepts on the nephrotoxicity of uranium compounds, first developed in the 1940s and 1950s, more recent studies using sensitive methods for the assessment of renal function have added considerably to the understanding of the renal effects of uranium compounds.

Binding to the brush border of proximal renal tubular cells, with special affinity for phospholipids, has been noted, as have penetration into tubular cells, accumulation in lysosomes, and mitochondrial changes, with adverse consequences for cellular respiration.

Reduced reabsorption of sodium, glucose, proteins, and amino acids, and increased transport of calcium into the cells (that may interfere with the ability of the cell to survive), have been described. Necrotic changes in tubular cells are not unusual and repair processes are incomplete; reduced glomerular filtration rate and loss in concentrating capacity of the kidney have been reported.

Higher exposure results in a larger fraction of absorbed uranium compounds being retained in the kidney. Retention time of uranium in the kidney also increases with exposure level.

The effects of long-term occupational uranium exposure have received much less attention. Although the kidney is recognized to be the critical site for organ damage from exposure to uranium metal, there are few studies on chronic renal effects in occupationally exposed workers. A recent study of health effects among workers of a uranium mill found significantly higher excretion of $\beta_2$-microglobulin; a quantitative relationship was noted with the length of time worked in the area with highest uranium exposure. In addition, a significantly increased urinary excretion of several amino acids was detected.

Recent reports from China on accidental overexposure of workers and long-term follow-up call attention to the possibility of relatively delayed deterioration in renal function several weeks to several months after exposure, and long persistence of proteinuria and increase in serum nonprotein nitrogen [28].

In light of current knowledge, the possible chronic renal effects of occupational exposure to soluble uranium compounds cannot be ignored, and the occupational standard for airborne uranium and uranium excretion in urine have to be carefully evaluated in order to appropriately protect workers.

### Indirect Renal Effects of Potent Hemolytic Agents

*Arsine.* Acute arsine ($AsH_3$) poisoning is a severe and life-threatening occupational hazard. Arsine is a colorless gas, without irritant warning properties, and is practically odorless when chemically pure. It usually is generated suddenly when metal ores or metals (such as lead, zinc, or cadmium) containing arsenic impurities come in contact with acid. Exposures also occur in the semiconductor industry, where arsine is used widely to "treat" crystals.

The major toxic effect of arsine is massive intravascular hemolysis. Arsine is the most potent hemolytic agent encountered in industrial processes (see Chap. 29).

Acute nephropathy is a major manifestation of arsine poisoning. Although previously attributed to renal tubular obstruction by hemoglobin precipitates, the mechanisms of acute arsine-induced renal failure are presently thought to be due to ischemic tubular injury (secondary to sudden-onset anemia and marked systemic hypotension) and also to a direct nephrotoxic effect of $AsH_3$ on the proximal tubular epithelium. Oliguria and anuria are the major manifestations of acute renal failure in arsine poisoning; hyperkalemia, metabolic acidosis, and increased BUN and creatinine can occur, especially in the most severe cases. Outcome is frequently fatal.

A 34-year-old chemical engineer had been working on the development of a method (pilot stage) for the extraction of cadmium from sludge. Analysis of the chemical reactions indicated that arsine could have been generated, since the mixture handled contained arsenic compounds. The patient was suddenly taken ill, with weakness, abdominal pain, unusual dizziness, and nausea. On admission, after several hours, she was markedly pale and jaundiced. Her red blood cell count fell rapidly and her bilirubin increased steadily for several days; oliguria was followed by anuria. All efforts to save this patient with acute arsine poisoning and renal failure (including dialysis) were unsuccessful; no recovery of her renal function occurred, indicating complete destruction of proximal tubular epithelium, including the basement membrane.

If a patient survives acute arsine nephropathy, urine flow returns to normal after an oliguric or anuric stage. Sometimes a polyuric stage ensues. Return of function may take many months, sometimes up to a year. Even in relatively mild cases of arsine poisoning, renal function tests indicate tubular dysfunction (due to direct nephrotoxicity of arsine) with markedly reduced concentrating capacity and reduced creatinine clearance.

*Stibine and Phosphine.* Stibine (antimony hydride; $SbH_3$) and phosphine (phosphorus hydride; $PH_3$) produce clinical manifestations similar (although generally less severe) to those of arsine poisoning.

## Solvent Nephrotoxicity

### Halogenated Aliphatic Hydrocarbons
Carbon tetrachloride ($CCl_4$) and chloroform ($CHCl_3$) are the best-known nephrotoxic agents in this large group of chemical compounds. Dibromochloropropane (DBCP), ethylene dibromide, ethylene dichloride, hexachloro-1,3-butadiene, 1,1,2-trichloroethane, allyl chloride, trichloroethylene, and perchloroethylene are halogenated aliphatic hydrocarbons with high-volume production and numerous industrial and agricultural applications. Inadequate information on their nephrotoxicity is available, and it derives mainly from animal studies.

Acute overexposure to carbon tetrachloride or chloroform, such as with the use of carbon tetrachloride as a degreaser or in the chemical industry,

can result in severe toxic nephropathy. Numerous such cases, due mostly to accidental inhalation *or* ingestion, have been documented. The proximal tubular epithelium is the principal target of aliphatic halogenated hydrocarbon renal injury; the severity of the lesion varies, but often includes tubular necrosis with acute oliguric or anuric renal failure. Concomitant hepatotoxicity may be a major complicating factor. Restoration of renal function generally occurs in 10 to 14 days as the tubular epithelium regenerates. In extreme cases proximal tubular necrosis with disruption of the basement membrane precludes regeneration.

Release of halogenated aliphatic hydrocarbons into the general environment occurs through industrial effluents and emissions and also through pesticide application. Generation of low molecular weight chlorinated chemicals in surface waters, as a result of water chlorination, has also received increasing attention. Cumulative nephrotoxic effects of such long-term, low-level exposure are yet unknown. Another issue of concern is the possible enhancement of halogenated hydrocarbon nephrotoxicity through concurrent absorption of chemical compounds, such as polychlorinated biphenyls (PCBs), which are inducers of mixed-function oxidases.

### Diethylenedioxide (Dioxan)
Inhalation of the vapor of the pesticide dioxan can result in acute or subacute poisoning characterized by toxic effects on the central nervous system (CNS), hepatotoxicity, and nephrotoxicity.

Several chemically related compounds, such as ethylene glycol, diethylene glycol, ethyl diethylene glycol, and ethylene glycol diacetate, have nephrotoxic effects similar to those of dioxan. Their low vapor pressure at normal temperatures explains why no acute nephropathy from their inhalation has been reported. Accidental ingestion (particularly of ethylene glycol, a major component of antifreeze) has resulted in severe and sometimes fatal cases of neurotoxicity, toxic pulmonary edema, and nephrotoxicity.

## Methanol (Methyl Alcohol)

Methyl alcohol ($CH_3OH$) is one of the most toxic organic solvents. Occupational exposure, with inhalation and skin contact, only rarely results in overt clinical poisoning since volatility is relatively low. Accidental ingestion, not unusual in industries where methyl alcohol is used, has resulted, however, in an important number of cases of severe poisoning, with a relatively high proportion of fatalities. Acute methyl alcohol poisoning is one of the most challenging medical emergencies; marked metabolic acidosis, neurotoxic effects with CNS depression and specific optic nerve injury, nephrotoxicity, hepatotoxicity, and injury of the pancreas can develop. In severe cases, toxic renal tubular injury can contribute significantly to fatal outcome. Correction of acidosis is important in management of such cases. Dialysis should be attempted in order to reduce methanol concentrations and allow return of renal function.

## Solvent Nephropathy (Other than Halogenated Aliphatic Hydrocarbons)

Numerous case reports have documented occurrence of glomerulonephritis with antibodies to glomerular basement membrane (anti-GM) after significant solvent exposure. In case-control studies, it has been shown that a significantly higher prevalence of solvent exposure is found in patients with glomerulonephritis than in control groups [29, 30]. The pathophysiologic mechanism of this nephropathy is not yet clarified. It has, however, been suggested that inhaled vapors of hydrocarbon solvents may bind to the pulmonary alveolar basement membrane, resulting in the generation of an antigenic compound. Antibodies to this solvent-induced antigen may then be produced. The similar chemical structures of the alveolar and renal basement membrane make the glomerular basement membrane vulnerable to these antibodies; thus, glomerulonephritis results. Cases of Goodpasture's syndrome as well as of acute autoimmune glomerulonephritis have been reported in persons exposed to solvents. An alternative possible pathophysiologic mechanism is that solvents may attach directly to the glomerular basement membrane, alter it, and thereby produce an antigenic compound that induces specific antibodies against the renal glomerular basement membrane. Chronic glomerulonephritis has been reported to develop following such a sequence of events. Solvent exposure by intentional sniffing of trichloroethylene, 1,1,1-trichloroethane, or toluene has been reported to cause acute tubular necrosis. Several cohort mortality studies so far have not detected increased mortality from renal disease in solvent-exposed refinery, oil distribution, or paint and varnish workers.

More recently, cross-sectional epidemiologic studies using sensitive indicators of renal dysfunction have been conducted on populations exposed to a variety of solvents: styrene, toluene, perchloroethylene, aromatic hydrocarbons, alkane petroleum distillates, and mixtures of solvents (refinery workers, printing workers, leather finishers, and painters).

Although the exposures and the methodology for assessing renal dysfunction varied, findings included:

- Increased albuminuria, excretion of a renal brush-border antigen (BB-50), and elevated titers of anti-albumin antibodies in refinery workers [31] with exposures lower than the current threshold limit values (TLV); these findings were interpreted as indicating glomerular dysfunction.
- Increased urinary NAG in women exposed to mostly aliphatic petroleum distillates and toluene in a shoe factory [32]. Total proteinuria was significantly higher in workers exposed to high petroleum naphtha concentrations (over 1,000 mg/m$^3$).
- Increased excretion of proteins, lysozymes, and beta-glucuronidase in shoemakers exposed to C5-C7 alkanes, suggesting slight tubular damage.

Significantly higher levels and increased prevalence of elevated RBP in paint manufacturing and spraying workers in Singapore, exposed mainly to toluene, when compared to matched control subjects. There was no significant difference in albumin excretion in the exposed group. RBP was significantly correlated with urinary o-cresol, a metabolite of toluene. The results were interpreted as indicating impaired proximal tubular function due to exposure to toluene and other solvents [33].

A recent collaborative European study [34] was conducted to assess the renal effects of occupational perchloroethylene (PCE) exposure in dry-cleaners by comparing results of a very comprehensive battery of about 20 markers of early nephrotoxic effects with those of matched control subjects.

Perchloroethylene-exposed workers excreted more high molecular weight proteins, such as albumin and tranferrin, brush-border antigens, fibronectin (FNU), and tissue nonspecific alkaline phosphatase (TNAP). Serum antiglomerular basement membrane (AGBM) antibodies and laminin fragments (LAM) were also significantly higher in PCE-exposed workers. The prevalence of low molecular weight proteinuria (RBP and $\beta_2$-M) and of increased immunoglobulin G (IgG), glucosaminoglycans (GAGs), and Tamm-Horsfall glycoprotein (THG) was significantly higher in PCE-exposed workers than in control subjects. In these PCE-exposed subjects, high molecular weight proteinuria (glomerular dysfunction marker) was frequently associated with markers of tubular dysfunction.

These results were interpreted as suggesting diffuse structural and functional renal changes, possibly resulting from generalized membrane disturbances. They were thought not to support the hypothesis of immunologically mediated renal abnormalities, although in susceptible individuals peak exposures could lead to autoimmune glomerular disease. Subtle diffuse abnormalities detected in PCE-exposed workers may represent an early stage of clinically silent but potentially progressive renal disease.

### Carbon Disulfide

Long-term low-level exposure to carbon disulfide ($CS_2$) has been associated with an atherosclerosis-potentiating effect (see Chap. 28). Increased incidence of ischemic heart disease, cerebral atherosclerosis ("sulfocarbonic encephalopathy"), and vascular chronic nephropathy have been found in workers with long-term exposure. Reduced concentrating capacity is the most frequently described renal functional abnormality.

## Occupational Exposure and Cancer of the Kidney and Urinary Tract

### Renal Cancer

The possible work-relatedness of primary renal cancer has not been adequately explored. Increased numbers of deaths from primary renal tumors have been reported among workers in the petroleum industry as well as in steelworkers exposed to coke oven emissions. Two case reports of renal cancer in lead workers have been noted. Lead has been shown to produce renal tumors in three species of experimental animals.

### Urinary Bladder and Urinary Tract Cancer

In the United States, the annual incidence of cancer of the bladder is 49,000 cases, and each year approximately 10,000 persons die of this neoplasm. Over the last decades incidence of bladder cancer in the United States rose 22 to 38 percent, varying with race and gender. Increases in incidence were more marked in the 1970s than in the 1980s, but during the same period mortality fell 16 to 23 percent. The observed increase in incidence may be, in part, due to earlier diagnosis; "carcinoma in situ" increased from less than 1 percent in 1969 to over 7 percent in the 1980s [35, 36].

Occupationally induced bladder cancer was first reported in 1895 among workers in Germany employed in the manufacture of synthetic aniline dyes. Subsequently, occupational bladder cancer spread worldwide following the international spread of the synthetic dyestuffs industry. The first cases of work-related bladder cancer in American chemical workers were reported in 1934.

Epidemiologic studies have identified about 40 high-risk occupations; strong evidence of increased risk is well documented for dye workers, aromatic amines manufacturing workers, leather workers, rubber workers, painters, truck drivers, and aluminum workers [37].

A large case-control study of over 2,200 bladder cancer cases and over 4,000 controls was conducted during the National Bladder Cancer Study in 10 areas of the United States. It was estimated that 21 to 25 percent of bladder cancer is attributable to occupational exposures in white men and a slightly higher proportion, 27 percent, in black men [37, 38].

The *aromatic amines* are the chemical compounds responsible for bladder cancer in dye workers. Carcinogenic aromatic amines initially identified as human carcinogens include benzidine, beta-naphthylamine, and 4-aminobiphenyl. In some occupationally exposed groups, a very high total mortality from bladder cancer has been reported.

Exposure to aromatic amines occurs in textile, fur, and leather dyeing. Workers in those trades have been shown to absorb synthetic dyes such as Direct Black 38, Direct Brown 95, and Direct Blue 6. Azo dyes have been shown to be metabolized to benzidine and to thus increase the risk of bladder cancer in these workers [39]. An unusually high mortality from bladder cancer in Mataro County, Spain, was linked to employment in the textile industry, especially in dyeing and printing using azo dyes [40].

An excess risk of bladder cancer in painters has been repeatedly reported. The possible role of ben-zidine-based azo dyes was emphasized in a recent report from Germany [41].

Aromatic amines are used also as antioxidants in rubber, and exposure to carcinogenic amines has been reported in rubber and cable manufacture. 4,4'-Methylene-bis-2-chloroaniline (MBOCA), an aromatic amine, is used as a stabilizer in plastics manufacture. MBOCA is an animal carcinogen, and cases of bladder cancer have recently been reported among workers in Michigan occupationally exposed to MBOCA [42]; it is now a confirmed human carcinogen.

The aromatic amine orthotoluidine (3,3'-dimethylbenzidine) has been shown, in recent epidemiologic studies, to be a human bladder carcinogen [42]. Two earlier epidemiologic studies had suggested it might be a human carcinogen and it was recognized as a carcinogen in animals.

Exposure to 4-chloro-*o*-toluidine was recently reported to have resulted in highly increased incidence (8 cases versus 0.11 expected) of urothelial carcinomas [43]. This compound had been shown to be genotoxic and carcinogenic in rodents, but no epidemiologic evidence of its human carcinogenicity had been available before 1988. It has been used in the manufacture of dyestuffs and pigments, and also of chlordimeform, an ascaricide and insecticide.

4,4'-Methylene-dianiline, an animal carcinogen, used as a curing agent for resins, is a probable human carcinogen.

The lag time between onset of occupational exposure to aromatic amines and bladder cancer ranges from 4 to over 40 years, with a mean of about 20 years. The minimum duration of exposure necessary to produce cancer is reported to be as short as 133 days.

Although the risk of bladder cancer from aromatic amines has been reduced, due to protective measures, mostly after the banning of beta-naphtylamine and benzidine in most industrialized countries, it has not been eliminated. Numerous reports of aromatic amine–induced bladder cancer continue to reveal the persistence of this hazard in countries such as China [44], Japan, Russia, and Poland. The long latency period for the development of aromatic-amine–induced bladder cancer is a factor that contributes to the persistence of risk in occupational groups with past exposure.

*Soots, tars,* and *polycyclic aromatic hydrocarbons* including *benzo-a-pyrene,* have been shown to cause bladder cancer. Elevated risks of bladder cancer have been reported in creosote manufacture (creosote is a tar-based wood preservative). The increased risk of bladder cancer in truck, bus, and cab drivers is thought to be related to polycyclic aromatic hydrocarbons (PAHs) present in motor exhaust. Exposure to PAHs seems also to be the causative agent for the increased bladder cancer risk of aluminum workers [45]; coal tar pitch could also produce aromatic amines. Coke plant workers and gas workers have similar exposures. Lubricating oils and coolants in metal machining processes contain some PAHs and nitrosamines; an increased risk of bladder cancer has been reported in metal workers.

Cigarette smoking has been shown to cause bladder cancer. Orthotoluidine and aniline are present in mainstream and sidestream cigarette smoke. They may play a role in the known excess risk of bladder cancer in smokers. A multiplicative interaction may exist between occupational exposure to aromatic amines and cigarette smoking in the causation of bladder cancer [46].

Previously, bladder cancers resulting from occupational exposures were considered indistinguishable from nonoccupationally related bladder cancers. However, it is now recognized that occupationally related bladder cancers differ in that they occur 15 years earlier on average than similar tumors in the general population. Also, occupationally induced malignancies appear more frequently to be preceded by carcinoma in situ.

There is some evidence that chemical carcinogens favor the development of the invasive, high-grade form of bladder cancer [47].

Although occupational and environmental carcinogens are major risk factors for urinary blad-

der cancer, variations in individual susceptibility have been recognized also to influence the outcome.

The critical role of hepatic mono-oxygenases in carcinogen metabolism and the possibility of genetic polymorphism in humans have been of considerable interest in recent years. Differences in metabolic activation of carcinogens are also related to differences in enzyme induction. Carcinogenic aromatic amines undergo hepatic microsomal N-hydroxylation that leads to the formation of highly reactive and mutagenic N-OH derivatives. Further oxidation yields nitrosamines.

Human liver microsomal preparations have been found to vary tenfold in their N-oxidation activity [48, 49].

Human liver-bound N-acetyltransferase plays a significant role in the metabolic detoxification of N-substituted aryl compounds. Rates of acetylation vary considerably between individuals, who can be categorized as being fast and slow acetylators. Heterogeneity is genetically controlled by two alleles at a single autosomal locus; rapid acetylation is dominant.

Dye manufacturing workers with bladder cancer were found to be slow acetylators in 22 of 23 cases [50]. The proportion of slow acetylators is higher in patients with bladder cancer who have had past exposure to aryl amines than in patients without such exposure. Acetylator status seems to have an influence on individual susceptibility to development of bladder cancer after exposure to aromatic amines [51].

Early detection is critically important in reducing morbidity and mortality from bladder cancer. Screening methods have generally relied on testing for hematuria (repeatedly, because hematuria is intermittent), using microscopic evaluation or dipstick assessment of hemoglobin in urine [52], in combination with cytology of the urinary sediment (Papanicolaou test).

Although the efficacy of early detection in curing and prolonging life of patients with bladder cancer has not yet been fully assessed, currently available data suggest that early detection may be lifesaving [46]. A positive finding of occult blood or abnormal urine cytology demands immediate cytoscopic examination.

In recent years, there has been considerable progress in the detection of premalignant changes at the cellular level and in the development of new markers for the detection of cancer at its earliest stages. Abnormal DNA ploidy is known to be characteristic of many cancer cells. Flow cytometry uses quantitative fluorescence to analyze DNA in single cells in urine; increases in DNA content signal malignant transformation. Quantitative fluorescence image analysis (QFIA) combines morphologic characterization of individual cells with DNA fluorescence measurement [53].

The possibility for quantitation of multiple tumor markers is currently being investigated. Monoclonal antibodies to tumor-associated antigens have been developed [54]. F-actin (a cytoskeletal marker of differentiation), tumor cell collagenase-stimulating factor (TCSF), urinary autocrine motility factor (uAMF), and human epithelial membrane antigen have been found to be potentially useful urine markers for bladder cancer [55].

Hemoglobin adducts with aromatic amines have been proposed as biologic markers; differences in DNA adduct formation between bladder tissue cultures obtained from different individuals are known to exist. DNA repair takes place after adduct formation and wide interindividual variation has been noted in tissue cultures. Excised DNA can be identified in the urine.

Some ongoing screening programs of workers with past exposure to aromatic amines have incorporated testing for such recently developed markers of malignant transformation [53, 55, 56]. This will allow evaluation of sensitivity and specificity of the individual tests and lead to recommendations for use in screening programs for the early detection of bladder cancer due to occupational chemical exposures.

## Occupational Urinary Tract Disease Resulting from Neurologic Impairment

Because the lower urinary tract is closely controlled by the autonomic nervous system, neurologic dysfunction may result in urinary tract disease. Urinary tract disease of neurologic origin is exemplified by the reported episodes of bladder paralysis in workers occupationally exposed to dimethylaminopropionitrile (DMAPN) (see Chap. 26).

## Diagnosis and Management

A thorough exposure history is an essential prerequisite to early detection and correct diagnosis of early renal and urinary tract effects due to occupational or environmental hazards. It is very important that health care providers be aware of patients' current and past occupational and environmental exposures (usual as well as accidental) and of the potentially toxic effects of those exposures, including nephrotoxic effects.

Acute nephropathy due either to direct toxicity or secondary to sudden renal ischemia always represents a serious medical emergency. It requires prompt diagnosis, intensive monitoring, and appropriate medical care. Hospital admission is an absolute necessity, since the possibility of rapidly developing acute renal failure exists. The most aggressive approach, including dialysis, might be necessary under such circumstances, and rapid intervention is crucial for a favorable outcome. In cases of severe overexposure to agents known to have potential for acute nephrotoxicity (such as metals, halogenated hydrocarbons, arsine, dioxan, ethylene glycol, or methyl alcohol), monitoring of urinary output is essential; proteinuria and, less often, hematuria are also significant alarm signals, as are rapid increases in serum creatinine, BUN, or potassium. The clinical picture is often complicated by simultaneous toxic effects on other organ systems, principally the CNS and the liver. Hemolysis is a major effect in arsine, stibine, or phosphine poisoning, and a sudden fall in the red blood cell count and hematocrit, together with increases in serum bilirubin and hemoglobin, are indicative of acute hemolysis.

Medical management of acute nephropathies caused by occupational or environmental agents is similar to that for acute severe nephropathies of other etiology. Discontinuing the hazardous exposure and, when possible, reducing the body burden of chemical toxins are the only specific components in the management of such cases. Chelation therapy, which is effective in some metal poisonings, for example, those due to lead, mercury, and arsenic, can rarely be used in the presence of nephrotoxicity, since most chelating agents can be nephrotoxic in large doses and could therefore compound the renal damage.

Documentation of increased urinary excretion or blood level of metals (lead, cadmium, mercury, and arsenic in the case of arsine) can significantly contribute to correct etiologic diagnosis. For acute nephropathies due to agents with a shorter half-life, identification of the etiologic agent can sometimes be made by exhaled breath analysis (for volatile solvents) soon after the accident or by detection of specific metabolites in blood or urine, or both, in the days following exposure. For example, oxalic acid is excreted in increased amounts in ethylene glycol poisoning; formic acid can be found in methyl alcohol poisoning.

### Early Detection and Prevention

The recent development of sensitive tests of renal dysfunction permits earlier detection than previously was possible of nephrotoxic effects due to long-term exposure to chemical compounds. Increased excretion of high molecular weight proteins, mainly albumin, is an early indicator of glomerular dysfunction. Still under development are tests for the detection of glomerular basement membrane antigens in blood and urine or of circulating antibodies against glomerular basement membrane for monitoring of workers exposed to chemical compounds (for example, solvents) that may produce an immune-type glomerular dysfunction. Increased excretion of low molecular weight proteins, such as $\beta_2$-microglobulin and RBP, is a sensitive indicator for proximal tubular dysfunction. These tests have been particularly useful in the detection of chronic cadmium nephropathy.

Increased urinary enzyme excretion, due to proximal tubular cell injury, is a sensitive test for early detection of nephrotoxicity; an assay for NAG has been most widely used in evaluation of renal injury following exposure to mercury, halogenated hydrocarbons, and cadmium. Tests for other urinary enzymes are still also added to the currently used tests for early detection of nephrotoxicity. Decrease in concentrating capacity, reduction in GFR, and increase in serum creatinine and BUN are found in more advanced cases of chronic toxic nephropathies and can be used to assess the extent of functional loss.

Prevention of occupational nephropathy relies on maintaining exposure to potentially nephrotoxic agents at levels well below hazardous limits; a safety margin is important, especially for agents for which information on a no-effect level is not yet available. Special caution is necessary for agents that have been shown to be nephrotoxic or carcinogenic in animal studies but for which no human data are yet available.

## References

1. Sugimoto T, Rosansky SJ. The incidence of treated end stage renal disease in the eastern United States: 1973–1979. Am J Public Health 1984; 74:14–7.
2. Landrigan PJ, et al. The work-relatedness of renal disease. Arch Environ Health 1984; 39:225–30.
3. Hook JB. ed. Toxicology of the kidney. New York: Raven, 1981.
4. Meyer BR, et al. Increased urinary enzyme excretion in workers exposed to nephrotoxic chemicals. Am J Med 1984; 76:989–98.
5. Bluhm RE, et al. Elemental mercury vapour toxicity, treatment, and prognosis after acute, intensive exposure in chloralkali plant workers. Part 11: Hy-

perchloraemia and genitourinary symptoms. Hum Exp Toxicol 1992; 11:211–5.

6. Goyer RA, et al. Lead dosage and the role of the intranuclear inclusion body. Arch Environ Health 1970; 20:705–11.

7. Lilis R, et al. Nephropathy in chronic lead poisoning. Br J Ind Med 1968; 25:196–202.

8. Lilis R, et al. Renal function impairment in secondary lead smelter workers: Correlations with zinc protoporphyrin and blood lead levels. J Environ Pathol Toxicol 1979; 2:1447–74.

9. Wedeen RP, et al. Occupational lead nephropathy. Am J Med 1975; 59:630–41.

10. Lilis R, et al. Kidney function and lead: Relationships in several occupational groups with different levels of exposure. Am J Ind Med 1980; 1:405–12.

11. Bernard A, Lauwerys R. Epidemiological application of early markers of nephrotoxicity. Toxicol Lett 1989; 46:293–306.

12. Mutti A, et al. Urinary excretion of brush-border antigen revealed by monoclonal antibody: Early indicator of toxic nephropathy. Lancet 1985; 26: 914–7.

13. Fowler BA, DuVal G. Effects of lead on the kidney: Roles of high-affinity lead-binding proteins. Environ Health Perspec 1991; 91:77–80.

14. Gourrier E, Lamour C, Feldmann D, Bensman A. Atteinte tubulaire precoce dans l'intoxication par le plomb chez l'enfant. Arch Fr Pediatr 1991; 48: 685–9.

15. Selevan SG, Landrigan PJ, Stern FG, Jones IH. Mortality of lead smelter workers. Am J Epidemiol 1985; 122:673–83.

16. Farhad KM, et al. Experimental model of lead nephropathy. II. Effect of removal from lead exposure and chelation treatment with dimercaptosuccinic acid (DMSA). Environ Res 1992; 58:35–54.

17. Van de Vyver FL, Wedeen RP, De Broe ME. Bone lead in dialysis patients. Kidney Int 1988; 33: 601–7.

18. Landrigan P. Strategies for epidemiologic studies of lead in bone in occupationally exposed populations. Environ Health Perspect 1991; 91:81–6.

19. Roels H, et al. Evolution of cadmium-induced renal dysfunction in workers removed from exposure. Scand J Work Environ Health 1982; 8:191–200.

20. Bernard AM, Roels H, Cardenas A, Lauwerys R. Assessment of urinary protein 1 and transferrin as early markers of cadmium nephrotoxicity. Br J Ind Med 1990; 47:559–65.

21. Mueller PW, Smith SJ, Steinberg KK, Thun MJ. Chronic renal tubular effects in relation to urine cadmium levels. Nephron 1989; 52:45–54.

22. Roels H, et al. A prospective study of proteinuria in cadmium workers. In PH Bach, EA Lock, eds. Nephrotoxicity: In vitro to in vivo, animals to man. New York: Plenum, 1987, pp. 33–36.

23. Mason HJ, et al. Relations between liver cadmium, cumulative exposure, and renal function in cadmium alloy workers. Br J Ind Med 1988; 45:793–802.

24. Thun MJ, et al. Nephropathy in cadmium workers: Assessment of risk from airborne occupational exposure to cadmium. Br J Ind Med 1989; 46:689–97.

25. Chia KS, Ong CN, Ong HY, Endo G. Renal tubular function of workers exposed to low levels of cadmium. Br J Ind Med 1989; 46:165–70.

26. Mueller PW, et al. Chronic renal effects in three studies of men and women occupationally exposed to cadmium. Arch Environ Contam Toxicol 1992; 23:125–36.

27. Lauwerys R, et al. Health effects of environmental exposure to cadmium: Objectives, design and organization of the Cadmibel study: A cross-sectional morbidity study carried out in Belgium from 1985 to 1989. Environ Health Perspect 1990; 87:283–89.

28. Su Lu, Fu-Yao Zhao. Nephrotoxic limit and annual limit on intake for natural U. Health Phy 1990; 58:619–23.

29. Churchill DN, Fine A, Gault MH. Association between hydrocarbon exposure and glomerulo-nephritis. An appraisal of the evidence. Nephron 1983; 33:169–72.

30. Nelson NA, Robins TG, Port FK. Solvent nephrotoxicity in humans and experimental animals. Am J Nephrol 1990; 10:10–20.

31. Viau C, et al. A cross-sectional survey of kidney function in refinery employees. Am J Ind Med 1987; 11:177–87.

32. Vyskocil A, et al. Urinary excretion of proteins and enzymes in workers exposed to hydrocarbons in a shoe factory. Int Arch Occup Environ Health 1991; 63:359–62.

33. Ng TP, et al. Urinary levels of proteins and metabolites in workers exposed to toluene. Int Arch Occup Environ Health 1990; 62:43–6.

34. Mutti A, et al. Nephropathies and exposure to perchloroethylene in dry cleaners. Lancet 1992; 340:189–93.

35. Matanowski GM, Elliot EA. Bladder cancer epidemiology. Epidemiol Rev 1981; 3:203–29.

36. Silverman DT, Hartge P, Morrison AS, Devesa SS. Epidemiology of bladder cancer. Hematol/Oncol Clin North Am 1992; 6:1–29.

37. Silverman DT, Levin LL, Hoover RN, et al. Occu-

pational risks of bladder cancer in the United States: 1. White men. J Natl Cancer Inst 1989; 81:1472–80.

38. Silverman DT, Levin LL, Hoover RN. Occupational risks of bladder cancer in the United States: 11. Non-white men. J Natl Cancer Inst 1989; 81:1480–3.

39. Lynn RK, et al. Metabolism of bisazobiphenyl dyes derived from benzidine, 3,3'-dimethylbenzidine or 3,3'-dimethoxybenzidine to carcinogenic aromatic amines in the dog and rat. Toxicol Appl Pharmacol 1980; 56:248–58.

40. Gonzales CA, Riboli E, Lopez-Abente G. Bladder cancer among workers in the textile industry: Results of a Spanish case-control study. Am J Ind Med 1988; 14:673–80.

41. Myslak ZW, Bolt HM, Brockmann W. Tumors of the urinary bladder in painters: A case-control study. Am J Ind Med 1991; 19:705–13.

42. Ward E, et al. Excess number of bladder cancers in workers exposed to orthotoluidine and aniline. J Natl Cancer Inst 1991; 83:501–6.

43. Stasik MJ. Carcinomas of the urinary bladder in a 4-chloro-o-toluidine cohort. Int Arch Occup Environ Health 1988; 60:21–4.

44. Xue-Yun Y, Ji-Gang C, Yong-Ning H. Studies on the relation between bladder cancer and benzidine or its derived dyes in Shanghai. Br J Ind Med 1990; 47:544–52.

45. Theriault GP, Tremblay CG, Armstrong BG. Bladder cancer screening among primary aluminum production workers in Quebec. J Occup Medicine 1990; 32:869–72.

46. Schulte PA, Ringen K, Hemstreet GP. Optimal management of asymptomatic workers at high risk of bladder cancer. J Occup Med 1986; 28:13–7.

47. Cartwright RA, et al. The influence of malignant cell cytology on the survival of industrial bladder cancer cases. J Epidemiol Community Health 1981; 35:35–8.

48. Vineis P, Caporaso N. Applications of biochemical epidemiology in the study of human carcinogenesis. Tumori 1988; 74:19–26.

49. Harris CC, Autrup H, Vahakangas K, Trump BG. Interindividual variation in carcinogen activation and DNA repair. Banbury Report no. 16:145–53, Cold Spring Harbor, 1984.

50. Cartwright RA, Glashan RW, Rogers HJ. Role of N-acetyl-transferase phenotypes in bladder carcinogenesis: A pharmacogenetic epidemiological approach to bladder cancer. Lancet 1982; 2:842–5.

51. Hanke J, Krajewska B. Acetylation phenotypes and bladder cancer. J Occup Med 1990; 32:917–8.

52. Messing EM, Vaillancourt A. Hematuria screening for bladder cancer. J Occup Med 1990; 32:838–45.

53. Hemstreet GP, Hurst RE, Bass RA, Rao JY. Quantitative fluorescence image analysis in bladder cancer screening. J Occup Med 1990; 32:822–8.

54. Guirguis R, et al. A new method for evaluation of urinary autocrine motility factor and tumor cell collagenase stimulating factor as markers for urinary tract cancers. J Occup Med 1990; 32:846–53.

55. Mason TJ, Vogler WJ. Bladder cancer screening at the DuPont Chambers Works: A new initiative. J Occup Med 1990; 32:874–7.

56. Marsh GM, et al. A protocol for bladder cancer screening and medical surveillance among high-risk groups: The Drake Health Registry experience. J Occup Med 1990; 32:881–6.

## Bibliography

Fowler BA. ed. Biological and environmental effects of arsenic. Amsterdam: Elsevier, 1983.
*This monograph is an excellent source of detailed information on the severe nephrotoxic effects of arsine.*

Friberg L, Nordberg GF, Vouk VB. eds. Handbook on the toxicology of metals. 2nd ed. Amsterdam: Elsevier, 1986. Vols. 1 and 2.
*Of particular interest is the chapter on cadmium, written by the world's most prominent experts on cadmium nephropathy, who first described the condition in the 1950s. There is also valuable information on nephrotoxicity of mercury and uranium.*

Hook IB. ed. Toxicology of the kidney. New York: Raven, 1981.
*An excellent book on renal toxicology. The use of renal function tests in the evaluation of nephrotoxic effects, including renal clearance and use of enzymuria assessment, is important for state-of-the-art evaluation of subclinical renal toxicity. A chapter on renal handling of environmental chemicals is very informative. The discussion of nephrotoxicity of low molecular weight alkane solvents, pesticides, and chemical intermediates includes valuable information on high-volume chemicals such as ethylene dibromide, ethylene dichloride, perchloroethylene, trichloroethane, and others.*

Landrigan PJ, et al. The work-relatedness of renal disease. Arch Environ Health 1984; 39:225–30.
*A review addressing the important issue of the largely unknown etiology (in most cases) of chronic renal disease; the possibility that occupational factors might make a larger contribution than currently recognized is considered. Methods for diagnosis of subclinical*

*nephrotoxicity, epidemiologic studies of populations exposed to compounds that have been shown to be nephrotoxic in animal experiments, as well as several other strategies, are proposed for the more complete assessment of the contribution of occupational exposures to chronic renal disease.*

Lauwerys RR, Bernard A. Early detection of nephrotoxic effects of industrial chemicals. State of the art and future prospects. Am J Ind Med 1987; 11:275–85.

*This paper discusses several tests that may permit the early detection of renal changes induced by long-term exposure to nephrotoxic industrial chemicals and may possibly serve as advance warning of pending renal damage. Some tests mainly attempt to assess the integrity of the glomerulus: high molecular weight proteinuria, glomerular basement membrane (GBM) antigens in blood and in urine, circulating anti-GBM antibodies, glomerular filtration rate after an acute oral load of proteins, and estimation of membrane negative charges (that is, glomerular polyanion). Others mainly attempt to identify functional and morphologic changes at the tubular level: low molecular weight proteinuria, aminoaciduria, glycosuria, hyperphosphaturia, hypercalciuria, enzymuria, tubular antigen excretion, kallikrein, and prostaglandin excretion. Some of these tests are already routinely used, although controversy may still persist with regard to their clinical significance. Recently, new tests have been developed that may open new perspectives for assessing the significance of the early renal changes induced by chemicals.*

Singhal RL, Thomas IA. Lead toxicity. Baltimore: Urban & Schwarzenberg, 1980.

*An excellent chapter is dedicated to a thorough review of lead nephrotoxicity. Early effects are well described as are the results of chronic low-level exposure and absorption. Pathologic changes are presented in great detail. This is based on the personal experiences of the authors.*

# V
# Selected Groups of Workers

# 32
# Women and Work

Margaret M. Quinn, Susan R. Woskie, and Beth J. Rosenberg

Women in the manufacturing industries, in the service sector, and in office work often report different health hazards and symptoms than men in these same workplaces. The fact that many job assignments are gender-based can explain much of this difference [1] and is the result of a complex web of social and economic factors that lead men and women into different occupations.

Since social and economic factors also determine many important aspects of an individual's work experience (such as income, the likelihood of being employed and remaining employed, opportunities for job advancement, and authority in workplace decisions), a woman who does the same job or a comparable job as a man is likely to have a different experience. The most well-documented manifestation of this difference is in wages. Despite a rhetoric of equality, as of 1991, women in the United States, in general, were earning 70 cents to every dollar earned by a man and the gap widens as one goes up the career ladder. For minority women, the gap is a lot greater; for example, African-American women and Latinas earn only 50 percent of white men's pay (Fig. 32-1).

Women who work outside of the home still do most of the household work in their homes as well. Added to the pressures of long hours of work inside and outside the home are the time conflicts that emerge when one is both homemaker—and usually family caretaker—and a wage earner. Sick children, school holidays, and ill elderly relatives all contribute to the challenges, in the context of inadequate social services and employer supports for working women. Additional problems include inflexible work schedules and the lack of good-quality, accessible, and affordable child and elder care. While the restructuring of work to include more part-time and "temporary" work has had some advantages for women, there are serious drawbacks as well. Part-time and temporary workers earn substantially less and have fewer employee benefits than their full-time counterparts; they are seldom thought to be as serious or dedicated to their work as those working full-time and therefore their job advancement is delayed. Finally, many working women are exposed to stresses and hazards particular to women in jobs and industries that have traditionally hired only men.

There were more than 54 million working women in the United States in 1993, comprising 45 percent of the entire U.S. workforce and 57 percent of all women 16 years of age and older. The number of wage-earning women has been steadily increasing since 1900 and this increase is expected to continue. Women are moving into heavy industrial jobs (Fig. 32-2), the building trades, and professional fields in small, but increasing, numbers. The number of families maintained by women grew by almost 90 percent between 1970 and 1985. In 1993 women headed 12 million families in the U.S. The percentage of families headed by black women has grown dramatically, more than doubling between 1970 and 1993. In 1993, 48 percent of all black families were headed by women compared with 25 percent of Latino families and 14 percent of white families. Over half of

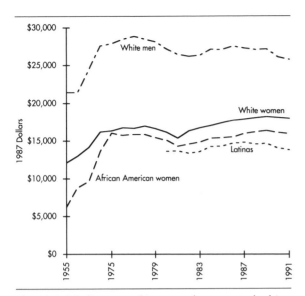

**Fig. 32-1.** Median annual income of women and white men, full-time year-round workers, 1955–1991 (in 1987 dollars). (From T Amott, *Caught in the crisis: Women and the U.S. economy today,* New York: Monthly Review Press, 1993.)

children in families with a female head of household lived below the poverty level. Over two-thirds of black and Latino children whose mothers supported them lived in poverty, primarily because black and Latino women maintaining families had lower median earnings, lower median ages, and higher unemployment rates than white women maintaining families.

## Sources of Occupational Stress

Stress can be defined as a physical or psychological stimulus that produces strain or disruption of the individual's normal physiologic equilibrium. Men and women may experience a wide range of stress reactions, including adverse health effects (see Chap. 19).

### Problems of Multiple Roles

As the distinction fades between women who marry and have families and women who work,

the major challenge of managing both aspects of life simultaneously emerges. Even though women frequently work outside the home for as many hours as their spouses, domestic duties are rarely shared equally. "A woman's work is never done" may be truer than ever. Working mothers sleep less, get sick more, and have less leisure time than their husbands [2]. Many working women, when interviewed by researchers, focus on sleep, how little they could survive on, and which of their friends needed how much sleep—and then they apologized for the amount that they needed. One researcher concluded: "These women talked about sleep the way a hungry person talks about food" [2].

Based on studies of time use that were done in the 1960s and 1970s, it was estimated that employed mothers worked approximately 15 hours longer each week than working fathers—which translates, over a year, to an extra month of 24-hour days! One study found that women who are employed full-time outside the home and whose youngest child is less than five years old spend an average of 47 hours a week on household work, while their male counterparts spend 10 hours per week [3]. Another study found that the average working woman works an estimated 80 hours a week in and outside the home and up to 105 hours if she has sole responsibility for children [4]. Although the situation may have improved somewhat over the last 10 years in the U.S., the stress and fatigue from balancing work life and home life remains a serious problem for women and their partners.

### The Structure of Women's Work: Part-Time, Temporary, and Home Work

In response to the shrinking economic pie of the 1980s, employers are increasingly using part-time and temporary workers ("temps," or contract workers). Often, this arrangement provides the desired flexibility in working hours. There are costs, however. The average part-time worker earns only 60 percent as much as a full-time worker on an hourly basis. Not only are they paid less, but their

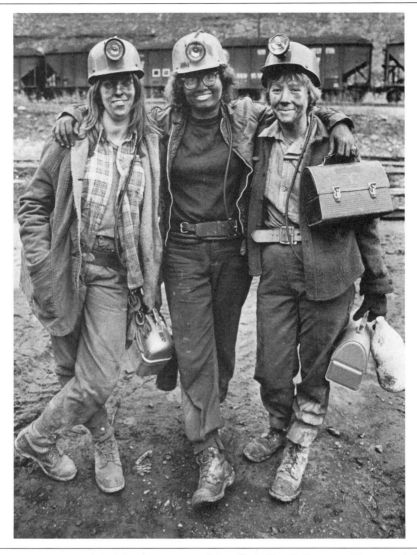

**Fig. 32-2.** Many women now work in jobs that were traditionally held only by men. (Photograph by Earl Dotter.)

benefits, such as health insurance, pensions, paid sick leave, and vacation, are substantially less than those of full-time workers. Fewer than 25 percent of part-timers have employer-paid health insurance, compared to nearly 80 percent of full-time workers. Sixty percent of full-time workers have pensions, while only 25 percent of part-timers have this coverage. In 1990 in the United States, there were nearly 5 million part-time workers who preferred to be employed full-time. Women make up more than two-thirds of all part-time workers in the U.S. and over half of them work less than full time, contrary to their wishes [5].

In addition "temps" often live with the stress of not knowing when they will be working. They also tend to work more overtime because they are often hired for "crunch periods" when intense work needs to be done to meet a deadline. Neither part-time workers nor temps "receive equal protection under government laws, including occupational safety and health regulations, unemployment insurance, and pension regulations. Few are represented by labor unions" [5]. A case study commissioned by the Occupational Safety and Health Administration (OSHA) of contract labor in the petrochemical industry showed that contract workers get less health and safety training and have higher injury rates than noncontract workers [6].

Another cost-cutting measure affecting women is the rise in home-based work—work to be done in workers' homes. In 1949 Congress passed a law making industrial home work illegal since it was so difficult to enforce labor standards, such as the minimum wage in home work. The Reagan administration made it legal again, which caused a growth in this type of work in the 1980s [5]. Typical female homeworkers are garment workers, clerical workers, independent contract workers, and entrepreneurs. Home garment workers and some clerical workers are usually paid not at hourly rates but rather by piece rates. Piece-rate payments lead to increased speed of performance of job tasks, long hours, and, combined with a repetitive and/or sustained posture, a high rate of injuries, many of which are due to poor workplace or workstation design.

Homeworkers also face hazardous chemical exposures. For example, in semiconductor manufacturing home work, workers and their family members are exposed to hazardous chemicals, which can also contaminate residential sewage systems. Trade unions, which have played a major role in improving working conditions, are weakened with home work because workers are isolated from each other.

## Discrimination

Racial, gender, and age discrimination all contribute to the stress experienced by working women (see also Chap. 33). These types of discrimination take many forms and affect women in economic terms (lower pay than men who do comparable work), social terms (alienation from supervisors and coworkers), and personal terms (low self-esteem and reduced creative growth). Women who work in occupations in which most workers are male are often seen as unwelcome intruders and many experience gender harassment. These working women may also feel excessive pressure to perform faultlessly to prove that they are good enough. These experiences, which are likely to be even more extreme for women who are part of racial or ethnic minorities, can have serious consequences for health and safety.

## Sexual Harassment

Women are the predominant targets of sexual harassment at work. Any unwanted verbal or physical sexual advance constitutes harassment, which can range from sexual comments and suggestions, to pressure for sexual favors accompanied by threats concerning one's job, to physical assault, including rape. Studies indicate that 40 to 80 percent of women have experienced some form of sexual harassment at work [7]. In a study of more than 500 cases of sexual harassment, 46 percent of the women said that it interfered with their work performance and 36 percent reported physical ailments that they associated with the harassment, including nausea, vomiting, depression, headaches, and drastic weight change [8] (see box on p. 623).

Sexual harassment is not only harmful to women's health, but it is also costly to business in terms of job turnover, sick time, impaired productivity, and the cost of legal claims. It was estimated that in 1988 the U.S. Government spent $189 million on the cost of sexual harassment. Almost one-third of the 500 largest U.S. companies spend $6.7 million a year because of this problem [7].

## Job Control

When the Framingham Heart Study examined the relationship between employment status and the incidence of coronary heart disease, it found that

## SEXUAL HARASSMENT ON THE JOB
Cathy Schwartz

### What Is It?
Sexual harassment is any unwanted verbal or physical sexual advance, ranging from sexual comments and suggestions, to pressure for sexual favors accompanied by threats (outright or subtle) concerning one's job, to physical assault including rape.

### How Widespread Is It?
Studies indicate that from 42 to 85 percent of working women report having been sexually harassed on the job.

### What Are the Effects of Sexual Harassment?
Psychological trauma and stress-related physical symptoms are the effects of sexual harassment. Both types of effects are compounded if the woman's job is in jeopardy, if she is forced to resign, or if she is fired as a result of the harassment situation.

### What Can Be Done?
Sexual harassment is illegal. It is a violation of rights under Title VII of the Civil Rights Act and of many state fair employment practice laws. A woman who is fired or resigns as a result of a harassment situation may be entitled to unemployment compensation. Organized protest against managers for sexual harassment is protected activity under the National Labor Relations Act.

### Getting Help
A woman can seek help from her union, coworkers, and local women's organizations. Talking to other people and getting assistance can help the woman feel less isolated and frustrated and is probably necessary to effectively deal with the situation. It may be necessary to seek legal help and to go to a local or state agency that deals with fair employment practices or the closest office of the federal Equal Employment Opportunity Commission (EEOC).

21 percent of female clerical workers develop coronary heart disease, a rate almost twice that of other nonclerical workers or housewives [3]. One study examined the widely held opinion that certain individuals are more prone to stress and that they are responsible for causing their own stress problems. Workers in typically female jobs were found to have much less control over decision making than those in typically male jobs. Female-dominated occupations, such as clerical work, electronics manufacturing, garment work, and poultry processing, are characterized by tedium, ergonomic hazards, and low job control. It may be the concentration of women in these jobs that accounts for the higher prevalence of stress-related disorders in women rather than their lack of ability to cope [8].

Recognizing the social, economic, and physical determinants of health effects related to occupational stressors—instead of focusing solely on personal pathology—is a first step in the complete and long-term management of stress-related problems. While many women may benefit from programs that provide individual coping and relaxation exercises, workplace stress management programs should also acknowledge the broader social and economic constraints that provide the context for the daily lives of working women (see Chap. 19).

## Ergonomic Hazards

Many workplaces are a haphazard layout of tools, machines, and workstations. Little thought is given to the fit of tools, the nature of the lifting tasks, or the fit of personal protective equipment (PPE) to the worker. This lack of thought results in injuries that could be prevented if basic guidelines for lifting and for job and tool design were used. Although these issues are not particular to women, this group often bears the brunt of poor workplace design because most tools, workstations, and PPE were manufactured for use by the "average" man.

Repetitive, forceful, and awkward motions have been associated with a number of occupational musculoskeletal disorders (see Chaps. 8 and 23). Neck, shoulder, and upper limb disorders (for example, cervicobrachial syndrome) have been associated with a number of jobs held largely by women, including keyboard operators of typewriters, telex, calculating machines, computers, and telephone exchangers; cash register operators; film roller and capper workers; cigarette rolling and packing workers; and scissors manufacture and assembly workers. Tenosynovitis has been reported among female assembly-line packers in a food production factory, female poultry-processing plant workers, and female scissors manufacture and assembly workers. Carpal tunnel syndrome (CTS) has been found among female garment workers, hotel cooks, maids, workers in the boning department of a poultry-processing plant, and cash register operators (including check-out counter workers who use bar-code readers). Packaging operations are particularly apt to produce musculoskeletal disorders because of the repetitive nature of the work.

Carpal tunnel syndrome has been reported to be 1.4 to 16.0 times more common in women than in men [9]. Hormonal changes following gynecologic surgery, especially hysterectomy with removal of the ovaries, have been related to increased risk of the disease [10]. Examination of CTS cases at one plant showed that workers in departments with repetitive-motion jobs had a very high risk of the disease while the risk attributed to gender, although elevated, was 20 times less than that attributed to having a job using repetitive motions [9]. Although women seem to be at a greater risk of developing CTS and related tendon disorders than

men, gender is probably less important than work pattern, segmental vibration, and hand stress. Since women are concentrated in jobs that require repetitive motions, such as bench assembly and small parts manufacturing, it is difficult to determine whether there are aspects of this disease that are solely related to gender.

Reduction of musculoskeletal injuries can be accomplished through careful consideration of the ergonomics of the work process. Improvements of tool and workstation design can contribute significantly to preventing musculoskeletal disorders (see Chaps. 8 and 23).

One company made improvements in the working conditions of cash register operators, including shortened operating time, development of a work-rotation system, and change from mechanical to electronic registers with lighter key touches. The result was a decrease in the workload on the arms and hands and a significant drop in complaints of pain, dullness, stiffness, or numbness in the hands, fingers, and arms [11].

When video display terminal (VDT) workers in an office were given an adjustable workstation that they could adapt to their preferred settings for a number of factors, including keyboard and screen height, viewing angle, and screen distance, they reported significantly fewer muscle complaints and significantly less impairment in the neck, shoulder, back, and wrist [12].

Heavy physical work is associated with low back pain (LBP). For example, among nurses and nurse's aides, those aged 20 to 29 who spent more time lifting had higher prevalence of LBP than those whose jobs did not require heavy lifting. This pain may also be related to child-bearing and child-rearing, which increase the load on the back even more [13]. Whereas only 5 percent of the women in light industry report ever having LBP lasting more than three days, 35 percent of the women in heavy industry report LBP. Only 7 percent of female office and postal clerks report LBP, compared to 17 percent of nurses. Low back pain is also common among working men (17 percent in nursing, 18 percent in light industry, and 19 percent in heavy industry), suggesting that much needs to be done to improve the ergonomic design of most jobs [14] (see box on p. 626).

## Problems with Personal Protective Equipment

Personal protective equipment should not be the primary method of controlling a worker's exposure to a workplace hazard, but it can be important in temporary situations, emergencies, or situations that cannot be controlled in other ways. However, for PPE to work, it must fit. In addition, PPE, such as gloves, that does not fit can increase the risk of accidents and increase the strength requirements for a task. For women, it is often difficult to find manufacturers who make equipment in women's sizes. Often small, medium, and large sizes of equipment are available, but even the small size is designed for small men, not small women. A survey of over 350 companies found that, in women's sizes, only 14 percent provided ear protection, 58 percent hand protection, 18 percent respirators, 14 percent head and face protection, 50 percent body protection, and 59 percent foot protection [15]. Many women end up purchasing men's PPE and try to modify it to fit, or they purchase women's equipment that is not up to safety standards. Until PPE is available in a variety of sizes for women, it may actually be contributing to the risk of workplace injuries.

## Reproductive Health Hazards

Occupational reproductive hazards are often viewed as a "woman's problem." As a result, the individual woman is left to bear the burden of the social, economic, and health consequences of reproductive hazards while the hazards faced by men are ignored. In fact, almost all occupational crises with documented adverse reproductive effects, such as exposure to dibromochloropropane (DBCP), chlordecone (Kepone), exogenous estrogens, and dimethylaminopropionitrile (DMAPN), have involved men (see Chap. 27). In situations in which men have been at risk, control of the hazard was achieved by elimination of the exposure. However, when even the potential for a reproductive health problem has existed for female workers, control of the "hazard" has often been achieved by eliminating women from the job, particularly if they are seeking a job in an industry that has not traditionally hired women. Both men and women will benefit if it is recognized that reproductive hazards may seriously compromise the health of all workers as well as the children they produce.

## The Pregnant Worker

Many organ system and musculoskeletal changes occur during pregnancy to accommodate the needs of the developing fetus. The most evident changes are modifications in cardiovascular, respiratory, and metabolic functions as well as shifts in the center of gravity associated with weight gain. These changes are normal and healthy, and may or may not affect a woman's ability to work. Pregnant women can usually continue to perform the physical activities to which they have been accustomed; however, pregnancy may not be the time to change to a new or unfamiliar level of work activity unless the woman undertakes a carefully supervised program of physical conditioning. Some medical conditions can be compromised by pregnancy; others predispose the pregnant woman to an increased likelihood of complications during pregnancy. The American Medical Association has developed guidelines for the continuation of various levels of work during pregnancy [16].

As with pregnancy, data about postpartum readiness to resume work are lacking. In 1977 the American College of Obstetricians and Gynecologists stated the following in their *Guidelines on Pregnancy and Work:* "The normal woman with

# THE STRENGTH OF WOMEN
Laura Punnett

## How Do Women Compare to Men?

Women's total body strength is, on average, about two-thirds that of men. However, the ratio of women's to men's static strength (ability to move a stationary weight) ranges from 35 to 85 percent, depending on the tasks and muscles involved. Women's average strength is closer to men's for static leg exertions and for certain dynamic lifting, pushing, and pulling activities.

Since muscle strength is greatest between the ages of 20 and 39, with a 20 percent decline by age 60, younger women and older men may have similar strength capabilities.

Despite these average differences, there is also substantial overlap in the strength distribution between men and women, as much as 50 percent or more for certain muscle groups. In fact, the factors of gender, age, weight, and height only explain about one-third of the variability in human strength data.

## Strength Testing

Evidence is inconclusive concerning the effectiveness of static strength testing to predict an individual's likelihood of injury. Worker selection based on general medical criteria is not effective in preventing musculoskeletal disorders. Although women are less strong than men on average, there is also no epidemiologic evidence that women suffer more work-related musculoskeletal injuries than men if they all perform the same task.

Strength testing may provide an alternative to blanket discrimination based on sex. Since there is a large overlap between the population distributions of the static strength abilities of men and women, selection of individuals able to lift a given weight will not exclude all prospective female employees. However, using this criterion may unnecessarily exclude persons who would not suffer injury. In addition, these tests do not measure endurance (aerobic capacity) or flexibility, both of which, on average, are greater in women than men, and which are protective against some aspects of strenuous work.

The best approach to eliminating musculoskeletal injuries from the workplace is the implementation of engineering controls. It has been estimated that the redesign of jobs to fit workers' capabilities could reduce injury rates by 67 percent.

## Pregnancy and Physical Exertion

The limited evidence available shows no change in muscle strength during pregnancy. Other studies indicate that a woman's aerobic capacity changes only in late pregnancy. However, it may be difficult to sustain high exertion levels if nausea or other health problems develop. Lifting capacity will be altered in later pregnancy as the center of gravity moves and as an increased body size prevents an object from being lifted close to the body. In addition, the ligaments and muscles of the back and abdomen are stretched, making lifting potentially more hazardous. There is evidence of increased risk of low back injury for pregnant women performing specific tasks such as heavy lifting, standing, and frequent climbing of stairs.

With regard to adverse pregnancy outcome, the epidemiologic evidence is still inconclusive. Heavy lifting, heavy industrial cleaning, and other strenuous exertions have been associated with spontaneous abortions, premature birth, and low birthweight. Long periods of standing at work appear to increase the risk of prematurity and low birthweight. These factors may also increase the frequency of uterine contraction during pregnancy. The effect of ergonomic stressors on the pregnancies of women working in the home has not been evaluated.

an uncomplicated pregnancy and a normal fetus in a job that presents no greater potential hazards than those encountered in normal daily life in the community may continue to work without interruption until the onset of labor and may resume working several weeks after an uncomplicated pregnancy" [17]. A woman's ability to work during pregnancy and return to work after pregnancy should be determined by the woman and her health care provider, considering the requirements of her job, her health status at the time she becomes pregnant, and her pregnancy experience.

### The First Trimester

During the first trimester, many women experience nausea and vomiting as well as fatigue and breast swelling and tenderness. There is a large increase in total blood volume, which results in an increased heart and metabolic rate. The ventilation rate begins to increase (from a nonpregnant average of 7 liters/min to an average of 10 liters/min by term). Glomerular filtration increases about 50 percent above the nonpregnant level.

These physiologic changes may affect a working woman in several ways. The vomiting and fatigue may decrease her capacity for work. Some women are particularly sensitive to bad odors that may increase their nausea. The increased metabolic rate raises body temperature, increasing sensitivity to hot and humid environments. The increased blood volume decreases the total percentage of red blood cells in the circulating blood and leads to an anemia, which is normal for a pregnant woman. However, it is especially important that a pregnant woman does not already have anemia caused by work factors, such as lead or benzene. Since the percentage of hemoglobin-carrying red blood cells is decreased, she will also be more vulnerable to environmental agents that interfere with the blood's ability to carry oxygen, such as carbon monoxide. The increased ventilation rate can result in increased absorption of any toxic materials in the air. Increased kidney function results in increased urination, making access to suitable bathroom facilities particularly important [17].

### The Second Trimester

While the body changes mentioned will persist throughout pregnancy, many of the symptoms will disappear and women often find they feel better during the second trimester. By the end of this period, there is a weight gain of approximately 7 kg (15 lb) and the uterus grows about 28 cm (11 in.) above the pelvis. As the uterus enlarges, its bulk tilts the body forward and the lower spine curves inward. The pelvic joints also become increasingly mobile. In addition to aggravation of any preexisting back problems, women often experience low back discomfort and stiffness. The change in the center of gravity may result in decreased ability to balance, and tolerance to physical exertion may vary widely. In general, women who are in good physical condition before pregnancy will have fewer problems and will be capable of greater exertion.

Along with these changes in body structure, there may be a greater tendency for the blood to pool in the legs. This can lead to dizziness and fainting with prolonged standing or working in hot environments, which increase the pooling. Varicose veins may also develop under these work conditions [17].

### The Third Trimester

During the third trimester, the uterus continues to enlarge and total body weight gain increases to an average of 11 kg (24 lb). Peripheral edema is common because there may be a decrease in venous return from the legs due to the pressure of the uterus on the pelvic veins. As the third trimester progresses, many women also experience increasing fatigue, insomnia, and shortness of breath. These symptoms may be caused by the uterus pushing on the diaphragm, increased respiratory demands with a tendency toward oxygen debt, and discomfort associated with weight gain. Near delivery, the uterus pressing on the bladder may cause women to be incontinent or to urinate frequently [17]. Prolonged standing or jobs requiring balance, endurance, exertion, and work in hot environments or in locations remote from bathroom facilities may become increasingly difficult.

### Breast-Feeding

Chemical exposures in the workplace may present a hazard to women and the infants they breastfeed. Toxic substances are passively transferred from plasma to breast milk if they are lipid soluble, polarized at body pH, and have a low molecular weight. These include many drugs, alcohol, some components of cigarette smoke, and many occupational and environmental toxins, such as lead, mercury, halogenated hydrocarbons, and organic solvents. The dose and duration of exposure to the infant also depend on how quickly the substance is metabolized or excreted by the mother. For chemicals such as dichloro-diphenyl-trichloroethane (DDT), polychlorinated biphenyls (PCBs), and related halogenated hydrocarbons, which are stored in body fat, breast milk can be a major route of excretion. The baby's dose may thus be as high as the mother's even after she has been removed from the exposure. However, solvents, though lipid soluble, are also metabolized or excreted through the liver, lung, and kidneys as well as breast milk, so maternal body burden rapidly decreases after removal from exposure [18].

### What the Health Care Provider Can Do

Information on a pregnant woman's work activity and that of her partner, including wage-earning work and work done at home, and chemical and physical exposures should be an essential part of the comprehensive perinatal health history. This information should be obtained from her at the first prenatal visit and reconfirmed by inquiry at each subsequent visit. This inquiry can often best be done by means of a questionnaire [16]. In some instances, it may be important to augment the questionnaire information, with the woman's permission, from the physician, nurse, or industrial hygienist in her employee health unit; from the plant safety director; or from the union representative. (See information on the occupational history in Chap. 3.)

### Legal Rights of Pregnant Workers

*When I told my new employer that I was pregnant, they lowered the amount of money they had offered to pay me, actually telling me I was worth less to them now. When my husband told his boss he was going to be a parent, he got a raise.*

The 1978 Pregnancy Discrimination Act, an amendment to Title VII of the 1964 Civil Rights Act, requires that women affected by pregnancy and related conditions must be treated the same as other employees and applicants for employment when an employer determines their probable ability or inability to perform a job. This law protects a woman from being fired or refused a job or promotion merely because she is pregnant. A woman unable to work for pregnancy-related reasons is entitled to disability benefits, sick leave, and health insurance (except for abortions) just like employees disabled for other medical reasons. Under the law, pregnant workers temporarily unable to perform their jobs must be treated in the same manner as other disabled employees, such as by modifying the task, changing the work assignment, or granting disability leave or leave without pay. An employer who assigns a pregnant woman to another job because she cannot perform her regular work or because the job represents a hazard, however, can reduce her pay to that of the new job (Fig. 32-3).

The employer cannot enforce a rule prohibiting a return after childbirth for a set period of time. The woman's ability to return to work is the only test. Unless the employee on leave has informed the employer that she does not intend to return to work, her job must be held open on the same basis as jobs are held open for employees on sick or disability leave for other reasons. During her pregnancy-related leave, the employee must receive equal credit for seniority, vacations, or pay raises.

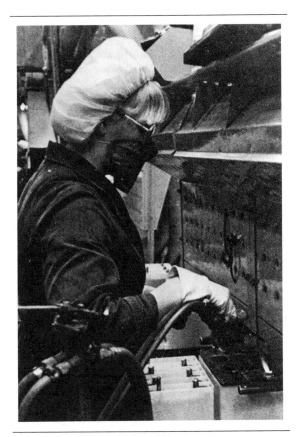

**Fig. 32-3.** Adequate control of lead exposure for *all* workers requires a high level of engineering control and may also include need for personal protective equipment. Since the U.S. law prohibits exclusion of pregnant women from lead work, controls must be sufficient to protect the fetus as well (see also Chaps. 13, 26, 27, and 29). (From C Zenz. Occupational Medicine: Principles and Practical Applications. Chicago: YearBook, 1975. Reproduced with permission.)

Pregnancy cannot have a role in the decision to hire an employee. If the applicant can perform the major functions required by the position, pregnancy-related conditions cannot be considered. The employer cannot refuse to hire her because of any real of imagined preference of coworkers, customers, or suppliers. In addition, the woman's request for maternity leave must be honored if the employer grants employees the rights to leaves of absence for such purposes as travel or education.

If a woman believes she has been discriminated against because of childbirth or pregnancy-related conditions, she may sue the employer. The law requires filing a complaint first with the state agency dealing with discrimination. If this state agency does not proceed with informal mediation or legal action under state law after 60 days, the woman can file a complaint with the federal Equal Employment Opportunity Commission (EEOC). The complaint must be filed within six months of the discriminatory event [19].

Legislation for the Family and Medical Leave Act of 1993 provides for a total of 12 weeks leave from work without pay and return to work at the same job or a job with equal pay, status, and benefits. Those eligible are men and women caring for a new baby and adoptive or foster child, or a sick child, spouse, or parent. The worker requesting the leave must have been employed with the same company for at least 12 months and have worked at least 1250 hours in the past year. In addition, the company must have at least 50 employees and have 50 employees who work within 75 miles of the work location where the leave is requested. This law provides only limited protection because many women are employed in workplaces with less than 50 employees. Additional information can be obtained from the Women's Bureau of the U.S. Department of Labor (see Bibliography).

## Specific Occupations

Although women are found in nearly every job category, they continue to be concentrated in those that have been traditionally female. More than one-half of all women employed outside the home are in two broad occupational categories: clerical and service. Nontraditional jobs for women are defined by the Women's Bureau as those in which women make up 25 percent or less of the total number of workers. In this regard, one of the most important shifts in the employment of women has been the influx of women into the skilled trades. In 1981 over 800,000 women were employed in these skilled trades in the United States, more than double the number in 1970 and almost four times the number in 1960. The number of women entering traditionally male occupations increased, at least in part, because of federal legislation and affirmative action programs.

### Household Work

The single largest type of work done by women in our society is that of unpaid household work. Despite the increasing number of women who work for wages, approximately one-third of married women in the United States are still full-time housewives, and most wage-earning women are responsible for work in their own households. In addition, over one million paid household workers are employed as servants, nannies, housekeepers, janitors, or cleaners. The exact number of paid household workers is very difficult to determine, however, because much of this work is undocumented. The vast majority of these workers are female and more than one-third are of racial or ethnic minorities. Few household workers, paid or unpaid, get sick days and many have no health insurance, Social Security, or workers' compensation.

Household work is thought of as "women's work," and is often not regarded as work at all. This perception devalues the labor involved and implies that there are no health and safety concerns of importance. In fact, a wide range of industrial substances and equipment is used and stored in the home under relatively uncontrolled conditions. There is growing recognition that certain home environmental conditions may pose important health problems, and that homes are significant small-source generators of hazardous waste.

Among the products used routinely in the home are drain cleaners, chlorine bleaches, scouring powders, ammonia, oven cleaners containing lye, furniture polish, furniture or paint strippers containing organic solvents, glues, paints, epoxies, and pesticides. There is an aerosol product containing ammonia, chlorine, organic solvents, acids, or detergents for every surface of the bathroom. All of these products are potential hazards and may become a problem, particularly when used in a confined space, such as an unventilated bathroom or attic, closet, crawl space, or the space beneath cabinets.

In well-insulated homes, potential health hazards may occur due to building, insulating, and decorating materials, such as formaldehyde emitted from particle board, plywood, carpeting, fabrics, and foam insulation; and asbestos in pipe lagging or furnace and boiler insulation. Toxic emissions from gas and wood stoves can accumulate in homes, as can radioactive radon.

In addition to hazardous chemical and physical agents in the home, some of the social factors that define the nature of housework can contribute to poor mental health. While many household workers enjoy their work and acquire a wide range of skills, their skills are largely unrecognized in the broader labor market, and they may have little long-term opportunity for job advancement or personal growth. For many, the work can be isolating and monotonous. In the industrial setting, it is recognized that such factors contribute to low job satisfaction. However, housewives are literally married to their jobs, and it can be difficult and threatening to grapple explicitly with low job satisfaction in this setting. The lack of support to directly address such dissatisfaction can lead to depression.

Sexual harassment and abuse are serious problems for women in the home. In fact, housework judged to be inadequate has been used as a pretext for wife battering. One police officer investigating an abuse case said, "If it had been my house, I would have beaten my wife for the condition it was in" [8].

An important step toward addressing the health and safety issues of women who work in the home is their recognition as legitimate workers with corresponding rights.

*Electronics Manufacturing*

Throughout the world most workers involved in the assembly production processes of the electronics industry are female (Fig. 32-4). Processes include precleaning and decreasing of fabrication materials with organic solvents, such as methylene chloride, l,l,l-trichloroethane, trichloroethylene, perchloroethylene, xylene, or mineral spirits; etching with acids; electroplating; soldering; and packaging.

Many electronics assembly processes involve rapid, repetitive motions of the wrists, hands, and arms. Assemblers may have to maintain uncomfortable postures throughout the work shift. Thus, repetitive trauma and other musculoskeletal disorders are a serious problem in the electronics industry.

Health and safety concerns have been raised concerning a particular subgroup of electronics: the semiconductor industry. Although this industry was originally concentrated in California and Massachusetts, rapid technologic and economic growth has fostered production facilities in most industrialized areas in the United States and much of the world. It is now estimated that microelectronics production will be the fourth largest industry in the United States by the end of the century.

According to employment statistics for Santa Clara County, California, the site of "Silicon Valley," more than 75 percent of the semiconductor production workers there are female and at least 40 percent of them are minorities, primarily Latinas and Asians. These workers are among the most poorly paid industrial workers in the United States today. This contrasts sharply with the large managerial and professional sector of this industry, which is nearly 90 percent white and male [8].

The major hazardous materials used in semiconductor manufacturing include hydrofluoric acid; solvents, such as freons and the glycol ethers (cellosolves); metals, such as antimony and gallium; and toxic gases, such as arsine and phosphine.

**Fig. 32-4.** Local exhaust ventilation successfully captures soldering fumes in a semiconductor assembly operation in China. (Photograph by Barry S. Levy.)

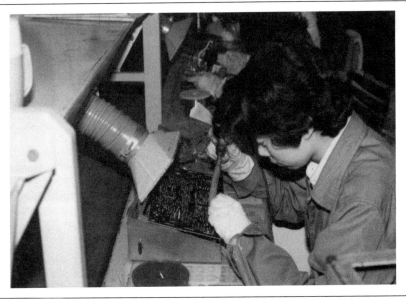

However, because the industry is relatively new, little is known about the chronic effects of the toxic materials used in this setting [20].

In 1980 the California Division of Labor Statistics and Research found that the rate of occupational illness among semiconductor workers was more than three times the rate among workers in the general manufacturing industry. The California workers' compensation statistics for 1980 through 1984 indicate that occupational illness in this industry accounted for 20 percent of all lost worktime injuries and illnesses, compared to 7 percent for the average of all manufacturing industries. These data also indicated that 47 percent of ill semiconductor workers experienced occupational illnesses attributable to exposure to toxic materials (called "systemic poisonings") as compared to 21 percent for all manufacturing industries [20].

Solutions for controlling hazards in the electronics industry include documentation of the nature and extent of materials used and integration of health and safety into the production process. The National Institute for Occupational Safety and Health (NIOSH) health hazard evaluations have repeatedly recommended installation of adequate local and general ventilation systems. The design of "clean rooms" should aim to minimize worker exposures as well as wafer contamination and, wherever possible, nonhazardous processes should be substituted for hazardous ones.

### Hospital Work

Over 2.3 million women work in hospitals and another 4.5 million in other health services. Women make up over 80 percent of the total workforce of these industries but less than 24 percent in "health-diagnosing" occupations, such as physician. In all health care occupations, women earn about 80 percent of what men earn, with the percentage decreasing as the skill level of the occupation increases.

Stress is a major problem for health care workers, who are often overworked and yet have responsibility for human life (see Chap. 19). Six of the top 27 occupations with the highest rate of mental health disorders are in the health care field [8]. Current cost-containment programs are expected to result in even more understaffing, as well as equipment maintenance problems and supply shortages. Rotating shifts, which are common among hospital workers, are another source of stress that can affect reproductive and cardiovascular health.

Nursing and personal care workers have an injury rate equal to that of agricultural workers. Hazards contributing to this high injury rate include electrical hazards from the extensive use of equipment to monitor and treat patients, needle sticks, slippery floors, and the movement of equipment and patients (Fig. 32-5).

Hospitals use a wide variety of chemicals for cleaning, sterilizing, laboratory analysis, and chemotherapy. A hospital worker can be exposed to chemicals or infectious agents through direct handling, cross-contamination of hospital areas due to poor ventilation design, the transport of waste, or the maintenance and cleaning of equipment or rooms.

Control methods have been developed for many of the hazardous substances to which hospital workers are exposed. For example, inexpensive scavenger systems are available to reduce exposures to anesthetic gases. Ventilation, substitution, and changes in work practices can minimize formaldehyde (formalin) exposures in autopsy, surgical pathology, and histology laboratories, and in renal dialysis units. The use of control procedures, such as complete evacuation of sterilizer units before opening, use of aeration cabinets and catalytic converters, and careful equipment maintenance, can reduce ethylene oxide exposures from sterilizers. Guidelines developed to minimize exposure to chemotherapeutic drugs include provisions for careful labeling of materials, use of biologic safety cabinets in drug preparation, and use of gowns and gloves.

Radiation exposures can result from portable x-rays, other diagnostic tests or therapies using radiation, and patients emitting radiation after ther-

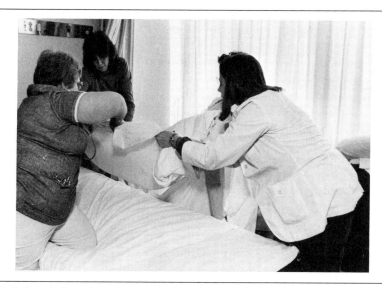

**Fig. 32-5.** Many female hospital workers are at risk of back strains from lifting patients. (Photograph by Marilee Caliendo.)

apeutic implants or diagnostic tests. Shielding and distance from the radiation source are the best protection along with regular maintenance, personal monitoring, reductions in unnecessary procedures, and careful labeling of materials, patients, and waste.

Hospital workers are exposed to a wide variety of infectious diseases, including hepatitis B, rubella, influenza, tuberculosis, meningitis, toxoplasmosis, cytomegalovirus disease, and acquired immunodeficiency syndrome (AIDS). To prevent infections, all blood, excretions, and secretions should be treated as infectious, and personal hygiene should be strictly maintained [21] (see Chap. 18).

### Office Work

*"For a year-and-a-half, I worked 3 feet from a copier . . . The fumes got so bad, I felt like I was being poisoned . . . It's important that I have won a workers' compensation claim . . . but I cannot place an order for another pair of lungs and I cannot wipe the worried look from the faces of the members of my family when I can't breathe,* *can't stop coughing, when I have to sit up to sleep. . . ."*—Former secretary before the House Subcommittee on Health

There are over 18 million clerical workers in the United States and nearly 80 percent of them are women. As illustrated by the above statement, despite its image of safe, clean white-collar work, there is a growing awareness of the hazards associated with office work. Among the more obvious safety hazards are slippery floors, open file cabinet drawers, electrical cords strung across the floor, swinging doors, and movement of bulky and heavy objects, such as cases of paper and office furniture.

The design of the office and its workstations is important in determining the extent to which noise, lighting, and ventilation are problems. The use of artificial fluorescent light can result in overillumination and flicker. By using desk blotters and task lighting controlled by the worker, the shadows and glare that are often the source of eye strain can be reduced. Once the ventilation system, copiers, typewriters, printers, and phones are operating in a modern, open office space occupied by many people, it is not uncommon for the noise level to exceed the 45 to 55 dBA recommended for easy office and phone conversation [22].

Many office buildings suffer from serious indoor air pollution (see Chap. 21). The combination of poor ventilation design, sealed buildings, the build-up of chemicals from building materials, office machines, and cigarette smoke has resulted in an office smog in many buildings. Photocopiers can produce ozone, nitropyrenes, and ultraviolet light. Duplicating machines emit ethanol, methanol, and ammonia. Formaldehyde is found in carbonless paper, building materials, carpets, and draperies. Several solvents, including trichloroethane, tetrachloroethylene, and trichloroethylene, are used in liquid eraser products. Pesticides used in the building can remain in the air for extended periods [8, 22].

In buildings constructed primarily between 1930 and 1976, asbestos was used as insulation for ducts and pipes, as fire retardant on the structural steel of the building, and as a spray-on ceiling material. Office workers can be exposed to asbestos when it degrades from age, water damage, or disruption during renovations and when computer, phone, or electrical lines are installed between floors in a building. Motor vehicle exhaust is a frequent air contaminant in buildings that have air ducts near busy streets, parking garages, or loading docks. Buildings made of granite, bricks, or cement may accumulate surprisingly high levels of radon emitted from these materials. Offices in the basements of buildings may also have radon gas exposures from the soil. Microorganisms can flourish in the air-conditioning and humidifying systems, evaporative condensers, and cooling towers in many office buildings. The result may be allergies and respiratory infections, such as legionnaires' disease, that sometimes can reach epidemic proportions. Perhaps the most common office air pollutant is cigarette smoke, which can increase the level of respirable particles in the air by five times that of a nonsmoking office. Since research has linked the cigarette smoking of a spouse with the increased lung cancer risk of a nonsmoking spouse, nonsmoking office workers may also be at risk.

Controlling the indoor air pollution of an office involves curtailing, alternating, or substituting some processes; isolating those sources of toxins that must be used; and improving the fresh-air ventilation of most buildings. For example, photocopiers should be kept in a separate room and vented, and substitutes should be used for carbonless copy paper containing sensitizing agents. Most office buildings have reduced fresh-air circulation to cut energy costs. The American Society of Heating, Refrigeration, and Air Conditioning Engineers recommends 20 cubic feet per minute (cfm) of fresh outdoor air per person where smoking is permitted (5 cfm where it is not) [23]. In addition, the relative humidity should be between 40 and 60 percent. By improving ventilation, the build-up of office smog can be avoided.

With the introduction of computers and VDTs into the office, a series of health problems have occurred. Among these problems are eye strain, headaches, neck and shoulder pain, and symptoms of carpal tunnel syndrome, and tenosynovitis.

Most VDTs in use today do not emit detectable levels of ionizing radiation (x-rays, gamma radiation). Nonionizing radiation, in the form of very low frequency (VLF) and extremely low frequency (ELF) radiation, can be emitted from VDTs that are not shielded; however, there is much scientific debate about the health significance of exposure to this form of radiation (see Chap. 17). In the early 1980s a series of miscarriage and birth defect clusters were reported among VDT users. There was some concern that they might be related to radiation leaks from VDT terminals. Since then, several studies have found inconsistent or inconclusive results regarding the association between VDT use and birth defects or miscarriages. However, these studies have been small and thus limited in their sensitivity. Several larger studies are currently being planned to examine this question.

Of the many recommendations made regarding VDTs, perhaps the most important is the need to provide workers with some control over their work patterns and environment. Many VDT data-entry positions have been set up with required hourly key-stroke rates that are constantly monitored. The combination of this pressure, poor workplace design, and few, if any, breaks all contribute to the health problems experienced by these workers. NIOSH has recommended a 15-minute break for every two hours of VDT work or 15 minutes every hour if the workload or visual demands are high [24].

A review of the literature on VDT design suggests that there is no consensus on the best ergonomic parameters for a VDT workstation. Adjustable chairs and VDT tables, with separate and adjustable platforms for keyboard and screen, should be used so that each worker can find the best fit of viewing angle, distance, and keyboard height.

Supports for palm, hand, wrist, and arm may be desirable for prolonged typing. Chairs should provide a high seat back with proper support for both the lower and upper back. The VDT screen should have a glare reduction device, where necessary, and background lighting should be low with a separate light for the hard copy. The VDT unit should be positioned in the office to minimize glare on the screen. Each worker should be able to adjust the lighting and layout of the workstation to his or her own comfort (Fig. 32-6).

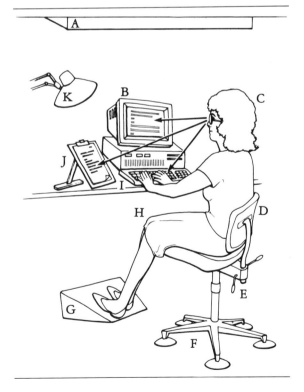

**Fig. 32-6.** A model video display terminal (VDT) workstation. In addition to specific features, indicated below, it has adequate ventilation, no excess noise or crowding, adequate privacy, relaxing colors and non-glare surfaces, and windows with blinds or curtains, and it allows adequate social contact with coworkers. The terminal should be regularly serviced and cleaned, and records should be kept easily accessible. The printer should be in a separate area; if located near the work area, it should be equipped with a noise shield. The specific features, as shown in the figure, are: (A) Indirect general lighting; moderate brightness (can be turned off if desired). (B) Screen about 1 to 2 feet away with midpoint slightly below eye level; characters are large and sharp enough to read easily; brightness and contrast controls present; adjustable height and tilt; glare-proof screen surface; no visible flicker of characters. (C) If necessary, special glasses for VDT viewing distance. (D) Adjustable backrest to support small of back. (E) Easily adjustable seat height and depth. (F) Swivel chair; safer with five-point base and casters. (G) Feet firmly resting on the floor; footrest available. (H) Thighs approximately parallel to the floor. (I) Movable keyboard on surface with adjustable height; arms approximately parallel to the floor. (J) Copy holder at approximately same distance as screen; adjustable space for copy holder and other materials. (K) Direct, adjustable task lighting. (From Office Technology Education Project [OTEP]. Drawn by Beth Maynard.)

### Construction Trades Work

Women who work in "nontraditional" jobs, where the workforce is predominantly male, face different health and safety hazards, in part because the work is different from traditionally female occupations and in part because of the stress of being an unwelcome minority. In the past decade, women entered the skilled trades through special apprenticeship programs developed to respond to hiring goals set by many federal government contracts. Yet even now only 1.6 percent of the workers in the construction trades in the United States are women, and it is not uncommon for there to be a single woman on a job site employing hundreds of construction workers. Both the isolation and animosity that many men direct toward a woman in the trades are sources of significant stress on the job. Tradeswomen may end up working in isolated areas of a job site, where they might be harassed or assaulted. This hostility may pressure women to attempt work that is unsafe in order to prove they can make the grade.

The most common injuries in construction involve slips and falls from scaffolds, ladders, and roofs; falls on the ground; being struck by objects; overexertion during movement of building materials or equipment; and injuries from hand tools [25]. Although none of these is a hazard for women in particular, tradeswomen are often less likely to stop work and insist that conditions be improved because men, with more seniority, are willing to do the work or are critical of their "pampered" attitude. However, tradeswomen also report they may be more likely to notice potentially hazardous conditions because they are new in the field.

The health hazards encountered in construction depend in part on the trade of a worker. However, since most trades operate concurrently at the same site, there is much crossover of exposures. Trades workers doing renovation or demolition work often are exposed to asbestos. Some of the other health hazards encountered by construction workers include lime and silica in cement, fumes from welding, diesel exhaust, organic solvents, wood dust, and fibrous glass. In addition, in most construction, there are potentially hazardous exposures to poison oak and poison ivy, chemical wastes in the soil, noise, extremes of heat and cold, and vibration from tools or equipment [25]. Authors of a recent U.S. Department of Labor study reported that safety instructions for the work being done were never given to approximately one-half of construction laborers injured on the job. Over three-fourths of these workers were never provided with any information on asbestos or hazardous chemicals in their work, and over two-thirds wanted more information on safety and health risks found in their jobs [26].

Many construction jobs are repetitive and require stressful postures. CTS, tenosynovitis, lower back injuries, and neck and shoulder pain are common problems for women as is the difficulty of finding tools and PPE that fits. Among tradeswomen, a common concern is the strength requirements for construction work. Tradeswomen are concerned about injuring themselves and at the same time they do not want to seek "special" treatment. In some cases, heavy lifting can be avoided by use of special tools or techniques, often used by older male workers, many of whom have been injured. In other cases, union agreements may define maximum lifting guides. Many tradeswomen lift weights or do other strength-conditioning exercises to prepare for work (see box on p. 626).

For pregnant construction workers, the heavy physical demands of nontraditional work may necessitate transfer to a job where the needs for good balance and stamina are not as great. The worker, in conjunction with her health care provider, can determine if and when this is desirable. No research has been done to look at the reproductive outcomes of construction workers, although some of the agents, such as noise, vibration, heat, cold, paints, and solvents, are thought to have potential adverse reproductive effects.

# References

1. Mergler D, Brabant C, Vezina N, Messing K. The weaker sex? Men in women's working conditions report similar health symptoms. J Occup Med 1987; 29:No. 5.

2. Hochschild A. The second shift: Working parents and the revolution at home. New York: Viking Press, 1989.

3. Bryant WK, Zick CD, Kim H. The dollar value of household work. Ithaca: Cornell University Press, 1992.

4. Warren-Gray B, Shapiro S. Hazards to women in the workplace. Department of Health, Education and Welfare, Health Resources Administration. Washington, D.C.: DHEW, 1979. (HRA contract no. 23278-0191.)

5. Amott T. Caught in the crisis: Women and the U.S. economy today. New York: Monthly Review Press, 1993.

6. Managing workplace safety and health: The case of contract labor in the U.S. petrochemical industry. Beaumont, TX: John Gray Institute, Lamar University, July 1991.

7. Spangler E. Sexual harassment: Labor relations by other means. New Solutions 1992; 3:24–9.

8. Chavkin W. ed. Double exposure: Women's health hazards on the job and at home. New York: Monthly Review Press, 1984.

9. Armstrong TJ. Carpal tunnel syndrome and the female worker. Transactions of the 43rd Annual Meeting of the American Conference of Governmental Industrial Hygienists. Cincinnati: ACGIH. 1981, p. 2635.

10. Cannon LJ, Bernacki EJ, Walter SD. Personal and occupational factors associated with carpal tunnel syndrome. J Occup Med 1981; 23:255–8.

11. Ohara H, Aoyama H, Itani T. Health hazards among cash register operators and the effects of improved working conditions. J Hum Ergonomics 1976; 5:31–40.

12. Grandjean E, Hunting W, Nishiyama K. Preferred VDT workstation settings, body posture and physical impairments. J Hum Ergonomics 1982; 11:45–53.

13. Videman T, et al. Low back pain in nurses and some loading factors of work. Spine 1984; 9:400–4.

14. Magora A. Investigation of the relation between low back pain and occupation. Ind Med 1970; 39:465–71.

15. Murphy DC, Henifin MS, Stellman JM. Personal protective equipment for women: Results of a manufacturers' and suppliers' survey. Transactions of the 43rd Annual Meeting of the American Conference of Governmental Industrial Hygienists. Cincinnati: ACGIH, 1981, pp. 62–72.

16. Kipen H, Stellman J. Core curriculum: Reproductive hazards in the workplace. White Plains, NY: March of Dimes, 1985.

17. National Institute for Occupational Safety and Health research report. Guidelines on pregnancy and work. The American College of Obstetricians and Gynecologists, U.S. Department of Health, Education and Welfare. Rockville, MD: NIOSH, 1977.

18. Welch LS. Decisionmaking about reproductive hazards. Semin Occup Med 1986; 1:97–106.

19. Goerth CG. Pregnant workers have discrimination protection. Occup Health Saf 1983:22–3.

20. LaDou J. ed. The microelectronics industry. Occup Med State of the Art Rev. Vol. I, no. 1, 1986.

21. Patterson WB, et al. Occupational hazards to hospital personnel. Ann Intern Med 1985; 102:658–90.

22. Stellman J, Henifin M. Office work can be dangerous to your health. New York: Pantheon, 1983.

23. American Society of Heating, Refrigeration, and Air Conditioning Engineers. Standard: Ventilation for acceptable indoor air quality. Atlanta, GA: ASHRAE, 1981. (ASHRAE publication no. 62-1981.)

24. Murray WE, Moss CE, Parr WH. Potential health hazards of video display terminals. Rockland, MD: National Institute for Occupational Safety and Health, 1981. (NIOSH publication no. 81-129.)

25. Bertinuson J, Weinstein S. Occupational hazards of construction. Labor Occupational Health Program. Berkeley, CA: University of California, 1978.

26. U.S. Department of Labor, Bureau of Labor Statistics. Injuries to construction laborers. Washington, D.C., 1986. Bulletin 2252.

# Bibliography

Chavkin W. ed. Double exposure: Women's health hazards on the job and at home. New York: Monthly Review Press, 1984.

*A thorough and well-documented selection of the social, economic, and scientific issues of women at work. Includes may important considerations that are often overlooked, including sections on household work, farm work, sexual harassment, and trade unions.*

Clark E. Stopping sexual harassment: A handbook. Labor Education and Research Project, P.O. Box 2001, Detroit, MI 48220.

*This handbook assists working women in identifying sexual harassment on the job and developing concrete strategies for change.*

Headapohl DM. Women workers. Occup Med, State of the Art Rev 1993; Vol. 8.

*This monograph presents a variety of medical and social issues related to women and the work environment. In addition to discussing reproductive risks, special attention is directed to cardiovascular, ergonomic, psychological, and psychosocial risks. Also considered are sexual harassment, gender discrimination, disability and problems associated with economic circumstances, and the mix of roles as worker and homemaker.*

Hunt VR. Work and the health of women. Boca Raton, FL: CRC, 1979.

*A comprehensive review of the physiologic, demographic, legal, and historical factors that affect the health and employment of women. Hazards of physical, chemical, and biologic environments are discussed including specific industries. Presents a concise summary of male reproductive hazards.*

MassCOSH Women's Committee. Our jobs, our health. Boston: Boston Women's Health Book Collective and Massachusetts Coalition for Occupational Safety and Health (MassCOSH), Boston, MA 02115 (1983).

MassCOSH Women's Committee. Confronting reproductive health hazards on the job. Massachusetts Coalition for Occupational Safety and Health (MassCOSH): Boston, MA, 1993.

*These are two handbooks written for female workers. The first is an overview of methods for recognition and control of workplace hazards. Chapters cover reproductive issues, stress, ergonomics, health and safety standards, toxic chemicals, legal rights, and accounts of women taking actions to correct workplace hazards. The second handbook focuses on reproductive hazard identification and problem-solving.*

Paul ME. Occupational and environmental reproductive hazards: a guide for clinicians. Baltimore, MD: Williams and Wilkins, 1993.

*This comprehensive guide for health care providers covers medical issues related to specific hazardous agents such as solvents. It also contains a useful chapter on legal and policy issues such as fetal protection and a regulatory framework.*

Stellman JM. Women's work, women's health. New York: Pantheon, 1977.

*An overview of the history of working women, including stress, health hazards on the job, and policy issues concerning protective legislation and reproductive hazards.*

U.S. Department of Labor. Facts of U.S. working women, 1986; Time of change: 1983 handbook on women workers, Bulletin 298; Weekly earnings in 1985: A look at more than 200 occupations, September 1986; Occupational injuries and illnesses in the U.S. by industry, Bulletin 2259.

*These publications were sources of the statistics on working women in this chapter. The Bureau of Labor Statistics publishes statistics on occupational safety, health, and wages, and the Women's Bureau has a wide variety of material on working women.*

# 33
# Minority Workers

Morris E. Davis, Andrew S. Rowland, Bailus Walker, Jr., and Andrea Kidd Taylor

Why does occupational disease among minority workers deserve special attention? Although it is accepted that the labor force is divided into subgroups of workers by industry or jobs and that different workers face different risks for occupational disease, not enough attention has been placed on studying the demographic characteristics, such as age, gender, and race, that may be linked to elevated risk for occupational disease. Such study may greatly broaden our understanding of the relationship between work and disease.

When populations can be demonstrated to be at high risk of occupational disease, clear social policy implications follow. For example, the whole concept of Equal Employment Opportunity in the United States would have to be re-evaluated if employers, in compliance with affirmative action guidelines, were hiring minority workers only into the most hazardous jobs—albeit at equal pay with other workers.

The purpose of this chapter is to document how disproportionate numbers of minority workers have been—and are—at increased risk of occupational disease, and to suggest ways in which the health professional can help to alleviate this problem. The chapter focuses on placement patterns of minority workers in American industry, providing data that associate these patterns with occupational injury and illness. Finally, the limitations in current social policy and the need for changes in such policy are presented.

For the purpose of this chapter, minority workers include African-Americans (blacks), Asian-Americans, Latinos (Hispanics), and Native Americans (American Indians), and the word *minority* is synonymous with nonwhite. Most of the examples chosen refer to African-American workers because, as poor as the data are for this group, occupational health data are effectively unavailable for the other minority groups covered here. In addition, African-Americans today constitute the majority of minority workers in the U.S., and the occupational health problems that they face are likely to represent the experience of other minority groups.

The distribution of the workforce into various job types within industry has often been based, directly or indirectly, on race and ethnicity. Historically, each immigrant group that arrived in the U.S. worked in some of the dirtiest, most demanding and dangerous jobs in industry only to be succeeded, within one or two generations, by the next immigrant group. In contrast to the experience of many of the white immigrant groups, however, racially motivated discriminatory hiring and employment patterns in many industries were used to prevent African-Americans, Asian-Americans, Latinos, and Native Americans from moving out of these entry-level jobs. Consequently, minority workers have been concentrated in the worst jobs in many industries as far back as the 1920s. In addition, discriminatory job placement practices have also resulted in elevated cancer incidence and death rates in African-Americans exposed to occupational carcinogens. Anyone assessing the impact of occupational exposures on the health of minorities needs to ask: "Where do minority workers work?"

## Placement Patterns
## of Minority Workers

Minorities continue to work disproportionately in higher-risk occupations. For example, in New York City, 30 percent of Latino workers and 18 percent of African-American workers work as operators, fabricators, and laborers, as compared with only 11 percent of white workers who work in these occupations. However, among lower-risk managerial and professional occupations there, only 11 percent of Latino workers and 15 percent of African-American workers, as compared to 30 percent of white workers, are employed in these jobs [1].

Nonwhite workers are concentrated in many of the most hazardous industries in the manufacturing sector; for example, they are concentrated in logging, "other primary iron and steel industries," and meat products, all of which have high injury and illness rates.

Minority workers have been documented to face greater on-the-job hazards. Forty-seven percent of African-American workers report themselves as exposed to at least one hazard, compared to 37 percent of white workers; the average number of significant hazards reported by blacks is 1.55, compared to 1.01 for whites. Of 13 hazards studied in one study, African-Americans were observed to be exposed significantly more often than whites in cases of extreme temperature, dirty conditions, loud noise, and risk of disease [14].

Ever since African-Americans were brought to the United States as slaves, they have been employed in the lowest paid and least desirable jobs. They have generally been denied entrance into many industries or into skilled trades and are often assigned the most dangerous jobs in the industries in which they have worked.

African-American women and other women of color have the lowest paid jobs and are mainly employed in domestic and service positions and blue-collar jobs. There are industries in the U.S. and elsewhere where large numbers of women of color are employed. Of the 240 poultry and meat processing plants in the U.S., with over 150,000 workers, nearly 75 percent are located in the southern part of the U.S., where communities are poor and many African-American women are employed. Conditions similar to those found in the Mexican maquiladoras exist. Working conditions are unsafe and unhealthy, minimum wages are paid, there are no health care benefits, and many plants are not unionized. Many Latina women are employed as farmworkers, especially in the western and southern parts of the U.S.

Often one particular minority group will be concentrated in performing the unskilled and semi-skilled jobs in a particular industry. For example, Latinos have been concentrated in these jobs in copper smelting and agricultural production in the western and southwestern U.S., Native Americans in such semiskilled jobs in uranium mining in the Southwest, and Asian-Americans in such jobs in the hotel and restaurant industry on the West Coast.

Not only are minority workers concentrated in the most dangerous sectors of the U.S. economy, but they are also overrepresented in the more dangerous occupations within these industries, even after controlling for education and experience (Table 33-1). The most significant occupational health problems faced by minority workers are related to patterns of their placement in the least desirable, semiskilled and unskilled jobs within industry. The author of one study estimated that African-American workers have a 37 percent greater chance than white workers of having an occupational injury or illness, and a 20 percent greater change of dying from one [2].

Is there evidence that minority workers are concentrated in the specific jobs where elevated rates of occupational disease have been documented? The answer is that evidence for this is incomplete. Three research practices common to many epidemiologic studies of occupational disease and injury are responsible for the paucity of solid data on occupational disease patterns among minority

**Table 33-1.** Employed blacks as a percent of all employed men and women in selected occupations and the lost workday rate due to occupational illness and injuries (1984)

| Occupation | Percent black | | Lost workdays[a] (rate/100 full-time workers) |
| --- | --- | --- | --- |
| | Men | Women | |
| Meat cutters and butchers | 9 | 19 | 181 |
| Waste collectors | 32 | [b] | 169 |
| Construction workers | 15 | [b] | 128 |
| Furnace workers | 25 | [b] | 109 |
| Farm laborers | 14 | 15 | 100 |
| Garage workers and gas station attendants | 8 | [b] | 47 |
| Laundry and dry-cleaners | 28 | 21 | 43 |
| Food service workers | 11 | 10 | 34 |
| Bank officials | 3 | 5 | 11 |
| Lawyers and judges | 3 | 7 | 5 |
| Insurance agents | 4 | 8 | 4 |
| Accountants | 4 | 9 | 3 |

[a]Lost workdays include days away from work and days of restricted work activity because of occupational injury or illness.
[b]Data not shown where numerator is less than 4,000 or denominator is less than 35,000.
Sources: U.S. Department of Labor, Bureau of Labor Statistics. Occupational injury and illness in the United States by industry. Washington, D.C.: U.S. Government Printing Office, 1984; and DN Westcott. Blacks in 1970s: Did they scale the job ladder? Monthly Labor Review 1982; 105:29–38.

workers: controlling for race so that no race-specific data are presented, focusing on whites only because they have a better national comparative database, and including race as a variable in the project design but not in the analysis of study results. While each of these practices can be defended on methodologic grounds, they have not been complemented by practices which are available that would permit race-specific risk information to begin to be developed.

The manner in which U.S. Government statistics are collected also contributes to the problem in the U.S., and similar practices may contribute to this problem in other countries. Although census and employment data are collected by race on broad groups of workers by industry, such as steelworkers, or by broad occupational categories, such as operatives in the steel industry, no one collects data by detailed job classification, such as coke oven workers. This means that when epidemiologic studies associate occupational disease with a particular job, such as cancer and coke oven workers, no national data are available to estimate the number of minority workers in that job classification.

## Evidence of Elevated Risk in Minority-Intensive Jobs

Presently, the most compelling evidence suggesting direct links between job placement patterns and occupational disease patterns among minority workers is a composite of selected race-specific epidemiologic studies, lawsuits, and industrial disasters that have attracted widespread public attention. The examples that follow describe situations in which African-Americans were concentrated in particular jobs that are now recognized to be linked with occupational disease. Although one can make inferences from these situations, the authors acknowledge the lack of direct evidence that work exposure caused disease in some of these specific situations. In many of these situations exposure data were not collected and appropriate comparisons were not done. Nevertheless, the authors believe that it is necessary to examine this type of evidence to appreciate occupational health problems among minorities since most people are not aware that these exposures occurred on such a widespread basis.

### In the 1930s and 1940s

Five thousand workers, mostly African-American, were recruited to tunnel through a mountain in West Virginia, during which time they were exposed to high concentrations of silica dust. Later a Congressional committee uncovered the fact that 1,500 of these workers had become disabled and another 476 died from silicosis [3]. More than half of the bituminous coal miners in Alabama were African-American as were about 25 percent of all coal miners in southern Appalachia [4]. Many of the workers were displaced during the Depression and never received compensation or medical treatment for the coal workers' pneumoconiosis they had developed.

In an investigation to determine the factors that contribute to high rates of pneumonia among steelworkers, the U.S. Public Health Service found that African-Americans employed in the blast furnace, coke oven, and open hearth departments had disproportionately high rates of pneumonia. The researchers believed that this problem was due to heat exposure, but steel industry representatives suggested that African-Americans have been "predisposed to the disease" [5].

In 1935 a total of 108 African-American steelworkers in Indiana sued subsidiaries of a large steel company for failing to provide healthful working conditions. The worker-plaintiffs were mostly furnace cleaners and coke oven workers who had been given the dirtiest jobs in the mill. They charged that their jobs had caused tuberculosis, silicosis, and other lung disease. The suit was settled out of court for an undisclosed amount of money in 1938 [6].

In the 1940s so many African-American automobile workers were hired in the foundry department that it became known as the "black department." A subsequent study has documented an increased cancer rate among foundry workers during this period [7].

During World War II, African-American workers were hired in record numbers in the shipbuilding and munitions industries. After the war, most were laid off [8]. Most African-American workers exposed to asbestos and other hazardous substances during the war have not received compensation for cancer and other occupational diseases they incurred.

### After World War II

A U.S. Public Health Service study of the chromate industry uncovered an occupational lung cancer epidemic. African-American workers in this industry were found to have 80 times the expected number of respiratory cancers—significantly higher than the 29-fold excess found for all chromate workers. The cause was identified as exposure to chromium-bearing dusts in the "dry end" of processing, where 41 percent of the African-American workers, as compared with 16 percent of the white workers, were employed [9].

In the 1960s a series of long-term mortality studies among American steelworkers began to be published, showing that African-Americans had been concentrated in the most dangerous areas of steel plants and had suffered disproportionately high rates of lung cancer. Of African-Americans assigned full-time to coke oven departments, 19 percent were employed in the most dangerous job of top-side coke oven worker, as compared with 3 percent of the white coke oven workers. This created a situation in which 80 percent of the full-time, top-side coke oven workers in the study were African-American. Full-time top-side coke oven workers were shown to have 10 times the expected risk of developing lung cancer [10].

Long excluded because of discriminatory hiring employment practices, over 90,000 African-American workers entered the textile mill industry between 1960 and 1979 (Fig. 33-1). An epidemiologic study of one of the largest textile corporations revealed that (1) the employment of African-American workers was being concentrated in the high-dust work areas, and (2) although African-American workers had been employed in the textile mills for fewer years, they were at higher risk of developing byssinosis [11].

A study of the rubber industry showed that employment of African-Americans was concentrated in the compounding and mixing areas, where elevation in cancer of the stomach, respiratory system, prostate, bladder, blood, and lymph nodes was found. In addition, African-American workers in these areas were found to have particularly high rates of respiratory and prostatic cancer when compared with white workers in the same work area [12].

African-American workers in lead smelters and paint and battery plants in three major cities instituted legal actions against their employers, charging them with responsibility for excessive exposure of workers to lead, falsification of medical monitoring records, and unethical and dangerous use of chelating drugs in attempts to prevent lead poisoning [13].

The NAACP instituted a class action suit against a shipyard on behalf of the African-American workers employed there. The suit alleged that virtually only African-American workers were as-

**Fig. 33-1.** Minority workers often are employed in the least desirable and most hazardous jobs, such as this worker opening bales of cotton—a job that has traditionally carried a high risk of byssinosis. (Photograph by Earl Dotter.)

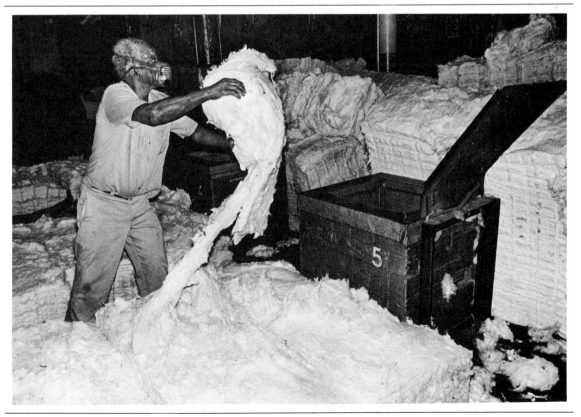

signed to sandblasting (with hazardous exposure to silica dust) and that workers were also being systematically denied workers' compensation benefits for resultant lung disease (silicosis).

Nonwhite workers experienced unemployment rates about double the national average during the 1970s and tended to remain unemployed longer than white. Two studies of unemployment written in the 1970s linked job loss with elevations in blood pressure, changes in mental health, and excess morbidity and mortality.

The devastating fire that occurred in 1991 in a chicken-processing plant in a small town in North Carolina is an example of dangerous working con-ditions for minority workers. Twenty-five male and female workers were killed in the fire because locked safety doors kept them from escaping. Two-thirds of the plant workforce were African-Americans.

Some of the evidence for higher occupational risks among minority workers relates to specific types of work. Farmworkers and their families are exposed to pesticides, and occupational injuries occur among them at very high rates. Of the work-force of migrant farmworkers (see Chap. 35), it is estimated that 50 percent are Latino, 30 percent African-American, and some of the rest Native American (Fig. 33-2). In parts of California, most

Fig. 33-2. Migrant farmworkers throughout the world, who are often members of minority groups, face many work-associated hazards, including physical stresses and exposure to pesticides. In the U.S. migrant farmworkers are often Latinos. (Photograph by Ken Light.)

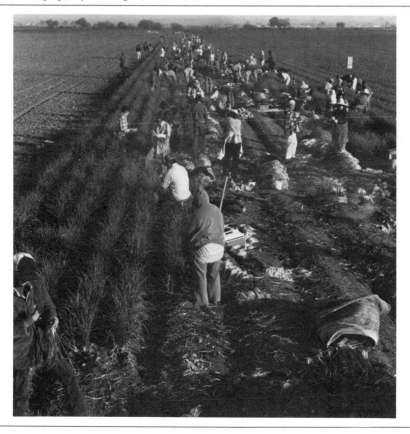

textile workers and apparel workers are Asian-American women who work in places that are often unsafe due to poor lighting, inadequate ventilation, and possible exposure to formaldehyde and other toxic substances (Fig. 33-3). Semiconductor workers, mainly Asian and Latina immigrant women, experience occupational illness at three times the rate of workers in general manufacturing. Construction is one of the most dangerous industries (see Chap. 36); in California, 62 percent of all construction workers are African-American or Latino.

Because minority workers have more reason to fear being fired they are less likely to question or complain about hazardous working conditions.

The average African-American worker is found to be in an occupation that is 37 to 52 percent more likely to result in a serious injury or illness than the occupation of the average white worker, and this overrepresentation in hazardous jobs holds strong, even after controlling for differences in education and on-the-job experience [14].

A study in California has demonstrated that African-American and Latino workers are at greater risk of occupational disease and injury than white workers. Latino men had more than double the risk of work-related illness and injury than white men, and African-American men had a 41 percent greater risk. Compared with white women workers, Latino women workers had 49 percent, and African-American women 31 percent, greater risk. At least part of the difference in risk cannot be explained by differences in education or number of years worked between ethnic groups.

For both sexes, African-Americans have greater rates of disabling injuries than whites. Fifteen percent of African-American workers are unable to work due to permanent or partial disabilities.

For male workers, there has been a dramatic narrowing of racial differences in exposure to occupational hazards since the 1960s. For female workers, no such narrowing of racial differences has occurred. African-American women now face

**Fig. 33-3.** Asian workers in the United States sometimes work in low-paying, monotonous jobs, such as in the garment industry, as shown here. (Photograph by Earl Dotter.)

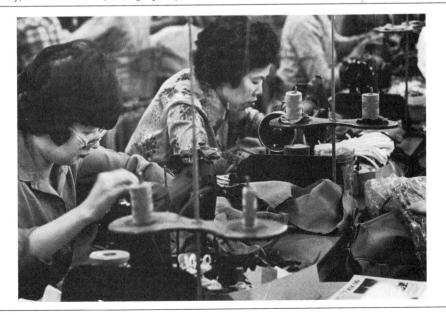

approximately the same risk of occupational injury as white men.

## General Health Status

African-Americans and other minorities have dramatically higher morbidity and mortality rates than whites for most major diseases. Almost 15 percent of the African-American workforce in the U.S. (1.5 million workers) are unable to work due to permanent or partial disabilities. The average life expectancy for African-Americans is about 7 years less than for whites, and between the ages of 25 and 44 hypertension-associated mortality is approximately 16 times higher among African-Americans than whites. Age-adjusted death rates for African-Americans are twice those of whites for pneumonia, influenza, diabetes mellitus, cirrhosis, and cerebrovascular disease, and five times that of whites for tuberculosis. In the working age population (between ages 17 and 64), the prevalence rate of heart disease is higher among nonwhites. Age-adjusted death rates for all malignancies for males are about 25 percent higher for nonwhites than whites, and for females about 10 percent higher for nonwhites than whites.

The causes of these large differences between white and nonwhite mortality and morbidity are not entirely understood. Nevertheless, these differences are unlikely to be explained solely by differences in genetic traits or in social class between the two populations. Given the minority group occupational exposures discussed earlier, all major health status indicators should be reviewed to determine whether there are any significant relationships between such indicators and occupational hazards and/or exposures.

## The Problem of Compensation

Although it is difficult to evaluate because race-specific data are not kept by any state workers' compensation program, some data suggest that minority workers may be receiving less compensation than other workers for work-related injuries. This seems to be true, even though minority workers as a group experience higher rates of occupational injury and disease. Workers who suffer severe job-related disabilities are more likely to receive welfare benefits than disability payments from state and federal workers' compensation programs, which suggests that workers as a group may be having difficulty receiving compensation for work-related injury and illness.

It is reasonable to assume that minority workers, who are concentrated in low-paying jobs with high job turnover, are even more likely to experience special difficulty receiving workers' compensation benefits, particularly for occupational *disease*. This assumption is supported by a Social Security Administration study of chronic disease and work disability that found that nonwhites were less likely to report disability but more likely to be disabled—particularly severely disabled—than whites. (Nonwhites in this study were found to be 1.5 times as likely as whites to be severely disabled, although they were younger on average.) The problems nonwhites may encounter in obtaining compensation benefits are also suggested by the long-term mortality study of steelworkers that indicated that employers were more likely to have information about the health status of white retirees than African-American retirees (see Chap. 11).

## Genetic Testing and Occupational Health

An increasing concern of minority workers and of health professionals who deal with minority health issues is the emphasis on genetic testing as a part of medical screening and monitoring in the workplace. Genetic testing is a collection of techniques used to examine workers for particular inherited genetic traits. It has been used by some major companies and utilities for medical evaluation and by others for research. Many more organizations have expressed an interest in incorporating genetic testing into occupational health programs (see Chap. 3).

Since many of the genetic traits sought in screening are found disproportionately among some races and ethnic groups, there is a heightened awareness among these groups that test results could be used for discrimination on the basis of race, sex, or ethnicity. There is also concern that genetic testing may direct attention away from other ways to address risk of occupational disease.

In this context, occupational health specialists question whether an employee's risk of future illness is an appropriate factor for job selection, even if screening or monitoring is highly predictive. They argue that employees have no control over their genetic make-up and generally have no control over previous exposures to harmful agents. In addition, their increased risk would not affect their current ability to do the job.

The counterarguments to these assertions include: (1) Society accepts immutable characteristics as possible proper criteria for employment selection, and (2) the autonomous interest of the individual should not be above the interest of society in reducing the economic and social cost of occupational illness.

The role of genes in disease is still not fully understood, however, and the identification of genetic factors that may contribute to the occurrence of job-related illness is a science still in its infancy. Data are most lacking concerning the correlation of genetic traits to occupational disease susceptibility. Clearly, genetic factors do not act in isolation from other biologic variables, such as nutritional status and preexisting disease, which affect a worker's susceptibility to a broad spectrum of occupational stressors. Thus, the assessment of factors that may increase the risk of occupational disease should not stop at quantification of inherited genetic traits but should also incorporate many other biologic variables.

A consequence of the public's concern about, and in some cases its opposition to, genetic testing has been an attempt to address a number of issues within the broad scope of employee-employer relations, ranging from the nature of the physician-employee relationship through the proper use of the test results.

One frequently advocated approach includes the following: (1) prohibit job exclusion on the basis of genetic make-up; (2) prohibit job transfer because of genetic make-up or genetic damage, unless the transfer is to a comparable job at comparable pay and benefits; (3) require strict confidentiality of medical information; and (4) require that employees be told of the results of testing and be given counseling.

This approach would protect the interest of workers, preventing serious consequences to individuals who have no control over the misuse of test results. It would also be consistent with many established legal principles governing the rights and duties of employers, employees, and company medical personnel.

## What Can Be Done

*"If society is seriously committed to reducing racial differences in health status, then it must consider active policies to reduce existing patterns of discrimination in the workplace"* [14].

Some experts have advocated using legal strategies, such as (1) Equal Employment Opportunity Commission complaints issued against employers for injuries or illnesses caused by discriminatory employment practices, and (2) unfair labor practice charges against employers who promote or acquiesce to discriminatory practices that result in injury or disease under the National Labor Relations Act.

There are at least the following three broad areas for action by health care providers, in general, and occupational health specialists, in particular:

1. *Recognition of occupational health problems among minorities.* Because minority workers are at increased risk of occupational disease, the

health professional should be even more alert to possible work-related medical problems among them.

2. *Documentation of occupational health risks of minorities.* Occupational health statistics on minority workers are not uniformly maintained. Nevertheless, considerable evidence suggests that minority workers, because they have been employed in many of the least desirable and more hazardous jobs, are at high risk for occupational disease and injury. Those who perform research should recognize the need for developing race-specific data so that the patterns of occupational disease among minority workers can be better understood.

3. *Facilitation of treatment and compensation.* Minority workers tend not to receive treatment or compensation for many occupationally related diseases and injuries. Therefore, health professionals can play an important advocacy role by making a special effort to follow these workers through the maze of the health care system to ensure that they receive the appropriate diagnosis, treatment, and compensation.

# References

1. U.S. Census, 1980, Public use microdata samples. Prepared for the Center for Puerto Rican Studies, Hunter College, New York, NY.
2. Davis ME. The impact of workplace health and safety on black workers: Assessment and prognosis. Labor Law J 1980; 31:723.
3. Cherniack M. The Hawk's Nest incident: America's worst industrial accident. New Haven, CT: Yale University Press, 1986.
4. Northrop H. Organized labor and the Negro. New York: Harper, 1944, pp. 156–57.
5. U.S. Public Health Service. Frequency of pneumonia among iron and steel workers. Public Health Bull, no. 202, November 1932.
6. Berman D. Death on the job. New York: Monthly Review Press, 1978, pp. 29–30.
7. Kotelchuck D. Occupational injuries and illnesses among black workers. Health PAC Bull April 1978, p. 33.
8. Weaver RC. Negro labor. Port Washington, NY: Kennikat Press, 1949. Reprinted in 1969.
9. Gafafer W. Health of workers in the chromate producing industry: A study. Washington, D.C.: U.S. Public Health Service, 1953.
10. Lloyd W. Long-term mortality study of steelworkers: V. Respiratory cancer in coke plant workers. J Occup Med 1971; 13:59.
11. Martin C, Higgins J. Byssinosis and other respiratory ailments: A survey of 6,631 cotton textile employees. J Occup Med 1976; 18:455.
12. McMichael AJ, et al. Mortality among rubber workers: Relation to specific jobs. J Occup Med 1976; 18:178.
13. Chicago Area Committee for Occupational Safety and Health News 4:1, 1976 and 4:1, 1977.
14. Robinson JC. Racial inequality and the probability of occupation-related injury or illness. Milbank Mem Fund Q 1984; 62:567.

# Bibliography

Davis ME. The impact of workplace health and safety on black workers: Assessment and prognosis. Labor Law J 1980; 31:723.
   *Overview of general health status, stress-related disease, and occupational cancer among black workers. Also includes a discussion of the policy issues and suggested strategies raised by the occupational health problems encountered by black workers.*
Davis ME, Rowland AS. Occupational disease among black workers: An annotated bibliography. Berkeley: Labor Occupational Health Program, University of California, 1980.
   *A useful source book.*
Rowland AS. Black workers and cancer. LOHP Monitor 1980; 8:14.
   *Discussion of the possible role of occupational exposures in the rise of cancer death rates among blacks. Links industrial placement patterns of black workers in the 1930s and 1940s with the rise in cancer incidence today. Available from the Labor Occupational Health Program, Institute for Industrial Relations, University of California, Berkeley, CA 94720.*
Coles R. Migrants, sharecroppers, mountaineers. Children of crisis, vol. 2. Boston: Little, Brown, 1971.
Florida Rural Legal Services. Danger in the field. 1980.
United States Commission on Civil Rights. The working and living conditions of mushroom workers. Washington, D.C.: U.S. Government Printing Office, 1977.

University of Wisconsin. Health care needs of Hispanic population in Dane, Doge, and Jefferson Counties. Madison, WI: Department of Rural Sociology, University of Wisconsin Extension, Dane County Mental Health Center, 1977.

*Important references on migrant and seasonal agricultural workers. Robert Coles studied the children of migrant workers who travel the eastern coast of this country. The survey from Florida Rural Legal Services, one of the best in the last 15 years, studies health status as self-reported and its relationship to pesticide overspraying. The mushroom workers studied by the U.S. Commission on Civil Rights are almost all Spanish speaking; they are among the lowest paid, most poorly housed, and most medically impoverished groups in the United States. The survey from the University of Wisconsin focuses on the health needs of permanent, year-round residents of the Hispanic community in south central Wisconsin.*

Friedman-Jimenez G. Occupational disease among minority workers: A common and preventable public health problem. AAOHN J 1989; 37:64–70.

Lillie-Blanton M, Martinez R, Taylor AK, Robinson BG. Latina and African American women: Continuing disparities in health. Int J Health Serv 1993; 23:555–84.

Morris LD. Minorities, jobs, and health: An unmet promise. AAOHN J 1989; 37:53–5.

Robinson JC. Racial inequality and the probability of occupation-related injury or illness. Health and Society 1984; 62:567–90.

Robinson JC. Trends in racial inequality and exposure to work-related hazards, 1968–1986. AAOHN J 1989; 37:56–63.

*These recent references further document the greater occupational health risks of minority workers.*

# 34
# Labor Unions and Occupational Health

Michael Silverstein

The history of industry and commerce has long been burdened with the loss of workers' lives. Events such as the Triangle Shirtwaist Fire of 1911, the Gauley Bridge silicosis disaster of the 1930s, the Farmington Mine explosion of 1968, and the malignant legacy of past asbestos exposures have taught generations of workers that survival to retirement age cannot be taken for granted [1].

It was not until the Occupational Safety and Health Act (OSHAct) of 1970 that the right to a safe and healthful workplace was guaranteed by law (see Chap. 9). Working people, therefore, have turned to their unions and other organizations for protection from the chemical and physical hazards that frequently accompany the earning of a living.

Personal and union involvement in health and safety programs is a moral imperative for workers. It is also a practical necessity for health care providers who seek to prevent job-related illness and injury. Just as clinical medicine cannot be practiced effectively without the participation of informed patients, occupational health and safety cannot be pursued successfully without the active involvement of the workers whose lives and health are at stake. Workers possess unique information about working conditions that is vital to the diagnostic process. Moreover, the health care provider does not have the independent ability to intervene to correct problems on the job once they have been identified.

Many health professionals have failed to recognize the potential for a mutually rewarding alliance with workers and their unions (see box), partly because of inadequate or misleading information that is generally available to health professionals about the role of unions and their commitment to health and safety—a problem this chapter addresses.

## Vehicles for Worker Involvement in Health and Safety

Labor unions are the major organizations that represent and pursue the collective interests of workers in health and safety. In addition to assisting their members with day-to-day needs, unions have actively worked for legislative and regulatory remedies for health and safety problems. Therefore, although only about 14 percent of workers in the United States are unionized, their influence has extended far beyond the workplaces where their members are employed.

Labor unions represent workers who share common work (trade or craft unions, such as the International Brotherhood of Carpenters) or who work in a common industry (industrial unions, such as the United Steelworkers of America). Employees at a specific workplace may be organized into several different unions. At a construction site, there may be more than a dozen unions representing groups of workers in the various building trades, such as the International Brotherhood of Painters and Allied Trades.

At the individual workplace, unions are called *local unions* or *lodges*. These local unions are generally part of an international union; in the United

651

## CHECKLIST FOR HEALTH AND SAFETY WORK WITH UNIONS

Health professionals who provide health and safety services for a union-organized workplace cannot be fully effective until they establish a working relationship with unions based on trust and mutual respect. The following steps will help prepare health professionals for this:

1. Determine which union(s) represents workers. Identify the local union leaders (presidents or chairs) and key representatives, such as health and safety or benefits representatives. Identify the representatives of the international union (servicing representatives or business agents) who are assigned to work with the local leaders.

2. Find out what kind of help the international union provides the local union on health and safety problems. Is there a health and safety department? Who is its director? Does the international union have staff professionals, such as industrial hygienists, safety engineers, or health educators?

3. Determine whether the local union or the international union has arrangements with outside experts for help on health and safety, such as those at academic institutions, COSH groups, and the Workers Institute for Safety and Health (WISH).

4. Establish communications with local union leadership before specific problems arise. The first contact should be with the elected leaders of the local, who can then make introductions to other key representatives. Ask about any outstanding issues of concern to the union.

5. Become knowledgeable about the nature of labor-management relations at the workplace. Read the collective-bargaining agreement with particular attention to any language on health and safety. Are there other written guidelines or procedures covering health and safety matters? For example, there should be a written respirator program under the terms of OSHA Standard 1910.134. How does the grievance procedure work for health and safety complaints? Does the union have the right to strike over health and safety? Is there a joint health and safety committee, a quality of work life program, or an employee assistance program?

6. Learn what procedures guard the confidentiality of workers with medical problems, and move immediately to strengthen them if they are inadequate.

7. Find out what types of health and safety training programs are provided for employees and seek to become directly involved with them.

8. Obtain and read copies of any health and safety studies that have been done at the workplace (industrial hygiene surveys, ventilation or other engineering studies, or medical surveillance or other epidemiologic reports). Make sure these have been made available to the union in accordance with legal requirements.

9. Visit the shop floor early and often. Establish a presence in the plant, independent of management or labor, but also be sure to tour the plant frequently while accompanied by union representatives. While observing jobs, be sure to talk with workers and listen carefully to their concerns.

States this usually refers to unions representing workers in Canada and the U.S. Most international unions in the U.S. are, in turn, affiliated with the American Federation of Labor—Congress of Industrial Organization (AFL-CIO), headquartered in Washington, D.C., and composed of unions that represent over 13 million members. Several important unions, most notably the Teamsters and the United Mine Workers, are independent of the AFL-CIO. On a regional or city-wide basis, local unions may work together in a group called a *central labor council.*

Local unions and their internationals enter directly into collective bargaining with employers. The AFL-CIO and local labor councils do not generally engage in collective bargaining but rather focus on political action and other public policy initiatives on behalf of workers.

Relationships between employers and unions are governed by labor laws, including the National Labor Relations Act (Wagner Act, 1935), the Labor-Management Relations Act (Taft-Hartley Act 1947), and the Labor-Management Reporting and Disclosure Act (Landrum-Griffin Act, 1959). These laws are designed to make employers bargain fairly with unions, to protect the rights of unions and union members in their relationships with employers, and to ensure democratic procedures and sound fiscal practices within unions. Labor law requires that employers bargain in good faith about concerns related to wages, hours, and conditions of employment. Bargaining must take place, therefore, over "conditions of employment" related to health and safety, such as the provision of ventilation, the use of personal protective equipment, or the operation of a plant medical clinic (Fig. 34-1).

Unions have represented their members on health and safety matters in four ways:

1. They bargain with employers for agreements aimed at improving working conditions. These agreements may include provisions for health and safety committees, union health and safety

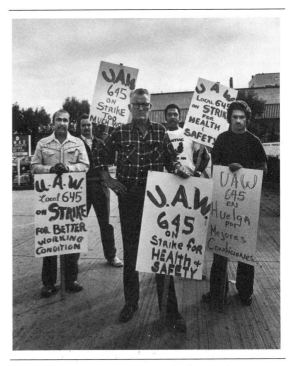

Fig. 34-1. Following the breakdown in local negotiations over health and safety conditions, a United Automobile Workers' local union went on strike at a California automobile assembly plant in an effort to secure improvements in the working environment. (Photograph by Robert Gumpert. Courtesy of United Automobile Workers.)

representatives, rights to refuse unsafe work, environmental improvements, and grievance procedures for members to use in pressing specific complaints.

2. They provide technical assistance to members facing chemical or safety dangers. Many international unions have health and safety departments with professionals, such as industrial hygienists or safety engineers. Other unions secure technical aid from committees on occupational safety and health (COSH groups, see below), the Workers Institute for Safety and Health

(WISH, a technical support group established by the Industrial Union Department of the AFL-CIO), academic programs, and government agencies.

3. They conduct educational and training programs so that members can better understand their legal and contractual rights and can more effectively recognize hazards and work for their elimination.

4. They work politically for laws, standards, and regulations (standards) designed to improve working conditions and worker health.

A number of organizations independent of the labor movement have been created by workers and sympathetic health professionals to educate and enlist the energies of workers on behalf of health and safety reforms and to apply pressure to employers, government agencies, and the scientific community. One of the earliest was the Workers' Health Bureau of America, which sought to assist labor unions with occupational health investigations, clinical services, education, and public policy agitation during the 1920s [2].

In the 1960s, the Black Lung Association (a coalition of mine workers and their families, union and community activists, and health professionals) used education, demonstrations, lobbying, and the media to raise awareness of the urgent need to eliminate the extreme hazards in the coal mines (Fig. 34-2). Special attention was focused on the risk of pneumoconiosis to underground coal miners. In conjunction with the United Mine Workers of America (UMWA), the Black Lung Association was instrumental in the passage of the federal Coal Mine Safety and Health Act of 1969 and later the Black Lung Benefits Reform Act. Dr. Lorin Kerr, director of the UMWA Occupational Health Department and, for many years, organized labor's only physician, was a major force in these proceedings. In a similar fashion, the Brown Lung Association and the Textile Workers Union (now called the Amalgamated Clothing and Textile Workers) drew public attention to the hazards of byssinosis in the cotton textile industry and suc-

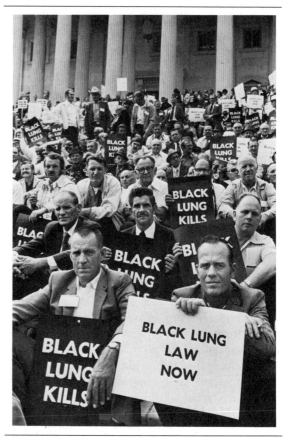

**Fig. 34-2.** Protest by union members that was part of the movement that led to the passage of the black lung legislation (Coal Mine Safety and Health Act) in 1969. (Photograph by Earl Dotter.)

cessfully pushed the Occupational Safety and Health Administration (OSHA) to promulgate its cotton dust standard in 1978.

Since early in the 1970s the most important nonunion support for health and safety has come from the loose network of COSH groups. The Chicago Area COSH group (CACOSH) was one of the early prototypes for these coalitions of local union activists with supportive health professionals, lawyers, and students. CACOSH generated excitement and action through worker education programs, provision of technical support to local unions, and political pressure for workers' compensation reform and stronger OSHA enforcement. By the late 1970s more than 25 COSH groups had developed across the U.S.

A significant out-growth of the COSH groups has been the Right-to-Know movement, initiated in the late 1970s by the Philadelphia Area COSH group (PHILAPOSH). It brought national attention to the need for workers to have full and accurate information on the composition and the hazards of chemicals on their jobs. Following a tumultuous Philadelphia City Council hearing, orchestrated by PHILAPOSH and the Delaware Valley Toxics Coalition, the nation's first local Right-to-Know ordinance was enacted in 1981. This city ordinance provided broad worker and community access to material safety data sheets (MSDSs) and other information on workplace chemicals (see box).

Under the leadership of Assistant Secretary of Labor and OSHA Director Dr. Eula Bingham, OSHA was preparing to issue a federal Right-to-Know standard. When President Reagan replaced Bingham in 1981 with Florida businessman Thorne Auchter, OSHA moved to dismantle the Right-to-Know proposal. As unions and COSH groups continued their successful work on state and local Right-to-Know bills, industry groups reluctantly decided that it would be preferable to have a single, uniform regulation rather than the evolving patchwork of local provisions. OSHA responded with a new, weaker proposal.

When OSHA issued its Hazard Communication Standard in late 1983, it was very much a compromise regulation. Despite concern with weak parts of the standard, organized labor has concentrated on the provisions that require employers to provide training on hazard recognition and control for all employees. Many unions, through collective bargaining, have secured the right to participate directly in the development and delivery of this training, which would otherwise be a unilateral employer prerogative.

## Health and Safety Issues of Importance to Workers and Unions

Union health and safety activities rest on a set of principles about rights and responsibilities in the workplace. Health professionals who intend to work with unions will be more effective if they understand and respect these premises.

*Premise 1: Workers and their union representatives are entitled to participate fully in the development and implementation of health and safety policies and programs because their lives and well-being are directly affected by the decisions made.*

This conviction about workplace democracy underlies worker demands for health and safety committees, upon review of new technology and equipment, and access to technical information and reports. Worker improvement in health and safety has taken many forms. In a Vermont battery plant, for example, the United Automobile Workers (UAW) negotiated an agreement for medical examinations to be performed by an independently based physician mutually acceptable to the company and union. In an Oklahoma assembly plant, there is a full-time union representative to work on ergonomics programs, which previously had been a unilateral management activity. National collective-bargaining agreements with major automobile manufacturers provide for union representation on hazardous materials control committees.

*Premise 2: All employees are equally entitled to safe working conditions and employers have an obligation, both legally and morally, to provide such conditions without resorting to discriminatory hiring and placement practices based on gender, ethnicity, genetic predispositions, or physical handicaps.*

This premise means that the employer must make a good-faith effort to design or alter the job to fit the worker rather than to limit jobs to those who are judged to be "fit." For example, the size and shape of tool handles should be adjustable so that workers of all sizes and shapes can work

WORKERS USE RIGHT-TO-KNOW
TO WIN JOB SAFETY
Peter Dooley

Federal, state, and local Right-to-Know laws and regulations have prompted many workers and their unions to participate in health and safety on the job. This activism has been displayed in several ways.

Individual workers have become informed about some of the health and safety hazards they face on the job. For example in a small machine shop in Michigan an experienced tool grinder received labels on the stock he was working with that warned about the health hazards associated with grinding on metals, such as cobalt and beryllium. He questioned the adequacy of the current ventilation system. An industrial hygiene inspection verified that it was poorly designed and maintained. Changes in ventilation were implemented based on his efforts.

Workers are participating in health and safety programs by exercising their Right-to-Know. This has occurred in several areas. Following completion of a class on the Right-to-Know, a union representative immediately requested to have a copy of her company's written program of compliance. After being denied her request, she produced a copy of the law and demanded it. On review, she found discrepancies in the written program. For instance, a "safety director" was designated to carry out compliance of the program, even though no such position existed at the plant. Following discussions with plant management, a new, more effective program was developed.

Another participant of Right-to-Know classes questioned his company's training and labeling program. After discussions in the joint health and safety committee, the company agreed to upgrade the labels by adding long-term chronic health effects and bringing in a union Right-to-Know training program to complement previous training.

*Workers and unions are winning solutions to health and safety problems through the Right-to-Know.* Warnings and information about chemical hazards have prompted new solutions to problems. For example, a workplace in Illinois was convinced to search for safer substitutes for extensively used chlorinated hydrocarbons, such as 1,1,1-trichloroethane. It had success in some areas using steam cleaning and other solvents as substitutes. Several machining plants have now experimented with vegetable oils as lubricants to replace hazardous metalworking fluids. Because of concerns about methanol exposures, a large office stopped all use of older duplicating machines that required use of this solvent. Many workers continue to discover the correct type of gloves or respirators to be used with chemicals they handle.

As is evident by these examples, an increasing number of workplaces have improved their health and safety programs by implementing effective Right-to-Know programs. Continuing efforts to improve the quality of Right-to-Know information and to educate workers and management about these programs are essential.

---

without fear of cumulative trauma disorders. Engineering controls and personal protective equipment should be used to reduce exposures sufficiently so that fertile or pregnant employees can work without discrimination. Return-to-work programs should be aimed at placing a worker back on the original job, even if the job must be adjusted to allow this (see Chaps. 6, 8, 11, and 23).

This principle of equal opportunity has several corollaries. First, medical examination programs should be used to guide environmental interventions rather than to determine hiring and personnel decisions. Second, procedures should be established to permit an employee to refuse to work without penalty on a job that is honestly believed to be unsafe until appropriate investigations and corrections can be made. Third, in the event that all feasible protections have been built into a job and a medical examination determines that it is still unsafe for a specific worker, the employer should have a "medical removal protection" program that entitles a worker to an alternative placement without loss of seniority, earnings, or other employment rights and benefits.

*Premise 3: Workers should not be asked to protect themselves from job hazards by employers who have not met their legal responsibility for making the workplace healthful and safe for all employees.*

For example, personal respirators are not an acceptable alternative to local exhaust ventilation to reduce harmful chemical exposure. Workers should not be lectured to "be careful" around automated powered machinery by an employer who wants to substitute warning signs for mechanical enclosures that completely prevent worker entry into danger zones.

*Premise 4: Workers have a fundamental need for and right to all information that is known to the employer, vendors, or suppliers about chemicals and physical hazards on the job.*

These needs exceed the provisions of the OSHA Hazard Communication Standard. For example, containers should be labeled with full chemical identities of all ingredients. Full disclosure of chemical ingredients should not be compromised by trade secret claims of chemical manufacturers.

Employers have argued that workers only need to be told how to protect themselves and can be provided this information without disclosure of detailed chemical data that are technically beyond worker comprehension. Unions respond that such policies are not only demeaning but also that workers cannot afford to defer vital judgments about their safety to company representatives whose interests may conflict with their own. Many

companies that use methylene chloride, for example, deny that evidence is sufficient to treat this solvent as a carcinogen. A data sheet that listed a mixture of chemicals that included methylene chloride as a "proprietary solvent" with irritant and other toxic properties, without mentioning potential cancer risks, would prevent workers from making an independent evaluation of risk and would seriously limit their ability to seek necessary protections.

*Premise 5: Workers who have been subjects in scientific studies are entitled to full notification about the results along with advice and support services to help them cope with their problems if they were found to be at high risk or to have a disorder.*

Worker notification is a particularly serious problem for thousands of workers who are the surviving members of cohort studies that were conducted by employers, universities, and government agencies and were found at high risk of cancer mortality. Unless these survivors are notified, they will be unlikely to seek whatever early diagnosis and treatment services may be available, they will not have the opportunity to make informed choices about their remaining years, they will not be able to take prompt advantage of any forthcoming advances in cancer prevention, and they will be kept ignorant of the need for protections on the job if the high-risk conditions persist.

*Premise 6: Workers who are temporarily or permanently disabled as a result of workplace injuries or illnesses deserve full, prompt compensation for any lost earnings and associated pain or suffering.*

State workers' compensation laws are antiquated. State-to-state differences in payment levels, diagnostic criteria, and filing and appeal procedures require substantial legislative reform including federal provisions that ensure equal treatment for all workers (see Chap. 10).

*Premise 7: Workers should not work with chemicals that have not been adequately tested for toxicity. There is a need for a substantial increase in occupational health and safety research and a national commitment to apply the results of research to the workplace.*

It is not acceptable to unions that thousands of potentially toxic chemicals are introduced into industrial use without adequate premarket toxicologic testing.

*Premise 8: Workers need a combination of health and safety laws and collective bargaining agreements to achieve maximum protection on the job. Neither legislation nor contracts alone are sufficient.*

Many serious health and safety problems are not covered by OSHA standards and require direct agreements with employers. For example, there are no federal standards governing control of ergonomic risk factors that are associated with musculoskeletal disorders. Most OSHA health standards consist only of a permissible exposure limit (PEL) and contain no provisions for worker training, medical surveillance, process design, and work practices.

On the other hand, even the strongest union contracts can only reach their full potential in the context of well-designed labor and public health laws. The UAW, for example, worked with a major employer to develop two training programs for hourly employees. One was hazard communication training and the other was safety training for skilled trades workers. After the first year of implementation, 95 percent of eligible employees had received the hazard communication training, which was required by law, but fewer than 50 percent had received the skilled trades training, which was not required by law.

The box on page 659 provides an example of how workers can use OSHA and their collective-bargaining relationship with the employer to solve health and safety problems.

*Premise 9: OSHA standards can be counterproductive if they are obsolete. Vigorous efforts are needed to bring many existing standards in line with current scientific knowledge.*

Almost all existing OSHA PELs for chemical exposure were adopted directly from the threshold limit value (TLV) list of the American Conference of Governmental Industrial Hygienists (ACGIH) in effect in 1968. Since that time many of the TLVs, which are only informal recommendations, have been revised yearly on the basis of new knowledge. Most TLVs are now much stricter than their corresponding OSHA-mandated PELs. The National Institute for Occupational Safety and Health (NIOSH) has also published numerous documents recommending more stringent PELs for dozens of chemicals.

The current situation is harmful to workers because most employers strongly resist demands that exposure levels be further reduced as long as the OSHA standards have been met, even though most scientists agree that many legal exposures, which are below the OSHA PEL, but above the ACGIH and NIOSH limits, are harmful.

*Premise 10: Workers are entitled to strict protections of confidentiality and privacy when they participate in occupational medical programs. This premise is particularly important because a violation of confidentiality can result in discrimination or job loss.*

All medical records should be maintained in locked files and restricted to the use of medical personnel unless authorized in writing by the employee or otherwise required by law. Unions strongly supported the passage of the OSHA Regulation on Access to Employee Exposure and Medical Records, which prohibits release of medical records to anyone without written authorization from the employee. However, this regulation makes it clear that personal air sampling and biological monitoring tests, such as blood-lead tests, are measures of environmental conditions and are to be more widely available.

Unions support the principle of the American College of Occupational and Environmental Medicine Code of Ethical Conduct, which permits physicians to counsel employers about the medical fitness of individuals to work but asks them not to provide the employer diagnoses or other clinical details [3] (see Chap. 12). There is a widespread perception among workers, however, that these guidelines are frequently violated by company

## AN ILLUSTRATION OF RESOURCES WORKERS CAN USE TO SOLVE PROBLEMS

At an aircraft instrument plant in Massachusetts, a vapor degreaser tank leaked a large pool of methylene chloride, which is a highly volatile solvent used to clean oily equipment. After being inhaled, it is converted to carbon monoxide in the blood and causes headache, dizziness, and, with prolonged exposure, unconsciousness and even death.

A worker at the plant, who was both a union shop steward and deputy chief of the plant's emergency crew, was requested to coordinate the emergency response to this leak. By the time he arrived at the scene, 50 people had left the building. He noted that the smell from the leaking solvent was overpowering, and that a few workers were ripping open 50-lb bags of an absorbent material and fabricating makeshift dams to contain the leak. There was no established emergency procedure for such a leak, and equipment and tools such as respirators and even brooms, which were necessary to respond to this emergency, were not available. Over the next two hours, the leak was soaked up with approximately 300 lb of the absorbent material, shoveled up, and hauled away. During this time the windowless plant was ventilated by opening the fire doors. Fortunately, no one was seriously injured.

Shortly after the accident, in response to a union complaint, OSHA inspected the plant and cited the company with four "serious" violations of its regulations: (1) failure to maintain the degreaser properly, (2) failure to locate eyewash and shower facilities near the tank, (3) failure to train workers in potential dangers of methylene chloride, and (4) failure to have clear-cut emergency procedures and to provide emergency crews with respirators and other necessary equipment. OSHA fined the company $2,240. The company contested these citations and appealed to the Occupational Safety and Health Review Commission, which has been established by Congress to hear such appeals. The union, in turn, exercised its right to participate in the appeals process.

Because there was an active and knowledgeable local union health and safety committee at this plant, and because OSHA had encouraged worker and union participation in the regulatory process, the union, with the support of the Solicitor of the U.S. Department of Labor, negotiated directly with the company. Management met several times with union officials over the next several months, and within seven months after the accident a settlement had been reached that produced dramatic changes in the plant.

In exchange for reducing the four "serious" violations to two "nonserious" ones and the fine from $2,240 to $500, the company and the union agreed to the following: a detailed inspection and maintenance procedure for the vapor degreaser including air-supplied respirators for clean-out crew and back-up, training of company medical personnel in recognizing symptoms of methylene chloride poisoning, informing present and new workers in the degreaser area of the health effects of methylene chloride, paying the workers who left the area during the emergency for time off the job (something that was originally denied), and installing a continuous monitor to measure airborne concentrations of methylene chloride near the degreaser. The monitor is equipped with a flashing light to indicate when methylene chloride levels represent a hazard (one-half the existing OSHA standard), and workers have been instructed to evacuate the area when this occurs. This spill evacuation procedure also requires that a trained emergency crew be established for all shifts.

Another result of this incident has been the realization by workers that they have the ability and expertise to stand up to the company in such situations and get results that improve conditions on the job. They have gained a great deal of confidence in the process and are prepared to continue their efforts to ensure the health and safety of their workplace.

This incident illustrates the variety of resources that workers can use to solve health and safety problems. In this case, there were two complementary resources: OSHA and the collective-bargaining relationship with the employer. In the absence of the union, workers would not have had the organizational resources that enabled them to participate in the appeals process. With this relationship, the workers were able to negotiate with the employer, with OSHA encouragement, and achieve substantial changes on the job. Without the OSHA citation, little of this would have been possible. It also reinforces the point that health professionals, in order to find out what is actually occurring on the job, must talk to workers.

Adapted with the assistance of Jim Weeks and Richard Youngstrom from R Howard. Do-it-yourself safety. In These Times 5:12, 1981.

physicians and nurses and that confidential medical information often ends up in the hands of supervisors and other management personnel. Substantial testimony was made to this effect during the public hearings on the OSHA access regulation.

## Union Health and Safety Activities: Examples

### Collective Bargaining

Before the passage of the OSHAct in 1970, collective-bargaining agreements typically contained general statements about health and safety. With the renewal of worker consciousness about health and safety in the late 1960s came the recognition that these agreements were insufficient and that stronger, more comprehensive contract language would be necessary to force employers to address serious hazards in a serious way. With a few unions leading the way, most notably the Oil, Chemical and Atomic Workers, a new generation of health and safety agreements began to emerge—often only in response to strike actions or other conflicts between labor and management. The most fully developed agreements today address five areas:

1. *Responsibility.* The OSHAct states that employers have the legal obligation for maintaining a safe and healthful working environment. Union contracts often restate this employer obligation and amplify it by enumerating specific responsibilities, such as providing appropriate medical examinations. The union role is typically expressed as a commitment to cooperate with and participate in programs aimed at fulfilling the employer's responsibility. The legal duty of the union is to represent its members fairly and fully with respect to the employer obligations and workers' rights spelled out in the contract. Courts have generally found that this duty does not mean that the union is responsible for the existence of unsafe conditions or the failure to correct them.

2. *Representation.* In many agreements, especially those that cover relatively small workplaces, it is part of the job of union stewards to handle health and safety matters along with their other duties. Some unions have been able to negotiate full-time positions for local union health and safety representatives in large plants appointed by the union and paid by the company. These representatives receive special technical training, conduct investigations, and handle health and safety complaints (Fig. 34-3).

Many unions have bargained for joint health and safety committees to which the company and

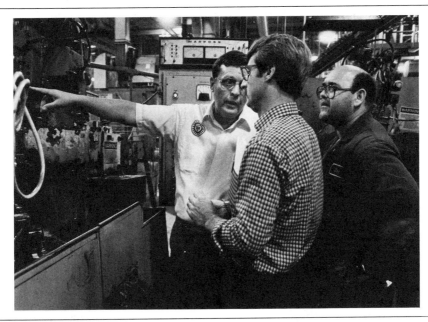

Fig. 34-3. A union health and safety representative (left) shows a supervisor (center) a dangling line that could get caught and cause a wheel to explode in a worker's face. This inspection led to the company correcting the problem and prohibiting use of the machine until this was done. (Photograph by Russ Marshall. Courtesy of United Automobile Workers.)

the union each appoint members. These committees are generally advisory in nature and have little authority to make environmental changes, enforce agreements, or shut down hazardous operations.

3. *Information and participation.* Some access to information is guaranteed by OSHA regulation, including the right of workers and union representatives under various circumstances to obtain MSDSs, industrial hygiene and biologic monitoring results, the "OSHA 200" logs (of work-related injuries and illnesses that are maintained by employers), company medical records, and copies of any specific analyses and reports prepared by or for the employer (see Chap 9). Unions have bargained for agreements that incorporate these provisions and go beyond them. For example, some unions have won the right to review plans for the introduction of new processes or equipment so that potential health and safety problems can be

identified and prevented before reaching the plant. Others have secured agreements to use air-monitoring equipment, to accompany company industrial hygienists during sampling, or to use the employer's computerized toxic materials database.

Many unions have secured company agreement to provide training for employees in hazards recognition and control beyond that required by law. The most comprehensive agreements to date were initiated in the mid-1980s between the UAW and General Motors (GM), Ford, and Chrysler. The centerpiece of these agreements is a fund for training activities, which is jointly administered by the company and the union. At GM, for example, four cents is put in this fund for every hour worked by a UAW member. The fund is used to develop training programs for skilled trades workers facing particularly dangerous risks, such as confined-space entry, and for local joint health and safety committees. While the funds do not pay for the employee hazard communication training required by law, the contracts do ensure that the training will include the union as a full participant in all phases of development and implementation.

4. *Grievance procedures.* Collective-bargaining agreements invariably contain procedures for the union to follow when it believes the company has violated the rights guaranteed to members. Grievance procedures typically call for a series of meetings in which progressively senior management and union representatives attempt to settle a complaint. Some agreements establish special expedited procedures for health and safety complaints. In the event that the parties find it impossible to agree, the contract will direct that disputes can ultimately be resolved by binding arbitration or by strike action.

5. *Environmental controls and other specific protections.* Some contracts go beyond general rights by specifying the way that particular problems will be handled. The company and union may agree that a new ventilation system will be installed, that a chemical will be eliminated, that medical examinations will be offered, or that a research project will be undertaken.

### Research

Unions have pressed employers, academic institutions, and government agencies to conduct high-quality occupational health research and to eliminate the inadequate and often self-serving research that has plagued the field for years. Two early leaders in this regard were the Oil, Chemical and Atomic Workers (OCAW) and the United Rubber Workers (URW).

During the 1970s OCAW was aggressively engaged in nearly all elements of health and safety activity, including campaigns for better standards and enforcement, access to information for workers, and improved research. With an OSHA New Directions grant, OCAW was able to hire several health professionals who provided technical assistance to local unions and who worked to stimulate needed research on potential hazards faced by OCAW members. For example, OCAW was able to challenge research of dubious value being conducted by petrochemical companies and to press NIOSH for the improvement and expansion of its Health Hazard Evaluation and Industry-wide Studies activities.

In 1970 the URW negotiated a research program of great vision and importance with the major tire manufacturers. Research funds were established with each employer contributing a sum of money, ranging from half a cent to two cents for each hour worked by a URW member. These funds, under joint labor-management control, were used to support university research into the hazards of the rubber industry. A series of epidemiologic and industrial hygiene studies were conducted by two schools of public health. Valuable information emerged about the relationship of stomach cancer and leukemia with solvent exposures in the rubber industry. Most important, manuals were prepared with information about how to reduce exposures to the chemicals of likely danger.

In the 1980s the UAW identified occupational health research as an area of major importance, expanding some of the earlier union initiatives. The UAW began to develop its own in-house epidemiology program. It established a mortality surveillance system, helped local unions undertake their own investigations, and completed a series of substantial mortality and morbidity studies [4, 5]. A number of work-related health risks continue to be identified, including associations between stomach cancer and work with metal-working fluids, lung cancer and nonmalignant respiratory disease with foundry work, and cumulative trauma disorders with various assembly jobs.

In addition to this independent activity, the UAW reached a series of agreements on research with employers. In 1982, the UAW and GM agreed to establish an Occupational Health Advisory Board of six mutually acceptable university-based scientists to assist in the development of research activities. The board's first major task was to sponsor a competitive peer review process to consider proposals for a comprehensive investigation of the health effects of exposure to metalworking fluids. This process resulted in a contract to a school of public health for a major mortality, pulmonary function, and industrial hygiene investigation. In 1984 the UAW negotiated occupational health research funds with GM, Ford, and Chrysler that totaled more than $5 million for an initial three-year period. Areas receiving support include the health effects of solvent and polymer systems, health and industrial hygiene surveillance for foundry workers, engineering controls for cutting fluids, and the mortality surveillance systems. Through 1993 these research funds have been renewed in collective-bargaining agreements every three years.

### OSHA Standards

Unions have consistently been the chief advocates for more protective OSHA standards, pressuring successive generations of OSHA administrators who have moved slowly on their own (and in some cases not at all). The history of the early OSHA standards (lead, vinyl chloride, asbestos, benzene, arsenic, and cotton dust) reveals that unions played a vital role at every step. They petitioned for emergency action, participated in public hearings, went to court to stop administrative delays, and filed complaints when employers failed to implement the provisions of new standards. For example, the regulatory agenda set by unions in the first year of the Clinton administration (1993) included such concerns as specific standards for glycol ethers, tuberculosis, fall protection, silica, and hexavalent chromium, along with standards for the more complex areas of ergonomics and indoor air quality, and generic standards on exposure monitoring and medical examinations. Unions have also supported the notion of innovative approaches to standard-setting, which would regulate large groups of similar materials, such as chlorinated solvents or pesticides, at one time rather than the current inefficient and time-consuming substance-by-substance approach (see Chap. 9).

### Legislation

Unions were deeply involved in activities necessary to secure passage of the federal Coal Mine Health and Safety Act in 1969 and OSHAct in 1970. Since then, much union energy has gone toward implementing these acts, protecting them from erosion, and supplementing the statutory protections with collective-bargaining protections. However, there is still a need for additional legal protection for workers. The major priority for the 1990s is reform of the OSHAct to better address the needs of protecting the health and safety of working people. Among the targets in the reform effort are the requirement for written comprehensive health and safety programs at every workplace, mandatory joint labor-management health and safety committee, increased criminal sanctions for rules violations, mechanisms for accelerated rule-making, expansion of authority to cover public employees, and reduction in the PELs. Other priorities include (1) establishment of procedures for the notification of workers at high risk and development of medical surveillance and related support programs for these workers and their families, (2) passage of state and federal laws that would provide uniform and improved workers' compensation protection for the victims of occupational illness and injury (see Chap. 10), and (3) legal action to preserve the ability of workers to seek just awards for the effects of negligent exposure to harmful conditions.

### References

1. Cherniack M. The Hawk's Nest incident: America's worst industrial accident. New Haven, CT: Yale University Press, 1986.
2. Rosner D, Markowitz G. Safety and health on the job as a class issue: The Workers' Health Bureau of America in the 1920s. Science and Society 1984; 48:466–82.
3. Code of Ethical Conduct for Physicians Providing Occupational Medical Services. Chicago: American Occupational Medical Association (now the American College of Occupational and Environmental Medicine), 1976.

4. Silverstein M, et al. Mortality among workers exposed to coal tar pitch volatiles and welding emissions: An exercise in epidemiologic triage. Am J Public Health 1985;75:1283–7.
5. The case of the workplace killers: A manual for cancer detectives on the job. Detroit: United Automobile Workers, 1981.

## Bibliography

AFL-CIO. Manual for shop stewards. Washington, D.C.: American Federation of Labor and Congress of Industrial Organizations, 1984.
*A basic guide for union representatives, including information about rights and responsibilities.*

Babson S. Working Detroit: The making of a union town. New York: Adama, 1984.
*An excellent chronicle of workers and unions in America's industrial heartland.*

Deutsch S. ed. Theme issue: Occupational safety and health. Labor Studies 6:1981.
*A collection of articles providing more details about several of the subjects covered in this chapter, including health and safety committees, collective bargaining, COSH groups, and workplace democracy.*

McAteer JD. Miner's manual: A complete guide to health and safety protection on the job. Washington, D.C.: Crossroads, 1981.
*A good example of a health and safety training publication designed with rank-and-file workers in mind.*

Melkin D, Brown M. Workers at risk: Voices from the workplace. Chicago: The University of Chicago Press, 1984.
*A powerful series of first-person accounts by workers faced with chemical hazards on the job.*

Mirer F. Worker participation in health and safety: lessons from joint programs in the American automobile industry. Am Ind Hyg Assoc 1989;50:598–601.
*A discussion of innovative collective-bargaining agreements that focus on health and safety programs designed to educate workers and management as well as to support the research necessary to identify and control work-related disease and injury.*

Page J, O'Brien M. Bitter wages. New York: Grossman, 1973.
*The best discussion available about the origins of the OSHAct, including substantial material about the political activity of labor unions in health and safety during the pre-OSHA era.*

Rashke R. The killing of Karen Silkwood: The story behind the Kerr-McGee plutonium case. Boston: Houghton Mifflin, 1981.
*An investigative reporter's probe into the tangled story of union activism, radiation hazards, the nuclear fuel industry, liability law, and, in the view of some, murder.*

Stein L. The Triangle fire. New York: Carroll & Graf, 1962.
*A historical re-creation of a workplace disaster that was linked to industry negligence and that led to important health and safety reforms in the early twentieth century.*

# 35
# Agricultural Workers

Richard Fenske and Nancy J. Simcox

Agriculture is the world's largest economic activity, involving an estimated 63 percent of the population in developing countries [1]. Its practice ranges from highly mechanized operations employing state-of-the-art technology to maintenance of subsistence plots.

The agricultural workplace may be a well-defined commercial enterprise that resembles an industrial setting, comprised of a workforce conducting specific tasks with assembly-line regularity, but it may also be virtually indistinguishable from the habits of everyday life, occurring in residential and community space, with family members helping in all phases of production.

The vast diversity of global agricultural activities represents a challenge to health care providers. The identification of occupational health hazards and the development of methods to evaluate, redress, and ultimately eliminate hazardous exposures and resultant illnesses and injuries are labor intensive and require wide knowledge in occupational health. This chapter includes discussion of the primary hazards, the health problems associated with these hazards, and the controls that are employed to reduce health risks for agricultural workers.

## Workforce Characteristics

In most countries, a substantial proportion of agricultural activity is controlled by farmers—that is, individuals who both own and work the land. While they may hire workers to assist in various aspects of production, the core of their workforce is their family. In the United States, family farm health and safety have been given long overdue attention by the convening of a national conference by the U.S. Surgeon General [2], and by the infusion of federal funds into regional research centers, surveillance programs, and a variety of outreach initiatives. While this chapter focuses primarily on agricultural workers who are now owners of the means of production, many of the health risks discussed here are also applicable to family farmers.

### The Hired Farmworker

"... Hired farmworkers are not adequately protected by federal laws, regulations, and programs; therefore, their health and well-being are at risk ..." and furthermore, "... their children—who may work in the fields because the families need the money or lack access to child care facilities—are subject to educational disadvantages and health risks from injuries and pesticides."
—U.S. Government Accounting Office, 1992 [3]

The number of agricultural workers in the world is difficult to estimate; in the United States, the number is estimated to be between 2.5 and 4.1 million, composed primarily of immigrants from Mexico, Puerto Rico, Haiti, Jamaica, and Central America as well as Native Americans and African-Americans [4]. Approximately one-half of all U.S. farmworkers are seasonal. These workers are at greatest risk for occupational hazards in agriculture because they are concentrated in high-risk crops and activities.

Agricultural labor has traditionally been treated as a "special case," both in the U.S. and elsewhere. In the U.S., workers are excluded from key labor laws, from many state and federal occupational health and safety laws, and, in one-half of the states, from workers' compensation [5]. This treatment of agriculture has even extended to basic rights, such as workplace sanitation. All other U.S. workers have been guaranteed rights to the provision of basic sanitation since 1971—that is, handwashing, potable water, and portable toilets. Not until 1987, however, did the U.S. Occupational Safety and Health Administration (OSHA) issue a field sanitation standard for agricultural fieldworkers. In many parts of the world, this same dichotomy between agriculture and other industries remains.

The occupational issues surrounding agricultural workers are not easily separated from other political, social, and ethical concerns related to the status and treatment of this labor group. In industrial societies, the living conditions of many agricultural workers more closely resemble those of families in developing countries (Fig. 35-1).

Deficiencies in nutrition, housing, sanitation, education, and access to health care all contribute to the general health status of these families and individuals, and frequently these deficiencies directly contribute to vulnerability to occupational health hazards. Housing in or near fields exposes workers and their families to pesticide spray drift. Inadequate sanitation is associated with an increased prevalence of parasitic and infectious disease among farmworkers. Inaccessible potable water in the fields and in some housing forces workers to drink irrigation water, which is frequently contaminated with pesticide run-off and is increasingly used as a direct method of pesticide application. Lack of education makes it difficult or impossible for workers to read pesticide labels and posted signs. Finally, the same economic and geographic factors that limit access to medical care for

**Fig. 35-1.** Migrant farmworkers typically suffer from housing and other socioeconomic problems, as illustrated by these workers sleeping under orange trees because no housing was provided. (Photograph by Ken Light.)

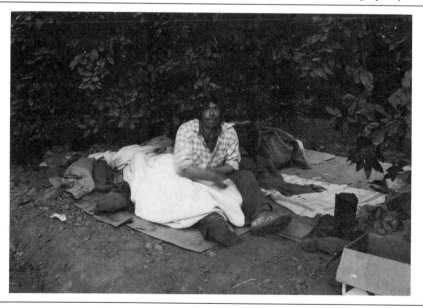

agricultural workers may also delay or prevent appropriate treatment for job-related injuries and illnesses.

### Child Labor

Child labor has become an important occupational and public health concern for the 1990s, and especially in agriculture [6]. The use of children as agricultural laborers can jeopardize their education and development, as well as place them at risk for injury, illness, and chemical exposures. In the United States, the minimum age for employment is 16 years old, and a child may not be employed in hazardous occupations or activities, such as mining, logging, or roofing, until reaching 18 years of age. Under the Fair Labor Standards Act, however, the minimum age for agricultural labor is 12 years, and 16-year-old children can participate in hazardous activities. For children on family farms, a full exemption has been granted from these age requirements. Allowable activities that are considered hazardous include operating tractors, using heavy machinery, climbing ladders, and mixing or applying acutely toxic pesticides.

Children under the age of 16 years are estimated to constitute as much as 16 percent of the agricultural workforce in the U.S. Children of hired farmworkers assist their parents with picking crops, carrying produce in bags and buckets, climbing ladders, caring for animals, and operating farm machinery. The risks posed by farm hazards may be increased for young workers due to their small size, inexperience, and inadequate safety training. Injuries that have occurred among children while at work include amputations, lacerations, and crush accidents from machinery, as well as trauma from animal and vehicular accidents. It is estimated that close to 300 children and adolescents die each year from farm injuries in the U.S., and that 23,500 suffer nonfatal trauma [7]. In addition to the physical hazards posed by machinery, noise produced by such equipment has been linked to early hearing loss in young agricultural workers.

Few injury and illness data are available regarding pesticide exposure. Children contact pesticides in much the same way as adults, and are exposed to the same concentrations of pesticide residues. In a recent study 48 percent of Mexican-American farmworker children reported working in fields still wet with pesticides, and 36 percent had been sprayed directly or indirectly by pesticide drift [7]. A recent report, *Pesticides in the Diets of Infants and Children,* published by the U.S. National Academy of Sciences, discusses differences in pesticide-related health risks for adults and children [8]. Differences in metabolic activity and a higher surface-area-to-weight ratio may place children at greater risk than adults following equivalent exposures. Also, research in animal models suggests that hormonal systems that are in development may be more susceptible to the toxic effects of some compounds. In general, however, the physiologic and clinical effects of pesticide exposure in children and adolescents are not fully documented.

## Morbidity and Mortality in Agriculture

Agriculture is among the most dangerous and physically demanding occupations (Fig. 35-2). Statistics available from the United States indicate that injury and death rates rank agriculture consistently among the three most hazardous industries. The death rate for U.S. agricultural workers in 1991 was 44 per 100,000 workers, in comparison with 31 per 100,000 workers in construction and 43 per 100,000 workers in mining. The injury rate for agricultural workers was greater than that for mining [9].

As with injury rates, illness rates place agriculture among the most hazardous occupations. Occupational illnesses per 10,000 full-time U.S. workers in 1990 were 43.0 for all industries combined, 127.7 for manufacturing, 56.4 for agriculture, 20.2 for mining, and 18.9 for construction [9]. While injury rates have been declining in the

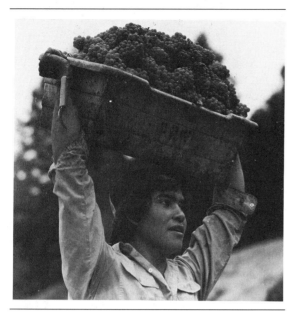

**Fig. 35-2.** Farmworkers, as illustrated by the work of this grape picker, face physically demanding jobs, which often predispose them to serious injury. (Photograph by Ken Light.)

U.S., occupational disease rates have not; they represent a rising proportion of all morbidity among agricultural workers. In public health terms, these statistics reflect the transition in environmental risk in developed industrial nations to patterns of mainly chronic disease. The health and safety risks faced by agricultural workers lead to pesticide-related illness, skin disorders, musculoskeletal problems, respiratory diseases, injuries, hearing loss, and other problems.

### Pesticide Poisonings

The World Health Organization (WHO) [1] estimates that acute pesticide poisonings have doubled in developing countries since the 1970s and are likely to increase further as the use of more toxic, less persistent, pesticides becomes widespread. Table 35-1 provides the major classes of pesticides from each group that are associated with pesticide-related illnesses and poisonings.

The use of organophosphates, a class of insecticides with neurotoxic properties, has resulted in more occupational acute pesticide poisonings and deaths than any other class. There are few state and national registries that document and report pesticide health problems. Estimates for acute pesticide poisoning are based on hospital visits and community-based surveys from various regions of the world.

Mortality and morbidity statistics related to pesticide exposure on a global level are difficult to uncover. In 1990 WHO [1] estimated that 1 million unintentional severe acute poisonings occur annually worldwide, resulting in 20,000 fatalities. WHO estimates that for every 500 symptomatic cases, there are 11 hospital admissions and one death. Authors of another study reported 24,731 worldwide cases of pesticide poisonings leading to 1,065 deaths between 1951 and 1990 [10].

Although the United States has arguably the most advanced regulatory requirements related to pesticide use, the full dimensions of pesticide-related illness are not well documented. The U.S. Environmental Protection Agency (EPA) estimates that farmworkers experience approximately 300,000 acute illnesses and injuries each year related to pesticides [3]. Only a few states, such as California and Washington, require mandatory reporting of pesticide illnesses. In 1990 almost 2,000 pesticide-related illnesses caused by occupational exposures were reported in California; more than 50 percent involved exposure during use such as in mixing and loading and 25 percent involved exposure to residues [11]. Why these poisonings occur and how they might be prevented are discussed in a separate section later in this chapter.

### Chronic Health Effects of Pesticides

In industrialized countries, reported cases of systemic pesticide illness in recent years have predominantly been in individuals or small groups of workers who have faced restricted-entry violations or accidental exposures. Exposure levels that were considered acceptable a decade ago are now being carefully evaluated for health risks. Industrialized

**Table 35-1.** Characteristics of pesticide poisoning

| Chemical basis (examples of compounds)* | Pharmacologic action or site of toxicity | Routes of absorption | Major acute signs and symptoms | Laboratory test |
|---|---|---|---|---|
| Chlorinated hydrocarbons (chlorobenzilate, Kelthane, Thiodan, methoxychlor, lindane, heptachlor, toxaphene, chlordane), endosulfan | Neurotoxin; CNS, kidney, liver | Ingestion, skin absorption, inhalation | Apprehension, dizziness, excitability, headache, disorientation, weakness, paresthesia, convulsions | Pesticide and/or metabolites measured in blood; concentration more important than mere presence |
| Organophosphates (diazinon, malathion, methyl parathion, parathion, Guthion, chlorpyrifos [Dursban], Di-Syston, dichlorvos, S-Seven), methamidophos, mevinphos (Phosdrin) | Irreversible inhibition of acetylcholinesterase enzyme | Ingestion, skin absorption, inhalation | *Mild:* fatigue, headache, blurred vision, dizziness, numbness of extremities, nausea, vomiting, excessive sweating and salivation, tightness in chest *Moderate:* weakness, difficulty talking, muscular fasciculations, miosis *Severe:* unconsciousness, flaccid paralysis, moist rales, respiratory difficulty, and cyanosis *Other:* cardiac arrhythmias | Red blood cell cholinesterase, plasma cholinesterase |
| Carbamates (aldicarb [Temik], methomyl, oxamyl, carbaryl [Sevin], carbofuran, Baygon) | Reversible inhibition of acetylcholinesterase enzyme | Ingestion, skin absorption, inhalation | Diarrhea, nausea, vomiting, abdominal pain, excessive sweating and salivation, blurred vision, difficulty breathing, headache, muscular fasciculations | Red blood cell and plasma cholinesterase may be normal and thus not reliable detectors of poisoning; carbamate metabolites in urine |

(continued)

**Table 35-1. (continued).**

| Chemical basis (examples of compounds)* | Pharmacologic action or site of toxicity | Routes of absorption | Major acute signs and symptoms | Laboratory test |
|---|---|---|---|---|
| Halocarbon and sulfuryl fumigants (methyl bromide, carbon disulfide, chloropicrin, ethylene dibromide, dibromochloropropane) | CNS, enzyme systems, liver, kidney, lungs | Ingestion, skin absorption, inhalation | Dizziness, headache, nausea, vomiting, abdominal pain, mental confusion, tremor, convulsions, pulmonary edema | Methyl bromide—blood bromide concentrations; carbon disulfides in urine |
| Phosphine fumigants (aluminum phosphide [Phostoxin]) | Lungs, CNS, liver, kidney | Inhalation, skin absorption, ingestion | Dizziness, headache, nausea, vomiting, dyspnea, pulmonary edema | None known; victim's breath may smell like garlic or acetylene |
| Cyanide fumigants (Cyclon) | Inactivates the cytochrome oxidase of cells in critical tissues, primarily the heart and brain | Ingestion, inhalation, skin absorption (rare) | *Large dose:* collapse and cessation of respiration<br>*Smaller dose:* headache, weakness, confusion, nausea, vomiting, dizziness, hyperpnea, apprehension, convulsions<br>*Other:* breath may smell like bitter almonds | Cyanide in blood and tissues; thiocyanate metabolite in urine and saliva |
| Nitrophenolic and nitrocresolic herbicides (dinitrocresol, dinoseb [Dinitro-3], dinitrophenol) | Liver, kidney, and nervous system; stimulation of oxidative metabolism in cell mitochondria | Ingestion, inhalation, skin absorption | Yellow staining of skin and hair; profuse sweating, headache, thirst, malaise, warm flushed skin, tachycardia, fever | Nitrophenols and nitrocresols in urine and serum |

| | | | | |
|---|---|---|---|---|
| Chlorophenoxy compounds (2,4-D, Silvex 2,4, 5-T, Dicamba) | Skin, eyes, respiratory, and gastrointestinal linings | Ingestion, skin absorption, inhalation | *Inhalation:* burning sensations in the nasopharynx and chest, dizziness. *Ingestion:* vomiting, esophagitis, abdominal pain, diarrhea, fibrillary muscle twitching, stiffness of muscles of extremities, metabolic acidosis in large doses | Chlorophenoxy compounds in blood and urine |
| Dipyridyls (diquat [Aquacide], paraquat [DextroneX]) | Injury of epithelial tissue: skin, nails, cornea, liver, kidney, and linings of gastrointestinal and respiratory tracts | Ingestion, skin absorption, inhalation | *Ingestion early:* nausea, vomiting, diarrhea, melena, pain (oral, substernal, abdominal) *48–72 hours after exposure:* oliguria, jaundice, cough, dyspnea, tachypnea, pulmonary edema, convulsions, coma | Paraquat and diquat in blood and urine |

Key: CNS = central nervous system.
*Use of trade names is for identification only and does not imply endorsement by the authors.
Source: J Brender et al. Tex Med 1988; 84:29–35; reprinted with kind permission of author.

countries are increasingly focusing their attention on long-term or chronic health effects of occupational pesticide exposure. Most epidemiologic studies have focused on manufacturing workers, pesticide applicators, and farmers rather than on hired farmworkers. Recent studies have suggested associations between pesticides and cancers of the lymphatic and hematopoietic systems, connective tissue, brain, prostate, skin, stomach, colon, and lip. Noncancer endpoints are also of concern, including those of the reproductive, nervous, and other organ systems [12].

### Dermatitis

Dermatitis is the most frequently reported occupational disease in agriculture, as it is in many occupations. In 1990 the incidence rate per 100 full-time U.S. workers for skin diseases and disorders was 0.38 for agriculture, 0.19 for manufacturing, 0.065 for construction, and 0.024 for mining [9]. Several large studies have been conducted on the prevalence of dermatitis in general populations from Western Europe and the United States [13].

Most agricultural dermatoses are due to plant exposures, although pesticide-related skin diseases often require extended periods of disability leave. It is usually difficult to distinguish the clinical presentation of plant dermatoses from pesticide dermatoses, be they irritant contact dermatitis, allergic contact dermatitis, or a photosensitivity reaction. Agricultural workers exposed to pesticides are four times more likely to develop a skin rash than is the average worker [14]. Environmental conditions, such as heat, sweating skin, clothing, and skin damage (sunburn), can exacerbate skin irritation. Recent pesticide-related dermatitis outbreaks have been reported in several regions of the U.S. [13]. According to the California Pesticide Incidence Reporting System, 677 cases of dermatitis associated with exposure to sulfur and 506 cases related to propargite (Omite-CR) were reported from 1974 to 1985. In 1986 one of the largest and more severe dermatitis outbreaks occurred among 114 orange pickers as a result of exposure to propargite [15].

The differential diagnosis of plant dermatosis versus pesticide dermatosis is made primarily through the history of a temporal association among work in a certain field or crop, the agricultural cycle and chemical applications, and symptoms. As examples, a recurrent rash in the early part of June may be related to a weed that flourishes then, or a rash occurring in July may result from exposure to an herbicide used on the crop at that stage of the cycle each year. Distribution of a rash on the arms or legs may also provide a clue; pesticide residues dislodged from foliage often irritate the face and neck in addition to the forearms, hands, and ankles, whereas contact with plants may produce irritation on the forearms, hands, and ankles alone. Patch testing with plant extracts or pesticide samples will frequently permit a definitive diagnosis in cases of allergic contact dermatitis (see Chap. 24).

### Musculoskeletal Diseases

Farmworkers are exposed to many of the risk factors that are associated with musculoskeletal disorders. Occupational factors include heavy lifting and carrying, forward bending, kneeling, bent-over positioning, and excessively fast-paced work. The physical strain and repetitive motions involved in farm work can lead to traumatic injuries, irritation of joint tissues, and accelerated degeneration of the joints. Descriptive survey data from U.S. states (New York, Florida, Michigan, and Wisconsin) report that musculoskeletal problems are one of the most frequently reported conditions among farmworkers, specifically back pain and vertebral sprain/strain [14].

Health surveys in the U.S. have further found that farmworkers have a higher prevalence of arthritis than white-collar, blue-collar, or service workers, and all workers combined; musculoskeletal conditions are the most commonly reported ailments among farmers and farm managers, and farmers report over 50 percent more musculoskeletal disorder than farm managers [16]. Musculoskeletal disorders are often ignored by clinicians, either because they look predominantly for signs of pesticide exposure or because they assume that musculoskeletal disease is an unavoidable result of farm labor. In fact, ergonomic strain associated with farm work can be minimized or entirely prevented with the appropriate redesign of equipment and labor practices. In forestry and construction occupations, related or similar to some in agriculture, such changes have significantly reduced the ergonomic problems of many tasks (see Chap. 8).

Traditional agricultural tools and labor practices exact a toll on the musculoskeletal system of lifelong farmers and workers. Modernization, in turn, has frequently brought more extensive use, and physiologically less adaptive uses, of traditional tools, such as "el cortito," the short-handled hoe. Replacing or modifying a tool can have a significant effect on the health of workers; for example, a 34 percent decrease in sprain and strain injuries occurred among California farmworkers as the use of the short-handled hoe declined. While California banned the short-handled hoe in 1975, other states did not do so until the 1980s.

The industrialization of agriculture has also introduced new equipment for harvesting and on-field packaging of many fruits and vegetables. This equipment, which has frequently been designed without the benefit of ergonomic analyses, leads to risks of musculoskeletal disorders and injury for farmworkers and operators.

### Other Occupationally Related Diseases

In addition to the occupational risks of pesticide intoxications, dermatitis, and musculoskeletal problems, agricultural work entails health and safety risks associated with the use of equipment, exposure to animal-borne infectious diseases (see Chap. 18), heat stress (see Chap. 17), and, from the operation of heavy equipment such as tractors and combines, hearing loss (see Chap. 16). Both acute and chronic lung disease have been associated with workplace exposures in agriculture (see Chap. 22). Airborne dusts, particularly those with high organic content, can produce acute hypersensitivity pneumonitis and organic dust toxic syndrome, a febrile illness associated with myalgias, malaise,

dry cough, chest tightness, and headache. Of special concern are exposures to mycotoxins and bacterial endotoxins, which are associated with many agricultural processes and products.

## Pesticide Exposures

On November 15, 1989, 81 fieldworkers were poisoned within the first hour of work tying leaves in a cauliflower field. The workers detected a strong odor upon entering the field and complained of feeling ill with nausea, fainting, vomiting, headache, extreme sweating, blurry vision, and dizziness; they were also noted to have bradycardia and elevated blood pressure. The field had been sprayed 16 hours earlier with a highly toxic organophosphorus insecticide, mevinphos (Phosdrin). The safe reentry interval for this EPA Toxicity I compound at the time was 24 hours (since extended to 48 hours). The workers were not informed of the application and no signs were posted to alert the crew of any hazard.

The workers went to the nearby migrant health and community clinic, where a system for decontamination was quickly established. This involved removing and bagging clothes, showering patients individually, and wrapping them in large sheets. The clinic, where 150 patients are seen daily, reported that it was not adequately prepared for the massive poisoning incident, even though a formal emergency response protocol for pesticide poisoning was available. The medical director of the clinic reported difficulty in obtaining the name of the chemical until he said that the clinic was faced with a crisis of major proportions. Forty-six workers were hospitalized. All of them received red blood cell and plasma cholinesterase tests at the time of hospitalization, as well as two subsequent tests to document the duration of inhibition of this enzyme. As many as 15 other workers continued to work in the cauliflower field the following day because they needed the wages to pay their bills and were afraid of losing their jobs [17].

Acutely toxic pesticides are used extensively in agriculture; it is estimated that the volume of organophosphorus insecticides used worldwide will double over the next decade [1]. The poisoning incident described above, one of the largest poisonings of a crew (team) documented in the U.S., illustrates many of the pesticide-related problems that farmworkers face. First, although health and safety standards prohibit early reentry into treated fields, such regulations may be overlooked or ignored. If workers are not provided with notification regarding applications, they have no means of protecting themselves in such circumstances. Second, even health care facilities that are aware of the potential for acute pesticide intoxications may be unprepared for outbreaks of this magnitude; in many such facilities, poisonings related to cholinesterase inhibition are still misdiagnosed. Finally, economic pressures often force workers to continue to work under hazardous conditions; support of one's family and even one's job may be at stake.

Large crew poisonings in the U.S. are not as common today as they were two decades ago, but this case indicates that even in societies with established health and safety laws and regulations, pesticide exposure continues to be a major health concern for agricultural workers. In countries where health and safety laws are virtually nonexistent and health care is often inaccessible, pesticide use can result in epidemics of severe poisoning.

### Worldwide Pesticide Issues

Pesticide use patterns have changed significantly during the past 20 years. Developed countries predominantly use herbicides and more selective insecticides and fungicides, while developing countries use mainly insecticides, many of which are acutely toxic [1]. Major pesticide groups and their global level of use in 1985 were as follows: herbicides (46 percent), insecticides (31 percent), and fungicides (18 percent). Highly toxic fumigants are also used in agriculture and are a serious hazard in some parts of the world. In terms of amounts applied per hectare (2.5 acres), pesticide consumption has been greatest in Japan, Europe, the United States, and China. Other major users of pesticides are Brazil, Mexico, Malaysia, Colombia, and Argentina.

The size of the population at risk for pesticide exposure is largest in developing countries, since the majority of the economically active members of the population work in agriculture. A recent report by the Pesticides Trust [18] considers that pesticide use is most hazardous in countries that have high rates of illiteracy, lack of protective equipment, lack of washing water, hot and humid climates, absence of medical facilities, and lack of trained workforce.

The WHO has identified Africa as the fastest-growing pesticide market, with pesticides almost tripling in sales between 1980 and 1984. This has serious implications for countries such as Benin, Senegal, and Togo because they lack pesticide legislation, have insufficient pesticide information on health effects and controls, and no monitoring systems to evaluate the health impact of pesticides. Although some trade control measures have been implemented during the late 1980s, developing countries continue to rely upon pesticides that have been restricted or banned for use in developed countries, such as carbofuran, methamidophos, parathion, and paraquat. Several explanations can be offered for the continued use of these compounds:

- The compounds are less expensive than the more selective pesticides.
- The compounds are broad spectrum and can be used for a variety of pest problems.
- Many chemical companies promote their safe use through strong marketing campaigns.
- Information regarding health effects is not always provided to the importing nation.
- Knowledge pertaining to integrated pest management practices and least toxic alternatives is lacking or not emphasized.

Developing nations are now focusing on many of the pesticide health and exposure problems experienced by industrialized countries during the 1970s. According to the few case reports and surveys from developing countries, pesticide poisoning is a major public health concern today (see box). The case studies presented here indicate that the problem is most likely underestimated by present statistics, especially since most statistics fail to account for mild poisonings. As illustrated in the case of Nicaragua, a comprehensive pesticide surveillance program can be instrumental in identifying and preventing pesticide poisonings. Cooperation among governments (especially those exporting pesticides), the agrochemical industry, and economic development institutions such as the World Bank is crucial to progress in this area.

### FAO International Code of Conduct

The United Nations Food and Agriculture Organization (FAO) adopted the International Code of Conduct on the Distribution and Use of Pesticides in 1985 as a means of addressing the growing number of illnesses, deaths, and environmental hazards caused by pesticides [19]. The Code received support from major pesticide manufacturers, governments, and nongovernmental organizations. The Code delineated a comprehensive set of international guidelines to assist governments with the registration and safe use of pesticides. An additional provision was passed in 1989, called Prior Informed Consent (PIC), which granted governments the right to refuse importation of pesticides that were already banned or severely restricted for health and environmental reasons by other countries. Countries also can apply this provision to those pesticides that have been identified as causing health or environmental problems in their own country. To date, 19 pesticides, including DDT, chlordane, ethyl parathion, toxaphene, and 2,4,5-T, have been granted PIC status, with others under consideration [18].

## Occupational Hygiene in Agriculture

Only recently have the principles of occupational hygiene been applied systematically to agriculture. The evaluation of pesticide use and exposure in ag-

riculture is complex for several reasons. First, the physical nature of the chemical can vary greatly: Workers may be exposed to pesticides in their concentrated form, as a dilute aqueous spray, as granules or pellets, or as a residue on crops and foliage. Second, workers are exposed to a wide variety of chemicals over a single season: An acutely toxic organophosphorus compound may be applied one day, a skin-irritating sulfur material the next day, and a mutagenic fungicide on the following day; or several compounds may be applied simultaneously. Third, chemical exposures occur under uncontrolled environmental conditions: Factors such as wind, rain, and sunlight can dramatically alter exposure potential. Finally, unlike exposures in many industrial settings, the major route of exposure to pesticides in agriculture is dermal rather than respiratory. For this reason, traditional occupational hygiene approaches, such as air sampling and adherence to threshold limit values (TLVs), have limited relevance. In considering the evaluation and control of agricultural pesticide exposures, it is useful to distinguish between workers who directly handle pesticides during application and those who are exposed primarily to residues following application.

### Mixers and Applicators

As the organophosphorus insecticides replaced organochlorines for many uses in the 1950s, it became evident that mixers and applicators were at high risk for acute intoxication. It was also determined at the time that the primary pesticide exposure pathway for agricultural workers was skin exposure and absorption. Investigators developed what has come to be known as the "patch technique," using absorbent pads as collection devices on various parts of the body to determine levels of deposition. Hand exposure was measured by rinsing the hands with water or alcohol and concentrating the residue collected. These methods were subsequently used throughout the world to assess worker exposure to pesticides, and form the basis of the WHO's current guidelines [20].

## CASE EXAMPLES FROM DEVELOPING COUNTRIES

Based on the limited case reports from developing countries, it is evident that pesticide poisoning is a major public health concern today. The case studies below indicate that the problem is most likely underrepresented by the present statistics and, therefore, warrants immediate attention by governments, the agrochemical industry, and other institutions, such as the World Bank. Furthermore, most statistics fail to account for the mild poisonings and chronic illnesses caused by pesticides. A comprehensive pesticide surveillance program can be instrumental in identifying and alleviating pesticide poisonings.

### Sri Lanka

One of the first surveys to indicate the severity of the pesticide problem among developing countries came from Sri Lanka in 1982. A study based on hospital surveys showed that approximately 13,000 patients were hospitalized and 1,000 died from acute pesticide poisoning. Twenty-five percent were attributed to occupational and accidental poisoning and 76 percent of the cases were due to organophosphates. The authors estimated that 5 of 1,000 agricultural workers are hospitalized each year for pesticide poisoning due to occupational exposures, and that ". . . the total number of poisoning episodes must be much greater than this figure" [30].

### Guatemala

Based on a doctor's report from Guatemala, a notable increase of pesticide poisonings occurred during the main agricultural spray season. The report showed that, on average, 1,100 cases of pesticide poisoning were treated in 18 hospitals between 1987 and 1990; 41 percent were due to occupational exposure in which skin was the major route of exposure. The agrochemical industry is targeting a pilot project in this country to promote the safe use of pesticides [18].

### Nicaragua

In the early 1980s Nicaragua implemented a national health surveillance system that included a regional pesticide poisoning registry for the northwest part of the country. During the 1987 growing season, an epidemic of 548 pesticide poisonings was reported through this system. Nineteen percent of the patients were less than 16 years of age. With an effective system in place, health care providers were able to identify the pesticides involved, carbofuran in 50 percent of cases and methamidophos in 33 percent. This allowed authorities to declare a regional health emergency and to conduct a worker education program to reduce future exposures and poisonings [31].

### Costa Rica

Costa Rica has an agricultural export-based economy in which pesticide use is widespread. It is one of the few developing countries that has documented cases of a chronic illness caused by the pesticide 1,2-dibromo-3-chloropropane (DBCP), a testicular toxicant. Over 1,500 workers, all banana plantation laborers, have been sterilized as a result of exposure to this compound, and more cases are reported each year. The transfer of health information from industrialized countries to the developing world is imperative to provide adequate care for the worker population and to prevent epidemics such as this one [32].

These methods have provided sufficient information to draw several important conclusions. First, the highest exposures usually occur during mixing and handling of the concentrated material. Second, wind is the single most important factor determining dermal exposure during application. Third, in most cases, exposure to the hands constitutes a major fraction of the total exposure. Fourth, the use of protective clothing can substantially reduce total dermal exposure. More recently, fluorescent tracers have been employed to visualize patterns of pesticide deposition on the skin (Fig. 35-3), allowing evaluation of protective clothing performance and effective worker education [21].

Efforts to reduce mixer and applicator exposures have focused on placing a barrier between the worker and the source of exposure. The primary method during pesticide mixing is an engineering control: the closed system that transfers the pesticide from its container to the mixing tank without direct handling by the worker. When functioning properly, these systems can reduce exposure considerably, but if a system failure occurs potential exposure is very high.

The most common engineering control for exposure reduction during the application of pesticides is the closed cab tractor. The closed cab normally provides an effective barrier to dermal contact; however, the efficiency of the air-filtration system is critical. If the cab is left partially open or if improper filters are employed, the utility of this approach is reduced drastically. Also, exposure may actually be higher inside the cab than outside if the worker enters the cab with boots and workclothes that have been contaminated during mixing procedures. A recent engineering control aimed at hand spraying, developed in Brazil, involves mounting the spray apparatus on bicycle wheels that are pushed ahead of the applicator. As the distance between the operator and the spray is increased, exposure is decreased substantially [22].

A supplemental but very important preventive measure for mixers and applicators is training:

**Fig. 35-3.** A. Fluorescent tracer evaluation of a pesticide applicator reveals deposition on the neck and on the chest beneath coveralls. The area around the mouth was protected by a respirator. B. The use of gloves while handling pesticides can reduce exposure dramatically. The right hand, in this photograph done with a fluorescent tracer, was not protected by a glove, as the left one was.

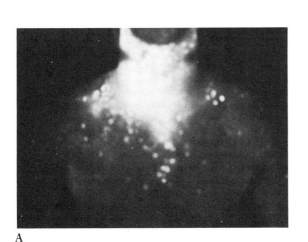

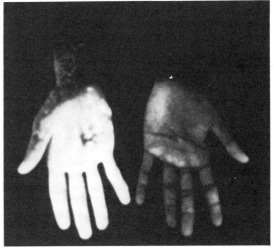

A                                                    B

Knowledge of the operation of closed systems, of the relative toxicity of compounds, of the proper handling and disposal of concentrated material, and of when to spray is required. (Since windy conditions will increase exposures and off-target drift substantially during application, many agricultural regions prohibit pesticide spraying at these times.)

The final control strategy for mixers and applicators is protective clothing. Protective gear, such as gloves, face shields, aprons, and boots, can effectively reduce exposure. If mixing is only an intermittent and short-term activity, such a strategy may prove practical, but skin contamination can still occur in the removal of the gear, in cases in which clothing is not properly cleaned before reuse, or when the barrier properties of the material fail. Regulatory agencies, such as the EPA, have increasingly turned to protective clothing as a primary strategy for exposure reduction in agriculture. Indeed, personal protection plays a prominent role in the EPA's recent Worker Protection Standard related to agricultural pesticides [23]. Personal protection has always been considered a control of last resort by occupational hygienists for a number of important reasons. First, such a control strategy requires continual training of personnel in the proper use and maintenance of clothing. Second, the clothing must be inspected periodically and replaced when necessary. Third, use of chemical protective clothing often reduces the comfort, agility, and dexterity of the worker and may contribute to heat stress under agricultural conditions. Thus, an effective control program based on protective clothing may prove to be more costly and more difficult to monitor than equally effective engineering and administrative approaches.

### Fieldworkers

The pesticide hazard that agricultural fieldworkers confront takes the form of residues on fruit, foliage, or soil. This hazard is complicated by workers generally being unaware of their potential for exposure and the consequent health risks they face. Since many of these workers are migratory and are not involved with other farm operations, they may not know what pesticides have been used or when they were sprayed. Furthermore, a substantial number of studies have demonstrated that residue levels on foliage are difficult to predict. In arid regions, such as California and the southwestern United States, high residue levels can remain for many weeks. Under certain environmental conditions, a number of organophosphorus compounds can even be transformed into their more toxic "oxon" derivatives; for example, the oxon derivative of parathion, paraoxon, is 10 times more acutely toxic than parathion.

The thinning and harvesting operations that fieldworkers perform require direct contact with foliage, and significant dermal exposure to any pesticide residues on the foliage is largely unavoidable. The hard physical labor and high temperatures typically encountered make protective clothing an even more unrealistic method for the prevention of exposure. Several decades of research point to the conclusion that the only practical means of minimizing exposure for fieldworkers is to make certain that toxic levels of residues have degraded or dissipated before workers are allowed into the fields. To achieve this goal, *restricted entry intervals* are derived from repeated studies of pesticide residue decay on specific crops. Under the new U.S. Worker Protection Standard, the EPA has established a minimum restricted entry interval of 12 hours for all pesticide applications, superseding the previous minimum interval of waiting "until sprays have dried and dusts have settled." A 48-hour restricted interval is now required for Toxicity I compounds and a 24-hour interval for Toxicity II compounds. In California, where extended reentry is an issue because of the arid climate and persistent residues, restricted entry intervals may extend up to 60 days for particular pesticide and crop combinations.

Traditional engineering controls used in occupational health are usually not feasible as a means of reducing pesticide residue exposures in agriculture. However, several prevention strategies with engineering aspects are useful. One strategy is the provision of handwashing facilities for the removal of pesticide residues before eating or using the bathroom and at the end of the workday. A second strategy is product substitution, in which a less toxic pesticide replaces a more hazardous one. A third approach is the development of alternative pest control technologies, such as biologic control, that reduce pesticide use. A final engineering possibility is the application of alternative cultivation practices, such as crop rotation and the cultivation of mixed varieties, that reduce the need for heavy pesticide use.

## Management and Prevention of Pesticide Illness

### Moderate to Severe Acute Illnesses

Acute pesticide-related illnesses are frequently recognized in the initial presentation of the patient to the clinician, although the specific chemical may be unknown (see Table 35-1). Most common among acute pesticide poisonings today are those caused by organophosphates with fairly typical symptoms, as illustrated in the case presented earlier in this chapter. As emergency life-support procedures are instituted, samples of vomitus, urine, and blood should be taken, and the patient should be rapidly decontaminated. Also, care must be taken to protect health workers from exposure because exposures in handling bodily fluids or contaminated clothing may be substantial, and emergency room personnel have become very ill while assisting pesticide-poisoned patients. Specific clinical treatment for acute and emergent pesticide exposure is comprehensively detailed in *Recognition and Management of Pesticide Poisonings* [24].

The clinical diagnosis of moderate or severe organophosphate poisoning is confirmed when a test dose of atropine does not result in symptoms of atropinization, including flushing, rapid heart rate, large pupils, and dryness of the mouth. Chemical tests for the presence of pesticide residues or their metabolites permit the subsequent identification of organophosphates and other compounds for medicolegal purposes, although usually not early enough to affect the course of clinical treatment. Because farmworkers who become ill at work often must obtain medical assistance on their own, it is important to inquire whether other workers were potentially exposed, so that public health investigators can attempt to locate them in order to both investigate the incident and offer medical care.

### Mild Acute Pesticide Illnesses

Mild acute organophosphate effects—those not severe enough to require treatment with atropine—have been associated with low-level occupational pesticide exposures in several descriptive epidemiologic studies [25]. These effects manifest themselves as one or more central nervous system symptoms that are easily mistaken for common nonoccupational diseases—headache, fatigue, drowsiness, insomnia and other sleep disturbances, mental confusion, disturbances of concentration and memory, anxiety, and emotional lability. It is extremely difficult to demonstrate a clinical association between symptoms and exposure under these circumstances, since the symptoms often occur at relatively slight levels of cholinesterase depression. Individual cases of such mild effects normally go undiagnosed and therefore unreported.

### Long-Term Effects of Acute Intoxications

Anecdotal reports and clinical case findings have long suggested that for some workers acute organophosphate intoxication is not a transient phenomenon. Rather, low-grade symptoms appear to linger for months and even years. Several recent studies employing neurobehavioral and neuropsychological test batteries have indicated that individuals with acute poisoning histories who appear normal on clinical evaluation exhibit deficits in one or more aspects of neurologic function [26, 27]. Such persistent effects have become the focus of substantial research aimed at understanding underlying mechanisms and dose-response relationships.

## Medical Surveillance

Measurements of cholinesterase inhibition have been used since the 1950s to evaluate acute poisonings and chronic exposure among pesticide applicators, and more recently to evaluate low-level exposure among farmworkers. Although plasma cholinesterase measurements are more widely used, the red blood cell (RBC) values are a more valid indicator of the pesticide's physiologic effect on the nervous system. There is a significant degree of intraindividual and interindividual variation for both types of cholinesterase; consequently, the reduction in cholinesterase activity required to diagnose pesticide-induced inhibition is relatively large even when preexposure baseline values are available for comparison.

Without baseline values, plasma activity levels usually must be 30 percent or more below the normal laboratory range to achieve statistical significance. When a baseline value is available, a 20 percent decline in plasma activity and 15 percent decline in red cell activity is significant. Unfortunately, mild, but persistent and disabling, symptoms may occur at levels of inhibition far less impressive than these. In a large study of California lettuce harvesters exposed to mevinphos (Phosdrin), for example, moderately severe symptoms were reported despite plasma and red cell cholinesterase inhibition averages of 16 percent and 6 percent, respectively. The frequency and duration of their symptoms is suggested by results shown in Fig. 35-4 [28].

Workers with probable pesticide-related symptoms or a cholinesterase inhibition of 30 percent or more, or both, should be withdrawn from work and retested; if the original test result is confirmed, the work situation and practices should be investigated. If the red cell or plasma cholinesterase activity declines from baseline are 40 or 50 percent,

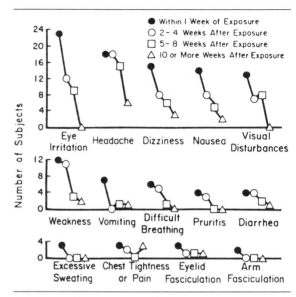

**Fig. 35-4.** The time course of symptoms reported by crew members exposed to organophosphates over the follow-up period (22–29 subjects examined at different times). (From MJ Coye et al. Clinical confirmation of organophosphate poisoning of agricultural workers. Am J Ind Med 1986; 10:399–409.)

respectively, the clinician should not release the worker to any risk of further exposure until both cholinesterase levels return to baseline. Release to work should depend on red cell cholinesterase activity. If a red cell value increases by more than 10 to 15 percent over the value one week earlier, the worker's normal baseline may not yet have been reached. However, farmworkers frequently return to work for economic reasons long before their red cell cholinesterase activity demonstrates complete recovery, or even before their symptoms have completely resolved.

Routine monitoring of cholinesterase levels is appropriate for workers handling organophosphate or carbamate pesticides on a regular basis, including applicators, mixer/loaders, flaggers, and equipment maintenance workers. Biologic monitoring for compounds other than the organophosphates and carbamates has been limited to a few chemicals that can be reliably detected in blood or urine, are relatively rapidly eliminated from the body, and are potentially toxic enough to merit surveillance. These chemicals include pentachlorophenol, methyl bromide, and chlordimeform. Although analytical methods exist for the detection of many other compounds in biologic samples, either intact or as metabolites, these tests are used primarily in research settings. In addition to research determining the absorption, metabolism, and excretion of pesticides, however, the tests are useful in research aimed at establishing restricted entry periods or evaluating the effectiveness of engineering controls and protective clothing.

### Prevention Strategies

The historic treatment of agriculture as a special case in regard to occupational safety and health has resulted in a failure to adequately protect the health of many agricultural workers. Health care providers, therefore, have a unique opportunity and responsibility to redress this inequity by offering these workers adequate information about occupational hazards and appropriate medical care. The experience of many agricultural workers has led them to believe that they must accept pesticide exposures as a price of employment. Without a thorough review, clinicians are never justified in assuming that workers are adequately informed about the hazards of their work, or that they are adequately protected.

Several techniques and approaches that may contribute to a pesticide exposure prevention strategy for agricultural workers are highlighted here in brief:

- *Reduced use or elimination policies for highly toxic pesticides.* The World Bank has recently promoted a shift to relatively low-toxicity pesticide formulations used in Bank-financed projects. This recommendation is based on the concept that complete protection of workers with personal protective equipment cannot be expected in hot climates [1].

- *Pesticide use and incident reporting systems.* Until pesticide-related illnesses can be enumerated and linked to specific pesticide use patterns, regulatory interventions will continue to be instituted on an ad hoc basis. Systems such as the California Pesticide Incident Reporting System can serve as models for such programs.

- *Improved hazard communication.* Workers should be provided with meaningful health and safety information. Fluorescent tracer evaluation of dermal exposures is one promising and inexpensive tool for improved worker education and training. Such an approach is particularly effective because it draws on the worker's own knowledge in analyzing the sources of exposure and the means for reducing them [21].

- *Routine medical surveillance.* Increased medical surveillance will be possible in many parts of the world as field-based systems for measuring cholinesterase inhibition are validated and made widely available. A field portable cholinesterase test kit has performed well in recent field trials and reduces the cost of such assays considerably [29].

- *Improved analytical procedures.* Residue monitoring and occupational exposure assessments can be simplified and costs reduced by use of new analytical techniques. Immunoassays for pesticide residue analysis show great promise in measuring low amounts of pesticides and their metabolites with great specificity.

- *Integrated pest management (IPM) programs.* IPM programs are gaining widespread acceptance in agriculture, and represent a shift in management practices from traditional chemical control to a mixture of control approaches. This approach recognizes pest control as a process requiring substantial knowledge of insect behavior within a broad agro-ecosystem context.

- *Safe use promotion programs.* Many pesticide manufacturers are voluntarily supporting the FAO Code. In addition, Groupement International des Associations Nationales de Fabricants de Produits Agrochimiques (GIFAP), a pesticide manufacturers' association, has begun a pilot project to promote the safe use of pesticides in Kenya, Thailand, and Guatemala [18].

# References

1. World Health Organization. The public health impact of pesticides used in agriculture. Geneva, 1990.
2. USDHHS/CDC/NIOSH. Papers and proceedings of the Surgeon General's Conference on Agricultural Safety and Health. Des Moines, Iowa, April 30–May 3, 1991. Washington, D.C.: U.S. Printing Office, (NTIS PB 93-114890).
3. United States General Accounting Office. Hired farmworkers: Health and well-being at risk. Washington, D.C. (GAO/HRD-92-46), 1992.
4. Commission on Agricultural Workers. Report of the Commission on Agricultural Workers. Washington, D.C., November 1992.
5. Moses M. Pesticide-related health problems and farmworkers. AAOHN J 1989; 37:115–130.
6. Pollack SH, Landrigan PJ, Mallino DL. Child labor in 1990: Prevalence and health hazards. Ann Rev Public Health 1990; 11:359–75.
7. Wilk V. Health hazards to children in agriculture. Am J Ind Med 1993; 24:283–90.
8. National Research Council. Pesticides in the diets of infants and children. Washington, D.C.: National Academy Press, 1993.
9. National Safety Council. Accident facts, 1992 ed. Chicago, 1992.
10. Levine RS, Doull J. Global estimates of acute pesticide morbidity and mortality. Rev Environ Cont Toxicol 1993; 129:29–44.
11. California Environmental Protection Agency, Department of Pesticide Regulation. Summary of illnesses and injuries reported by California physicians as potentially related to pesticides in 1990. HS-1666, March 1, 1993.
12. Maroni M, Fait A. Health effects in man from long-term exposure to pesticides. Toxicology 1993; 78:1–180.
13. Mobed K, et al. Cross-cultural medicine: A decade later. West J Med 1992; 157:368–73.
14. Wilk V. The occupational health of migrant and seasonal farmworkers in the United States. Washington D.C.: The Farmworker Justice Fund, 1986.
15. Outbreak of severe dermatitis among orange pickers—California. MMWR 1986; 35:465–7.
16. NIOSH. Musculoskeletal disease in agricultural workers. Cincinnati: NIOSH, 1983. Internal Document. Information extracted for this chapter courtesy of Shiro Tanaka, M.D., Industry Wide Studies Branch, Division of Surveillance, Hazard Evaluations and Field Studies.
17. Ryder RE. Florida clinic handles massive pesticide poisoning. Migrant Health Clin Suppl 1989; 6: 66–7.
18. Dinham B. The pesticide hazard: A global health and environmental audit. Zed Books, London and New Jersey: The Pesticides Trust, 1993.
19. International Code of Conduct on the Distribution and Use of Pesticides (amended version). Rome: FAO, 1990.
20. WHO. World Health Organization field surveys of exposure to pesticides standard protocol. Toxicol Lett 1986; 33:223–35.
21. Fenske RA. Visual scoring system for fluorescent tracer evaluation of dermal exposure to pesticides. Bull Environ Contam Toxicol 1988; 41:727–36.
22. Machado N, Matuo JG, Matuo YK. Dermal exposure of pesticide applicators in staked tomato crops: Efficiency of a safety measure in the application equipment. Bull Environ Contam Toxicol 1992; 48:529–34.
23. Environmental Protection Agency. Worker protection standard, hazard information, hand labor tasks on cut flowers and ferns exception; final rule and proposed rules (40 CFR Parts 156 and 170). Fed Register 57:38102–76, 1992.
24. Morgan D. Recognition and management of pesticide poisonings. 4th ed. Washington, D.C.: Environmental Protection Agency, 1989. (EPA-540/9-88-001)
25. Coye MJ. The health effects of agricultural production: 1. The health of agricultural workers. J Public Health Policy 1985; 6:349–70.
26. Savage EP, et al. Chronic neurological sequelae of acute organophosphate pesticide poisoning. Arch Environ Health 1988; 43:38–44.
27. Rosenstock L, et al. Chronic central nervous system effects of acute organophosphate pesticide intoxication. Lancet 1991; 338:223–6.
28. Coye MJ, Barnett PG, Midtling JE. Clinical confirmation of organophosphate poisoning of agricultural workers. Am J Ind Med 1986; 10:399–409.
29. McConnell R, Cedillo L, Keifer M, Palamo M. Monitoring organophosphate insecticide exposed workers for cholinesterase depression: New technology for office or field use. J Occup Med 1992; 1:34–7.
30. Jeyaratnam J, Seneviratne de Alwis RS, Copplestone JF. Survey of pesticide poisoning in Sri Lanka. Bull WHO 1982; 60:615–9.
31. McConnell R, Hruska AJ. An epidemic of pesticide

poisoning in Nicaragua: Implications for prevention in developing countries. Am J Public Health 1993; 83:1559–62.

32. Thrupp LA. Sterilization of workers from pesticide exposure: The causes and consequences of DBCP-induced damage in Costa Rica and beyond. Int J Health Serv 1991; 21:731–57.

## Bibliography

Environmental Protection Agency. Worker protection standard: Final rule and proposed rules. Fed Register 57:38102–76, 1992.
*This document provides a comprehensive rationale for current regulations designed to protect agricultural workers from pesticide-related health risks, as well as the U.S. Environmental Protection Agency's final standard. It is available from the Occupational Safety Branch (H7506C), Environmental Protection Agency, 401 M St., SW, Washington, D.C. 20460 (phone: 703-305-7666).*

Maroni M, Fait A. Health effects in man from long-term exposure to pesticides. Toxicology 1993; 78:1–180.
*A thorough review of all the scientific literature related to chronic health effects of pesticides in humans. Excellent source for references.*

Morgan D. Recognition and management of pesticide poisonings. 4th ed. Washington, D.C.: Environmental Protection Agency, 1989. (EPA-540/9-88-001)
*The most authoritative source for clinical aspects of pesticide poisonings. Used throughout the world as a handbook.*

Wilk V. The occupational health of migrant and seasonal farmworkers in the United States. Washington, D.C.: The Farmworker Justice Fund, 1986.
*This book provides an excellent overview of the wide range of health issues related to agricultural workers in the United States.*

World Health Organization. The public health impact of pesticides used in agriculture. Geneva, 1990.

Dinham B. The pesticide hazard: A global health and environmental audit. Zed Books, London and New Jersey: The Pesticides Trust, 1993.
*These two monographs provide a global review of pesticide use. Work-related aspects of pesticide exposures are a small but important section of these monographs.*

# 36
# Construction Workers

Knut Ringen, Anders Englund, and Jane Seegal

Construction workers build highways, stadiums, industrial plants, office buildings, and homes. They also repair or renovate roads, bridges, and other structures and demolish or clean up former building sites and hazardous waste sites. The work is hard physical labor, often under difficult conditions, including hot, cold, or wet weather. Construction workers—drawn largely from immigrants and members of other low-income groups—face predictable occupational illnesses and injuries, including the vibration white finger of the jackhammer operator, silicosis of the tunnel builder, low back pain of the bricklayer, skin allergies of the mason, carpal tunnel syndrome of the iron worker or electrician, solvent-related kidney disorders of the painter and roofer, lead poisoning of the bridge rehabilitation worker, asbestosis of the building demolition worker, and heat stress (from wearing "moon suits") of the hazardous waste clean-up worker [1] (Fig. 36-1).

The causes of work-related injuries are well defined, while the risks of chronic occupationally related disorders are poorly defined, as are the relationships between exposures and chronic diseases.

## Epidemiologic Overview

The construction industry in the U.S. employs 5 to 6 percent of the labor force, but has 15 percent of the fatal injuries and more than 9 percent of the days lost to work-related injuries. National Safety Council estimates for 1992 show a death rate among construction workers of 22 per 100,000

workers; 5 or more workers are killed by injuries sustained on the job in the U.S. during each workday. This rate of traumatic deaths in construction is 11,000 times higher than the rate of one death per million workers over a 45-year work life, which the Occupational Safety and Health Administration (OSHA) defines as a significant risk for a carcinogen.

Lost-time injuries affect 6.6 per 100 full-time workers in the U.S. yearly, according to the U.S. Bureau of Statistics. That rate and the time taken off to recover have been slowly increasing since 1975. Experience is a factor, with the rate of injuries "decreasing substantially as length of service increases" [2]. Familiarity with a job site also is a consideration. For laborers, who suffer some of the highest injury rates, the U.S. Bureau of Labor Statistics reports that 12 percent of lost-time injuries occur during the first day on a job site; this pattern appears to hold for most of the trades.

Construction workers disabled or killed each year by work-related illnesses are believed to number in the tens of thousands, but there are no firm data to support this estimate.

For a mix of reasons—work-related and not, and many still poorly understood—the average age at death for construction workers is substantially lower than that for members of low-risk groups, such as teachers or physicians (Fig. 36-2). The chart of standardized mortality ratios (SMRs) for selected occupations in California shows how many construction-related occupations have SMRs that are 1.5 to 3.0 times greater than the average for all professions, and 4 to 5 times higher

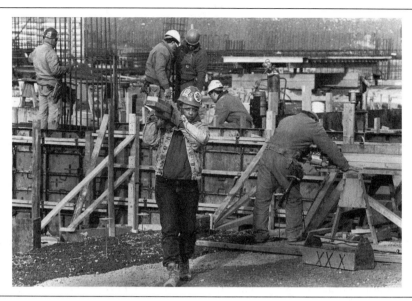

**Fig. 36-1.** Construction workers building a large sewage treatment plant. Women remain a small minority of the construction workforce in most countries. (Photograph by Marvin Lewiton.)

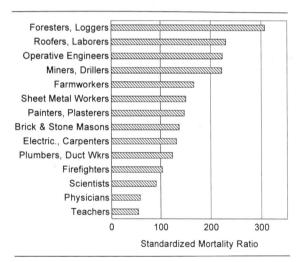

**Fig. 36-2.** Standardized mortality ratio for selected occupations. (Data from California Department of Health Services. *California Occupational Mortality, 1979–1981.* Sacramento, March 1987. Table 7A.)

than for low-risk occupations. These data translate to an average age at death for construction workers that is 8 to 12 years less than for low-risk occupations.

Protection of the construction workforce in some other industrialized countries is more effective than in the U.S. International comparisons are difficult to make, but the death rate for construction workers in the U.S. appears to be substantially higher than it is elsewhere, including Germany (the former West Germany), the Netherlands, Sweden, and Ontario, Canada. Since 1970 the rate of deaths from worksite injuries has been reduced 75 percent in Sweden; since 1965 it has declined 83 percent in Ontario. One reason for the disparity between the U.S. and these other nations is that the other nations have a history of focused safety and health programs.

## Organization of the Work

Several factors contribute to the grim picture for safety and health in construction. All are related to

## THE SWEDISH LONGITUDINAL STUDY

In the late 1960s the construction unions and employers in Sweden established Bygghälsan, the Swedish Construction Industry's Organization for Working Environment, Occupational Safety, and Health. The organization has had as its objective the identification of safety and health risks and the development of strategies to reduce them. Physicians, nurses, physical therapists, safety engineers, and industrial hygienists provide an integrated program focusing on safety and health from the perspectives of exposures on the worksite and medical problems of the worker. One of the critical contributions made by Bygghälsan has been the systematic study of health status of construction workers.

### Two Cohorts

Bygghälsan in 1969 began offering, on a voluntary basis, preventive and occupational medical examinations to all construction workers. Starting in 1971 it began establishing a cohort of all construction workers who participated. By 1979 more than 225,000 workers had been registered. This longitudinal study has used the medical examination results of the cohort and its listings in the national cancer incidence registry and the national mortality registries.*

Bygghälsan has simultaneously followed a smaller cohort of *all* male union painters and certified plumbers and insulators (approximately 50,000). This cohort was divided into those who did participate (approximately two-thirds) and those who did not participate (one-third) in the voluntary medical examinations.

Both cohorts have been followed through 1988 for mortality and through 1987 for cancer incidence. For the larger cohort, 18,659 deaths have been reported and 9,940 cancer cases were diagnosed after the first medical examination (Table 36-1). As expected, cardiovascular disease was the main cause of death, but the death rate from this cause was lower than the national rate. Cancer incidence, on the other hand, was at 90 to 95 percent of the rate for the overall population. The lower cardiovascular mortality is thought to be a combination of selection mechanisms, as well as preventive programs on hypertension, smoking, diet, and exercise.

### The Nonparticipant Factor

One notable finding in the smaller cohort was the observation that nonparticipants showed an overall mortality 72 percent greater than that of participants. Similar results were obtained for cancer incidence. These differences were more marked for those diseases associated with poor health behaviors. Prostate cancer was in significant excess for participants, however, a finding that might reflect better diagnosis resulting from the regular use of preventive services.

In addition to what these studies tell us about the health of construction workers, the findings call attention to the need to seek new and better ways to identify and reach nonparticipants. Equally important is the need to be careful about conclusions drawn based on data from voluntary health programs because of the large selection bias (see Chap. 5).

---

*Engholm G. Prospective follow-up of a medical surveillance programme. Danderyd, Sweden: Bygghälsan, 1992.

**Table 36-1.** Selected excess mortality and incidence for cancer and other causes of death, Swedish construction workers[a,b]

| Trade | Cause of death (n) | SMR | Incident cancers (n) | SIR |
|---|---|---|---|---|
| Bricklayer | — | — | Peritoneum (2) | 12.5 |
| Carpenter | — | — | Nose (11) | 2.2 |
| Driver (truck/heavy equipment)[c] | — | — | Lip (6) | 3.6 |
| | | | Multiple myeloma (7) | 2.7 |
| Electrician | Bladder cancer (13) | 2.3 | [Bladder (39)] | 1.3 |
| Insulator | Pneumoconiosis (2) | 40 | Peritoneum (2) | 200 |
| Laborer | Accidental falls (67) | 1.5 | Lip (41) | 1.8 |
| | | | Stomach (152) | 1.2 |
| Maintenance worker[c] | Other accidents (7)[d] | 8.4 | Colon (11) | 2.5 |
| | Drowning (5) | 4.7 | | |
| Plumber | Pneumoconiosis (4) | 4.4 | Pleura (15) | 6.3 |
| | | | Lung (105) | 1.3 |
| Sheet metal worker | Accidental falls (11) | 2.4 | Lung (26) | 1.6 |
| Tunnel worker | Prostate cancer (20) | 1.9 | [Prostate (33)] | 1.1 |
| | Other accidents (10)[d] | 6.1 | | |
| | Violent death (69) | 1.5 | | |

SMR = standardized mortality ratio; SIR = standardized incidence ratio.
[a]Ratios are based on comparison with the white male Swedish population. The cohort of more than 225,000 workers was established in 1971 to 1979. Mortality was followed through 1988. Cancer incidence was followed through 1987.
[b]All values are statistically significant unless in brackets.
[c]Compared with the other construction trades, drivers and maintenance workers have a risk of death from heart disease of 1.37 and 1.40, respectively.
[d]Other accidents were predominantly work-related injuries.
Source: Data from Göran Engholm.

how the industry operates or how the work is performed.

Construction rarely provides steady employment; construction workers are always working themselves out of their jobs. Although some projects may last several years, many last only a few months. Many assignments on a project, such as roofing or painting, may last only a few days each, with several trades working on the site simultaneously. Thus, a construction worker may have four, five, or more employers in a year. Because of bad weather and layoffs between assignments, an individual may clock only 1,200 to 1,500 hours of work yearly in construction, compared with 2,000 hours in other industries. (Therefore, to permit comparisons among industries, construction employment statistics are based on full-time equivalents—the total number of hours worked divided by 2,000. There are 7 million construction workers in the U.S., which equals 3 million to 4 million full-time equivalents.)

Just as the work assignments change throughout a construction project, so do the topography of the worksite and the cast of employers. Each trade may work for a different contractor.

In addition, the universe of contractors is marked by high turnover. The only official estimate of the number of employers in construction, from the U.S. Department of Commerce, found 1.9 million establishments in 1987. Many of the contractors are self-employed individuals or mom-and-pop operations; an estimated 80 percent or more of construction firms have 10 or fewer employees. Less than 20 percent of all firms belong to a construction trade association.

These features all create public health problems. With so many job changes and small and short-lived firms, it is difficult to monitor an individual's work history. It is even more difficult to monitor injuries or exposures to hazards (see the following section, *Exposure-Related Problems*). The recording of injuries (except those that can be handled with first aid) in a log—as required by OSHA—has proved virtually unenforceable. A 1987 study commissioned by the National Academy of Sciences noted the difficulties in obtaining injury and illness data for construction. Among other things, the study cited poorly defined responsibility for reporting injuries and illnesses [3].

The constantly changing worksite has another marked effect on safety and health. Unlike in an industrial setting, where the tasks are often repetitive and controlled by the location of machinery, the construction site allows—and requires—extensive movement by the worker from moment to moment. This means that the worker is much more responsible for his or her own protection.

In addition to risk of injuries and exposures to hazardous substances, construction workers face long-term risk from the stress of on-and-off employment. Stress may be caused by the fear of not having a paycheck. Further, because construction jobs can be few and far apart, construction workers may have to travel long distances daily to work or may need to move their families frequently. The need to constantly move work location also takes its toll.

A lack of comprehensive employer organizations with which to work hampers some public health efforts. Labor-management organizations have served as the vehicles for the successful safety and health programs in Germany, the Netherlands, Sweden, and Ontario, Canada. In some sectors of all construction in the U.S., only 20 to 30 percent of the workers are unionized; the percentage is much higher for nonresidential construction. Having a multitudinous industry makes it difficult to implement preventive safety and health programs, including training programs.

## Exposure-Related Problems

### Measurement Technology

Industrial hygienists and researchers have been stymied in their efforts to develop a reliable system for measuring exposures in construction. In addition to the common problems of identifying and measuring exposures to substances at a worksite, there are problems tied to the logistics of worksites and available technology. (The use of *material safety data sheets* also presents problems; see Appendix A.)

Because each construction worker moves about a site, the worker's position in relation to exposure sources may change constantly. At some moments, a worker may be directly exposed while using a hazardous substance, but at other times the worker may be exposed to another substance as a bystander 10 feet downwind. It is thus difficult to anticipate all the substances and degrees of exposure a worker will encounter on a given day.

To measure exposures in manufacturing, integrated samples are collected to determine 8-hour time-weighted averages. Such an approach may not tell the whole story about health effects in construction, however. Brief, high-level exposures may have different and significant health effects compared with longer-term, low-level exposures. In addition, construction work is marked by types of exposures for which time-weighted averages cannot account—through skin absorption and, to a lesser extent, ingestion.

### Personal Protective Equipment

Workers may not know when they need to use specific personal protective equipment. If they do know, they may lack the equipment or needed training. And the use of some controls may create problems. For instance, construction workers often perform as teams, yet respirators may prevent coworkers from communicating with each other. Full-body protective clothing (moon suits) can contribute to heat stress.

Having protective gear without knowing its limitations can do more harm than good, by giving the worker or employer the illusion that the worker is protected. For example, no gloves protect for more than 2 hours against methylene chloride, which is contained in mixtures used in paint stripping. Solvent mixtures, such as those containing both acetone and toluene or both methanol and xylene, seep through gloves in less than one work shift.

A lack of eating and sanitary facilities may also present problems. Often, workers cannot wash up before meals and must eat in the work zone. A lack of changing facilities may result in transport of contaminants from the workplace to a worker's home.

**Table 36-2.** Distribution of lost-time injuries (fatal and nonfatal) among roofers and laborers

| Cause of injury | Roofers | Laborers |
|---|---|---|
| Falls from elevations | 23% | 11% |
| Overexertion | 23% | 22% |
| Struck by an object | 14% | 25% |
| Contact with temperature extremes | 9% | 2% |
| Struck against | 7% | 10% |
| Falls from same level | 6% | 7% |
| Bodily reaction[a] | 5% | 3% |
| Caught in/under/between (including cave-ins) | 3% | 8% |
| Rubbed/abraded | 3% | 7% |
| Contact with radiation, caustics, etc. | 2% | 3% |
| Other[b] | 5% | 2% |

[a]Includes, for instance, slipping and twisting body to catch oneself or twisting an ankle while climbing a ladder.
[b]Includes transport and nonclassifiable injuries.
Source: For laborer injuries: Bureau of Labor Statistics, Injuries to construction laborers. Washington, D.C., March 1986. Bulletin 2252, p. 8.; for roofer injuries: Martin E. Personick, Bureau of Labor Statistics, based on workers' compensation data, selected states.

## Major Health Outcomes

### Traumatic Injuries

Construction workers are at great risk of injury partly because of where they work—from scaffolding hundreds of feet up to trenches underground (Table 36-2). Specific hazards and overall risk vary by trade. Based on what is known in the U.S., iron workers appear to have the highest risk of work-related deaths [4]; in other countries, roofing may be the most dangerous trade because of the danger of falls and exposures to hot tar [5].

The rankings of causes of fatal and nonfatal injuries appear to differ, however. For example, falls from elevations tend to be so serious that they are responsible for most traumatic deaths on-site. For nonfatal injuries, however, most studies list "struck by an object" and "overexertion" as most important. The leading causes of lost-time injuries vary by trade. (In regions where a large proportion of the construction labor force consists of immigrants, the worker's inability to understand the national language may increase the risk of injury.)

### Musculoskeletal Disorders

Some musculoskeletal disorders result from traumatic injuries, but many others develop incrementally. These stem from repetitive tasks and awkward body positions. The bricklayer lifts an estimated 3 to 4 tons daily, with 1,000 trunk-twist flexions. The iron worker tying intersections of the perpendicular rods used to reinforce concrete may bend over more than half the workday, repeatedly twisting the wrist under pressure. In building construction, much of the finishing work involves areas above shoulder height or below knee level.

Although musculoskeletal disorders are not fatal, they are significant. According to data for construction in Ontario, Canada, about 66 percent of all workers' compensation claims and 90 percent of all days lost are the result of soft tissue injuries. In the U.S., these disorders are believed to account for 40 to 65 percent of workers' compensation costs in construction. A 3-year study in the state of Washington found that laborers, carpenters, roofers, and electricians generally have higher rates of musculoskeletal disorders.

Very little detailed analysis has been done of the problems of each trade. Since 1989 Bygghälsan (Sweden's Construction Industry's Organization for Working Environment, Occupational Safety, and Health) has collected questionnaires from more than 83,000 construction workers, including more than 19,000 carpenters. One-fifth of the carpenters responded "often" to questions on kneeling, working with hands above the shoulders, heavy lifting, and stooping. The following musculoskeletal disorders were also frequently reported by respondents: disorders of the knee, 21 percent; shoulder, 22 percent; lower back, 27 percent; and neck, 16 percent.

*The Holmström Study.* The most detailed scientific report on musculoskeletal disorders in construction workers included a sample of 1,773 construction workers in Malmö, Sweden [6]. Low back pain was found to be correlated with increasing age, construction trade personal habits, and psychosocial factors. Only 8 percent of the workers studied reported no musculoskeletal problems in the preceding year. For the preceding year, low back pain was reported by 72 percent, knee problems by 52 percent, and neck-shoulder pains by 37 percent.

The prevalence of most musculoskeletal symptoms increased with age. Low back pain correlated with frequent handling of handheld machines, handling of bricks and roofing materials, and awkward postures, such as stooping or kneeling for more than an hour a day. The prevalence and type of disorder varied by trade, however. Roofers, carpet and tile layers, and scaffolding erectors had the highest prevalence of low back pain, compared with the other construction trades.

Reported low back pain was 2.7 times more prevalent for smokers than for nonsmokers. Psychosocial factors also contributed significantly to "explain" low back pain, when other factors were kept constant.

Workers who reported no low back problems were generally in better physical condition, were more involved in recreational activities, smoked less, and had a more positive outlook than other workers. They reported fewer psychosomatic symptoms and were more active participants in worksite decision making. The average length of employment in construction for this group was 15 years.

Both groups of workers were found to have the same maximum abdominal and back muscle strength. Workers who reported severe low back problems had significantly reduced back muscle endurance.

### Chronic Illnesses

Some work-related illnesses appear to be correlated with specific construction trades (Table 36-3). For several reasons, including long latencies, however, it has often been difficult to relate chronic diseases to an individual's employment history.

*Pulmonary Diseases, Including Lung Cancers, and Bystander Exposures.* Construction sites are generally dusty—as powdered bags of cement are emptied for mixing, as wood is sawed, as heavy machinery lumbers across uneven terrain, and as pneumatic tools are used on quartz, drywall, and concrete. Fumes are produced by such activities as welding, roofing, and paving. Thus, construction workers' lungs are exposed to toxic hazards in several ways.

Asbestos and silica are the two best-documented hazards. Recent research by the National Institute for Occupational Safety and Health (NIOSH) has found that the highest proportionate mortality ratios (PMRs) for white male construction workers under age 65 are for asbestosis (PMR = 393) and silicosis (PMR = 327). These findings, from un-

**Table 36-3.** Common toxic hazards on the construction site

| Substance | Key source of exposure | Substance | Key source of exposure |
|---|---|---|---|
| Dusts | | Solvents | |
| Asbestos* | Demolition, maintenance, insulation | Benzene* | Hazardous waste clean-up, petrochemical plant sites |
| Cement | Foundations, sidewalks, floors | Methylene chloride | Paint strippers |
| Synthetic vitreous fibers, other insulation | Insulation on pipes, air conditioning | Toluene | Varnishes, paints, adhesives, cleaners |
| Silica | Sandblasting, tunneling | Trichloroethylene | Varnishes, paints, adhesives, cleaners |
| Wood dust* | Remodeling, demolition, sawing | Other chemicals | |
| | | Epoxy resins | Impermeable paints, wood floor primers |
| Metals (dusts and fumes) | | | |
| Cadmium* | Welding, cutting pipe | Polyurethanes (isocyanates) | Seam sealers, insulation, electrical wire coats |
| Hexavalent chromium* | Welding, cutting pipe | | |
| Copper | Welding, cutting pipe | Coal tar pitch* | Roofing, road work |
| Lead | Demolition, work on lead-paint surfaces | | |
| Magnesium | Welding, cutting pipe | | |
| Zinc | Welding, cutting pipe | | |

*Human carcinogen.
Source: Adapted from Workplace Hazard and Tobacco Education Project. Construction workers' guide to toxics on the job. Berkeley: California Public Health Foundation, 1993.

derlying cause-of-death codes on death certificates for 1984 to 1986, compare with a PMR for falls of 177.

In 1964 the first of a number of studies documented a clear pattern of lung cancer among insulation (asbestos) workers, along with risk for other neoplasms and a suggestion that workers who produced or handled asbestos were also at risk [7]. The research showed almost a sevenfold greater risk of death from bronchogenic carcinoma and mesothelioma than that for the general U.S. population, which led the authors to express con-

cern about "bystander" exposure (". . . the floating fibers do not respect job classifications . . .") on a worksite. Although the spray application of asbestos insulation has been stopped in the U.S. since 1973 and most other uses of asbestos are well controlled, construction workers involved in demolition continue to be exposed to asbestos installed many years ago.

Similarly, although OSHA has set permissible exposure limits for respirable silica, new cases of silicosis are still reported. Those at risk include tunnel workers, sandblasters, workers in trades using concrete and mortar—laborers, masons, concrete finishers, tile setters, and plasterers—and bystanders [8]. Depending partly on the percentage of silica in the materials used, a wide range of tasks can prove hazardous, such as drilling holes, grinding concrete surfaces, power-cleaning concrete forms, or cutting through concrete block, walls, or pipe. The risks are not limited to new construction. For example, powered grinders may be used to remove mortar for restoration.

*Other Cancers.* Potential exposures to carcinogens are common in all types of construction. Some sources are well-known, such as hydrocarbons in roofing tar. Welding can produce carcinogenic fumes, such as nickel and hexavalent chromium from stainless steel welds. Other carcinogenic exposures, however, are of recent origin. The use of plastics has been multiplying, and the health effects of their use remain unknown. Many specialty paints include metals and dangerous solvents, such as benzene and mercury. Among resins, acrylonitrile in acrylics, epichlorhydrin in epoxies, and isocyanates in polyurethanes all pose potential, but poorly documented, risks. Benzene and vinyl chloride are among the substances commonly found at Superfund sites.

*Central Nervous System Disorders.* Lead poisoning continues to be a particular concern for construction workers. Although lead has been restricted to trace amounts in residential plants in the U.S. since 1978, it is still allowed for industrial uses, including signs, road paints, and steel structures. The California Occupational Lead Registry found that construction workers accounted for 18 percent of the workers who had peak blood-lead levels of 80 $\mu g/dL$ (this is well above the level requiring removal) [9]. Exposures to lead occur during rehabilitation or demolition of lead-painted structures, including (particularly) housing built before 1950. These exposures can occur during scraping, cutting with torches, sandblasting—and welding. Welders may be exposed to fumes containing lead, but also epoxy resins,

manganese, nickel, polyurethane, and vinyl chloride.

Threats to the nervous system commonly found by hazardous waste clean-up workers include toluene, trichloroethylene, tetrachloroethylene, arsenic, benzene, lead, and mercury.

On a lesser scale, painters and laborers are at risk of mercury exposure from latex paints—through skin contact, ingestion, or inhalation of vapor or dust. As a result of U.S. Environmental Protection Agency efforts, the paint industry stopped adding mercuric compounds to latex paints used for interiors after August 1990 and manufacturers agreed to stop selling phenylmercuric acetate to paint companies for use in exterior latex paints after 1991 [10]. Existing stocks of this material can still be used, however.

*Skin Disorders.* Bricklayers, masons, and others who handle cement are prone to allergic and irritant dermatitis on the hands and other exposed areas. The symptoms can be severe enough to necessitate early retirement. The allergic dermatitis is believed to be caused by water-soluble hexavalent chromium (see Chap 24).

*Hearing Loss.* Noise levels on construction sites commonly exceed 95 dB around heavy machinery, such as bulldozers or front-end loaders. Noise levels of 95 to 105 dB have been measured around power tools, such as saws. Bygghälsan found that bilateral normal hearing among construction workers decreased gradually with age, so that only about 26 percent of those examined at ages 38 to 40 had hearing in the normal range. At the same time, approximately 3.6 percent of construction workers aged 38 to 40 suffered bilateral, severe, high-frequency hearing loss (4,000 Hertz or above). Among other things, this problem endangers workers who cannot be warned of immediate dangers or hear an approaching vehicle (see Chap. 16).

*Temperature Extremes.* Some of the most difficult hazards faced by construction workers are those presented by the extremes of temperature that occur, particularly in summer and winter. Consequences of overexposure to heat are similar to those documented for other working groups (see Chap. 17). While the same is true for the consequences of cold temperatures, there is the added hazard of increased risk of traumatic injury or other types of accident that can result from reduced ability to handle tools and equipment properly.

*Family Contact Disease.* It is believed that asbestos fibers have been transported, in some cases in asbestos products carried home to show family members and inadvertently on clothing, in hair, and on skin. A similar risk may exist for lead poisoning among construction workers' family members—particularly children, whose systems are more vulnerable to lead exposure.

## What is Being Done

In recent years construction safety and health in the U.S. have received increased attention. Several changes under way could prove critical in site safety and health planning and management, worker and supervisor training, safer construction technologies, and health monitoring.

### Regulation
Since 1989 OSHA has issued three regulations that are giving new direction to the construction industry.

*Hazardous Waste Operations and Emergency Response Standard.* This standard, governing all work where hazardous wastes exist, was the first regulation to require site safety and health plans, extensive specialized training of workers and supervisors, and health monitoring, recordkeeping, and reporting. It is gradually becoming a model for general construction in the U.S.

*Process Safety Management of Highly Hazardous Chemicals Standard.* This standard was adopted to prevent catastrophic explosions, especially when construction and maintenance are performed at such places as refineries and chemical plants. This standard also focuses on worker training and site safety and health planning by requiring contractors at industrial facilities to identify the hazards associated with construction tasks and to provide training. The standard also requires that owners evaluate a contracting firm's safety record before hiring it.

*Lead Exposure in Construction.* In 1993 OSHA established an interim lead standard for construction patterned on the existing standard for general industry. Permissible airborne levels at the worksite are 50 $\mu g/m^3$, averaged over 8 hours. A blood-lead level of 50 $\mu g/dL$ (measured twice, over 2 weeks) is enough to trigger medical removal, and a level of 40 $\mu g/dL$ triggers an annual medical examination. It is generally agreed, however, that the levels are not stringent enough. A consortium of public health, labor, government, and industry representatives has taken this move a step further. Because much of the problem of poorly controlled exposures occurs among bridge rehabilitation and demolition workers, model specifications for a lead protection program for these workers have been prepared for inclusion in appropriate bid documents [11].

### Site Safety and Health Planning and Management
There is widespread agreement that planning is a key to better safety and health on the worksite [12, 13]. This involves all details of logistics and begins well before the first shovelful of earth is turned. A critical element is assigning responsibility for safety and health, while improving coordination among subcontractors and the trades.

### Education and Training
Safety training and worker and manager education have long been provided in the U.S. by some

## CONSTRUCTION WORK IN DEVELOPING COUNTRIES: THE EXPERIENCE IN EAST AFRICA

Occupational health and safety hazards facing construction workers in developing countries are even greater than those facing their counterparts in industrialized countries. The experience in the East African countries of Kenya, Tanzania, and Uganda is illustrative.

In these developing countries, the hazards that are inherent in construction work are compounded by hot and humid conditions, inadequate training of workers, and shortages or inadequacies of construction tools, scaffolding, and helmets and other basic personal protective equipment. There is a great variety of inconsistency in equipment and processes. Among major construction hazards cited in Kenya, for example, are excavation work, inadequate scaffolds and electric equipment, and lack or inadequacy of lifting equipment. In these and other countries, hand tools and diesel engines at construction sites generate much noise; dusts and fumes are also major problems, especially in confined spaces.

In East African countries, well over half of construction workers are casual workers who are employed on a daily basis and do not belong to unions, as many other construction workers do. In these countries, construction workers are often paid on a piece-rate basis, which encourages rapid work and often unsafe work practices. Clean water and nutritious food, taken for granted at many workplaces in industrialized countries, are often not available to construction workers in the countries of East Africa. The same is true for basic health and safety services.

Data for work-related injuries and illnesses of construction workers in East Africa are even more incomplete than comparable data for these workers in industrialized countries. Nevertheless, available data provide some useful descriptions of the situation. Reporting is highly variable; for example, in Zanzibar, Tanzania, 44 construction accidents were reported between 1983 and 1989, with the number varying from 0 to 19 annually. In Kenya in 1989, according to workers' compensation data, there were 1,117 reported accidents among the approximately 60,000 building and engineering construction workers. Of these accidents, 43 were fatal and 52 caused permanent total incapacity.

The rate of reported fatal accidents for construction workers (72 per 100,000 workers per year) was three times the estimated rate in the U.S. and 12 times the rate in Denmark. Of the 618 accidents that could be classified, 40 percent were caused by "stepping on or being struck by objects" and 31 percent were caused by transportation vehicles. Ministries of Labor in the East African countries, with assistance from the International Labour Organization, the Finnish Institute of Occupational Health, and other organizations and groups, are attempting to improve health and safety in the construction industry by improving training of workers, establishing better means of surveillance and evaluation of hazards, and instituting better measures for prevention, often using low-cost, readily available materials and methods.

Adapted from East African Newsletter on Occupational Health and Safety, December 31, 1990.

companies and some trade unions. The training programs cover such topics as rigging, trenching, stretching exercises, and substance abuse recovery. Many training programs include instruction about dangerous substances that is mandated under OSHA's Hazard Communication Standard.

The same concern in Germany has led to development of the Gefahrstoff-Informationssystem der Berufsgenossenschaften der Bauwirtschaft (GIS-BAU) program. GISBAU works with manufacturers to determine the content of all substances used on construction sites. Equally important, it provides the information in a form to suit the differing needs of health staff members, managers, and workers. The information is available through training programs, in print, and on computer terminals at worksites. GISBAU gives advice about how to substitute for some risky substances and tells how to safely handle others.

### New Technologies

Technological improvements are reducing the risks of musculoskeletal and other health problems. Many of the changes are straightforward. For example, a two-handed screwdriver with a longer handle that is used in Sweden increases torque and reduces stress on the wrist(s).

To make lifting easier for the bricklayer, in Germany, bricks now are designed with holes or handles (Fig. 36-3). Regulations require that bricks weighing more than 25 kg (55 lbs) be lifted only by machine. In the Netherlands, brick manufacturers, unions, and management have developed a different system in which bricks are packaged in sets that are easily moved about the worksite on dollies and lifted by levers to a convenient height.

Tower crane cabins are being redesigned in Germany and Sweden. One change extends the window to the cabin floor. This enables the operators to see below without having to lean forward constantly. As a result, they report less chronic neck pain.

A new Swedish tool is reportedly reducing back injuries to iron workers. The *Najomat*, which looks like a giant pogo stick, lets workers tie rebar

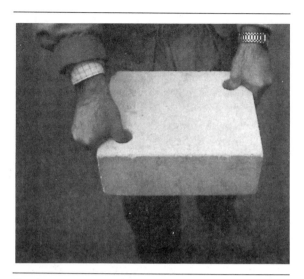

Fig. 36-3. A variety of handholds can be designed to assist in lifting bricks of different sizes and shapes. (Photograph by Bau-Berufsgenossenschaft, Frankfurt.)

rods while standing up (Fig. 36-4). The worker operates it by pushing down on the handles.

To reduce the risk of silicosis by about 90 percent, researchers in Germany have turned to wet blasting—using water to dampen the sand as it is being sprayed and thus minimize dust. Nevertheless, throughout Europe, silica sand blasting is being banned, except where essential.

In Denmark, Sweden, Finland, and more recently Germany, researchers have found that adding small amounts of ferrous sulfate to cement—begun in the mid-1980s—changes water-soluble hexavalent chromium to trivalent chromium. This change appears to explain the substantial decline in allergic dermatitis among construction workers in the Nordic countries and requires only an added cost of $1 per ton of cement.

Some efforts to improve worker health combine technologies and training. Bygghälsan is reducing noise on-site and instructing workers in hearing conservation. By 1986 to 1990, 42 percent of workers had normal bilateral hearing at age 38 to 40. Severe high-frequency loss had been reduced to 2.2 percent for the same age level.

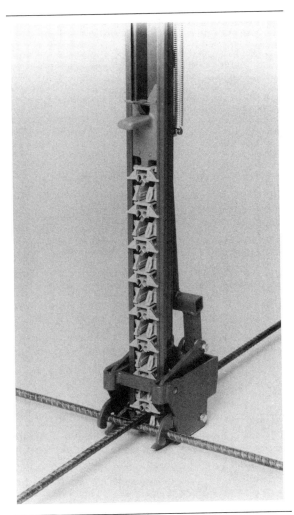

Fig. 36-4. This tie rod device replaces the need for workers to undertake the ergonomically and physically demanding tasks of hand-tying the metal rods required for concrete construction. (Photograph by Glim Betongprodukter AB, Norrköping, Sweden.)

## Opportunity and Responsibility of the Clinician

Construction is a field in which the occupational health professions can play major roles. To be effective, however, health professionals must first understand the organizational and sociologic aspects of construction work—and the risks workers face on the job—so that effective medical delivery systems can be put into place. Second, health professionals must develop protocols and programs appropriate to the needs of construction workers and their families.

### Delivery Systems

There are numerous opportunities to provide improved health programs for construction workers by working with health and welfare plans, workers' compensation carriers, employers, and unions. Structured care systems are needed that are based on close cooperation among clinicians and experts in physical therapy, occupational hygiene, and safety engineering.

Few employers provide their own medical staff. Therefore, existing community or academic occupational health clinics generally have a large volume of building trades activities—evaluating and treating individual workers who have been referred or self-referred and also investigating special problems in the worker population. This pattern, however, does not reflect industry-wide use of health services. Because of the episodic nature of construction employment and the high cost of health care, most construction workers have not had continuous medical care and a long-term relationship with a medical provider who knows his or her work situation.

A partial exception has been in the unionized sector, which for 40 years has provided health insurance through health and welfare funds that are jointly trusteed (with employers). There are about 750 such funds of varying size in the U.S., most of them local. To address the episodic employment question, the health and welfare funds have established hour "banks" in which workers can accumulate hours worked to qualify for coverage. Workers can thus maintain group coverage through as much as 3 to 6 months of unemployment, by drawing on their bank reserves. This system has its limitations, however. With erratic employment, some workers still are not able to build up reserve hours. And, even with health care coverage, medical care usage has been poor.

Despite this spotty record, construction may be unique in the strong incentives it offers employers and workers to support public health efforts. The excessive costs of workers' compensation in the U.S. mean that most safety and health programs are likely to have positive economic impacts, beginning in the short term. Although workers' compensation premiums vary widely depending upon trade and jurisdiction, the workers' compensation premium for three trades—carpenters, masons, and structural iron workers—averaged $28 per $100 of payroll nationally in mid-1993 [14].

### Preventive Services

Targeted preventive services are needed in most health insurance plans that cover construction workers and their families. These should include discussing with patients the precautions to take around the hazardous substances their trades are most likely to encounter.

*Development of Protocols.* One experiment in preventive medicine is being conducted with a health and welfare fund in the Pacific Northwest of the U.S. A protocol was designed comprising procedures, history forms, data reporting, and frequency for periodic examinations. It was based on the experience of Bygghälsan, recommendations of the U.S. Preventive Services Task Force, and local medical practice patterns. An outpatient preferred provider organization (PPO) network serving this health and welfare fund identified providers best suited to provide the examinations. Selection criteria included special medical expertise, interest in workers, and a willingness to submit data. The health and welfare office verifies worker eligibility for the examination. The PPO clinical director's office performs quality control, collects and enters data, and assures continuity between examinations.

This program is exceptional, however. Few occupational medicine protocols have been developed and validated for use for construction groups, even for preventive medicine in general. Issues include whether there is a role for chest x-rays in periodic preventive medical examinations and whether liver enzyme tests have a useful role in predicting fitness for work in hazardous waste clean-up.

*Targeted Medical Monitoring.* Because of the difficulties of reliably establishing work histories and exposures, medical monitoring is especially important, particularly in hazardous waste clean-up and lead abatement. Only a few types of exposures require medical monitoring in the U.S., whereas German law specifies medical monitoring for a large number of potentially toxic substances in any work setting. Checkups are required before work is begun, at specified intervals, and, even after exposure ceases, checkups are required at regular intervals following known exposure to carcinogenic substances. The preemployment checkup provides a baseline for future examinations. Information from the checkups that can be used to improve workplace conditions is given to the employers. Employers are responsible for continuing medical monitoring according to a schedule begun with a different employer. However, if a worker is unemployed for an interval longer than the scheduled interval for checkups, the examination schedule usually begins over again with a baseline examination at the time of next employment.

*Screening for Disease.* Although there has been a long history of screening programs for asbestos-related diseases, little is known in the U.S. about the prevalence or incidence of hearing loss, most musculoskeletal disorders, dermatitis, or other chronic diseases. And, as the first and second waves of asbestos disease reach their conclusion, it will be useful to study whether overall incidence is in decline.

## Determination of Disability and Support for Rehabilitation

*Medical Panels.* Better medical support to determine disability under workers' compensation and help workers return to work as early as possible are needed. Newly forming closed medical panels for disability determination can help make the systems in the U.S. more responsive to the needs of disabled workers. The occupational health physician can also help identify light-duty tasks that match a worker's level of disability.

*Standards-Setting.* Occupational health care workers can help with the setting and implementation of health-related standards. Most OSHA standards are inadequate in terms of medical monitoring requirements for construction workers. The medical monitoring requirements of the OSHA Hazardous Waste Operations Standard, for instance, are vague. The recently issued OSHA Final Rule for Lead Exposure in Construction has clear medical requirements for monitoring and actions, but is impractical for implementation in the construction sector. For instance, a worker with a high blood-lead level is supposed to be provided another job removed from the lead exposure and at the same pay. If a project is completed, however, the contractor no longer is required to provide a job. The worker then may have difficulty finding another job until the blood-lead level goes down.

## Research

Issues such as the measurement of and consequences of toxic exposures are poorly understood largely because of inadequate past research on work-related safety and health in construction. The problems have partly been tied to funding. As recently as 1988 federally funded safety research averaged $2.16 per manufacturing worker and $0.08 per construction worker. The investment in construction research, however, has been increasing.

For health professionals interested in research, construction is largely unexplored terrain. Areas that have not been addressed are exposure characterization, epidemiology, health services, interventions, and policy.

*Exposure Characterization.* An exposure assessment model is needed that addresses the unique nature of construction work. The model should efficiently collect descriptive and quantitative data on exposures so that they can be predicted before each job starts. The model should be in a form that construction workers can use easily on-site. It should also be part of a system that permits storage of data for reference years later.

Given the limits of existing technology, the best approach may be to develop estimates of the range of exposures for given tasks—such as rod tying, riveting, and welding—taking into account such factors as the substances used, duration, and ventilation. For welding, for example, an estimate would consider the welding method, the welding rod used, and materials welded, including any coatings, but should also include ingestion and dermal exposures.

Exposures worth special attention include noise, dusts, vibration, manual lifting, and work postures. For instance, back belts are in widespread use, but no study has determined whether they are effective.

*Epidemiology.* The U.S. does not have good epidemiologic surveillance systems, and estimates based on different data sets show major inconsistencies. Descriptive studies are needed. There is a shortage of reliable data on the morbidity patterns of the different trades. Virtually no research has been done on patterns of disability for the trades.

*Health Services.* No research has been done on the delivery of occupational or general medical services for construction workers in the U.S., and little is known about construction workers' patterns of health care use. If one accepts that continuity of care is a key determinant of the effectiveness of medical care, the episodic nature of construction appears to be a major barrier.

*Interventions.* Studies are needed in four types of intervention. First, different approaches to the delivery of preventive services should be tested. Second, information is needed on a host of preventive measures. These include training, certification of workers and contractors, use of personal protective equipment, and technologies that may reduce exposures. Third, no studies have been performed on the best systems for monitoring the health of construction workers, including exposure monitoring, medical monitoring, and the tracking of workers in a transient industry. Fourth, experiments should be performed to reduce the sequelae of disability and to return injured workers to gainful employment.

*Policy.* Little consideration has been given to the economics of improved safety and health in construction. There have been no geographically defined projects to characterize the construction industry and to intervene in its basic characteristics of small employers, transient work, temporary worksites, and multi-employer worksites. In addition, there have been no valid studies to examine the effects of disability on workers and their families.

## References

1. Burkhart G, et al. Job tasks, potential exposures, and health risks of laborers employed in the construction industry. Am J Ind Med, 1993; 24:413–25.
2. Culver C, Marshall M, Connolly C. Construction accidents: The workers' compensation data base, 1985–1988. Office of Construction and Engineering, OSHA, April 1992.
3. Pollack ES, Keimig DG. eds. Counting injuries and illnesses in the workplace: Proposals for a better system. Washington, D.C.: National Academy Press, 1987.
4. Sorock GS, Smith EO'H, Goldoft M. Fatal occupational injuries in the New Jersey construction industry, 1983 to 1989. J Occup Med, 1993; 35:916–21.
5. Helander MG. Safety hazards and motivation for safe work in the construction industry. Int J Ind Economics 1991; 8:205–23.
6. Holmström E. Musculoskeletal disorders in construction workers. Lund, Sweden: Lund University, Department of Physical Therapy, 1992.
7. Selikoff IJ, Churg J, Hammond EC. Asbestos exposure and neoplasia. JAMA, 1964; 188:22–6.
8. Lofgren DJ, Silica exposure for concrete workers and masons. Appl Occup Environ Hyg, 1993; 8:832–6.
9. Waller K, Osorio AM, Maizlish N, Royce S. Lead exposure in the construction industry: Results from the California Occupational Lead Registry, 1987 through 1989. Am J Public Health 1992; 82:1669–71.
10. Hefflin BJ, et al. Mercury exposure from exterior latex paint. J Appl Occup Environ Hyg, 1993; 8:866–70.
11. Center to Protect Workers' Rights, Washington, D.C., and Steel Structures Painting Council, Pittsburgh, PA.
12. Construction Industry Institute. Zero injury techniques. Austin, TX, May 1993. Publication 32-1.
13. An Agenda for Change: Report of the National Conference on Ergonomics, Safety, and Health in Construction. Washington, D.C.: Center to Protect Workers' Rights, 1993.
14. Costs keep climbing. ENR. September 17, 1993, pp. 32–3, based on figures from Marsh & McLennan Inc. Insurance Brokers.

## Bibliography

Construction Safety Association of Ontario. Construction health and safety manual. Toronto: Construction Safety Association of Ontario, 1992. 343 pp.
*This is the most complete and concise compendium of recommended construction safety and health practices published in English. Guidelines provided include (1) general information about responsibilities on-site, personal protective equipment, and ways to avoid back injuries, and (2) trade-specific safety and health information for carpenters, drywallers, and others.*
Pollack ES, Ringen K. Risk of hospitalization for specific non-work-related conditions among laborers and their families. Am J Ind Med, 1993; 23:417–25.

*This is the only study to attempt a population-based morbidity measurement for a construction trade and dependents.*

Schneider S, Susie P. Final report: An investigation of health hazards on a new construction project. Washington, D.C.: The Center to Protect Workers' Rights, 1993. Report OSH1-93. 78 pp.

*This is the most complete report on safety and health hazards encountered in all phases of a construction project. The authors, industrial hygienists, spent a year regularly visiting a building construction site. They observed the work; measured sound levels, fumes, and other exposures; and interviewed workers about possible ergonomic hazards on the job. The report provides detailed listings of hazards found.*

An Agenda for Change: Report of the National Conference on Ergonomics, Safety, and Health in Construction. Washington, D.C.: The Center to Protect Workers' Rights, 1993.

*Findings and recommendations of groundbreaking 4-day meeting of 750 decisionmakers in industry, government, and science from the U.S. and other industrialized countries.*

# Appendixes

# A

# How to Research the Toxic Effects of Chemical Substances

## Stephen Zoloth and David Michaels

In taking work histories, you are likely to discover that many of your patients are exposed to one or more substances that have toxic properties that are unknown or unfamiliar to you. It is necessary to investigate the potential toxicity of these products. The following is a systematic approach to important resources in this area. These are resources with which you should become familiar, since they will be useful in providing information necessary for determining if your patients' health problems are work-related. (The sources listed are mainly in the United States; similar sources exist in other countries.)

## Step 1: Set Priorities

It is often impractical to research every substance and process to which your patients are exposed. A few common sense guidelines may help focus your efforts on the more important exposures—those most likely to cause disease.

*Ask the patient for guidance.* Workers are usually well aware of the most potentially toxic substances to which they are exposed; the products that particularly concern them warrant your attention. In many cases, workers have themselves obtained useful information about chemical hazards, often from labels on containers, their unions, or other sources, and they will share it with you.

Furthermore, by observing health and disease patterns among themselves, workers are often able to identify clusters of work-related disease—often for acute disease occurring shortly after exposure, but sometimes for chronic disease as well. Inquire if your patients suspect that their health problems, or those of coworkers, are work-related.

*Consider the magnitude of exposure.* If your patient has more intensive or prolonged exposure to a few substances, these should be investigated first. It is vital to remember, however, that even low-dose exposure to a carcinogen is cause for concern (see Chap. 14).

*Consider toxicologic information.* Your background reading will alert you to the toxicity of certain classes of chemicals; it should help you be "selectively suspicious" and direct your research accordingly. For example, halogenated hydrocarbons, organochlorine pesticides, and heavy metals should generally be given priority in your research since they may be extremely toxic.

*Consider clinical-toxicologic correlations.* If the onset of symptoms in your patient dates from the introduction of a new chemical in the workplace, this product certainly deserves further investigation.

*Consider epidemiologic correlations.* If your patient and his or her coworkers share the same symptoms or diseases, discover what exposures they have in common.

## Step 2: Obtain the Generic Name

Many chemicals used in the workplace are known by their trade names. It can be extremely difficult to investigate a substance without knowing its generic, or chemical, name or ingredients.

*ions.* Now
vate sector
Safety and
d Commu-
tion about
rk from their
on, many public
Its under Right-to-
tes. Under these reg-
rovide workers with in-
ous chemicals used in the
workplace through proper labeling of containers, distributing material safety data sheets (MSDSs), and conducting training programs. The MSDS for a product, generally prepared by its manufacturer, is of particular importance to health care providers since it lists the product's generic ingredients, their toxic properties, recommendations for safe use, and other important information.

If your patient is working with a product under suspicion, he or she can request the MSDS from the employer and provide you with it. Your patient has the right to make this request—you do not, and your contacting the employer may jeopardize your patient's job. *Never* contact your patient's employer without his or her permission.

It is important to remember, however, that MSDSs can be incomplete or out of date. While MSDSs are valuable as sources of generic names and chemical constituents of a product, the toxicity information they contain should be confirmed, when possible, in other sources; do not rely on MSDSs alone. In addition, if your patient is no longer employed or no longer working with the substance, it may be difficult to obtain the appropriate MSDS. Another source of MSDSs is the Canadian Center for Occupational Health and Safety, which produces an MSDS database of more than 65,000 Canadian and U.S. products (access through STN International, Columbus, OH; 800-848-6533).

Finally, it should be noted that in many states and localities, community residents, firefighters, and others have the same rights to information about chemicals used by local employers, under community Right-to-Know regulations.

*Contact the manufacturer.* You should not call your patient's employer, but you may decide to contact the manufacturer of the substance in question. Product labels usually contain the manufacturer's name and often an address as well. If the address is not listed, use *Thomas' Register of American Manufacturers,* available at many public libraries (Thomas Publishing Co., New York, 1994; also available on-line via Dialog Information Services, Palo Alto, CA). In contacting a manufacturer, request the MSDSs on the substances of interest. Calls from physicians and other health care providers generally receive quick responses from manufacturers, who may be concerned about potential liability.

*Contact the poison control center.* Poison control centers are a vital source of data on both the generic ingredients and acute toxic properties of chemical substances, and one is located in every region of the United States.

*Contact the National Institute for Occupational Safety and Health (NIOSH).* NIOSH has a computerized data bank of the ingredients of trade-name substances from both the National Occupational Hazard Survey (1972–1974) and the National Occupational Exposure Survey (1981–1983). While these data banks are incomplete, NIOSH continues to update them and is able to provide the generic names of approximately one-third of the trade-name products requested. Contact Hazard Surveillance Section, NIOSH, Mailstop R-19, 4676 Columbia Parkway, Cincinnati, OH 45226. The phone number is (513) 841-4491.

*Check reference books.* Several are useful sources of generic ingredient information. For example, the *Clinical Toxicology of Commercial Products,* 5th ed. (R Gosselin, R Smith, H Hodge, Baltimore: Williams & Wilkins, 1984), available in all medical libraries, lists the ingredients of over 17,500 trade-name products. If you encounter what may be a synonym or trade name of a chemical, use the *NIOSH Registry of Toxic Effects of*

*Chemical Substances,* commonly known as RTECS (1985–1986 edition, NIOSH publication no. 87-114). If neither of these is sufficient, try one of the several chemical dictionaries or collections of synonyms that list common trade names.

## Step 3: Research the Chemical

Information provided on an MSDS or a label on the toxic effects of the chemical is often incomplete. It is important to obtain the most accurate and current toxicologic information. There are many sources that provide detailed toxicity data. Several chapters of this book review the effects of chemicals on specific organ systems, and the bibliographies in these chapters are good starting points for obtaining information. In addition, major textbooks of industrial hygiene, toxicology, and pharmacology generally have chapters devoted to specific chemicals or families of chemicals (see bibliography of Chap. 13). In addition to these sources, the following approaches may be useful in researching the toxic effects of chemicals.

### Chemical Fact Sheets

Toxicologic data on specific chemicals can be found in chemical fact sheets. Similar to MSDSs, chemical fact sheets are brief summaries of toxicologic data. For example, NIOSH published *Occupational Health Guidelines for Chemical Hazards* (NIOSH publication no. 81-123). This three-volume set of fact sheets covers more than 300 substances for which there are federal occupational safety and health regulations. Among the topics included for each chemical are a description of symptoms and signs of exposure, recommended medical surveillance protocols, and a summary of the toxicology data.

In addition, many state health and labor departments also publish chemical fact sheets or serve as resources for information on hazardous chemicals. For example, the New Jersey and New York state health departments both have developed well-researched fact sheets on industrial chemicals.

In addition to these sources, two NIOSH publications also provide summaries of chemical toxicity. The *Pocket Guide to Chemical Hazard* (NIOSH publication no. 90-117) lists major industrial chemicals and provides a statement on their toxicity, protective equipment, and exposure limits. The RTECS is much more extensive, covering more than 80,000 chemicals, and provides a gateway into the toxicologic literature. The entries in RTECS are telegraphic and unevaluated summaries of recent toxicology data. RTECS is best used to identify references to the toxicologic literature. RTECS can be a useful reference. The last print edition was in 1986; now RTECS can only be accessed as a computerized database.

Finally, the Agency for Toxic Substances and Disease Registry (ATSDR) publishes the *Toxicological Profile* series, which provides information concerning the health effects of 275 hazardous substances that are commonly found at Superfund sites and that pose the most significant potential threat to human health. These profiles undergo periodic review and are updated at least once every three years. Contact ATSDR, Centers for Disease Control, Mail Code E-28, 1600 Clifton Road, Atlanta, GA 30333; (404) 693-0720 for more information.

### Using Computers to Research Chemicals

The rapid growth of the microcomputer industry, telecommunications, and public and private databases provides another method of researching toxic properties of chemicals. Bibliographic databases, such as the National Library of Medicine (NLM) MEDLINE, TOXLINE, and TOXNET, contain references to the published medical and toxicologic literature. MEDLINE contains references to approximately 500,000 citations from 3,000 biomedical journals and provides health professionals rapid access to the most recently published information on any biomedical subject. MEDLINE is searched using key words or names to scan the database. When the search is completed, references to articles in the database that contain the key words or names will be listed. The author, title, journal name, and abstract for each reference can be printed out immediately or printed off-line and mailed to you from NLM.

Occupational and environmental health references are also accessible through TOXLINE. This database contains over 3,000,000 citations, covering human and animal toxicity studies, effects of environmental chemicals and pollutants, adverse drug reactions, and analytical methods. TOXLINE is available through the National Library of Medicine.

Finally, TOXNET is a comprehensive database containing both factual information and references covering several thousand chemicals. One advantage of TOXNET is that statements on toxicity and biomedical effects undergo scientific peer review. TOXNET is actually an integrated system of databases, and provides search and retrieval of records from RTECS, the Chemical Carcinogenesis Research Information System, the Hazardous Substances Databank, and other services.

Until recently, searching these computerized databases had to be done at a medical library. The reference librarian developed a search strategy and consulted the database while you waited. While most medical libraries still provide this service and reference librarians are the best source of information on how to use the databases, it is now possible to use microcomputers and telecommunication packages to search NLM and other databases from your home or office.

If you have a personal computer and a modem, access to the NLM can be accomplished using the NLM's inexpensive software package *Grateful Med*. The *Grateful Med* package, which is extremely easy to use, formats the search with your prompting. The results of the search can be printed directly, downloaded to your disk, or mailed to

you from the NLM. Information about MEDLINE, TOXLINE, TOXNET, and *Grateful Med* can be obtained from the Medlars Management Section, National Library of Medicine, Building 38, Room 4N421, 8600 Rockville Pike, Bethesda, MD 20894; (800) 638-8480.

In addition to *Grateful Med*, several commercial telecommunications networks provide access to the NLM databases. For example, BRS Colleague, Compuserve, and Dialog Information Systems all allow on-line access to NLM as well as to a wide range of other databases. Generally, billing is a combination of an hourly connect-time charge and a print fee. Information about these and other privately run databases are available in most personal computing magazines.

*NIOSH* also maintains its own occupational safety and health database, *NIOSHTIC*, which covers 150 journals and includes toxicology, epidemiologic studies, ergonomics, and other information about health and safety in the workplace. Access to *NIOSHTIC* can be arranged through NIOSH (800-35-NIOSH), or through Dialog.

### CD-ROMs

Another new technology that is currently revolutionizing database searching is the development of affordable and efficient CD-ROMs. These removable storage devices for personal computers have rapidly changed the nature of database searching. No longer do you have to connect to an on-line database; much of the same information is now available on CD-ROMs. For example, Silver Platter (Norwood, MA; 800-874-1130) offers OSHROM, a compilation of four databases covering occupational health and safety information in the U.S. and the United Kingdom and from the International Labour Organization (ILO). Silver Platter also produces CHEM-BANK, five databases, including RTECS, which cover the hazardous effects of chemicals.

## Databases for Chemical Research

| NAME | CONTENTS | FORMAT |
|---|---|---|
| MEDLINE[1,8] | Medical references | On-line, CD-ROM |
| NIOSHTIC[2,4] | Occupational health literature | On-line, CD-ROM |
| RTECS[2,4] | Toxicity data | On-line, CD-ROM |
| TOXNET[1,2,8] | Toxicity data (includes several databases) | On-line, CD-ROM |
| TOXLINE[1,2,8], TOXLIT[1,2,8] | Bibliographic information on chemicals | On-line, CD-ROM |
| REPROTOX[9] | Summaries of reproductive/ developmental data | On-line |
| Hazardous Substances Databank[1,2] | Emergency procedures, toxicity | On-line, CD-ROM |
| Chemical Carcinogenesis Research Information System[1] | Mutagenicity, carcinogenicity | On-line |
| TERIS[10] | Summaries/risk ratings for drugs and chemicals | On-line |
| ETICBACK (through 1988) DART (since 1989)[11] | Bibliographic database on agents causing birth defects | On-line |
| Pesticide Products Database[2] | Composition, toxicity warning | CD-ROM |
| Pesticide Information System[5] | Monitoring inventory, usage, chemical index | On-line |
| MSDS Reference Files— Pesticides[2,6] | MSDSs for pesticides | On-line, CD-ROM |
| MSDS—Canadian Center[7] | MSDS for > 65,000 chemicals | CD-ROM |

1. National Library of Medicine, Bethesda, MD (800-638-8480)
2. Silver Platter, Inc., Norwood, MA (800-874-1130)
3. Dialog Information Services, Palo Alto, CA (800-334-2564)
4. NIOSH, Cincinnati, OH (800-35-NIOSH)
5. U.S. EPA, Washington, D.C. (703-557-1919)
6. Center for Environmental and Regulatory Information Systems (CERIS), NPIRS User Services, West Lafayette, IN (317-494-6616)
7. STN International, c/o Chemical Abstract Services, Columbus, OH (800-848-6533)

8. *Grateful Med,* Personal Computer access to MEDLINE, National Library of Medicine, Bethesda, MD (800-638-8480)
9. Reproductive Toxicology Center, Washington, D.C. (202-293-5137)
10. Teratogen Information System, Seattle, WA (206-543-2465)
11. Toxicology Information Program, National Library of Medicine, Bethesda, MD (301-496-3147)

# B
## Other Sources of Information
### Compiled by Marianne Parker Brown

The following resources can be obtained or contacted for additional information:

## General Resources

### 1. Emergency Services
Telephone numbers are listed to call for technical, medical, regulatory, or reporting information in the event of an exposure-related problem or medical emergency.

CHEMTREC
(800) 424-9300

24-hour hotline operated by the Chemical Manufacturers' Association relays information to manufacturers about a spill involving their products or employees and will rapidly determine for the caller the contents of a spilled container and suggest appropriate action for containment. The non–emergency services number is (800) 262-8200.

National Pesticide Telecommunications Network
(800) 858-7378

Provides information on pesticide products, safety and health concerns, and disposal procedures.

National Response Center
(800) 424-8802; (in Washington, D.C., only, call 202-426-2675)

First federal point of contact for reporting of, and guidance on, oil and hazardous spills. 24-hour hotline relays information on regulatory and response agencies and immediately contacts appro-

priate federal on-scene coordinators to respond to the spill.

NIOSH Technical Information Service
(800) 35-NIOSH (800-356-4674)

Provides information and technical assistance on workplace hazards.

Occupational and Environmental Reproductive
  Hazards Center
  (508) 856-6162

Provides advice on how to address concerns of reproductive hazards among pregnant women or couples seeking to become pregnant.

Office of Hazardous Materials and
  Transportation, U.S. Department of
  Transportation
  (202) 366-4488

Provides information on HAZMAT transportation regulations.

Organization of Teratology Information Services
(617) 466-8474

Will provide telephone numbers of pregnancy hotlines in U.S. and Canada.

OSHA Technical Support Directorate
(202) 219-7031

Central number for federal OSHA provides rapid technical and occupational medical support and will notify, in the event of a significant emergency, the OSHA Salt Lake Technical Center Health Response Team (801-487-0267). Also provides phone numbers for regional technical support offices for further assistance.

Poison Control Centers

Each state or region has a 24-hour poison control center offering expert emergency medical information and referrals. Centers are listed on the inside cover of local phone directories. They can also be reached by dialing 911 and asking for the Poison Control Center or by calling the National Response Center, listed above.

Tox-Center
(619) 320-9401
(800) 682-9000 (California only)

Responds to nationwide calls, providing 24-hour, immediate information on toxic incident containment and control, sampling, protective measures for on-scene personnel, evaluation, and medical treatment advice.

### 2. Guides, Catalogs, and Directories

*NIOSH Bookshelf*, 4676 Columbia Parkway, Cincinnati, OH 45226

List of all NIOSH publications, including criteria documents, manuals, reports, health hazard evaluations, and others.

OSHA Computerized Information System (OCIS) U.S. Government Printing Office, Washington, D.C. 20402-9325
(202) 783-3238

The OCIS on CD-ROM contains agency documents, technical information, and training materials files. More than half the audiovisual materials listed can be borrowed from the OSHA Office of Training and Education. A catalog of items can be obtained from: Librarian, OSHA Office of Training and Education, 1555 Times Drive, Des Plaines, IL 60018.

*A Directory of Academic Programs in Occupational Health* (1987), NIOSH, Division of Training, 4676 Columbia Parkway, Cincinnati, OH 45226

### 3. Films and Other Audiovisuals

*Audiovisual Material Catalogue* (1987), NIOSH, 4676 Columbia Parkway, Cincinnati, OH, 45226

Describes 49 NIOSH-produced films available either for purchase or loan.

*BNA Communications Safety Catalog*, Bureau of National Affairs, 9439 Key West Avenue, Rockville, MD 20850
(800) 233-6067

Produces and distributes safety, environmental, and regulatory compliance videos, including a Right-to-Know package and a Hazardous Waste Management series for purchase or rental.

*Film and Video Finder,* Access Innovations, Inc., NICEM, P.O. Box 40130, Albuquerque, NM 87196

Exhaustive compilation of educational media categorized by subject and title. Available at most research libraries. On-line through Dialog Information Services and the Human Resource Information Network. Also on CD-ROM.

*Films and Video Tapes for Labor,* Film Division, AFL-CIO Department of Education, 815 16th Street, NW, Washington, D.C. 20006

Lists a number of films and videos on occupational health and safety, including training on regulations, workers' rights, and union strategies. For rental only.

*Media Resource Catalog.* National Audiovisual Center of the National Archives Records Administration, 8700 Edgeworth Drive, Capitol Heights, MD 20743

Includes over 200 health and safety training programs developed by 28 federal agencies, including OSHA, FDA, FEMA, and DOD. Materials include videos, slide and tape shows, and audiocassettes. For purchase only.

*Occupational Health Resource Guide,* Resource Center of the Environmental and Occupational Health and Safety Institute, Public Education

and Risk Communication Division, 681 Frelinghuysen Road, P.O. Box 1179, Piscataway, NJ 08855-1179
(908) 932-0110

University of Medicine and Dentistry of New Jersey (UMDNJ) and New Jersey Department of Health, 1989. Invaluable guide to occupational health–related books, journals, pamphlets, audiovisual materials, databases, organizations, vendors, and more. Resources on hazard identification and control, legislation and regulations, occupational diseases, specific industries and processes, and more. Can be obtained for $15.

*Safety and Health Video Catalog,* International Film Bureau, 332 South Michigan Ave., Chicago, IL 60604
(800) 432-2241

Videos for safety and health training in industrial hygiene, personal protection and operational safety, hazardous materials handling, and other areas. Some are available in Spanish.

National Clearinghouse on Occupational and Environmental Health Training for Hazardous Materials, Waste Operators and Emergency Response, George Meany Center for Labor Studies, 10000 New Hampshire Avenue, Silver Spring, MD 20903
(301) 431-5425

Ask for their catalog of information on hazardous waste worker training programs. The National Clearinghouse also maintains a library of curricula developed and used by organizations involved in the training of hazardous waste workers and emergency responders.

## Organizations

### 1. Federal Government

#### National Institute for Occupational Safety and Health (NIOSH)
1600 Clifton Road, N.E. Atlanta, GA 30033 (Headquarters)

Robert A. Taft Laboratories, 4676 Columbia Parkway, Cincinnati, OH 45226-1998

Appalachian Laboratory for Occupational Safety and Health, 944 Chestnut Ridge Road, Morgantown, WV 26505-2888

#### NIOSH Regional Offices

In 1986 NIOSH consolidated the number of regional offices from 10 to 3. The 3 regional offices now cover 20 states. West Virginia is covered by the Morgantown office and the remaining 29 states are handled by the Cincinnati office (see addresses above).

Boston Regional Office (CT, MA, ME, NH, RI, and VT), JFK Federal Building, Room 1401, Boston, MA 02203

Atlanta Regional Office (AL, FL, GA, KY, MS, NC, SC, and TN) 101 Marietta Tower, Atlanta, GA 30323

Denver Regional Office (CO, MT, ND, SD, UT, and WY), Federal Building, Room 1185, 1961 Stout Street, Denver, CO 80294

### Occupational Safety and Health Administration (OSHA)
U.S. Department of Labor, 200 Constitution Avenue, NW, Washington, D.C. 20210

#### OSHA Regional Offices

Region I (CT, MA, ME, NH, RI, and VT), 133 Portland Street, First Floor, Boston, MA 02114

Region II (NJ, NY, Peurto Rico, and Virgin Islands), 201 Varick Street, Room 670, New York, NY 10014

Region III (DC, DE, MD, PA, VA, and WV), Gateway Building, Suite 2100, 3535 Market Street, Philadelphia, PA 19104

Region IV (AL, FL, GA, KY, MS, NC, SC, and TN), 1375 Peachtree Street, NE, Suite 587, Atlanta, GA 30367

Region V (IL, IN, MI, MN, OH, and WI), 230 South Dearborn Street, 32nd Floor, Room 3244, Chicago, IL 60604

Region VI (AR, LA, NM, OK, and TX), 525 Griffin Street, Room 602, Dallas, TX 75202

Region VII (IA, KS, MO, and NE), 911 Walnut Street, Room 406, Kansas City, MO 64106

Region VIII (CO, MT, SD, ND, UT, and WY), Federal Building, Room 1576, 1961 Stout Street, Denver, CO 80294

Region IX (AZ, CA, HI, NV, American Samoa, Guam, and Trust Territories of the Pacific), 71 Stevenson Street, 4th Floor, San Francisco, CA 94105

Region X (AK, ID, OR, and WA), 1111 Third Avenue, Suite 715, Seattle, WA 98101

### 2. State Agencies

States with approved plans are listed below. Unless indicated, plans cover public and private workers.

### OSHA State—Plan States

ALASKA
Alaska OSHA
    P.O. Box 21149
    Juneau, AK 99802-1149
    (907) 465-2700

ARIZONA
State of Arizona OSHA
    800 West Washington
    P.O. Box 19070
    Phoenix, AZ 85007
    (602)542-5795

CALIFORNIA
CAL/OSHA
    455 Golden Gate Avenue
    Room 5202
    San Francisco, CA 94102
    (415) 703-4341

CONNECTICUT*
Connecticut Department of Labor
    Occupational Safety and Health Division
    200 Folly Brook Boulevard
    Wethersfield, CT 06109
    (203) 566-5123

HAWAII
State of Hawaii Department of Labor and
    Industrial Relations
    Division of Occupational Safety and Health
    830 Punchbowl Street
    Honolulu, HI 96813
    (808) 548-3150

INDIANA
Indiana Department of Labor
    1013 State Office Building
    100 North Senate Avenue
    Indianapolis, IN 46204
    (317) 232-2655

IOWA
Iowa Division of Labor Services
    1000 East Grand Avenue
    Des Moines, IA 50319
    (515) 281-3447

KENTUCKY
Kentucky Occupational Safety and Health
    Program
    U.S. Highway 127 South
    Frankfort, KY 40601
    (502) 564-3070

MARYLAND
State of Maryland—MOSH
    Division of Labor and Industry
    501 St. Paul Place
    Baltimore, MD 21202-2272
    (301) 333-4179

MICHIGAN
Michigan Department of Public Health
    Division of Occupational Health
    3423 North Logan Street

Lansing, MI 48909
(517) 335-8022
Michigan Department of Labor
309 North Washington
Lansing, MI 48909
(517) 373-9600

MINNESOTA
Minnesota Occupational Health and Safety
443 Lafayette Road
St. Paul, MN 55101
(612) 296-2342

NEVADA
Department of Industrial Relations
Division of Occupational Health and Safety
1370 South Curry Street
Carson City, NV 89710
(702) 885-5240

NEW MEXICO
New Mexico Occupational Health and Safety
Bureau
1190 St. Francis Drive—N2200
Santa Fe, NM 87503-0968
(505) 827-2850

NEW YORK*
New York State Department of Labor
Public Employees Safety and Health Program
One Main Street
Brooklyn, NY 11201
(518) 457-3518

NORTH CAROLINA
North Carolina Department of Labor
Division of Occupational Safety and Health
4 West Edenton Street
Raleigh, NC 27603
(919) 733-7166

OREGON
Occupational Safety and Health Division
(OR-OSHA)
160 Labor and Industries Building
Salem, OR 97310
(503) 378-3304

PUERTO RICO
Department of Labor and Human Resources
Occupational Safety and Health Offices
505 Munoz Rivera Avenue
Hato Rey, PR 00918
(809) 754-2119-22

SOUTH CAROLINA
South Carolina Department of Labor
3600 Forest Drive
Columbia, SC 29211-1329
(803) 734-9594

TENNESSEE
Tennessee Department of Labor
Division of Occupational Safety and Health
501 Union Building, Suite A—2nd Floor
Nashville, TN 37219
(615) 741-2582

UTAH
Utah OSHA
Industrial Commission
160 East 300 South
Salt Lake City, UT 84110-5800
(801) 530-6900

VERMONT
Vermont Occupational Safety and Health
Administration
120 State Street
Montpelier, VT 05602
(802) 828-2765

VIRGIN ISLANDS
Department of Labor
2131 Hospital Street
Christiansted, St. Croix, VI 00828-4660
(809) 773-1994

VIRGINIA
Commonwealth of Virginia
Department of Labor and Industry
P.O. Box 12064
Richmond, VA 23241
(804) 786-2376

WASHINGTON
Washington State Department of Labor and
  Industries
  General Administration Building
  Room 334—AX-31
  Olympia, WA 98504-0631
  (206) 253-6307

WYOMING
Wyoming Occupational Health and Safety
  Herschler Building, 2nd Floor, East Wing
  Cheyenne, WY 82002
  (307) 777-7786

*Connecticut and New York have public sector
  programs only.

### 3. Other Federal Agencies
Agency for Toxic Substances and Disease
  Registry (ATSDR), ATSDR-Chamblee, 1600
  Clifton Road, N.E., Atlanta, GA 30333

U.S. Public Health Service agency that implements
the health-related sections of the "Superfund" Act
and its amendments and the Resource Conservation and Recovery Act (RCRA). Involved in the
areas of emergency response, health assessments,
health effects research, literature inventory/dissem-
ination, exposure and disease registries, toxicologic profiles, health professional training, and
worker health. Maintains a list of toxic waste sites
closed to the public.

Environmental Protection Agency (EPA), Public
  Information Center, PM-211B, 401 M Street,
  SW, Washington, D.C. 20460

The Public Information Center (PIC) provides
nontechnical information about environmental issues and the EPA. Information is available from
the PIC on drinking water, air quality, pesticides,
radon, indoor air, Superfund, wetlands, and many
other environmental topics.

Mine Safety and Health Administration (MSH
  Ballston Towers #3, 4015 Wilson Boulevard,
  Arlington, VA 22203

Regulates health and safety in the mining industry.

National Cancer Institute (NCI), National
  Institutes of Health, Public Health Service, U.S.
  Department of Health and Human Services,
  Bethesda, MD 20205

Supports various types of research related to occupational cancer hazards, including epidemiologic studies and carcinogenesis assays of industrial chemicals.

National Institute of Environmental Health
  Sciences (NIEHS), National Institutes of
  Health, Public Health Service, U.S. Department
  of Health and Human Services, P.O. Box
  12233, Research Triangle Park, NC 27709

Principal federal agency for biomedical research
on the effects of chemical, physical, and biologic
environmental agents on human health and well-
being. Supports and conducts basic research focused on the interaction between humans and potentially hazardous agents. Administers hazardous
waste training and research grants programs.

National Toxicology Program (NTP), M.D. B2-
  04, P.O. Box 12233, Research Triangle Park,
  NC 27709

Established in 1978 to develop scientific information needed to determine the toxic effects of chemicals and to develop better, faster, and less expensive test methods.

Nuclear Regulatory Commission (NRC),
  Washington, D.C. 20555-0001

Regulates the commercial use of nuclear materials
and issues licenses for such use.

### 4. Professional Organizations in the United States
American Association of Occupational Health
  Nurses (AAOHN), 50 Lenox Pointe, Atlanta,
  GA 30324-3176

Professional organization of registered nurses engaged in occupational health and safety and oc-

cupational health nursing. Major activities are the following: formulating and developing principles and standards of occupational health nursing practice; promoting, by means of publications, conferences, continuing education courses, and symposia, educational programs designed specifically for the occupational health nurse; and impressing on managers, physicians, and others the importance of integrating occupational health and safety services into employee activities.

American Cancer Society (ACS), 1599 Clifton Road NE, Atlanta, GA 30329

Voluntary health organization; in part, funds research projects on occupationally related cancer.

American College of Preventive Medicine (ACPM), 1015 15th Street, NW, Suite 403, Washington, D.C. 20005

The American College of Preventive Medicine is the national professional society for physicians committed to disease prevention and health promotion. ACPM seeks to advance the science and practice of preventive medicine by providing educational opportunities for its members; advocating public policies consistent with scientific principles of the discipline; supporting the investigation and analysis of issues relevant to the field; participating in national forums to address important professional and public health concerns; and communicating developments in the specialty through a peer-reviewed journal, newsletter, and other timely publications.

American College of Occupational and Environmental Medicine, 55 West Seegers Road, Arlington Heights, IL 60005

Largest society in the United States of physicians (6,000) in industry, government, and academia, who promote the health of workers through clinical practice, research, and teaching. Cosponsors with AAOHN the annual American Occupational Health Conference; sponsors state-of-the-art occupational health conference, coupled with a series of free-standing programs in Basic Curriculum Occupational and Environmental Medicine, Americans with Disabilities Act, medical review officer training, and other multifaceted physician CME activities. Publishes the monthly *Journal of Occupational Medicine,* the *ACOEM Report,* the *ACOEM Self Assessment Program in Occupational Medicine,* and other materials.

American Conference of Governmental Industrial Hygienists (ACGIH), 6500 Glenway Avenue, Cincinnati, OH 45211

Organization of industrial hygiene and occupational health and safety professionals who are engaged in occupational health and safety services, consultation, enforcement, research, or education. Publishes information for all occupational health and safety workers to assist them in providing more adequate health and safety services for workers. Publications focus on specific areas of industrial hygiene, health and safety, environment, laboratory/quality control, toxicology, medical, hazardous materials, hazardous waste, controls, physical agents, ergonomics, safety, computer, and professional development.

American Industrial Hygiene Association (AIHA), 2700 Prosperity Avenue, Suite 250, Fairfax, VA 22031

Professional organization of industrial hygienists and allied specialists. Publishes *AIHA Journal* and extensive literature on all phases of industrial hygiene. Promotes information on career opportunities in industrial hygiene.

American Lung Association (ALA), 1740 Broadway, New York, NY 10019

The ALA offers literature and films on occupational lung diseases, chronic obstructive pulmonary disease, tuberculosis, adult and pediatric lung disease, air conservation, and smoking. Publishes *American Review of Respiratory Disease*. Its medical section is the American Thoracic Society. Local branches conduct a variety of activities directed at a more limited geographic area.

American Medical Association, Group on Science, Technology, and Public Health, 515 North State Street, Chicago, IL 60610

Conducts projects, prepares reviews, and comments on federal documents and proposed regulations; responds to professional queries on medical and health issues. These activities are designed to attract, motivate, and educate physicians. Encourages and supports medical societies, assists governmental agencies and allied health organizations, and informs the public. Some literature and position statements available.

American Medical Student Association (AMSA), Task Force on Occupational and Environmental Health, 1890 Preston White Drive, Reston, VA 22091

Publishes a quarterly newsletter, *The Task Force Quarterly;* develops and publicizes educational materials; and facilitates student participation in occupational and environmental health projects.

American National Standards Institute (ANSI), 11 West 42nd Street, New York, NY 10036

Coordinates the voluntary development of national standards. Serves as a clearinghouse and information center for national and international safety standards. ANSI is the official U.S. member of the International Organization for Standardization (ISO) and the International Electro-Technical Commission (IEC), via the U.S. National Committee.

American Public Health Association (APHA), Occupational Health and Safety Section, 1015 15th Street, NW, Washington, D.C. 20005

Presents numerous sessions at annual APHA meeting each fall, develops public policy statements on occupational health and safety issues, and publishes a newsletter. Develops links between occupational health and public health.

American Society for Safety Engineers (ASSE), 1800 East Oakton, Des Plaines, IL 60018

Publishes *Professional Safety.* Supports safety professionals in accident, injury, and illness preven-

tion. Offers certification and training, technical publications, and an annual convention.

Association of Teachers of Preventive Medicine (ATPM), 1015 15th Street, NW, Suite 405, Washington, D.C. 20005

Promotes and supports teaching of preventive medicine, including occupational medicine, in medical schools.

The Ergonomics Society, Devonshire House, Devonshire Square, Loughborough, Leics., LF11 3DW, Great Britain UK

Original society for ergonomics, which has special interest in industrial ergonomics. Publishes *Ergonomics* and *Applied Ergonomics* and holds annual meeting.

Human Factors and Ergonomics Society, P.O. Box 1369, Santa Monica, CA 90406

Professional organization of ergonomics and human factors professionals. Holds annual meeting and its technical groups hold regular meetings. Publishes *Human Factors, Ergonomics in Design,* and the proceedings of the annual meeting. Its Industrial Ergonomics Technical Group is of special interest.

National Safety Council (NSC), 1121 Spring Lake Drive, Itasca, IL 60143-3201

A not-for-profit, nongovernmental, international public service organization offering occupational safety and health training programs and literature. The Council library is available for safety and health research, and experts in safety, industrial hygiene, and occupational health offer consultations.

Society for Occupational and Environmental Health (SOEH), 6728 Old McLean Village Drive, McLean, VA 22101

Actively seeks to improve the health quality of the workplace by holding open forums that focus public attention on scientific, social, and regulatory problems.

### 5. U.S. Occupational Health Clinics

Association of Occupational and Environmental Clinic (AOEC), 1010 Vermont Avenue, NW, Suite 513, Washington, D.C. 20005

Organization of clinics to aid in identifying, reporting, and preventing occupational/environmental health hazards nationwide; to increase communication among such clinics concerning issues of patient care; and to provide data for occupational/environmental research projects.

### 6. Committees on Occupational Safety and Health (COSH Groups)

COSH groups are grassroots voluntary advocacy organizations in the U.S. consisting of health professionals, legal professionals, and labor representatives who work to improve health and safety in the workplace through education and policy change.

### Committees on Occupational Safety and Health (COSH Groups)

ALASKA
Alaska Health Project
   1818 W. Northern Light Boulevard
   Anchorage, AK 99517
   (907) 276-2864/Fax: (907) 279-3089

CALIFORNIA
San Francisco Labor Council
   Fran Schrieberg, c/o Worksafe
   510 Harrison Street
   San Francisco, CA 94105
   (415) 543-2699/Fax: (415) 433-5077
LACOSH (Los Angeles COSH)
   5855 Venice Boulevard
   Los Angeles, CA 90019
   (213) 931-9000/Fax: (213) 380-9274
SA-COSH (Sacramento COSH)
   c/o Fire Fighters, Local 522
   3101 Stockton Boulevard
   Sacramento, CA 95820
   (916) 442-4390/Fax: (916) 446-3057

SCCOSH (Santa Clara COSH)
   760 N. 1st Street
   San Jose, CA 95112
   (408) 998-4050/Fax: (408) 998-4051

CONNECTICUT
ConnectiCOSH (Connecticut)
   32 Grand Street
   Hartford, CT 06106
   (203) 549-1877/Fax: (203) 728-0287

DISTRICT OF COLUMBIA
Alice Hamilton Occupational Health Center
   410 Seventh Street, SE
   Washington, D.C. 20003
   (202) 543-0005 (DC); (301) 731-8530 (MD)/
   Fax: (202) 546-2331; (301) 731-4142

ILLINOIS
CACOSH (Chicago area)
   37 South Ashland
   Chicago, IL 60607
   (312) 666-1611/Fax: (312) 243-0492

MAINE
Maine Labor Group on Health
   Box V
   Augusta, ME 04330
   (207) 622-7823/Fax: (207) 622-3483

MASSACHUSETTS
MassCOSH (Massachusetts)
   555 Amory Street
   Boston, MA 02130
   (617) 524-6686/Fax: (617) 524-3508
Western MassCOSH
   458 Bridge Street
   Springfield, MA 01103
   (413) 731-0760/Fax: (413) 732-1881

MICHIGAN
SEMCOSH (Southeast Michigan)
   2727 Second Street
   Detroit, MI 48206
   (313) 961-3345/Fax: (313) 961-3588

MINNESOTA
MN-COSH
  c/o Lyle Krych M330
  FMC Corp. Naval System Division
  4800 East River Road
  Minneapolis, MN 55421
  (612) 572-6997/Fax: (612) 572-9826


NEW HAMPSHIRE
NHCOSH
  c/o NH AFL-CIO
  110 Sheep Davis Road
  Pembroke, NH 03275
  (603) 226-0516/Fax: (603) 225-7294


NEW YORK
ALCOSH (Alleghany COSH)
  100 East Second Street
  Jamestown, NY 14701
  (716) 448-0720
CNYCOSH (Central New York)
  615 W. Genessee Street
  Syracuse, NY 13204
  (315) 471-6187/Fax: (315) 422-6514
ENYCOSH (Eastern New York)
  c/o Larry Rafferty
  121 Erie Boulevard
  Schenectady, NY 12305
  (518) 372-4308/Fax: (518) 393-3040
NYCOSH (New York)
  275 Seventh Avenue, 8th Floor
  New York, NY 10001
  (212) 627-3900/Fax: (212) 627-9812
  (914) 939-5612 (Lower Hudson)
  (516) 273-1234 (Long Island)
ROCOSH (Rochester COSH)
  797 Elmwood Avenue, #4
  Rochester, NY 14620
  (716) 244-0420
WYNCOSH (Western NY)
  2495 Main Street, Suite 438
  Buffalo, NY 14214
  (716) 833-5416/Fax: (716) 833-7507

NORTH CAROLINA
NCOSH (North Carolina COSH)
  P.O. Box 2514
  Durham, NC 27715
  (919) 286-9249/Fax: (919) 286-4857


OREGON
c/o Dick Edgington
  ICWU-Portland
  7440 SW 87 Street
  Portland, OR 07223
  (503) 244-8429


PENNSYLVANIA
PhilaPOSH (Philadelphia POSH)
  3001 Walnut Street, 5th Floor
  Philadelphia, PA 19104
  (215) 386-7000/Fax: (215) 386-3529


RHODE ISLAND
RICOSH (Rhode Island COSH)
  741 Westminster Street
  Providence, RI 02903
  (401) 751-2015


TENNESSEE
TNCOSH (Tennessee COSH)
  309 Whitecrest Drive
  Maryville, TN 37801
  (615) 983-7864


TEXAS
TexCOSH
  c/o Karyl Dunson
  5735 Regina
  Beaumont, TX 77706
  (409) 898-1427


WASHINGTON
WASHCOSH
  c/o Anna Bachmann
  2800 First Avenue, Room 206
  Seattle, WA 98121
  (206) 762-8337

WISCONSIN
WisCOSH (Wisconsin COSH)
   734 North 26th Street
   Milwaukee, WI 53230
   (414) 342-1996 (ATU 998)

CANADA
Ontario
   WOSH (Windsor OSH)
   547 Victoria Avenue
   Windsor, Ontario N9A 4N1
   (519) 254-5157/Fax: (519) 254-4192

### 7. University Labor Education Programs

#### University and College Labor Education Association (UCLEA)

Labor Education Department and Labor Relations, Attn: Sue Shurman, Institute of Management and Labor Relations, Rutgers State University, Ryders Lane and Clifton Avenue, New Brunswick, NY 08903

The UCLEA is an organization of academic-based labor education programs in the U.S. and Canada. Expertise in health and safety varies among the programs, but they can be good sources of background information on general labor issues and can help in the design of worker education programs.

ALABAMA
University of Alabama at Birmingham, Center for Labor Education and Research, School of Business, University Station, Birmingham, AL 35294

CALIFORNIA
University of California-Berkeley Labor Occupational Health Program (LOHP), 2515 Channing Way, Berkeley, CA 94720
University of California-Los Angeles Labor Occupational Safety and Health Program (UCLA-LOSH), Center for Labor Research and Education, Institute of Industrial Relations, 1001 Gayley Avenue, 2nd Floor, Los Angeles, CA 90024

ILLINOIS
University of Illinois, Institute of Labor and Industrial Relations, 504 East Armory, Champaign, IL 61870

LOUISIANA
Labor Studies Program/LA Watch, Loyola University, Box 12, New Orleans, LA 70118

MAINE
University of Maine, Bureau of Labor Education, Maine Tech Center, 16 Godfrey Drive, Orono, ME 04473

MARYLAND
Antioch, George Meany Center for Labor Studies, 10000 New Hampshire Avenue, Silver Spring, MD 20903

MICHIGAN
The Labor Studies Center, Institute of Labor and Industrial Relations, 303 Victor Vaughan, 1111 E. Catherine, Ann Arbor, MI 48109-2054

NEW JERSEY
Rutgers, The State University Labor Education Department and Labor Education Center, Institute of Management and Labor Relations, Ryders Land and Clifton Avenue, New Brunswick, NJ 08903

WEST VIRGINIA
Institute of Labor Studies, 710 Knapp Hall, West Virginia University, Morgantown, WV 26506

### 8. University Professional Training Programs

NIOSH funds 14 university programs that train occupational health professionals, conduct research, and provide service in this area. A number of other programs have been awarded NIOSH training funds to support graduate studies in the different disciplines (occupational medicine, occupational nursing, industrial hygiene, occupational ergonomics, and occupational safety). A complete list of these programs can be obtained from NIOSH (see table on p. 723).

### Educational Resource Centers

Alabama Educational Resource Center, Birmingham, AL 35294, University of Alabama at Birmingham

California Educational Resource Center–Northern, School of Public Health, University of California, Berkeley, CA 94720

California Educational Resource Center–Southern, Department of Preventive Medicine, University of Southern California, Los Angeles, CA 90089

Cincinnati Educational Resource Center, Department of Environmental Health, University of Cincinnati, Cincinnati, OH 45267-0056

Harvard Educational Resource Center, Occupational Health Program, Harvard School of Public Health, Boston, MA 02115

Illinois Educational Resource Center, School of Public Health, University of Illinois, Chicago, IL 60680

Johns Hopkins Educational Resource Center, School of Hygiene and Public Health, Johns Hopkins University, Baltimore, MD 21205

Michigan Educational Resource Center, School of Public Health, University of Michigan, Ann Arbor, MI 48109

Minnesota Educational Resource Center, School of Public Health, University of Minnesota, Minneapolis, MN 55455

New York/New Jersey Educational Resource Center, Department of Community Medicine, Mt. Sinai School of Medicine, New York, NY 10029

North Carolina Educational Resource Center, School of Public Health, University of North Carolina, Chapel Hill, NC 27514

Texas Educational Resource Center, School of Public Health, University of Texas Health Science Center, Houston, TX 77225

Rocky Mountain Center for Occupational and Environmental Health, University of Utah, Salt Lake City, UT 84112

Washington Educational Resource Center, Department of Environmental Health, University of Washington, Seattle, WA 98195

### 9. Industry-Sponsored Advisory and Research Groups

American Petroleum Institute, 1220 L Street, NW, Washington, D.C. 20005

Conducts research programs on occupational health and industrial hygiene aspects of all phases of the petroleum industry. These projects may result in manuals or guides or in research reports, which are available to interested parties.

American Welding Society, 550 NW LeJeune Road, P.O. Box 351040, Miami, FL 33135

Offers seminars and home-study courses designed specifically to relate welding and cutting operations to plant environmental safety and health.

Chemical Industry Institute of Toxicology (CIIT), P.O. Box 12137, Six Davis Drive, Research Triangle Park, NC 27709

Conducts basic toxicologic research to provide an improved scientific basis for understanding and assessing the potential adverse effects of chemicals, pharmaceutical, and consumer products on human health. Acquires, interprets, and disseminates technical information and test data. Trains toxicologists and scientists in related fields.

Chemical Manufacturers Association, 2501 M Street, NW, Washington, D.C. 20037

Publishes monthly newsletter, *ChemEcology*. Has a committee that deals with occupational safety and health matters. Has over 200 member companies. Sponsors projects and occasionally publishes educational materials.

## Other Graduate Degree Programs

| UNIVERSITY | INDUSTRIAL HYGIENE | OCCUPATIONAL MEDICINE | OCCUPATIONAL NURSING | ERGONOMICS SAFETY | OTHER |
|---|---|---|---|---|---|
| University of Arizona | x | x | | | |
| Catonsville Community College | | | | | x |
| Central Maine Technical College | | | | | x |
| Colorado State University | x | | | | |
| East Carolina | x | | | x | |
| Eastern Kentucky | | | | x | |
| Emory University | | x | | | |
| University of Hawaii | x | | | | |
| University of Iowa | x | x | | | |
| University of Kentucky | x | x | | | |
| University of Massachusetts Lowell | x | | x | x | x |
| Meharry Medical College | | x | | | |
| Montana Technical College | x | | | | x |
| Murray State University | | | | | x |
| University of Oklahoma | | x | | | x |
| University of Pennsylvania | | | x | | |
| University of Puerto Rico | x | | | | |
| University of Pittsburgh | | x | | | |
| St. Augustine College | | | | | x |
| San Diego State University | x | | | | |
| University of South Carolina | x | | | | |
| University of South Florida | x | | | | |
| Temple University | x | | | | |
| Texas Tech University | | | | x | |
| Virginia Polytechnic Institute | | | | x | |
| West Virginia University | | x | | x | |
| Western Kentucky | | | | | x |
| University of Wisconsin–Stevens Pt. | | | | | x |
| University of Wisconsin–Stout | | | | x | |
| Yale University | | x | | | |

Chlorine Institute, 2001 L Street, NW, Suite 506, Washington, D.C. 20037

Promotes safety in manufacturing and handling of chlorine products. Provides educational materials to over 200 member companies and to the public.

Industrial Health Foundation, 34 Penn Circle West, Pittsburgh, PA 15206

Conducts engineering plant visits to review industrial hygiene and health and safety aspects, publishes extensive abstracts, provides toxicology consultation, conducts training courses in occupational health and safety, and performs analytical testing of environmental and biologic samples.

International Lead-Zinc Research Organization, 2525 Meridian Parkway, P.O. Box 12036, Research Triangle Park, NC 27709

Conducts occupational and environmental health research on such subjects as pediatric lead absorption, occupational lead and cadmium exposure, and biologic interactions. Publishes annual lead/cadmium research digest.

Joint Labor Management Committee of the Retail Food Industry, 2120 L Street, NW, Washington, D.C. 20037

Studies and recommends programs to provide safe working conditions and to protect employees in all phases of retail food operations from exposure to hazardous working conditions.

Plastics Education Foundation, 14 Fairfield Drive, Brookfield, CT 06804

Provides audiovisual materials, including films and videotapes, on occupational health and safety in plastics and manufacturing industries.

## 10. Labor-Oriented Advisory/Research Groups

American Labor Education Center (ALEC), 2000 P Street, NW, Washington, D.C. 20036

Provides education and educational materials to workers about health and safety.

Center for Safety in the Arts, 5 Beekman Street, Suite 1030, New York, NY 10038

National clearinghouse for research and information on health hazards in the arts, including the visual arts and crafts, theater, and museum conservation. Has lecture and consultation program, art hazards newsletter, and an art hazards information center.

Environmental Defense Fund, 1875 Connecticut Avenue, NW, Suite 1016, Washington, D.C. 20009

Toxic Chemicals Program seeks to establish public policy that minimizes human and environmental exposure to toxic chemicals. Current projects focus on both occupational and general consumer exposure to toxic chemicals, especially lead and dioxin. Prior actions involved DDT, endrin, chlordane/heptachlor, 2,4,5-T, asbestos, benzene, TRIS, and hair dye chemicals.

Farmworker Health and Safety Institute (FHSI), Director: Mark Lyons, 2001 S Street, NW, Suite 210, Washington, D.C. 20009

FHSI is a consortium of the George Washington University School of Medicine, CATA (Farmworkers Support Committee), the Farmworker Association of Central Florida, and the Farmworker Justice Fund. FHSI trains clinicians and farmworkers about farmworker health and safety issues, including pesticides, workplace injuries, and women's health using "popular education" methods. FHSI develops training materials in English and Spanish at appropriate literacy levels.

Health Research Group, Public Citizen, 2000 P Street, NW, Suite 700, Washington, D.C. 20036

Public interest group that studies many subjects, including occupational health hazards, and disseminates information to the working public. Has numerous publications and other informational resources that are of value to medical students and physicians. In certain circumstances, it can also investigate specific hazardous situations.

Highlander Research and Education Center, 1959 Highlander Way, New Market, TN 37820

Major labor education center, which, among other things, conducts educational conferences on occupational safety and health for labor activists, health science students, and others.

The Labor Institute, 853 Broadway, Room 2014, New York, NY 10003

Specializes in developing economic analyses of the problems workers face and presents them in easy-to-understand language from the workers' point of view. Has produced workbooks and videotapes on Hazardous Waste Training, Hazards of the Modern Office, Electromagnetic Fields, Sexual Harassment, and Multiple Chemical Sensitivity.

Migrant Legal Action Program (MLAP), 2001 S Street, NW, Suite 310, Washington, D.C. 20009

MLAP, a Legal Services Corporation–funded national support center, represents migrant and seasonal farmworkers in numerous areas, including health and safety, housing, health care, and child labor.

Occupational Health Foundation, 815 16th Street, NW, Suite 608, Washington, D.C. 20006

Labor-supported organization that provides technical, scientific, and educational services in occupational health and safety to unions. Responds to requests for information.

9–5 Working Women Education Fund, 614 Superior Avenue, NW, Cleveland, OH 44113

National association that works to win rights and respect for female office workers. Engaged in a specific effort to address health and safety problems of office workers with research and education.

Scientists' Institute for Public Information (SIPI), 355 Lexington Avenue, New York, NY 10017

Publishes newsletter containing information on environmental hazards. Past articles have been on subjects including asbestos, fibrous glass, pesticides, and polychlorinated biphenyls (PCBs). Other published materials also available. Also provides information to journalists in the U.S. and internationally.

## 11. International Organizations

International Commission on Occupational Health (ICOH) c/o Jerry Jeyaratnam, Secretary/Treasurer ICOH, Community, Occupational & Family Medicine, National University Hospital, Lower Kent Ridge Road, Singapore, 0511

International scientific society that fosters scientific progress, knowledge, and development of all aspects of occupational health on an international basis. Holds a triennial international congress, maintains scientific committees, and collects and disseminates information on occupational health.

International Labour Organization (ILO), CH-1211, Geneva 22, Switzerland

Focuses on the prevention of occupational accidents and diseases; promotion of safety, health, and well-being in all occupations; and identification and elimination of problems of working environments. Involvement in occupational safety and health is articulated in its International Programme for the Improvement of Working Conditions and Environment (PIACT). Modes of action include adoption of international conventions and recommendations, the establishment of model codes of practices, convening of tripartite meetings, collection and dissemination of information (including the *Encyclopedia of Occupational Health and Safety*), and technical cooperation.

World Health Organization (WHO), Office of Occupational Health, Avenue Appia, CH 1211, Geneva 27, Switzerland

Offers a wide range of services in occupational health and safety, including publishing documents and sponsoring a variety of educational programs.

## 12. Labor Organizations

The following list of labor organizations is not all-inclusive but includes some of those with the most active health and safety departments.

American Federation of Labor and Congress of Industrial Organizations (AFL-CIO), 815 16th Street, NW, Washington, D.C. 20006

Confederation of labor unions that serves as their advocate in health and safety matters. The Building and Construction Trades Department, Industrial Union Department, and Food and Allied Services Trades Department are trade and industrial departments of the AFL-CIO that work extensively on safety and health issues for unions in their respective sectors. These departments are at the same address as the AFL-CIO.

American Federation of Government Employees, 1325 Massachusetts Avenue, NW, Washington, D.C. 20005

American Federation of State, County and Municipal Employees (AFSCME), 1625 L Street, NW, Washington, D.C. 20036

Communication Workers of America (CWA), 501 3rd Street, NW, Washington, D.C. 20001

International Brotherhood of Painters and Allied Trades, United Unions Building, 1750 New York Avenue, NW, Washington, D.C. 20006

International Chemical Workers Union (ICWU), 1655 West Market Street, Akron, OH 44313

International Union of Automobile, Aerospace and Agricultural Implement Workers (UAW), 8000 East Jefferson Avenue, Detroit, MI 48214

Oil, Chemical and Atomic Workers International Union (OCAW), P.O. Box 2812, Denver, CO 80201

Service Employees International Union (SEIU), 2020 K Street, NW, Washington, D.C. 20006

United Mine Workers of America (UMWA), 900 15th Street, NW, Washington, D.C. 20005

# Index

# Index